Valvular Heart Disease

CONTEMPORARY CARDIOLOGY

CHRISTOPHER P. CANNON, MD
SERIES EDITOR
ANNEMARIE M. ARMANI, MD
EXECUTIVE EDITOR

Valvular Heart Disease

Edited by

Andrew Wang, MD

Division of Cardiovascular Medicine
Duke University Medical Center
Durham, NC
USA

Thomas M. Bashore, MD

Division of Cardiovascular Medicine
Duke University Medical Center
Durham, NC
USA

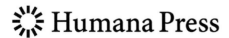 Humana Press

Editors
Andrew Wang, MD
Division of Cardiovascular Medicine
Duke University Medical Center
Durham, NC
USA
wang0016@mc.duke.edu

Thomas M. Bashore, MD
Division of Cardiovascular Medicine
Duke University Medical Center
Durham, NC
USA
basho001@mc.duke.edu

ISBN 978-1-58829-982-6   e-ISBN 978-1-59745-411-7
DOI 10.1007/978-1-59745-411-7
Springer Dordrecht Heidelberg London New York

Library of Congress Control Number: 2009931797

Cover illustration: Duke University Echocardiography Lab (Durham, NC); Dr. William Edwards, Dept of Laboratory Medicine and Pathology, Mayo Clinic (Rochester, MN); Atlas of Valvular Heart Disease: Clinical and Pathologic Aspects (eds: Willerson, Cohn, McAllister, Manabe, Yutani), Churchill Livingstone, 1998.

Printed on acid-free paper

Humana Press is part of Springer Science+Business Media (www.springer.com)

Preface

Prior to the invention of the stethoscope by Laennec in 1816, valvular heart disease was predominantly diagnosed by post-mortem examination. With advancements in our diagnostic tools, such as cardiac catheterization and non-invasive imaging, the diagnosis and assessment of valvular heart disease has improved to the point where the cause, severity, and hemodynamic consequences of these lesions can now be accurately defined. The recognition of heart valve abnormalities at an earlier stage has led to better understanding of the progression of these lesions and their effects on patient outcome. Surgical treatment options have also markedly advanced in the last half-century, with improvements in surgical risk assessment, surgical techniques, and outcome. As the number of older adults continues to increase, the prevalence of valvular lesions also rises. Current and future challenges for the treatment of valvular heart disease include the development of effective yet less invasive interventions and therapies to treat and attenuate the progressive nature of these conditions. Major new therapeutic options are on the close horizon.

In this book, a highly respected and internationally recognized group of cardiologists, cardiac surgeons, and researchers have contributed their insights into the pathology, hemodynamic, and clinical effects of heart valve conditions and the contemporary management of these patients. The content within these chapters is intended to offer a broad perspective on these diseases and to complement and expand upon the recent guidelines on valvular heart disease developed by the major heart societies in the United States and Europe.

Andrew Wang, MD
Thomas M. Bashore, MD

Contents

Contributors

LUKAS ALTWEGG, MD, *Division of Cardiology, St. Paul's Hospital, University of British Columbia, Vancouver, British Columbia*

B. ZANE ATKINS, MD, *Division of Cardiothoracic Surgery, Duke University Medical Center, Durham, NC*

THOMAS M. BASHORE, MD, *Division of Cardiovascular Medicine, Duke University Medical Center, Durham, NC*

ROBERT O. BONOW, MD, *Division of Cardiology, Northwestern University Feinberg School of Medicine, Chicago, IL*

CHARLES J. BRUCE, MBCHB, *Division of Cardiovascular Diseases and Internal Medicine, Mayo Clinic and Mayo Foundation, Rochester, MN*

CHRISTOPHER H. CABELL, MD, *Quintiles Transnational Corporation, Durham, NC*

BLASE A. CARABELLO, MD, *Department of Medicine, Baylor College of Medicine, Houston, TX*

HEIDI M. CONNOLLY, MD, *Division of Cardiovascular Diseases and Internal Medicine, Mayo Clinic and Mayo Foundation, Rochester, MN*

SAPAN S. DESAI, MD, PhD, *Division of Cardiovascular and Thoracic Surgery, Duke University Medical Center, Durham, NC*

JEAN G. DUMESNIL, MD, *Research Center of Laval Hospital, Quebec Heart Institute, Quebec, Canada*

MAURICE ENRIQUEZ-SARANO, MD, *Division of Cardiovascular Diseases and Internal Medicine, Mayo Clinic and Mayo Foundation, Rochester, MN*

TED FELDMAN, MD, *Division of Cardiology, Evanston Northwestern Healthcare, Evanston, IL*

LISA FORBESS, MD, *Division of Cardiology, University of Texas Southwestern Medical Center, Dallas, TX*

THOMAS R. GEHRIG, MD, *Division of Cardiovascular Medicine, Duke University Medical Center, Durham, NC*

DONALD D. GLOWER, MD, *Division of Cardiovascular and Thoracic Surgery, Duke University Medical Center, Durham, NC*

BRIAN P. GRIFFIN, MD, *Cardiovascular Medicine, Cleveland Clinic Lerner College of Medicine, Cleveland, OH*

CARMEL M. HALLEY, MD, *Cardiovascular Medicine, Cleveland Clinic Lerner College of Medicine, Cleveland, OH*

J. KEVIN HARRISON, MD, *Division of Cardiovascular Medicine, Duke University Medical Center, Durham, NC*

STEPHEN A. HART, BS, *Cardiovascular Medicine, Cleveland Clinic Lerner College of Medicine, Cleveland, OH*

HOWARD C. HERRMANN, MD *Cardiovascular Medicine Division, University of Pennsylvania Medical Center, Philadelphia, PA*

G. CHAD HUGHES, MD, *Division of Cardiovascular and Thoracic Surgery, Duke University Medical Center, Durham, NC*

ANDRA H. JAMES, MD, *Department of Obstetrics and Gynecology, Duke University Medical Center, Durham, NC*

JONG MI KO, BA, *Baylor Heart and Vascular Institute, Baylor University Medical Center, Dallas, TX*

NEAL D. KON, MD, *Division of Cardiothoracic Surgery, Wake Forest Baptist University Medical Center, Winston-Salem, NC*

RICHARD A. KRASUSKI, MD, *Cardiovascular Medicine, Cleveland Clinic Lerner College of Medicine, Cleveland, OH*

ANDREW J. LODGE, MD, *Division of Cardiovascular and Thoracic Surgery, Duke University Medical Center, Durham, NC*

JULIEN MAGNE, Bsc, *Research Center of Laval Hospital, Quebec Heart Institute, Quebec, Canada*

HECTOR I. MICHELENA, MD, *Division of Cardiovascular Diseases and Internal Medicine, Mayo Clinic and Mayo Foundation, Rochester, MN*

NAZANIN MOGHBELI, MD, MPH, *Cardiovascular Medicine Division, University of Pennsylvania Medical Center, Philadelphia, PA*

RICK A. NISHIMURA, MD, *Division of Cardiovascular Diseases and Internal Medicine, Mayo Clinic and Mayo Foundation, Rochester, MN*

VUYISILE T. NKOMO, MD, *Division of Cardiovascular Diseases and Internal Medicine, Mayo Clinic and Mayo Foundation, Rochester, MN*

PATRICK T. O'GARA, MD, *Cardiovascular Division, Brigham and Women's Hospital, Boston, MA*

SAHIL A. PARIKH, MD, *Cardiovascular Division, Brigham and Women's Hospital, Boston, MA*

PATRICIA A. PELLIKKA, MD, *Division of Cardiovascular Diseases and Internal Medicine, Mayo Clinic and Mayo Foundation, Rochester, MN*

GAIL E. PETERSON, MD, *Division of Cardiology, University of Texas Southwestern Medical Center, Dallas, TX*

PHILIPPE PIBAROT, DVM, PhD, *Research Center of Laval Hospital, Quebec Heart Institute, Quebec, Canada*

NALINI M. RAJAMANNAN, MD, *Division of Cardiology, Department of Medicine and Department of Pathology, Northwestern University Feinberg School of Medicine, Chicago, IL*

VERA H. RIGOLIN, MD, *Division of Cardiology, Northwestern University Feinberg School of Medicine, Chicago, IL*

WILLIAM CLIFFORD ROBERTS, MD, *Baylor Heart and Vascular Institute, Baylor University Medical Center, Dallas, TX*

CARLOS E. RUIZ, MD, PhD, *Department of Interventional Cardiology, Lenox Hill Heart and Vascular Institute, New York, NY*

LAURENCE M. SCHNEIDER, MBBCH, *Department of Interventional Cardiology, Lenox Hill Heart and Vascular Institute, New York, NY*

PAUL SORAJJA, MD, *Division of Cardiovascular Diseases and Internal Medicine, Mayo Clinic and Mayo Foundation, Rochester, MN*

ASLAN T. TURER, MD, *Division of Cardiovascular Medicine, Duke University Medical Center, Durham, NC*

ANDREW WANG, MD, *Division of Cardiovascular Medicine, Duke University Medical Center, Durham, NC*

CARY WARD, MD, *Division of Cardiovascular Medicine, Duke University Medical Center, Durham, NC*

JOHN G. WEBB, MD, *Division of Cardiology, St. Paul's Hospital, University of British Columbia, Vancouver, British Columbia*

1

Morphologic Aspects of Valvular Heart Disease

William Clifford Roberts and Jong Mi Ko

CONTENTS

SOURCES FOR MORPHOLOGIC STUDIES

Before 1960, the only source to study the heart itself was the autopsy. The early years of cardiac valve replacement provided a rich source of necropsy "material" until valve techniques and artificial heart valves became more refined. During the 1960s and 1970s, many thousands of patients with rheumatic heart disease underwent replacement of one or more cardiac valves. By the 1980s, most of this rheumatic heart disease pool of patients had undergone operation and additionally the frequency of rheumatic fever and subsequently rheumatic heart disease had dropped dramatically. Also, in the 1950s and 1960s, most physicians attributed valvular heart disease in adults at that time to rheumatic heart disease. By the 1970s, the congenitally malformed aortic valve was found to be frequent in adults with aortic stenosis (AS), and mitral valve prolapse (MVP) was being recognized as a common cause of pure (no associated stenosis) mitral regurgitation (MR). Also, by the 1990s, the frequency of autopsies in hospitals in the United States had dropped enormously compared to the 1950s, and operatively excised cardiac valves were becoming the major source of anatomic study. Although established by the 1980s, cardiac transplantations were rarely performed because of valvular heart disease.

FREQUENCY OF VARIOUS VALVULAR DISORDERS IN NECROPSY STUDIES

Roberts *(1)* personally studied 1,010 hearts at necropsy in patients with fatal valvular heart disease (Table 1). All had died between 1955 and 1980 and the specimens were retrieved from a number of different hospitals, most of which were located in the Washington, DC, area. As shown in Table 1, these cases were given both a *functional* [valve stenosis with or without regurgitation or pure regurgitation (no element of stenosis)] and an *anatomic* classification. A number of these patients had only one dysfunctional valve but in addition had one or more anatomically abnormal valves (normal function). (A valve may be anatomically abnormal yet function normally.) Aortic stenosis (AS) was the most common functional disorder (29%); in 35 (12%) of these 292 patients, the mitral leaflets were diffusely

From: *Contemporary Cardiology: Valvular Heart Disease*
Edited by: Andrew Wang, Thomas M. Bashore, DOI 10.1007/978-1-59745-411-7_1
© Humana Press, a part of Springer Science+Business Media, LLC 2009

Table 1
Functional and Anatomic Classification of Valvular Heart Disease in 1010 Necropsy Patients Aged ≥15 Years*

Functional class	Patients	Anatomic class				
		AV	MV	MV–AV	TV–MV	TV–MV–AV
1. Aortic stenosis (AS)	292 (29%)	256 (88%)	0	35 (12%)	0	1 (0.3%)
2. Mitral stenosis (MS)	189 (19%)	0	117 (62%)	40 (21%)	13 (7%)	19 (10%)
3. MS + AS	152 (15%)	0	0	120 (79%)	0	32 (21%)
4. Aortic regurgitation (AR)†	119 (12%)	107 (90%)	0	10 (8%)	0	2 (2%)
5. Mitral regurgitation (MR)	97 (10%)	0	85 (88%)	8 (8%)	1 (1%)	3 (3%)
6. MS + AR	65 (6%)	0	52 (80%)	0	0	13 (20%)
7. MR + AR	45 (4%)	0	0	39 (87%)	0	6 (13%)
8. AS + MR	23 (2%)	0	0	21 (91%)	0	2 (9%)
9. Tricuspid stenosis + MS ± AS	28 (3%)	0	0	0	4 (14%)	24 (86%)
Totals	1010 (100%)‡	363 (36%)	254 (25%)	273 (27%)	18 (2%)	102 (10%)

AV = aortic valve; MV = mitral valve; TV = tricuspid valve.

*Excludes patients with mitral regurgitation secondary to coronary heart disease (papillary muscle dysfunction), carcinoid heart disease, hypertrophic cardiomyopathy, and those with infective endocarditis limited to one or both right-sided cardiac valves. Tricuspid valve regurgitation was present in many patients in most of the nine functional groups. All patients were in functional class III or IV (New York Heart Association), and more than half had one or more cardiac operations.

†In many patients, the aortic valve cusps were normal or nearly normal and the regurgitation was the result of disease of the aorta (Marfan and Marfan-like syndrome, syphilis, systemic hypertension, healed aortic dissection).

‡The hearts in all 1010 patients were examined and classified by WCR.

Reproduced with permission from Elsevier (Am J Cardiol 1983;51:1005–1028).

thickened (rheumatic heart disease) but there was no clinical evidence of mitral dysfunction. Most of the 256 patients with AS and anatomically normal mitral valves had congenitally unicuspid or bicuspid aortic valves. Mitral stenosis was the next most common functional valve disease but 72 (38%) of these 189 patients also had anatomic involvement of one or more other cardiac valves. All patients with MS, whether isolated or associated with a functional disorder of another cardiac valve, had the valvular disease attributed to rheumatic heart disease. Combined MS and AS was the third most common functional valvular disease (15%) and 32 (21%) of these 152 cases also had anatomic disease of the tricuspid valve leaflets. The purely regurgitant lesions [aortic regurgitation (AR), MR, or both] were less common. Tricuspid stenosis of rheumatic etiology occurred in only 3% of the 1,010 cases and all had associated MS with or without associated AS. No other large series of patients with valvular heart disease studied at necropsy has been reported in the last 25 years and it is unlikely that such a large series, all studied by the same physician (namely, WCR), will be accumulated in the future because of the low autopsy rates in most hospitals today and also because few specimens are retained indefinitely after autopsy.

CHANGING FREQUENCY OF VARIOUS VALVULAR DISORDERS IN RECENT DECADES IN THE WESTERN WORLD

Today the most frequently studied operatively excised valve is the stenotic aortic valve followed by the excision of a portion of posterior mitral leaflet in patients with MR secondary to mitral valve prolapse (MVP) (Table 2). Operatively excised purely regurgitant aortic valves with or without excision of portions of ascending aorta are also common. Purely regurgitant mitral valves, which are replaced usually, yield only anterior mitral leaflets as specimens; the posterior leaflet usually is not excised. Rarely is a tricuspid valve operatively excised today.

Table 2

Type of Valvular Dysfunction in Patients* Having Aortic Valve Replacement and/or Mitral Valve Replacement or Repair at Baylor University Medical Center (Dallas), 1993–2006

Valve dysfunction	Number of patients (%)
1. Aortic stenosis (AS)	985 (53)
2. Mitral stenosis (MS)	129 (7)
3. MS + AS	54 (3)
4. Aortic regurgitation (AR)[†]	326 (17)
5. Mitral regurgitation (MR)	313 (17)
6. MS + AR	10 (<1)
7. MR + AR	28 (1)
8. AS + MR	27 (1)
9. Tricuspid stenosis + MS + AS	0
Totals	1872 (100%)[‡]

*Excludes patients with mitral regurgitation secondary to coronary heart disease (papillary muscle dysfunction), carcinoid heart disease, hypertrophic cardiomyopathy, and those with infective endocarditis limited to one or both right-sided cardiac valves. Tricuspid valve regurgitation was present in many patients in most of the nine functional groups.

[†]In many patients, the aortic valve cusps were normal or nearly normal and the regurgitation was the result of disease of the aorta (Marfan and Marfan-like syndrome, syphilis, systemic hypertension, healed aortic dissection).

[‡]The operatively excised valves in all 1872 patients were examined and classified by WCR.

SPECIFIC VALVULAR DISORDERS

Aortic Stenosis (with or without Regurgitation)

Frequency and causes. If systemic hypertension is not considered, AS is the second most common potentially fatal or fatal heart disease after coronary heart disease. There are three major causes of AS: *atherosclerosis* (formerly called degenerative), *congenitally malformed valves*, and *rheumatic heart disease*.

That atherosclerosis is a cause of AS is derived primarily from five pieces of evidence: (1) that patients with familial homozygous hyperlipidemia usually develop calcific deposits on the aortic aspects of their aortic valve cusps at a very young age, usually by the teenage years (These individuals have serum total cholesterol levels >800 mg/dl from the time of birth.) (2); (2) that progression of AS can be slowed by lowering total and low-density lipoprotein cholesterol levels by statins (3); (3) that patients >65 years of age with AS involving a three-cuspid aortic valve (unassociated with mitral valve disease) usually have extensive atherosclerosis involving the major epicardial coronary arteries and usually other systemic arterial systems (4); (4) that serum total cholesterol levels and concomitant coronary bypass grafting tend to be higher in patients with AS involving three-cuspid aortic valves than in patients of similar age and sex without AS or with congenitally bicuspid aortic valves (5); and (5) that histologic study of three-cuspid stenotic aortic valve demonstrates features similar to those in atherosclerotic plaques (2).

The unicuspid aortic valve appears to be stenotic from the time of birth (6, 7). The congenitally bicuspid valve, however, infrequently is stenotic at birth but becomes stenotic as calcific deposits from on the aortic aspects of the cusps (8). Rheumatic heart disease never involves the aortic valve anatomically without also involving the mitral valve (9). Although the mitral valve may be diffusely abnormal anatomically, its function can be normal and consequently a patient with rheumatic heart disease can present initially with only aortic valve dysfunction and therefore rheumatic heart disease has to be considered a cause of functionally isolated AS (with or without AR) or pure AR (9).

Valve Structure: In patients with isolated AS (with or without AR) (only cardiac valve anatomically abnormal), the aortic valve may be unicuspid, bicuspid, tricuspid, or quadricuspid. The congenitally *unicuspid valve* is of two types: acommissural and unicommissural (7, 10). The acommissural valve, which represents <10% of the unicuspid valves, has a central orifice and no distinct commissures. The unicommissural valve, which constitutes most of the unicuspid valves, has one commissure and

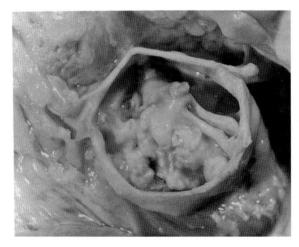

Fig. 1. *Aortic stenosis. Congenitally unicuspid unicommisured aortic valve* in a 48-year-old man. The heart weighed 750 g. (Reproduced with permission from Ref. *(7)*).

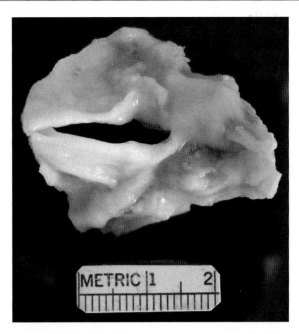

Fig. 2. *Aortic stenosis.* Operatively excised *unicuspid unicommissural aortic valve* in a 41-year-old man. The valve weighed 5.42 g. The mean transvalvular pressure gradient was 51 mmHg.

usually two other rudimentary commissures and a vertical orifice extending out from the only true commissure (Figs. 1 and 2) *(9)*.

The *congenitally bicuspid valve* (Figs. 3 and 4) of course has two cusps and they are usually of slightly unequal size in both cuspal surface area and weight. Usually one of the two cusps contains a raphe (rudimentary commissure) in its central portion. Often the raphe cusp has free

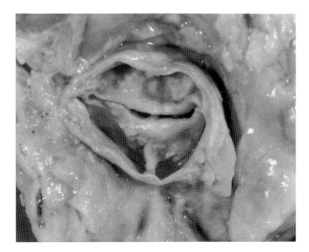

Fig. 3. *Aortic stenosis. Congenitally bicuspid aortic valve* in a 61-year-old man. At catheterization 2 years before his death, the peak systolic transvalvular pressure gradient was 45 mmHg when the cardiac index was 2.6 l/min/m^2. He had complete heart block secondary to the destruction of the atrioventricular bundle by calcium. The heart weighed 700 g.

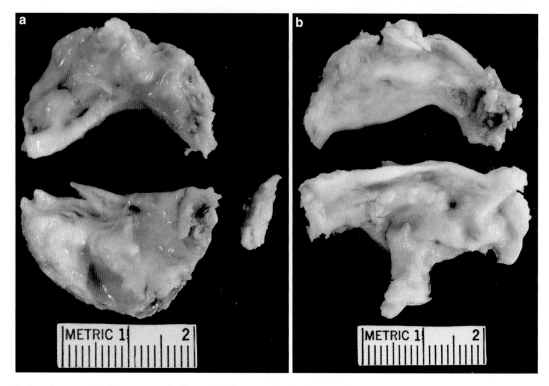

Fig. 4. *Aortic stenosis.* Two operatively excised *congenitally bicuspid aortic valves.* **(a)** Valve in a 60-year-old man. The valve weighed 4.65 g. The patient had severe heart failure. **(b)** Valve in a 66-year-old man. The valve weighed 4.79 g and the peak systolic transvalvular gradient was 84 mmHg.

margins that are V-shaped with the apex of the V pointing to the raphe producing a concave configuration. The nonraphe cusp in this circumstance commonly has a convex configuration that fits nicely into the concave shape of the raphe cusp such that associated regurgitation is absent or minimal. These bicuspid valves with a concave configuration of the raphe cusp and a convex appearance of free margin of the nonraphe cusp are often confused with tricuspid valves with fusion of one of three commissures. In other bicuspid valves the free margins of both cusps are relatively straight.

The *tricuspid aortic valve* is common in older patients with AS (atherosclerotic origin) and in patients in whom the AS is of rheumatic etiology. [These latter patients always have mitral leaflets that are diffusely fibrotic (with or without focal calcific deposits) or at least the margins of both leaflets are everywhere thickened by fibrous tissue.] In patients with AS of rheumatic etiology, one or more of the three commissures are often fused and the cusps may be either diffusely or focally fibrotic with or without commissural fusion or calcific deposits. The stenotic tricuspid aortic valve in older persons contains calcific deposits on the aortic surfaces, usually involving the sites of cuspal attachments, and the commissures are not characteristically fused (Fig. 5). Thus, operative excision produces three cusps, none of which are attached to another (Fig. 6). Older patients with AS often also have calcified mitral anomaly. Figure 7 shows how calcium might develop in both the aortic valve and the mitral annulus.

The *quadricuspid aortic valve* is rare (*11*). When present and if dysfunctional, the dysfunction is usually pure AR. AS with a quadricuspid valve is exceedingly rare, seen by Roberts (*12*) in 1 of 1,112 operatively excised stenotic aortic valves.

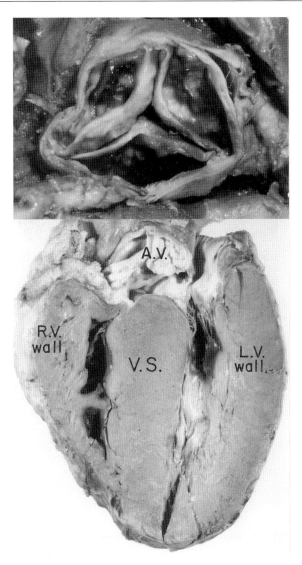

Fig. 5. *Aortic stenosis*. Three-cuspid aortic valve (*upper*) and longitudinal section of heart in an 89-year-old man whose heart weighed 440 g. None of the three aortic valve commissures are fused. The mitral annulus contains calcific deposits. (Reproduced with permission from Elsevier and *Am J Cardiol (4)*).

NECROPSY STUDIES OF PATIENTS WITH ISOLATED AORTIC STENOSIS (WITH OR WITHOUT) AND NEVER A CARDIAC OPERATION – NATURAL HISTORY

During a 32-year period at the National Institutes of Health, Roberts collected (mainly from hospitals in the Washington, DC, area) the hearts of 192 adults (aged 16–99 years) with isolated AS and none of them had ever had a cardiac operation (unpublished data). Of the 192 patients, 139 (72%) were men and 53 (28%) women (Table 3). The average age of the men was 61 years and that of the women, 71 years, the same average ages of death as in coronary heart disease. The weight of the hearts was 610 ± 135 g (normal <400 g) in the men and 486 ± 111 g (normal <350 g) in the women. The aortic valve was congenitally unicuspid in 17 patients (9%), congenitally bicuspid in 89 patients (46%), and tricuspid in 86 patients (45%) (Table 4). Other observations in these 192 patients are shown in Tables 3 and 4.

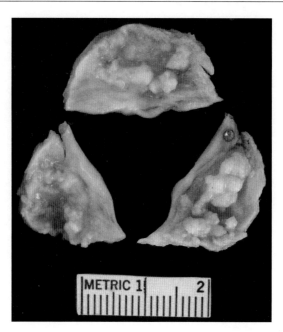

Fig. 6. *Aortic stenosis.* Operatively excised aortic valve in a 70-year-old man. The valve weighed 1.69 g and the peak systolic transvalvular gradient was 55 mmHg, and left ventricular function was normal (ejection fraction = 60%).

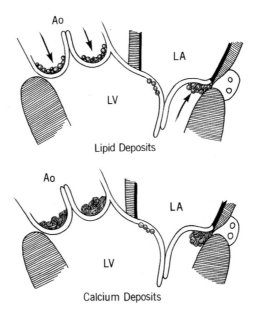

Fig. 7. *Aortic valve and mitral annular calcium.* Commonly calcific deposits are present in the aortic valve cusps, mitral annulus, and epicardial coronary arteries. Roberts has referred to this condition as "the senile cardiac calcification syndrome" (*Am J Cardiol* 1986; 58:572–574). The cause of the calcific deposits in these locations is speculative but atherosclerosis seems to be the most reasonable. In younger individuals, lipid deposits are usually present on the aortic aspects of the aortic valve cusps and on the ventricular aspects of the posterior mitral leaflet and to a much less extent on the ventricular aspect of the anterior mitral leaflet. The lipid in these locations is usually both intracellular and extracellular. Degeneration of the lipid probably leads to the calcific deposits in these locations.

Table 3
Findings at Necropsy in Isolated Aortic Valve Stenosis in Men vs Women (*n*= 192)

Variable	Men [*n* = 139 (72%)]	Women [*n* = 53 (28%)]
Ages (Years): Range (mean)	16–99 (61)	32–90 (71)
Symptomatic	103/129 (80%)	41/49 (84%)
Total cholesterol (mg/dl)	206 ± 63	161 ± 26
Severity of stenosis		
1+	24 (17%)	7 (13%)
2+	22 (16%)	9 (17%)
3+	93 (67%)	37 (70%)
Coronary narrowing		
0	73 (53%)	20 (38%)
≥1	66 (47%)	33 (62%)
Mitral annular calcium		
0	101 (73%)	23 (43%)
1+–3+	38 (27%)	30 (57%)
Heart weight (g)	610 ± 135	486 ± 111
Aortic valve		
Unicuspid	16 (12%) ⎫ 82	1 (2%) ⎫ 24
Bicuspid	66 (47%) ⎬ (59%)	23 (43%) ⎬ (45%)
Tricuspid	57 (41%) ⎭	29 (55%) ⎭
Left ventricular		
Fibrosis	57 (41%)	13 (25%)
Necrosis	13 (9%)	5 (9%)

WEIGHTS OF OPERATIVELY EXCISED STENOTIC AORTIC VALVES

The weight of operatively excised stenotic aortic valves is useful in quantitating the severity of the stenosis because the weight is determined primarily by the quantity of calcific deposits and the larger the calcific deposits, the greater the transvalvular pressure gradient *12–23*. Roberts and colleagues (*21*) reported weights in 1,849 operatively excised stenotic valves in patients aged 21–91 years without concomitant mitral valve replacement or mitral stenosis. These authors found that the weight of the stenotic valves varied inversely with the number of aortic valve cusps (*13*). The unicuspid valves were the heaviest, the bicuspid valves the next heaviest, and the tricuspid aortic valves the lightest. The men had heavier valves than did the women (Fig. 8), and the younger patients had heavier valves than did the older patients. The mean weights of the valves were similar in patients whose body mass index was <25, 25–30, and >30 kg/m^2. Mean valve weights were also heavier in the patients who *did not* undergo simultaneous coronary artery bypass grafting vs those who did.

Table 5 shows various clinical findings in the 1,849 patients whose stenotic aortic valves were studied by Roberts and colleagues (*21*). The patients underwent aortic valve replacement at three different institutions: National Institutes of Health (NIH) during 1963–1989; Georgetown University Medical Center (GUMC) during 1969–1992; and Baylor University Medical Center (BUMC) during 1993–2004. All 1,849 operatively excised stenotic valves were examined and classified by WCR. Patients having simultaneous mitral valve replacement or mitral stenosis were excluded. The valves excised at NIH and at GUMC from 1963 to 1992 were heavier than the valves excised at BUMC from 1993 to 2004: men 4.05 ± 1.91 (NIH), 4.36 ± 1.83 (GUMC), and 3.11 ± 1.51 g (BUMC); women 2.80 ± 1.26 (NIH), 3.02 ± 1.26 (GUMC), and 1.89 ± 0.87 g (BUMC).

Table 4
Underlying Structure of the Aortic Valve in Patients Studied at Necropsy With Isolated
Aortic Valve Stenosis With or Without Associated Aortic Regurgitation (n= 192)

Variable	Unicuspid [$n = 17$ (9%)]	Bicuspid [$n = 89$ (46%)]	Tricuspid [$n = 86$ (45%)]
Ages (years): Range (mean)	25–73 (46)	16–87 (62)	36–99 (64)
Males	16 (94%)	66 (74%)	57 (66%)
Symptomatic	15 (88%)	73/84 (87%)	57/78 (73%)
Total cholesterol (mg/dl)	216	203	173
Mode of death			
Sudden (outside hospital)	1 (6%)	15 (17%)	11 (13%)
Sudden (inside hospital)	1 (6%)	13 (15%)	6 (7%)
Nonsudden (cardiac)	14 (82%)	47 (53%)	45 (52%)
Vascular	0	2 (2%)	4 (5%)
Noncardiovascular	1 (6%)	12 (14%)	20 (23%)
Severity of stenosis			
1^+	1 (6%)	11 (12%)	19 (22%)
2^+	0	14 (16%)	17 (20%)
3^+	16 (94%)	64 (72%)	50 (58%)
Coronary narrowing			
0	15 (88%)	57 (64%)	41 (48%)
≥ 1	2 (12%)	32 (36%)	45 (52%)
Mitral annular calcium			
0	12 (71%)	72 (81%)	40 (47%)
1^+–3^+	5 (29%)	17 (19%)	46 (53%)
Heart weight (g) (mean)	617	578	573
Left ventricular			
Fibrosis	8/15 (53%)	34/88 (39%)	28/85 (33%)
Necrosis	1/16 (6%)	8/87 (9%)	9/85 (11%)

Not only did the valve weights vary according to valve structure (unicuspid > bicuspid > tricuspid), but often there was variation in individual cusps among patients with bicuspid valves and among patients with tricuspid valves (14–15). Of 200 operatively excised stenotic congenitally bicuspid valves, the two cusps in 152 patients (76%) differed in weight by >0.2 g, and the cusps in 48 patients (24%) were of similar weight ($\leq$0.2 g difference) (14). In 161 of the 200 patients, a raphe was present in one of the two cusps: the raphe and nonraphe cusps differed in weight in 120 patients (74%) with the raphe cusps being heavier in 89 patients (55%), lighter in 31 patients (19%), and of similar weight in 41 (26%). Of the 39 patients without a raphe in one cusp, the two cusps were of different (>0.2 g) weight in 32 patients and of similar weight ($\leq$0.2 g) in 7 patients (18%).

Of 260 operatively excised stenotic three-cuspid aortic valves, all three cusps differed (by >0.1 g) in weight in 71 patients (27%); all three cusps were similar ($\leq$0.1 g difference) in weight in 33 patients (13%); and in 156 patients (60%), one cusp differed from either of the other two cusps, which were similar in weight (15).

Why might cusps of operatively excised stenotic valves differ in weight? The most likely explanation would appear to be that the cusps differ in size, that is, in surface area, from the time of birth. The cusps with the largest surface area has, of course, the larger area on which calcium can be deposited, and the weight of a cusp is determined primarily by the amount of calcium deposited on its aortic surface.

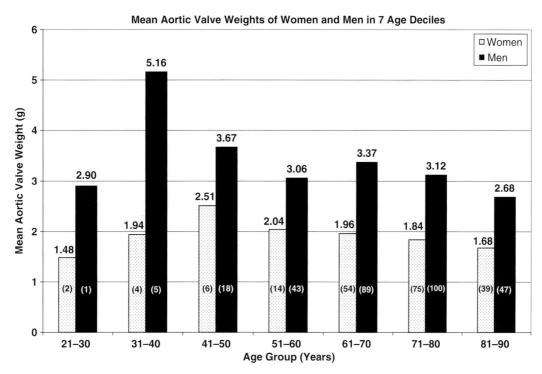

Fig. 8. Bar graph showing aortic valve weights in men and women in each of seven decades. All had aortic stenosis. (Reproduced with permission from Elsevier Ref. *(13)*).

RELATION OF AORTIC VALVE WEIGHT TO TRANSVALVULAR TO PEAK SYSTOLIC PRESSURE GRADIENT

The best determinant of the magnitude of obstruction in patients with AS has been a topic of debate. Determinants considered have been aortic valve area or index, mean transvalvular systolic gradient, and peak transvalvular systolic gradients. Roberts and Ko *(16)* compared the weights of operatively excised stenotic aortic valves to peak transvalvular systolic pressure gradient and to aortic valve area. The results of these studies in 201 men and in 123 women with isolated AS are shown in Table 6. In both men and women the weights of the stenotic aortic valves increased significantly as the peak left ventricular-to-aortic systolic gradient increased but valve weight had essentially no relation to aortic valve area. Women had significantly lower valve weights with peak gradients similar to those in men. In men with valve weights from 1 to 2 g the peak transvalvular gradient averaged 36 mmHg and the valve areas 0.86 cm^2; in the men with valve weights >6 g the peak gradients averaged 87 mmHg, whereas the valve area was 0.71 cm^2. In women with valve weights ≤1 g the peak gradient averaged 28 mmHg and the valve area 0.83 cm^2; in women whose valve weighed from >3 to 4 g the peak gradients averaged 85 m Hg and the valve area 0.51 cm^2 (Table 6).

Relatively few operatively excised aortic valves in adults with AS are ≥5 g and those that are are usually congenitally malformed. Of unicuspid valves, 37 (30%) of 124 valves in men and 5 (11%) of 44 in women reached this weight; of bicuspid valves, 96 (18%) of 521 valves in men and 4 (2%) of 236 valves in women reached this weight (unpublished data). In contrast, only 15 (4%) of 361 tricuspid valves in men and only 2 (0.72%) of 281 valves in women reached this weight. Of 1,038 operatively excised stenotic aortic valves in men, 161 (16%) were ≥5 g, and of 571 valves in women, only 13 (2%)

Table 5
Data in Patients Having Isolated Aortic Valve Replacement For Aortic Stenosis (± Aortic
Regurgitation) at Three Different Medical Centers

Variable	NIH (1963–1989)	GUMC (1969–1992)	BUMC (1993–2004)
Valve structure			
Unicuspid			
Men	84/342 (25%)	56/255 (22%)	36/601 (6%)
Women	14/110 (13%)	24/145 (17%)	12/356 (4%)
Bicuspid			
Men	158/342 (46%)	129/255 (50%)	316/601 (53%)
Women	53/110 (48%)	68/145 (47%)	153/356 (43%)
Tricuspid			
Men	47/342 (14%)	63/255 (25%)	242/601 (40%)
Women	28/110 (25%)	48/145 (33%)	186/356 (52%)
Indeterminate			
Men	53/342 (15%)	7/255 (3%)	7/601 (1%)
Women	15/110 (14%)	5/145 (3%)	5/356 (1%)
Ages: Range (mean ± SD) (years)			
Men	21–82 (54 ± 12)	24–88 (64 ± 11)	25–91 (69 ± 12)
Men ≥65	62/331 (19%)	124/251 (49%)	424/601 (71%)
Women	33–86 (57 ± 11)	22–89 (67 ± 12)	27–91 (70 ± 11)
Women ≥65	27/104 (26%)	94/142 (66%)	273/356 (77%)
Gender			
Men	342/452 (76%)	255/400 (64%)	601/957 (63%)
Women	110/452 (24%)	145/400 (36%)	356/957 (37%)
Aortic valve weight (g)			
Men	0.70–10.2 (4.05 ± 1.91)	1.20–11.0 (4.36 ± 1.83)	0.89–11.30 (3.11 ± 1.51)
Women	0.55–5.50 (2.80 ± 1.26)	0.40–6.70 (3.02 ± 1.26)	0.45–4.97 (1.89 ± 0.87)
Left ventricular to aortic peak systolic gradient (mmHg)			
Men	10–145 (69 ± 30)	10–160 (69 ± 25)	10–141 (52 ± 23)
Women	10–165 (76 ± 34)	30–170 (81 ± 32)	10–133 (54 ± 28)
Aortic valve area (cm^2)			
Men	0.20–1.90 (0.66 ± 0.32)	0.27–1.97 (0.75 ± 0.31)	0.20–1.90 (0.78 ± 0.26)
Women	0.23–1.10 (0.53 ± 0.21)	0.20–1.30 (0.57 ± 0.21)	0.18–1.49 (0.67 ± 0.22)
Cardiac index (l/min/m^2)			
Men	1.10–5.00 (2.58 ± 0.72)	1.00–7.30 (2.87 ± 0.93)	–
Women	1.60–4.50 (2.68 ± 0.69)	1.60–6.20 (2.79 ± 0.81)	–
Simultaneous coronary bypass			
Men	21/238 (9%)	77/198 (39%)	332/601 (55%)
Women	6/74 (8%)	29/118 (25%)	167/356 (47%)

AV=aortic valve; BUMC=Baylor University Medical Center; GUMC=Georgetown University Medical Center; NIH=National Institutes of Health.

Reproduced with permission from Lippincott Williams & Wilkins (*Circulation* 2005;112:3919–3929).

Table 6

Ages, Body Mass Index, and Concomitant Coronary Artery Bypass, Left Ventricular to Aortic Peak Systolic Gradients, and Aortic Valve Areas in Seven Aortic Valve Weight Groups in Men and Women

AV weight (g)	No. of patients	Ages (years) Range (average)	BMI (kg/m²) Range (average)	AV weights (g) Range (average)	LV–aorta PSG (mmHg) Range (average)	AV area (cm²) Range (mean)	Coronary bypass	UAV or BAV	Ejection fraction (%) No.	Range (mean)	No. (%) <= 40	No. (%) >40
Men												
<= 1	0	–	–	–	–	–	–	–	–	–	–	–
> 1–2	41	47–90 (72)	19–37 (27)	1.16–2.00 (1.64)	11–81 (36)	0.27–1.43 (0.86)	27 (66%)	11 (27%)	37	15–78 (48)	13 (35%)	24 (65%)
> 2–3	60	29–87 (69)	20–43 (29)	2.01–3.00 (2.58)	15–97 (45)	0.42–2.25 (0.89)	32 (53%)	24 (40%)	52	10–85 (51)	14 (27%)	38 (73%)
> 3–4	50	37–84 (69)	17–40 (27)	3.03–4.00 (3.40)	20–100 (56)	0.20–1.63 (0.75)	26 (52%)	30 (60%)	44	15–80 (53)	7 (16%)	37 (84%)
> 4–5	29	42–87 (69)	18–45 (28)	4.01–4.84 (4.40)	20–108 (64)	0.32–1.06 (0.67)	11 (38%)	25 (86%)	26	15–70 (53)	5 (19%)	21 (81%)
> 5–6	12	49–90 (70)	24–36 (28)	5.03–5.93 (5.60)	50–116 (71)	0.40–0.88 (0.60)	3 (25%)	10 (83%)	10	20–65 (43)	4 (40%)	6 (60%)
> 6	9	38–84 (58)	21–38 (28)	6.24–11.30 (7.92)	35–141 (87)	0.39–1.23 (0.71)	2 (22%)	8 (89%)	8	15–70 (51)	2 (25%)	6 (75%)
Women												
<= 1	10	55–85 (74)	21–44 (30)	0.69–0.95 (0.83)	15–62 (28)	0.34–1.28 (0.83)	7 (70%)	2 (20%)	9	30–70 (47)	4 (44%)	5 (56%)
> 1–2	73	19–88 (71)	17–51 (29)	1.02–1.99 (1.46)	10–119 (49)	0.18–1.49 (0.72)	40 (55%)	14 (19%)	66	15–80 (56)	9 (14%)	57 (86%)
> 2–3	29	30–87 (70)	18–50 (28)	2.04–3.00 (2.42)	26–113 (63)	0.27–1.09 (0.58)	15 (52%)	12 (41%)	23	30–80 (54)	4 (17%)	19 (83%)
> 3–4	10	47–85 (73)	17–35 (26)	3.14–4.00 (3.42)	53–131 (85)	0.23–0.78 (0.51)	3 (30%)	9 (90%)	9	45–75 (53)	0	9 (100%)
> 4–5	1	83	29	4.27	53	0.75	0	1 (100%)	1	50	0	1 (100%)
> 5–6	0	–	–	–	–	–	–	–	–	–	–	–
> 6	0	–	–	–	–	–	–	–	–	–	–	–

AV = aortic valve; BAV = bicuspid aortic valve; BMI = body mass index; LV = left ventricular; No. = number; PSG = peak systolic gradient; UAV = unicuspid aortic valve.

Reproduced with permission from Elsevier (*J Am Coll Cardiol* 2004;44:1847-55).

reached this weight. Seven operatively excised stenotic valves weighted ≥ 10 g: all were in men and all seven were either unicuspid or bicuspid and the peak pressure gradient across them ranged from 80 to 143 mmHg (average 101) (unpublished data).

ASSOCIATED CORONARY ARTERIAL NARROWING

Patients with operatively excised congenitally unicuspid and bicuspid valves have significantly less epicardial coronary arterial narrowing than do patients with tricuspid aortic valves (Table 7). Concomitant coronary artery bypass grafting (CABG) also varies according to the era during which the AVR was done and depending on the institution where it was done. Also, criteria for performing CABG in patients having AVR have changed with time.

Table 7
Frequency of Concomitant Coronary Artery Bypass Grafting Among Patients
Having Isolated Aortic Valve Replacement for Aortic Stenosis at Three Different
Institutions[*]

Valve structure	NIH 1963–1989 ($n = 259$)	GUMC 1969–1992 ($n = 308$)	BUMC 1993–2007 ($n = 1351$)
Unicuspid	2/61 (3%)	13/55 (24%)	13/83 (16%)
Bicuspid	13/140 (9%)	42/162 (26%)	280/646 (43%)
Tricuspid	10/58 (17%)	47/91 (52%)	390/622 (63%)

[*]Excludes cases in which the number of valve cusps was unclear (indeterminate).

BUMC = Baylor University Medical Center; GUMC = Georgetown University Medical Center;

NIH = National Institutes of Health.

RELATION TO LEFT BUNDLE BRANCH BLOCK AND/OR COMPLETE HEART BLOCK

At one time, patients with AS and left bundle branch block or complete heart block were believed to have the conduction disturbance because of associated severe coronary arterial narrowing from atherosclerosis. Study at necropsy, however, of many patients with combined AS and left bundle branch block or complete heart block has indicated that the conduction disturbance was due not to the associated coronary narrowing but to the destruction of the left bundle branches or the atrioventricular bundle by calcific deposits, which had extended caudally from the aortic valve (Roberts unpublished data). Most of these patients had congenitally malformed aortic valves – not tricuspid valves – and severe degrees of hemodynamic obstruction as a result of heavy calcific deposits.

Pure Aortic Regurgitation

There are two major causes of pure (no element of stenosis) aortic regurgitation (AR): (1) conditions affecting primarily the valve and (2) conditions affecting the aorta and only secondarily causing the valve to be incompetent. Roberts and Ko (*24*) recently reviewed the cause of pure AR in 268 patients having isolated AVR at BUMC from 1993 to 2005. As shown in Table 8, conditions affecting primarily the valve was the cause of the AR in 122 patients (46%), and nonvalve conditions was the cause in 146 patients (54%). Among the former, the *congenitally bicuspid valve* unassociated with infective endocarditis was the problem in 59 patients, 22 (37%) of whom had resection of portions of the dilated ascending aorta. Eleven of the 22 patients with resected aortas had severe loss of medial elastic fibers. Infective endocarditis was the cause in 46 patients, 15 (33%) of whom had congenitally bicuspid aortic valves. Thus, of the 122 with valve conditions causing the AR, 74 (61%) had congenitally bicuspid aortic valves. Why one congenitally bicuspid aortic valve becomes stenotic (8, 25) and another purely regurgitation without superimposed infective endocarditis (26), why another becomes severely dysfunction only when infective endocarditis appears (27), and why some congenitally bicuspid valves function normally an entire lifetime are unclear (8). Of 85 patients, aged 15–79 years, with congenitally bicuspid aortic valves studied at autopsy by Roberts (8), 61 (72%) valves were stenotic, 2 (2%) were purely regurgitation without superimposed infective endocarditis, 9 (11%) had AR because of infective endocarditis, and 13 (15%) functioned normally during the patients' 23–59 years of life (mean 45 years).

Rheumatic heart disease is a relatively infrequent cause of pure AR in patients with normally functioning mitral valves (9). All such patients (by our definition of rheumatic heart disease) have diffuse fibrosis of the mitral leaflets or at least diffuse thickening of the margins of these leaflets. In this circumstance, mitral valve function would be normal despite the anatomic abnormality.

Infective endocarditis more commonly involves a three-cuspid aortic valve rather than a two-cuspid one because the tricuspid valve is so much more common than the bicuspid valve (27).

Rheumatoid arthritis is a rare cause of AR. The anatomic abnormality is specific for this condition and consists of rheumatoid nodules within the aortic valve cusps (28, 29).

Conditions affecting the ascending aorta causing it to dilate cause AR more commonly than those conditions affecting primarily the aortic valve. Of 146 patients having pure AR and isolated AVR, the cause of the AR was not determined after examination of the operatively excised aorta and aortic valve (24). Many of these patients had *systemic hypertension* but only mild dilation of the aorta and all had normal or nearly normal three-cuspid aortic valves. It is likely that systemic hypertension in some way played a role in the AR (30, 31).

Aortic dissection usually produces acute AR due to the splitting of the aortic media behind the aortic valve commissures, resulting in prolapse of one or more cusps toward the left ventricular cavity (32).

Diffuse thickening of the tubular portion of the central ascending aorta with sparing of the wall of aorta behind the sinuses is characteristic of *cardiovascular syphilis* (33). These patients generally undergo a cardiovascular operation because of diffuse aneurysmal dilatation of the tubular portion of ascending aorta, not as a rule because of severe AR. *Granulomatous (giant cell) aortitis* grossly mimics cardiovascular syphilis but is far less common. During the past 10 years, 15 patients have had resection of aneurysmally dilated syphilitic aortas with or without simultaneous aortic valve replacement at BUMC (unpublished). The characteristic histologic feature of cardiovascular syphilis is extensive thickening of the aortic wall due to fibrous thickening of the intima and of the adventitia (Fig. 9). The medial elastic fibers and smooth-muscle cells are also replaced focally by scars due to narrowings in the vasa "vasora". Focal collections of plasma cells and lymphocytes are present in the adventitia. Giant-cell aortitis is similar to syphilitic aortitis except for the presence of multinucleated giant cells.

The AR in patients with *the Marfan syndrome* and forme fruste varieties of it is the result of severe dilatation of the sinus portion and proximal tubular portion of the aorta (34). The consequence of the "aortic root" dilatation is stretching of the aortic valve cusps in roughly a straight line between the commissures leading to a wide-open central regurgitant stream. In contrast to cardiovascular syphilis, the aortic wall in the Marfan syndrome is thinner than normal due to the massive loss of medial elastic fibers and lack of thickening of either the intima or the adventitia.

There is one condition that causes AR by involving both valve cusp and the portion of aorta behind and adjacent to the lateral attachments of the aortic valve cusps. That condition is *ankylosing spondylitis* (35, 36). About 5% of patients with this form of arthritis develop AR. The bases of aortic valve cusps become densely thickened by fibrous tissue, which is also present on the ventricular aspect of anterior mitral leaflet and on the left ventricular aspect of the membranous ventricular septum. Varying degrees of heart block may be a consequence of this subaortic deposit of dense fibrous tissue. The AR

Table 8

Causes of Aortic Regurgitation in Patients Having Isolated Aortic Valve Replacement at Baylor University Medical Center (1993 - 2005)

Causes of Aortic Regurgitation	Total	Ages (Yrs) at Operation Range (mean)	M	F	Acute	Chronic	SH	CABG	Excised	Examined Histologically	"CMN" (3+,4+)	BAV	Calcium Deposits on AV Cusps	Men	Women
Congenital Malformation Without Infective Endocarditis															
Bicuspid	59 (22%)	22-77 (55)	49	10	0	59	39 (66%)	18 (31%)	22	22	11	59	31	0.52-2.99 (1.42)	0.68-1.80 (1.24)
Quadricuspid	2 (1%)	53, 79 (66)	0	2	0	2	0	1 (50%)	0	0	0	0	0	–	0.57, 1.13 (0.85)
Tricuspid	5 (2%)	33-48 (40)	3	2	0	5	2 (40%)	0	1	1	0	0	0	1.11-1.40 (1.23)	0.34, 0.66 (.050)
Infective Endocarditis	46 (17%)	21-82 (45)	31	15	27	19	29 (63%)	7 (15%)	6	4	0	15	8	0.77-2.31 (1.53)	0.44-2.50 (0.98)
Rheumatic ?	8 (3%)	25-63 (47)	6	2	0	8	6 (75%)	2 (25%)	0	0	0	0	3	1.10-2.45 (1.81)	1.31, 1.83 (1.57)
Miscellaneous	2 (1%)	24, 42 (33)	1	1	0	2	2 (100%)	1 (50%)	0	0	0	0	0	0.55	–
Aortic Dissection	28 (10%)	25-78 (58)	20	8	21	7	22 (79%)	5 (17%)	28	20	5	3	4	0.51-1.19 (0.81)	0.37-0.90 (0.59)
Marfan or Forme Fruste	15 (6%)	21-71 (47)	9	6	0	15	10 (67%)	1[†] (7%)	15	13	13	0	2	0.73-1.01 (0.94)	0.35-0.85 (0.66)
Aortitis	12 (4%)	35-82 (66)	5	7	0	12	10 (83%)	5 (42%)	12	12	12	0	2	0.63-0.79 (0.70)	0.35-0.70 (0.54)
Etiology Unclear	91 (34%)	50-84 (66)	58	33	0	91	83 (91%)	46 (51%)	7	7	0	0	26	0.48-2.13 (1.08)	0.31-1.74 (0.73)
Total	268 (100%)	21-84 (57)	182 (68%)	86 (32%)	48 (18%)	220 (82%)	203 (76%)	86 (32%)	91 (34%)	76	41	77 (29%)	76/263 (29%)	0.48-2.99 (1.22) 151‡	0.31-2.50 (0.81) 75‡

122 (46%) VALVE

146 (54%) NONVALVE

AV=aortic valve; BAV=bicuspid aortic valve; CABG=coronary artery bypass grafting; "CMN"=cystic medial necrosis"; F=female; M=male; SH=systemic hypertension
"Cystic medial necrosis" is used here to refer to the magnitude of loss of elastic fibers in the aorta's media.
[†]Four other patients had CABG due to extension of the aortic dissection into a coronary artery.
[†]One additional patient had CABG due to extension of the aortic dissection into a coronary artery.
[‡]Number of cases with aortic valve weight
Reproduced with permission from Lippincott Williams & Wilkins *Circulation* 2006;114:422-429)

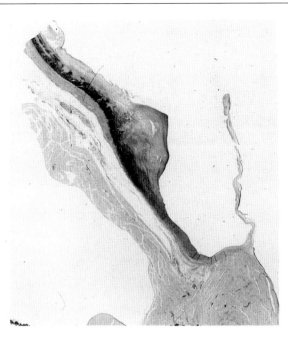

Fig. 9. *Cardiovascular syphilis.* Photomicrographs of an aortic valve cusp, sinus portion of aorta (behind the cusp), and proximal tubular portion of ascending aorta, which is thickened by intimal and adventitial fibrous tissue. Many medial elastic fibers have been destroyed. The location of the process in the tubular portion of aorta with sparring of the sinus portion of aorta is characteristic of cardiovascular syphilis. Elastic tissue stain, 4.5×.

associated with ankylosing spondylitis is usually severe with diastolic pressures in both aorta and left ventricle often being similar. The histologic appearance of the aorta in ankylosing spondylitis is similar to that in syphilitis but the syphilitic process never extends onto the aortic valve cusps or subvalvular and rarely involves the wall of aorta behind the sinuses.

Various conditions affecting the aortic valve are shown in Fig. 10.

Mitral Stenosis

Of the 1,010 patients aged ≥15 years of age with functionally severe valvular cardiac disease studied at necropsy by Roberts up to 1980, 434 (44%) had mitral stenosis (MS) (*1*). MS occurred alone in 189 (44%) patients and in combination with other functional valve lesions in the other 245 (56%) patients. MS was of rheumatic etiology in all 434 patients.

Rheumatic heart disease may be viewed as a disease of the mitral valve; other valves also may be involved both anatomically and functionally, but anatomically the mitral valve is always involved (*37, 38*) (Fig. 11). *Aschoff bodies* have never been reported in hearts without anatomic disease of the mitral valve (*38*). Of the first 543 patients with severe valvular heart disease that Roberts and Virmani (*39*) studied at necropsy, 11 (2.7%) had Aschoff bodies, and all had anatomic mitral valve disease. The 11 patients ranged in age from 18 to 68 years (mean 38) and 9 had a history of acute rheumatic fever; 9 had MS with or without dysfunction of one or more other cardiac valves; 1 had isolated AR and 1 had both AR and MR. All 11 had diffuse fibrous thickening of the mitral leaflets and all but 1 had diffuse anatomic lesions of at least two other cardiac valve. Thus, among patients with chronic valve disease, Aschoff bodies, the only anatomic lesion pathognomonic of rheumatic heart disease, usually indicate diffuse anatomic lesions of >1 cardiac valve, and the most common hemodynamic lesion is MS with or without MR.

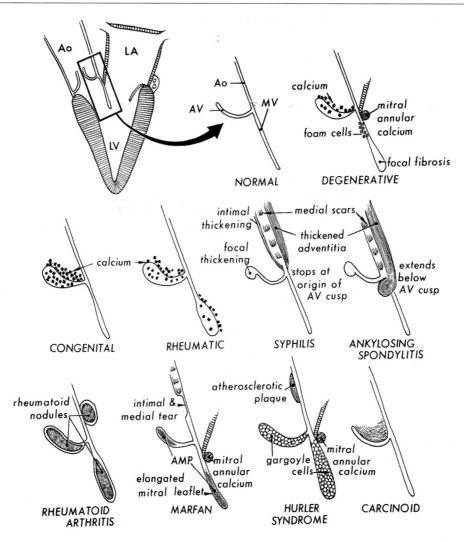

Fig. 10. Diagram of some of the conditions affecting the aorta or aortic valve or mitral valve. [Reproduced with permission from Roberts WC and Perloff JK *(37)*].

Although rare at necropsy in patients with fatal chronic valve disease, Aschoff bodies are fairly common in the heart of patients having mitral commissurotomy for MS. Among 481 patients having various valve operations, Aschoff bodies were found by Virmani and Roberts *(40)* in 40 (21%) of 191 operatively excised left atrial appendages, in 4 (2%) of 273 operatively excised left ventricular papillary muscles, and in 1 (6%) of 17 patients in whom both appendage and papillary muscle were excised. Of these 45 patients with Aschoff bodies, 44 had MS (Fig. 12) and only one, a 10-year-old boy, had pure MR. Sinus rhythm was present preoperatively in 38 (84%) and atrial fibrillation in 7 (16%).

Rheumatic heart disease is a disorder of the cardiac valves, and it may also affect mural endocardium, epicardium, and myocardium. The atrial walls virtually always have increased amounts of fibrous tissue in both myocardial interstitium and mural endocardium, atrophy of some and hypertrophy of other myocardial cells, and hypertrophy of smooth muscles in the mural endocardium. In all patients with rheumatic MS, the leaflets are diffusely thickened by either fibrous tissue or calcific

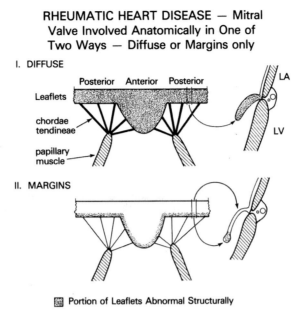

RHEUMATIC HEART DISEASE — Mitral
Valve Involved Anatomically in One of
Two Ways — Diffuse or Margins only

I. DIFFUSE

II. MARGINS

▦ Portion of Leaflets Abnormal Structurally

Fig. 11. *Rheumatic heart disease.* Diagram showing the two types of anatomic involvement of the mitral valve in rheumatic heart disease.

deposits or both, the two commissures are usually fixed, and the chordae tendineae are usually (but not always) thickened and fused (Figs. 13 and 14).

The amount of calcium in the leaflets of stenotic mitral valves varies considerably (Fig. 15). Generally, the calcific deposits are more frequent and in larger quantities in men than in women, in older than in younger patients, and in those with higher pressure gradients compared to those with lower pressure gradients between left atrium and left ventricle (Fig. 14). The rapidity with which calcium develops also varies considerably: it is present at a younger age in men than in women. Lachman and Roberts (*41*) determined the presence or the absence and the extent of calcific deposits in operatively excised stenotic mitral valves in 164 patients aged 26–72 years. The amount of calcific deposits in the stenotic mitral valves correlated with *sex* and the *mean transvalvular pressure gradient* (Fig. 16), but it did not correlate with the patients' age (after 25 years), cardiac rhythm, pulmonary arterial or pulmonary arterial wedge pressure, previous mitral commissurotomy, presence of thrombus in the body or the appendage of left ventricle, or the presence of disease in one or more other cardiac valves. Of the 164 patients, radiographs of the operatively excised valve showed no calcific deposits in 14 of them and only minimal deposits in 43 of them. Of the 57 patients, however, 37 had moderate or severe MR. The remaining 20 in an earlier era would have been ideal or near ideal candidates for mitral commissurotomy (*42*).

A major complication of MS is *thrombus formation in the left atrial cavity.* The thrombus may be limited to atrial appendage (by far most common) or be located in both the appendage and the body of left atrium. Left atrial "body" thrombus was observed in 5% of the 1,010 necropsy patients with fatal valvular heart disease studies by Roberts and all had severe MS (unpublished data). Left atrial "body" thrombus was not found in any of the 165 patients with pure MR. All patients with left atrial "body" thrombus had atrial fibrillation. In contrast, of 46 patients with MS having cardiotomy at NHLBI and thrombus in the left atrial "body," 42 (91%) had atrial fibrillation and 4 (9%) had sinus rhythm. *Thrombus appears to occur in the body of left atrium only in patients with MS, and atrial fibrillation in the absence of MS is incapable of forming thrombus in the left atrial body.*

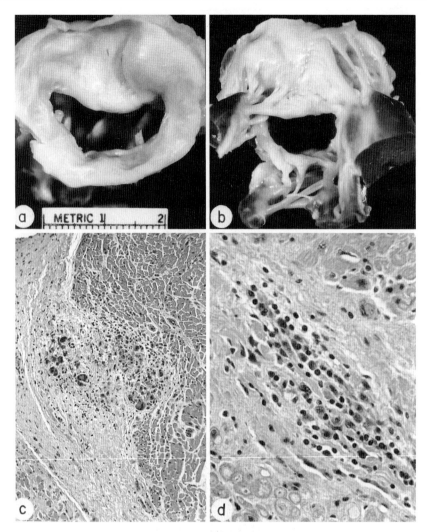

Fig. 12. Acute rheumatic fever and mitral stenosis. Excised mitral valve in a 23-year-old Indian woman with mitral stenosis (13 mmHg mean diastolic pressure gradient between pulmonary artery wedge and left ventricle) and regurgitation. She had had acute rheumatic fever initially at age 7 and recurrence of migratory polyarthritis at age 22. During the early postoperative course after mitral valve replacement, she had swelling and pain in one knee and one ankle and erythema in about two joints. Shown are the excised valves viewed from the left atrium **(a)** and from the left ventricle **(b)** and Aschoff bodies **(c)** and **(d)**, which were numerous in both excised left ventricular papillary muscles. (hematoxylin and eosin; 110 **[c]**, 400× **[d]**) (Reproduced with permission of Virmani R and Roberts WC *(40)*).

Calcific deposits on the mural endocardium of left atrium almost certainly are indicative of previous organization of left atrial thrombi (*43*). Histologically, the "calcific thrombi" also contain cholesterol clefts and are identical to atherosclerotic plaques. The observation that left atrial thrombi can organize into lesions identical to atherosclerotic plaques supports the view that atherosclerotic plaques may in part be the result of organization of thrombi.

Nonrheumatic causes of MS include *congenital anomalies (37, 38)*; *large mitral annular calcific deposits associated with left ventricular outflow obstruction (44, 45)* (Fig. 17); *neoplasms* (particularly myxoma) protruding through the mitral orifice (*46*); *large vegetations from active infective*

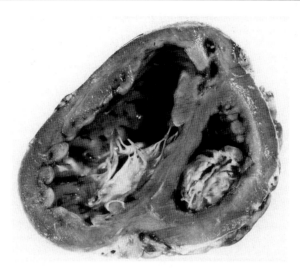

Fig. 13. *Mitral stenosis.* Heart in a 16-year-old boy who had acute rheumatic fever at age 6 and chronic heart failure beginning at age 10. He had severe mitral stenosis and tricuspid valve regurgitation. At cardiac catheterization 10 hours before death, the right ventricular pressure was 100/20 and the left ventricular pressure, 100/10 mmHg. By left ventricular angiogram, the left ventricular cavity was of normal size and there was no mitral regurgitation. At necropsy, the heart weighed 450 g (the patient weighed 43 kg). The right ventricular cavity was greatly dilated and both ventricular walls were of similar thickness. Both mitral and tricuspid valve leaflets were diffusely thickened and free of calcific deposits. No Aschoff bodies were found. (Reproduced with permission from Roberts WC *(38)*).

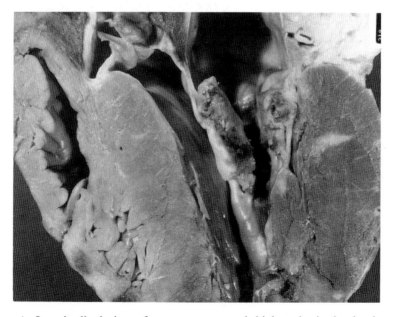

Fig. 14. *Mitral stenosis.* Longitudinal view of a very narrow and thickened mitral valve in a 55-year-old man with equal peak systolic pressures in the right and left ventricles and no associated mitral regurgitation during cannulation of the aorta for planned mitral valve replacement. Both anterior and posterior mitral leaflets are heavily calcified. (Reproduced with permission from Roberts WC *(38)*).

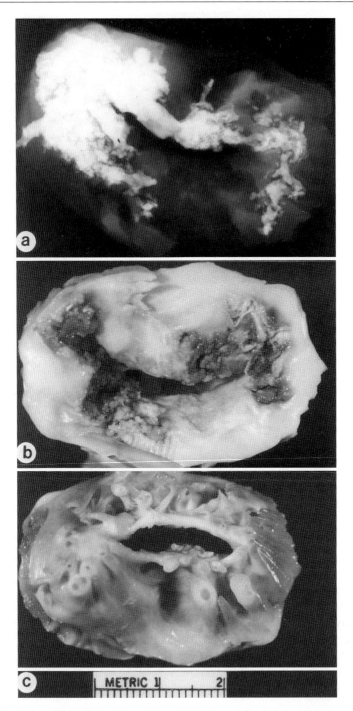

Fig. 15. *Mitral stenosis.* Operatively excised heavily calcified stenotic mitral valve in a 57-year-old man with combined mitral stenosis (12 mmHg means transvalvular diastolic gradient) and aortic stenosis. **(a)** Radiograph of the excised valve. **(b)** View of valve from the left atrial aspect. Thrombi are present near and at the commissures. **(c)** View from the left ventricular aspect. The orifice is severely narrowed.

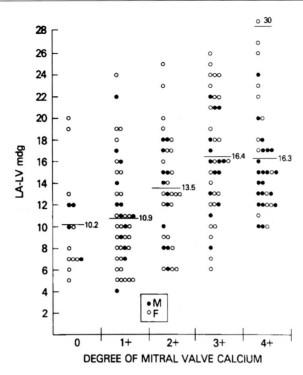

Fig. 16. *Mitral stenosis.* Diagram comparing the relation of the mean left atrial–left ventricular mean diastolic gradient to the quantity of mitral valve calcium graded by radiograph of the operatively excised mitral valve. The greater the quantity of mitral calcium, the greater the transvalvular gradient (Reproduced with permission from Lachman AS and Roberts WC *(41)*).

endocarditis (47), and of course a mechanical prosthesis or a bioprosthesis used to replace a native mitral valve *(48)*.

Histologic examination of sections of stenotic mitral valves when stained for elastic fibers shows the mitral leaflet to have lost most or all of its spongiosa element such that the leaflet itself consists entirely or nearly entirely of the fibrosa element. The leaflet (as are the chordae) is outlined by an elastic fibril (which stains black by an elastic tissue stain) and covering it on both atrial and ventricular aspects is dense fibrous tissue containing focally some vascular channels. Similar dense fibrous tissue surrounds the chordae and the chordae themselves appear normal.

Patients with MS usually have distinct pulmonary vascular changes secondary to the pulmonary venous and arterial hypertension. These anatomic changes consist of thickening of the media of the muscular and elastic pulmonary arteries and focal intimal fibrous plaques. Plexiform lesions never occur in the lungs as a result of MS. The alveolar septa also thicken due to dilatation of the capillaries, proliferation of lining alveolar cells, and some increase of alveolar septal fibrous tissue.

Pure Mitral Regurgitation

Pure MR (no element of MS) is the most common dysfunctional cardiac valve disorder, and, in contrast to MS, it has many different causes. If patients with MR due to left ventricular dilatation from any cause (ischemic cardiomyopathy, idiopathic dilated cardiomyopathy, anemia, etc.) are excluded, the most common cause of MR treated operatively in the Western World today is *mitral valve prolapse* (MVP) (Figs. 18 and 19). This condition, which was described initially in the 1960s by Barlow and

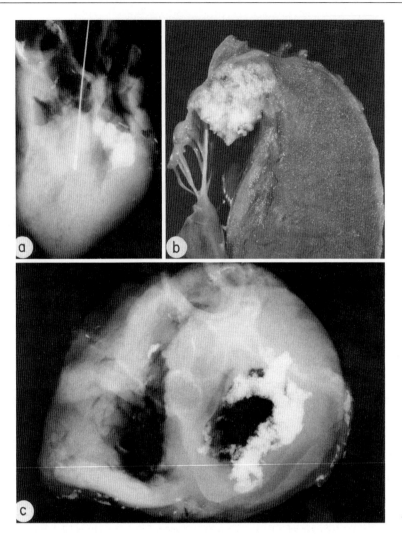

Fig. 17. *Mitral annular calcium.* Heavily calcified mitral annulus in a 71-year-old woman with previous second-degree heart block and a pacemaker for 23 months. She died of acute myocardial infarction complicated by the rupture of the left ventricular free wall. **(a)** Radiograph of the heart at necropsy showing mitral annular calcium and the pacemaker leads. **(b)** Longitudinal section showing heavy calcific deposits behind the posterior itral leaflet. **(c)** Radiograph of the base of heart after removing its apical one-half showing the circumferential extent of the mitral annular calcific deposits. (Reproduced with permission from Roberts WC, Dangel JC, Bulkley BH *(33)*).

colleagues *(49)* and by Criley and colleagues *(50)*, is now recognized to occur in approximately 5% of the adult population, and if this condition is considered a congenital deficiency of mitral tissues – which we do – it is the most common congenital cardiovascular disease. Among 97 patients having mitral valve replacement for pure MR from 1968 to 1981 at the NHLBI, MVP was responsible in 60 patients (62%), papillary muscle dysfunction from coronary heart disease in 29 (30%), infective endocarditis in 5 (5%), and possibly rheumatic disease in 3 (3%) *(51)*.

Although several authors have attempted to do so, defining MVP has not been easy *(1)*. The following have proved useful in separating the valve affected by MVP from other conditions affecting the mitral valve:

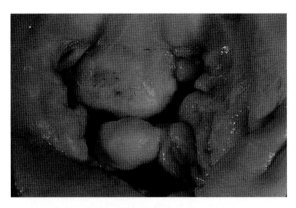

Fig. 18. *Mitral valve prolapse.* View from above shows prolapse of both anterior and posterior cusps in a man who died from consequences of an acute myocardial infarction.

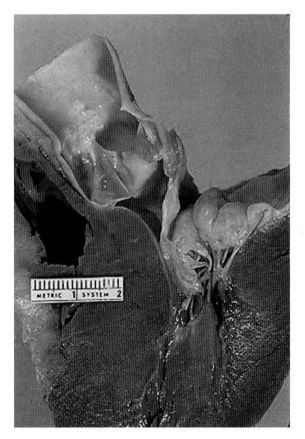

Fig. 19. *Mitral valve prolapse.* View of prolapsed posterior leaflet in a 74-year-old woman who during life was found to have a precordial murmur but never had symptoms of cardiac dysfunction.

(1) *Focal lengthening of the posterior and/or the anterior mitral leaflets from their site of attachment to their distal margins.* Normally, the length of the posterior leaflet from its attachment to distal margin is about 1 cm. In MVP, this leaflet focally often is as long as the anterior leaflet (*51*).
(2) *Elongation and thinning of chordae tendineae.*

(3) *Focal thickening of the posterior and/or the anterior leaflet.* This finding is particularly prominent on the portion of leaflet that prolapses toward or into the left atrium during ventricular systole. The atrial surface is uniformly smooth. The thickening of the leaflet produces a spongy feel.

(4) *The mitral leaflet is increased in area, either focally or diffusely (51).*

(5) *Loss of chordae tendineae on the ventricular aspect of posterior mitral leaflet.* It is rare to see actually a ruptured chorda but what is seen are areas where chordae should be attached but none are there. They presumably ruptured in the past and with time were matted down on the leaflets' ventricular aspect, giving this surface a "bumpy" appearance and feel. Chordae are nearly uniformly missing (previously ruptured) in portions of posterior mitral leaflet excised during mitral valve repair or during replacement. Indeed, MVP appears to be by far the most common cause of ruptured chordae tendineae. Infective endocarditis is the next most frequent cause (52).

(6) *Dilatation of the mitral annulus.* Annular dilatation probably is the major cause of development of severe MR in the presence of MVP (51, 53). (The other is the rupture of chordae tendineae.) Normally, the mitral annulus in adults averages about 9 cm in circumference. In patients with left ventricular dilatation from any cause, with or without MR, the mitral circumference usually dilates slightly, usually to about 11 cm or <25% above normal (54). Among patients with MVP associated with severe MR, this annular circumference generally increases >50% to 12–18 cm. Acute rupture of chordae tendineae may occur in patients with MVP in the absence of mitral annular dilatation.

(7) *An increase in the transverse dimension of the mitral leaflets such that the length of the mitral circumference measured on a line corresponding to the distal margin of the posterior leaflet is much larger than the circumference measured at the level of the mitral annulus (51).* In the normal mitral valve, the two are the same. It is analogous to a skirt gathered at the waist. The leaflets of the opened normal mitral valve are flat or smooth on the atrial aspect (like the mucosa of the ileum), whereas those of the opened floppy mitral valve are undulating (like those of the duodenum or jejunum).

(8) *Focal thickening of mural endocardium of left ventricle behind the posterior mitral leaflet.* Salazar and Edwards (55) called these fibrous thickenings "friction lesions" to indicate that they are believed to be the result of friction between the overlying leaflets and chordae and the underlying left ventricular wall. Lucas and Edwards (56) observed these "friction lesions" in 77 (75%) of 102 necropsy cases of MVP, and Dollar and Roberts (57) found them in 23 (68%) of 34 necropsy cases of MVP.

(9) *Fibrinous deposits on the atrial surface of the prolapsed portion of mitral leaflet and particularly at the angle formed between prolapsed leaflet and left atrial wall* (mitral valve – left atrial angle). These fibrin deposits may be a source of emboli.

Histologically, the MVP valve is distinctive. Utilizing elastic tissue stains the mitral leaflet and chordae are surrounded by a single thick elastic fibril. The underlying leaflet generally – but not always – contains an excess amount of the spongiosa element and this causes the leaflet itself to be a bit thicker than normal. Most of the leaflet thickening, however, is due to superimposed fibrous tissue on both its atrial and ventricular aspects. The covering on the atrial side of the leaflet contains numerous elastic fibers, whereas that on the ventricular aspect contains few or no elastic fibrils. Often on the ventricular aspect, previously ruptured and now "matted" chordae tendineae are covered by fibrous tissue. The spongiosa element within the leaflet itself appears normal – just increased in amount – and therefore the phrase "mucoid degeneration" appears inappropriate.

Ultrastructural studies of mitral valves grossly characteristic of MVP have disclosed alterations of the collagen fibers in the leaflets and in the chordae tendineae (58). These changes have included fragmentation, splitting, swelling, course granularity of the individual collagen fibers, and also spiraling and twisting of the fibers. These alterations in the structure of the collagen are probably far more important than the excess acid mucopolysaccharide material in the leaflet in that they lead to focal weakness of the leaflets and chordae and their subsequent elongation. The left ventricular systolic pressure exerted against these weakened areas may account for the prolapse.

Just as the frequency of MVP varies clinically depending on the age and sex group being examined and in the clinical criteria employed for diagnosis (ausculatory, echocardiographic, angiographic), its frequency at necropsy is quite variable and the variation is determined by several factors such as (1) age and sex group of population being examined; (2) type of institution where necropsy is performed (general hospital, referral hospital for cardiovascular disease, or medical examiner's (coroner's) office); (3) expertise in cardiovascular disease of the physician performing the necropsy or reporting the findings; (4) percent of total deaths having autopsies at the particular hospital; (5) presence or absence of evidence of cardiac disease before death; (6) whether the patient underwent mitral valve replacement or repair; and (7) whether the percentage of patients being examined had a high frequency of the Marfan syndrome, infective endocarditis, atrial septal defect, and so on.

No study shows better how bias alters the finding in necropsy studies than the one performed by Lucas and Edwards (Table 9) (56). These investigators, in one portion of their study, determined the frequency of and complications of floppy mitral valves observed at necropsy in one community (non-referral) hospital for adults. Of 1,376 autopsies performed, 7% or 102 patients had morphologically floppy mitral valves at necropsy. Their mean age at death was 69 ± 12 years; 62 (61%) were men and 40 (39%) were women. Of the 102 patients, MVP was the cause of death in only 4. Of the 102 patients, one leaflet had prolapsed in 34 patients and two leaflets in 68. Only 18 had anatomic evidence of previous MR; 7 had infective endocarditis; 7 had ruptured chordae tendineae (without infection); 1 had the Marfan syndrome; and 3 had secundum atrial septal defect. No patient died suddenly. In contrast, in the other portion of their study, these authors described complications in 69 necropsy patients whose hearts had been sent to Edwards for his opinion and interest. Among these 69 patients, 16 (23%) had died suddenly and unexpectedly; 19 (28%) had ruptured chordae tendineae (without infection); 7 (10%) had infective endocarditis; 20 (29%) had the Marfan syndrome; and 9 (13%) had secundum-type atrial septal defect. Thus, in contrast to their infrequency in their community hospital series, most cases submitted to their cardiovascular registry from other institutions had ruptured chordae, infective endocarditis, sudden unexpected and unexplained death, or the Marfan syndrome.

The earlier studies by Pomerance (59) and by Davies and colleagues (60) can also be compared to the community hospital series of Lucas and Edwards (56) (Table 9). The study by Dollar and Roberts (57) (Table 9) is comparable to the study of Lucas and Edwards and their selected cases. These authors studied at necropsy 56 patients, aged 16–70 years (mean 48) and compared findings in the 15 who died suddenly and unexpectedly to the other 41 who did not. Compared with the 34 patients without associated congenital heart disease and with non-MVP conditions capable in themselves of being fatal, the 15 patients who died suddenly with isolated MVP were younger (mean age 39 vs 52 years), more often women (67% vs 26%), had a lower frequency of MR (7% vs 38%), and less likely to have ruptured chordae tendineae (29% vs 67%).

The frequency of atrial fibrillation is different in patients with MVP and those with MS immediately before a mitral valve replacement or "repair." Among 246 patients aged 21–84 (mean 61) (66% men) who had mitral valve repair or replacement for MR secondary to MVP, Berbarie and Roberts (61) found only 37 patients (15%) (mean 60) with atrial fibrillation and 209 patients (88%) with sinus rhythm. In contrast, of 104 patients aged 33–80 (12% men) with rheumatic MS severe enough or symptomatic enough to warrant MVP, Sims and Roberts (62) found atrial fibrillation by electrocardiogram immediately preoperatively in 47 (45%) and sinus rhythm in 57 (55%).

OTHER CAUSES OF PURE MITRAL REGURGITATION

Cleft Anterior Mitral Leaflet. Partial atrioventricular "defect" includes a spectrum of five anatomic anomalies (63). Some patients have all five and others have only one or two. The five are the following: (1) defect in the lower portion of the atrial septum, the so-called primum atrial septal defect; (2) defect in, or absence of, the posterobasal portion of ventricular septum; (3) cleft, anterior mitral

Table 9
Reported Necropsy Cases of Mitral Valve Prolapse

Authors	Year of publication	Number With MVP	Ages (years)	Male/Female	MVP cause of death	Number of mitral leaflets prolapsed 1/2	MR	RCT	IE	SD	MS	ASD*	MAC	HW increased	DMA
Pomerance	1969	35†	51–98 (mean 74)	23/12	4	12/23	8	2‡	2	1	0	1	9	13	–
Davies et al.	1978	90§	<40–100	44/46	6	69/21	23	–	9	13	0	0	3	8‖	6
Lucas and Edwards	1982	102¶	69 ± 12	62/40	4	34/68	18	7‡	7	0	1	3	–	–	–
Lucas and Edwards	1982	69**	–	–	–	–	–	19‡	7	16	20	9	–	–	–
Dollar and Roberts	1991	56**	16–70 (mean 48)	33/23	29	50/6	32	18‡	0	15	2	4	12	30††	40

ASD = atrial septal defect; DMA = dilated mitral annulus; HW = heart weight; IE = infective endocarditis; MAC = mitral annular calcium; MR = mitral regurgitation;

MS = the Marfan syndrome; MVP = mitral valve prolapse; RCT = ruptured chordae tendinae; SD = sudden death.

– = no information available.

*Secundum-type atrial septal defect.

†Thirty cases from a single hospital (1% of autopsies).

‡Unassociated with infective endocarditis.

§Cases acquired from four different hospitals (4.5% of autopsies).

‖Heart weight >300 g.

¶Cases seen in a single community hospital (7% of autopsies).

**Cases "whose hearts had been sent to Edwards or Roberts for his opinion and interest."

††Heart weight >350 g in women and >400 g in men.

leaflet; (4) anomalous chordae tendineae from the anterior mitral leaflet to the crest of the ventricular septum; and (5) partial or complete absence of the septal tricuspid valve leaflet. There are at least four potential functional consequences of these five anatomic anomalies: (1) shunt at the atrial level, (2) shunt at the ventricular level, (3) MR, and (4) obstruction to left ventricular outflow. Well over 95% of patients with partial atrioventricular defect have a primum-type atrial septal defect, and most of those without a primum defect have a shunt at the ventricular level. The occurrence of MR from a cleft in the anterior mitral leaflet unassociated with a defect in either atrial or ventricular septa is rare, but such has been the case in several reported patients (*64*).

Left-Sided Atrioventricular Valve Regurgitation Associated with Corrected Transposition of the Great Arteries. *Corrected transposition* is an entity that has produced much confusion (65, 66). Corrected transposition and complete transposition are quite different; the only thing they have in common is the word "transposition." Complete transposition is essentially one defect: The great arteries are transposed so that the aorta arises from the right ventricle and the pulmonary trunk from the left ventricle. In corrected transposition, the great arteries are also transposed, but, in addition, the ventricles, atrioventricular valves, epicardial coronary arteries, and conduction system are inverted. Patients with complete transposition die because they have inadequate communications between the two circuits. Patients with corrected transposition theoretically should be able to live a full lifespan, but usually this is not the case because associated defects – namely ventricular septal defect or regurgitation of the left-sided atrioventricular valve or both – cause the heart to function abnormally. The left-sided valve anatomically is a tricuspid valve (in the case of the situs solitus heart) and its most frequent abnormality is the Ebstein-type abnormality (Fig. 20). Although most patients with corrected transposition present with excessive pulmonary blood flow because of the left-to-right shunt via the ventricular septal defect, an occasional patient with corrected transposition had no defect in the cardiac septa and has evidence of pure "MR," occasionally mistaken for other type causes of MR (*67*).

Infective Endocarditis

The most common cardiac valve affected by infective endocarditis is the aortic valve and the mitral valve is most commonly affected by vegetations growing down the anterior mitral leaflet from the regurgitant aortic valve causing mitral leaflet damage and chordal rupture (*68, 69*). Infection isolated to the mitral valve is far less common and when this situation occurs the vegetations are on the atrial aspects of the mitral leaflets (*70*).

Coronary Heart Disease

The MR in patients with coronary heart disease is due to myocardial infarction, which may acutely cause necrosis of one or more left ventricular papillary muscles (usually the posteromedial one) with or without rupture of the entire muscle or far more commonly rupture of a portion of the "tip" of the papillary muscle (*37, 71–72*) (Fig. 21). Rupture, either partial or complete, of a papillary muscle during acute myocardial infarction is far less common a cause of acute MR than is necrosis of a papillary muscle and the free wall beneath it. When it occurs late after acute myocardial infarction, the MR is usually the result of dilatation of the left ventricular cavity and severe scarring of a papillary muscle, which tends to pull the mitral leaflets laterally preventing proper coaptation of the two mitral leaflets during ventricular systole.

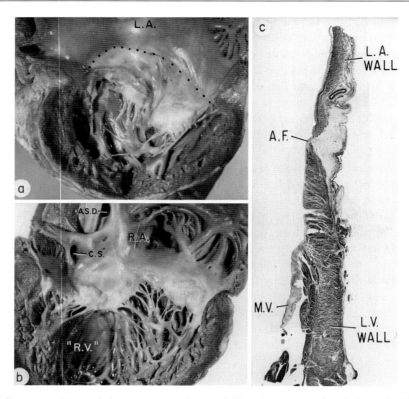

Fig. 20. *Corrected transposition of the great arteries and Ebstein's anomaly of the left-sided atrioventricular valve* in a 38-year-old woman who was cyanotic from birth and in heart failure periodically all of her life. She also had severe pulmonic valve stenosis and ventricular septal defect. She died shortly after operative insertion of a conduit between the left subclavian and left main pulmonary arteries. (**a**) Opened left atrium (LA) and anatomic right ventricle. The normal annulus is shown by the *dotted line*. (**b**) Opened right atrium (RA) and anatomic left ventricle (R.V.). ASD, atrial septal defect; CS, ostium of coronary sinus. (**c**) Histologic section of left atrial and left ventricular (LV) walls showing the normal annulus fibrosis (AF) and insertion of the mitral valve (MV) considerably caudal to the annulus and directly from the ventricular wall. Verhoeff-von Gieson stain X4. (Reproduced with permission from Berry WB, Roberts WC, Morrow AG, Braunwald E. *(66)*).

Cardiomyopathy

Most patients with idiopathic dilated cardiomyopathy (*73*), ischemic cardiomyopathy (74, 75) and hypertrophic cardiomyopathy (*76*) have MR at some time in their course. The first two conditions of course are associated with dilatation of the left ventricular cavity primarily in a lateral or right-to-left direction – not in a caudal – cephalad direction – and the consequence is abnormal papillary muscle "pull" on the mitral leaflets during ventricular systole with resulting incomplete coaptation of the mitral leaflets. Evidence that mitral annular dilation is the prime cause of MR in patients with dilated cardiomyopathy is lacking (*54*). The cause of MR in patients with hypertrophic cardiomyopathy is entirely different from that in patients with dilated cardiomyopathy and results at least in part to anterior movement of the anterior mitral leaflet toward the ventricular septum during ventricular systole (*76*). Patients with chronic anemia, e.g., sickle-cell anemia, usually also have MR from papillary muscle fibrosis and left ventricular cavity dilatation (*77*).

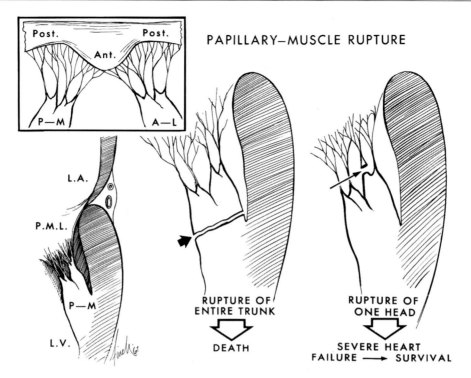

Fig. 21. Papillary muscle rupture secondary to acute myocardial infarction. Diagrammatic representation of the possible consequences of papillary muscle rupture during acute myocardial infarction. Rupture of the entire trunk is incompatible with survival (*left*). With rupture of an apical "head" (*right*), survival depends on the extent to which function of the left ventricle has been impaired by the infarct. With severely impaired left ventricular function, the additional burden of even modest MR may be intolerable. If the left ventricle is less severely compromised, survival is possible for weeks or months but heart failure will almost invariably develop. (Modified from Morrow AG, Cohen LS, Roberts WS, Braunwald NS, Braunwald E. (*71*)).

Tricuspid Valve Disease

Tricuspid regurgitation: The most common cause of pure tricuspid regurgitation (TR) is dilation of the right ventricular cavity – from any cause – the most common being left ventricular dilatation and, next, parenchymal lung disease. In contrast to mitral annular dilatation, which is severe only in patients with MVP, tricuspid annular dilatation is by far the most common cause of TR. The tricuspid valve is the only cardiac valve with a true annulus bordering its entire circumference, whereas the mitral valve has a true annulus only for its posterior leaflet and its anterior leaflet is braced, so to speak, by its connection to ascending aorta. Usually patients with functional TR also have functional MR because both ventricular cavities are so commonly dilated together.

Infective endocarditis on the right side of the heart usually (90%) attacks the tricuspid valve and TR of course may be the consequence (*78*). Operative treatment of active IE involving the tricuspid valve has initially been total tricuspid valve excision (to remove the source of infective pulmonary emboli) with later valve replacement (*79*).

Tricuspid valve stenosis: This hemodynamic lesion is rare and probably still is most commonly the result of rheumatic heart disease. If the tricuspid valve is made stenotic on the basis of rheumatic heart disease, the mitral valve is also always stenotic, never purely regurgitant (*1*). Carcinoid heart disease affects the right side of the heart by producing pulmonic stenosis and usually pure TR (although some degree of tricuspid stenosis may occur as well) (*80, 81*). The combination of pulmonic stenosis and tricuspid regurgitation usually results in considerable heart failure, and, indeed, a good experimental method to produce right-sided heart failure is to place a tight band on the pulmonary trunk (pulmonic stenosis) and partially destroy the tricuspid valve by a surgical instrument (tricuspid regurgitation). This combination is seen in carcinoid heart disease (80, 81). A tumor or vegetation on rare occasions has also produced tricuspid valve obstruction (*46*).

Pulmonic Valve

Pulmonic stenosis is usually the result of congenital heart disease – either isolated or associated with one or more other major cardiovascular congenital defects (*33*). In isolated PS the valve is usually acommissural unicuspid with a central very stenotic orifice. These valves by adulthood collect calcific deposits on their ventricular aspect rather than on the arterial aspect as occur with the left-sided semilunar valve. In a rare patient with rheumatic heart disease, pulmonic stenosis has occurred and in this circumstance all four cardiac valves have been affected. Tumors in the right ventricular outflow tract or pulmonary trunk also have produced "pulmonic stenosis" (*82*).

Pulmonic regurgitation is usually of iatrogenic origin but also occurs as a consequence of pulmonary hypertension or other causes of dilation of the main pulmonary artery.

SUMMARY

Morphologic characteristics of the heart valves have yielded important early insights into the causes of valvular heart disease. These characteristics have subsequently been correlated with clinical aspects of these diseases.

REFERENCES

1. Roberts WC. Congenital cardiovascular abnormalities usually silent until adulthood. In *Adult Congenital Heart Disease* edited by Roberts WC, Philadelphia: FA Davis, 1987:631–691.
2. Sprecher DL, Schaefer EJ, Kent KM, Gregg RE, Zech LA, Hoeg JM, McManus B, Roberts WC, Brewer HB Jr. Cardiovascular features of homozygous familial hypercholesterolemia: Analysis of 16 patients. *Am J Cardiol* 1984; 54:20–30.
3. Moura LM, Ramos SF, Zamorano JL, Barros IM, Azevedo LF, Rocha-Goncalves F, Rajamman NM. Rosuvastati affecting aortic valve endothelium to slow the progression of aortic stenosis. *J Am Coll Cardiol* 2007; Feb. 6; 49(5):554–561.
4. Roberts WC, Perloff JK, Costantino T. Severe valvular aortic stenosis in patients over 65 years of age: A clinicopathologic study. *Am J Cardiol* 1971; 27:497–506.
5. Stephan PJ, Henry AC III, Hebeler RF Jr, Whiddon L, Roberts WC. Comparison of age, gender, number of aortic valve cusps, concomitant coronary artery bypass grafting, and magnitude of left ventricular-systemic arterial peak systolic gradient in adults having aortic valve replacement for isolated aortic valve stenosis. *Am J Cardiol* 1997; 79:166–172.
6. Roberts WC, Morrow AG. Congenital aortic stenosis produced by a unicommissural valve. *Br Heart J* 1965; 27:505–510.
7. Falcone MW, Roberts WC, Morrow AG, Perloff JK. Congenital aortic stenosis resulting from unicommissural valve: Clinical and anatomic features in twenty-one adult patients. *Circulation* 1971; 44:272–280.
8. Roberts WC. The congenitally bicuspid aortic valve: A study of 85 autopsy cases. *Am J Cardiol* 1970; 26:72–83.
9. Roberts WC. Anatomically isolated aortic valvular disease. The case against its being of rheumatic etiology. *Am J Med* 1970; 49:151–159.
10. Roberts WC, Ko JM. Clinical and morphologic features of the congenitally unicuspid acommissural stenotic and regurgitant aortic valve. *Cardiology* 2007; 108:79–81.
11. Hurwitz LE, Roberts WC. Quadricuspid semilunar valve. *Am J Cardiol* 1973; 31:623–626.
12. Roberts WC, Ko JM, Filardo G, Henry AC, Hebeler RF Jr, Cheung E H-K, Matter GJ, Hamman BL. Valve structure ad survival in *sexagenarians* having aortic valve replacement for aortic stenosis (and/or aortic regurgitation) with versus without coronary artery bypass grafting at a single US medical center (1993–2005). *Am J Cardiol* 2007; 100:1287–1292.

13. Roberts WC, Ko JM. Weights of operatively-excised stenotic unicuspid, bicuspid, and tricuspid aortic valves and their relation to age, sex, body mass index, and presence or absence of concomitant coronary artery bypass grafting. *Am J Cardiol* 2003; 92:1057–1065.

14. Roberts WC, Ko JM. Weights of individual cusps in operatively-excised stenotic congenitally bicuspid aortic valves. *Am J Cardiol* 2004; 94:678–681.

15. Roberts WC, Ko JM. Weights of individual cusps in operatively-excised stenotic congenitally three-cuspid aortic valves. *Am J Cardiol* 2004; 94:681–684.

16. Roberts WC, Ko JM. Relation of weights of operatively excised stenotic aortic valves to preoperative transvalvular peak systolic pressure gradients and to calculated aortic valve areas. *J Am Coll Cardiol* 2004; 44:1847–1855.

17. Roberts WC, Ko JM. Frequency by decade of unicuspid, bicuspid, and tricuspid aortic valves in adults having isolated aortic valve replacement for aortic stenosis, with or without associated aortic regurgitation. *Circulation* 2005; 111:920–925.

18. Roberts WC, Ko JM, Matter GJ. Isolated aortic valve replacement without coronary bypass for aortic valve stenosis involving a congenitally bicuspid aortic valve in a nonagenarian. *Am J Geriatr Cardiol* 2006; 15(6):389–391.

19. Roberts WC, Ko JM, Garner WL, Filardo G, Henry AC, Hebeler RF Jr, Matter GH, Hamman BL. Valve structure and survival in *octogenarians* having aortic valve replacement for aortic stenosis (and/or aortic regurgitation) with versus without coronary artery bypass grafting at a single US medical center (1993–2005). *Am J Cardiol* 2007; 100:489–498.

20. Roberts WC, Ko JM, Filardo G, Henry AC, Hebeler RF Jr, Cheung EH, Matter GJ, Haman BL. Valve structure and survival in *septuagenarians* having aortic valve replacement for aortic stenosis (and/or aortic regurgitation) with versus without coronary artery bypass grafting at a single US medical center (1993–2005). *Am J Cardiol* 2007; 100:1157–1165.

21. Roberts WC, Ko JM, Hamilton C. Comparison of valve structure, valve weight, and severity of the valve obstruction in 1849 patients having isolated aortic valve replacement for aortic valve stenosis (with or without aortic regurgitation) studied at 3 different medical centers in 2 different time periods. *Circulation* 2005; 112:3919–3929.

22. Roberts WC, Ko JM, Filardo G, Henry AC, Hebeler RF Jr, Cheung EH, Matter GJ, Haman BL. Valve structure and survival in *quinquagenarians* having aortic valve replacement for aortic stenosis (and/or aortic regurgitation) with versus without coronary artery bypass grafting at a single US medical center (1993–2005). *Am J Cardiol* 2007; 100:1584–1591.

23. Roberts WC, Ko JM, Filardo G, Kitchens BL, Henry AC, Hebeler RF Jr, Cheung E H-K, Matter GJ, Haman BL. Valve structure and survival in *quadragenarians* having aortic valve replacement for aortic stenosis (and/or aortic regurgitation) with versus without coronary artery bypass grafting at a single US medical center (1993 to 2005). *Am J Cardiol* 2007; 100:1683–1690.

24. Roberts WC, Ko JM, Moore TR, Jones WH III. Causes of pure aortic regurgitation in patients having isolated aortic valve replacement at a single US tertiary hospital (1993–2005). *Circulation* 2006; 114:422–429.

25. Roberts WC. The structure of the aortic valve in clinically-isolated aortic stenosis. An autopsy study of 162 patients over 15 years of age. *Circulation* 1970; 42:91–97.

26. Roberts WC, Morrow AG, McIntosh CL, Jones M, Epstein SE. Congenitally bicuspid aortic valve causing severe, pure aortic regurgitation without superimposed infective endocarditis. Analysis of 13 patients requiring aortic valve replacement. *Am J Cardiol* 1981; 47:206–209.

27. Roberts WC, Oluwole BO, Fernicola DJ. Comparison of active infective endocarditis involving a previously stenotic versus a previously nonstenotic aortic valve. *Am J Cardiol* 1993; 71:1082–1088.

28. Carpenter DF, Golden A, Roberts WC. Quadrivalvular rheumatoid heart disease associated with left bundle branch block. *Am J Med* 1967; 43:922–929.

29. Roberts WC, Kehoe JA, Carpenter DF, Golden A. Cardiac valvular lesions in rheumatoid arthritis. *Arch Intern Med* 1968; 122:141–146.

30. Waller BF, Zoltick JM, Rosen JH, Katz NM, Gomes MN, Fletcher RD, Wallace RB, Roberts WC. Severe aortic regurgitation from systemic hypertension (without aortic dissection) requiring aortic valve replacement. Analysis of four patients. *Am J Cardiol* 1982; 49:473–477.

31. Waller BF, Kishel JC, Roberts WC. Severe aortic regurgitation from systemic hypertension. *Chest* 1982; 82:365–368.

32. Roberts WC. Aortic dissection: Anatomy, consequences, and causes. *Am Heart J* 1981; 101:195–214.

33. Roberts WC, Dangel JC, Bulkley BH. Non-rheumatic valvular cardiac disease: A clinicopathologic survey of 27 different conditions causing valvular dysfunction. *Cardiovasc Clin* 1973; 5:333–446.

34. Roberts WC, Honig HS. The spectrum of cardiovascular disease in the Marfan syndrome: A clinico-morphologic study of 18 necropsy patients and comparison to 151 previously reported necropsy patients. *Am Heart J* 1982; 104:115–135.

35. Bulkley BH, Roberts WC. Ankylosing spondylitis and aortic regurgitation. Description of the characteristic cardiovascular lesion from study of eight necropsy patients. *Circulation* 1973; 48:1014–1027.

36. Roberts WC, Hollingsworth JF, Bulkley BH, Jaffe RB, Epstein SE, Stinson EB. Combined mitral and aortic regurgitation in ankylosing spondylitis. Angiographic and anatomic features. *Am J Med* 1974; 56:237–243.

37. Roberts WC, Perloff JK. Mitral valvular disease. A clinicopathologic survey of the conditions causing the mitral valve to function abnormally. *Ann Int Med* 1972; 77:939–975.

38. Roberts WC. Morphologic features of the normal and abnormal mitral valve. *Am J Cardiol* 1983; 51:1005–1028.
39. Roberts WC, Virmani R. Aschoff bodies at necropsy in valvular heart disease. Evidence from an analysis of 543 patients over 14 years of age that rheumatic heart disease at least anatomically, is a disease of the mitral valve. *Circulation* 1978; 57:803–807.
40. Virmani R, Roberts WC. Aschoff bodies in operatively excised atrial appendages and in papillary muscles. Frequency and clinical significance. *Circulation* 1977; 55:559–563.
41. Lachman AS, Roberts WC. Calcific deposits in stenotic mitral valves. Extent and relation to age, sex, degree of stenosis, cardiac rhythm, previous commissurotomy and left atrial body thrombus from study of 164 operatively-excised valves. *Circulation* 1978; 57:808–815.
42. Roberts WC, Lachman AS. Mitral valve commissurotomy versus replacement. Considerations based on examination of operatively excised stenotic mitral valves. *Am Heart J* 1979; 98:56–62.
43. Roberts WC, Humphries JO, Morrow AG. Giant right atrium in rheumatic mitral stenosis. Atrial enlargement restricted by mural calcification. *Am Heart J* 1970; 79:28–35.
44. Hammer WJ, Roberts WC, de Leon AC Jr. "Mitral Stenosis" secondary to combined "massive" mitral annular calcific deposits and small, hypertrophied left ventricles. *Am J Med* 1978; 64:371–376.
45. Theleman KP, Grayburn PA, Roberts WC. Mitral "annular" calcium forming a complete circle "O" causing mitral stenosis in association with a stenotic congenitally bicuspid aortic valve and severe coronary artery disease. *Am J Geriatr Cardiol* 2006; 15:58–61.
46. Roberts WC. Neoplasms involving the heart, their simulators, and adverse consequences of their therapy. *Proc (Bayl Univ Med Cent)* 2001; 14:358–376.
47. Roberts WC, Ewy GA, Glancy DL, Marcus FI. Valvular stenosis produced by active infective endocarditis. *Circulation* 1967; 36:449–451.
48. Roberts WC, Bulkley BH, Morrow AG. Pathologic anatomy of cardiac valve replacement: A study of 224 necropsy patients. *Prog Cardiovasc Dis* 1973; 15:539–587.
49. Barlow JB, Pocock WA, Marchand P, Denny M. The significance of late systolic murmurs. *Am Heart J* 1963; 66:443–452.
50. Criley JM, Lewis KB, Humphries JO, Ross RS. Prolapse of the mitral valve: Clinical ad cine-angiocardiographic finding. *Br Heart J* 1966; 28:488–496.
51. Waller BJ, Morrow AG, Maron BJ, Del Negro AA, Kent KM, McGrath FJ, Wallace RB, McIntosh CL, Roberts WC. Etiology of clinically isolated, severe, chronic, pure mitral regurgitation: Analysis of 97 patients over 30 years of age having mitral valve replacement. *Am Heart J* 1982; 104:276–288.
52. Roberts WC, Braunwald E, Morrow AG. Acute severe mitral regurgitation secondary to ruptured chordae tendineae. Clinical, hemodynamic, and pathologic considerations. *Circulation* 1966; 33:58–70.
53. Roberts WC, McIntosh CL, Wallace RB. Mechanisms of severe mitral regurgitation in mitral valve prolapse determined from analysis of operatively excised valves. *Am Heart J* 1987; 113:1316–1323.
54. Bulkley BH, Roberts WC. Dilatation of the mitral annulus. A rare cause of mitral regurgitation. *Am J Med* 1975; 59:457–463.
55. Salazar AE, Edwards JE. Friction lesions of ventricular endocardium. Relation to chordae tendineae of mitral valve. *Arch Pathol* 1970; 90:364–376.
56. Lucas RV Jr, Edwards JE. The floppy mitral valve. *Curr Probl Cardiol* 1982; 7(4):1–48.
57. Dollar AL, Roberts WC. Morphologic comparison of patients with mitral valve prolapse who died suddenly with patients who died from severe valvular dysfunction or other conditions. *J Am Coll Cardiol* 1991; 17:921–931.
58. Renteria VG, Ferrans VJ, Jones M, Roberts WC. Intracellular collagen fibrils in prolapsed ("floppy") human atrioventricular valves. *Lab Invest* 1976; 35(5):439–43.
59. Pomerance A. Ballooning deformity (mucoid degeneration) of atrioventricular valves. *Br Heart J* 1969; 31:343–351.
60. Davies MJ, Moore BP, Braimbridge MV. The floppy mitral valve. Study of incidence, pathology and complications in surgical, necropsy, and forensic material. *Br Heart J* 1978; 40:468–481.
61. Berbarie RF, Roberts WC. Frequency of atrial fibrillation in patients having mitral valve repair or replacement for pure mitral regurgitation secondary to mitral valve Prolapse. *Am J Cardiol* 2006; 97:1039–1044.
62. Sims JB, Roberts WC. Comparison of findings in patients with vs. without atrial fibrillation just before isolated mitral valve replacement for rheumatic mitral stenosis (with or without associated mitral regurgitation). *Am J Cardiol* 2006; 97:1035–1038.
63. Braunwald E, Ross RS, Morrow AG, Roberts WC. Differential diagnosis of mitral regurgitation in childhood: Clinical pathological conference at the National Institutes of Health. *Ann Int Med* 1961; 54:223–1242.
64. Barth CW III, Dibdin JD, Roberts WC. Mitral valve cleft without cardiac septal defect causing severe mitral regurgitation but allowing long survival. *Am J Cardiol* 1985; 55:1129–1231.
65. Schiebler GL, Edwards JE, Brchell HB, DuShane JW, Ongley PA, Wood EH. Congenital corrected transposition of the great vessels: A study of 33 cases. *Pediatrics* 1961; 27(5) Suppl:851–888.

66. Berry WB, Roberts WC, Morrow AG, Braunwald E. Corrected transposition of the aorta and pulmonary trunk: Clinical, hemodynamic and pathologic findings. *Am J Med* 1964; 36:35–53.

67. Roberts WC, Ross RS, Davis FW Jr. Congenital corrected transposition of the great vessels in adulthood simulating rheumatic valvular disease. *Bull Johns Hopkins Hosp* 1964; 114:157–172.

68. Buchbinder NA, Roberts WC. Left-sided valvular active infective endocarditis. A study of forty-five necropsy patients. *Am J Med* 1972; 53:20–35.

69. Arnett EN, Roberts WC. Active infective endocarditis: A clinicopathology analysis of 137 necropsy patients. *Curr Probl Cardiol* 1976; 1(7):1–76.

70. Fernicola DJ, Roberts WC. Clinicopathologic features of active infective endocarditis isolated to the mitral valve. *Am J Cardiol* 1993; 71:1186–1197.

71. Morrow AG, Cohen LS, Roberts WC, Braunwald NS, Braunwald E. Severe mitral regurgitation following acute myocardial infarction and ruptured papillary muscle. Hemodynamic findings and results of operative treatment in four patients. *Circulation* 1968; 37(4) Suppl II:124–132.

72. Barbour DJ, Roberts WC. Rupture of a left ventricular papillary muscle during acute myocardial infarction: Analysis of 22 necropsy patients. *J Am Coll Cardiol* 1986; 8:558–565.

73. Roberts WC, Siegel RJ, McManus BM. Idiopathic dilated cardiomyopathy: Analysis of 152 necropsy patients. *Am J Cardiol* 1987; 60:1340–1355.

74. Virmani R, Roberts WC. Quantification of coronary arterial narrowing and of left ventricular myocardial scarring in healed myocardial infarction with chronic eventually fatal, congestive cardiac failure. *Am J Med* 1980; 68:831–838.

75. Ross EM, Roberts WC. Severe atherosclerotic coronary arterial narrowing and chronic congestive heart failure without myocardial infarction: Analysis of 18 patients studied at necropsy. *Am J Cardiol* 1986; 57:51–56.

76. Klues HG, Maron BJ, Dollar AL, Roberts WC. Diversity of structural mitral valve alterations in hypertrophic cardiomyopathy. *Circulation* 1992; 85:1651–1660.

77. Berezowski K, Roberts WC. Scarring of the left ventricular papillary muscles in sickle-cell disease. *Am J Cardiol* 1992; 70:1368–1370.

78. Roberts WC, Buchbinder NA. Right-sided valvular infective endocarditis. A clinicopathologic study of twelve necropsy patients. *Am J Med* 1972; 53:7–19.

79. Barbour DJ, Roberts WC. Valve excision only versus valve excision plus replacement for active infective endocarditis involving the tricuspid valve. *Am J Cardiol* 1986; 57:475–478.

80. Roberts WC, Sjoerdsma A. The cardiac disease associated with the carcinoid syndrome (carcinoid heart disease). *Am J Med* 1964; 36:5–34.

81. Ross EM, Roberts WC. The carcinoid syndrome: Comparison of 21 necropsy subjects with carcinoid heart disease to 15 necropsy subjects without carcinoid heart disease. *Am J Med* 1985; 79:339–354.

82. Shmookler BM, Marsh HB, Roberts WC. Primary sarcoma of the pulmonary trunk and/or right or left main pulmonary artery. A rare cause of obstruction to right ventricular outflow. Report on two patients and analysis of 35 previously described patients. *Am J Med* 1977; 63:263–272.

2 Cellular Pathogenesis of Degenerative Valvular Heart Disease: From Calcific Aortic Stenosis to Myxomatous Mitral Valve Disease

Nalini M. Rajamannan

CONTENTS

INTRODUCTION

Valvular heart disease is the third most common form of cardiovascular diseases. Heart valve degeneration is the most common pathologic valve disease in the United States and Europe. The number of surgical valve replacements and surgical valve repairs is increasing in the United States due to rapidly aging population. For years, valvular heart disease was thought to be due to degenerative or passive phenomena causing the valves to thicken or become stenotic. In the past decade, experimental studies have further defined the mechanisms by which heart valve disease develops. Results from these studies have provided the foundation for the cellular mechanisms of this disease process. The most common location of degenerative valves is the left side of the heart including the mitral valve and the aortic valve. Aortic stenosis develops secondary to calcified lesions along the aortic surface of

From: *Contemporary Cardiology: Valvular Heart Disease*
Edited by: Andrew Wang, Thomas M. Bashore, DOI 10.1007/978-1-59745-411-7_2
© Humana Press, a part of Springer Science+Business Media, LLC 2009

the aortic valve. Myxomatous mitral valve lesions are a thickened glistening white lesion that develops along the atrial surface of the mitral valve and causes progressive mitral regurgitation. There have been a growing number of studies that are currently defining the diseases of the heart valve according to the etiology of this disease process. This chapter will review the cellular pathways important in the development of the most common valvular heart disorders such as calcific aortic stenosis and myxomatous mitral valve disease.

HISTORICAL PERSPECTIVE OF VALVULAR HEART DISEASE

The first case report of calcific aortic stenosis was described in 1663 by a French physician Lazare Riviere *(1)*. He described a patient who was noted to have cardiac palpitations and an irregular heartbeat. Over time, the patient's symptoms became progressively worse, concurrently his pulse diminished and subsequently the patient died. At autopsy, the outflow tract was noted to have large mass along the stenosed aortic valve. This is the first clinical description demonstrating the pathophysiologic effect of calcific aortic stenosis and the subsequent clinical effects of outflow track obstruction secondary to this disease process. William Stokes *(2)*, in his textbook in 1845 on the heart, further described the pathogenesis of calcification in the heart valve as an extreme ossific growth surrounding the orifice and stretching into the ventricle. Historically, calcium deposits along the aortic valve and myxoid accumulation along the surface of the mitral valve have clearly been implicated in the pathogenesis of these disease processes. Figure 1 demonstrates the development of degenerative valve lesions in the aortic and mitral position.

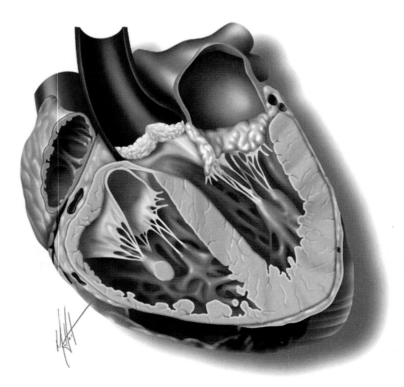

Fig. 1. Aortic valve disease and mitral valve disease. Diagram demonstrates the development of degenerative valve lesions in the aortic and mitral position.

GROSS PATHOLOGY OF AORTIC VALVE DISEASE

The cellular biology of the aortic valve has recently undergone progress toward the understanding of the mechanisms and signaling pathways involved in this disease. For years, degenerative calcific aortic stenosis was thought to be due to a passive accumulation of calcium along the surface of the valve leaflet. Figure 2 demonstrates the nodules that develop along the aortic surface of the aortic valve *(3)*. As the calcified nodules develop along the valve surface, obstruction of blood flow from the left ventricle to the aorta occurs. The obstruction may be at the valve, above the valve (supravalvular), or below the valve (subvalvular). Supravalvular aortic stenosis results from a congenital lesion. Subvalvular aortic stenosis results either from a discrete fibromuscular obstruction, which is a congenital lesion, or from a muscular obstruction (hypertrophic cardiomyopathy).

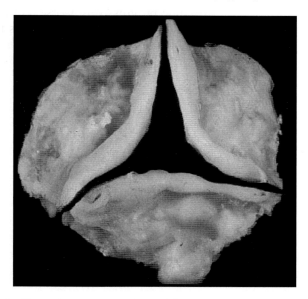

Fig. 2. Calcific aortic stenosis. Photo demonstrates the nodules that develop along the aortic surface of the aortic valve *(3)*. Used with permission.

The most common causes of aortic stenosis are congenital bicuspid, rheumatic, and calcific (degenerative). Calcific aortic stenosis is found in patients 35 years of age or older and is the result of calcification of a congenital or rheumatic valve or of a normal valve that has undergone calcific changes. Rare causes of aortic stenosis include obstructive, infective endocarditis, Paget's disease, renal failure, drug induced, familial hypercholesterolemia, systemic lupus erythematosus, irradiation, and ochronosis *(3)*. As the valves stenosis, valvular abnormality produces turbulent flow, which traumatizes the leaflets and eventually leads to progressive cell proliferation, extracellular matrix production, and calcification of the valve.

In the last decade, many laboratories have performed studies to demonstrate that the aortic valve has an active cellular biology and not a passive process. These studies are providing the future evidence that this surgical disease may be targeted with medical therapies similar to that of vascular atherosclerosis and that these medical therapies may slow the progression of this disease.

GROSS PATHOLOGY OF MITRAL VALVE DISEASE

Degenerative mitral valve disease presents with a different pathologic process. Degenerative myxomatous mitral valve disease is associated with mitral valve prolapse and abnormal movement of the leaflets into the left atrium during systole due to inadequate chordal support (elongation or rupture), excessive valvular tissue. There is a spectrum of pathologic changes found in the development of myxomatous mitral valve disease from a marked increase in valve area and length to secondary ruptured chordae. Microscopically, the valves are myxomatous, with deposition of mucopolysaccharides and glycosaminoglycans in a thickened spongiosa layer encroaching on the fibrosa layer *(4)*. Annular myxomatous changes may lead to dilation and calcification of the annulus. Figure 3 demonstrates a mitral valve removed at the time of surgical valve replacement *(5)*. The valve appears thickened with a white appearance along the atrial surface of the valve leaflet. This lesion presents with various clinical presentations including prolapse, retraction, and redundancy of the leaflet. Although there is a spectrum of presentation of this valve lesion, over time this valve lesion uniformly develops progressive regurgitation.

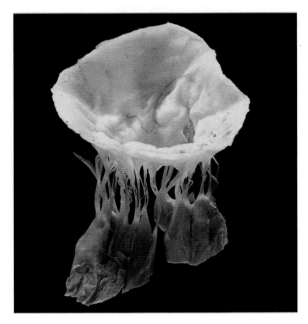

Fig. 3. Degenerative mitral valve disease. Photo demonstrates a mitral valve removed at the time of surgical valve replacement *(5)*. Used with permission.

The complexity of the mitral valve apparatus provides the foundation for the different pathologic manifestations of mitral valve prolapse in many conditions that affect one or more of the components of the apparatus (e.g., ruptured mitral chordae). There is growing evidence that the disorder of the mitral valve leaflets exists in which there are pathologic changes causing redundancy of the mitral leaflets and their prolapse into the left atrium during systole. This is the primary form of mitral valve prolapse. In primary mitral valve prolapse, there is intrachordal hooding due to leaflet redundancy. The height of the interchordal hooding usually exceeds 4 mm and involves at least one-half of the anterior leaflets or at least two-thirds of the posterior leaflet. The basic microscopic feature of primary mitral valve prolapse is marked proliferation of the interstitial cells in the spongiosa, the delicate connective tissue between the atrialis (a thick layer of collagen and elastic tissue forming the atrial aspect of the leaflet), and the fibrosis, or ventricularis, which is composed of dense layers of collagen and forms the basic support of the leaflet. In primary mitral valve prolapse, increase in the synthesis of acid mucopolysaccharides and glycosaminoglycans containing spongiosa tissue causes focal interruption of the fibrosa. Secondary pathologic findings of primary mitral valve prolapse include thickening of the surfaces of the mitral valve leaflets, thinning and/or elongation of chordae tendinae. The entire syndrome of mitral valve prolapse and the subsequent mitral valve regurgitation can be thought of as a continuum of the same underlying cellular disorder that presents with varying degrees of penetrance and pathologic findings.

RISK FACTOR HYPOTHESIS FOR VALVULAR HEART DISEASE

In the past half century, studies in the field of vascular biology have clearly indicated that targeting specific cellular targets can slow the disease progression of this disease. Understanding the cellular mechanisms of valvular heart disease will also provide the important foundation for the future understanding of medical therapy for this patient population. The importance of research in vascular atherosclerosis was summarized in 1942 by Dr. James B. Herrick. He wrote a textbook on the short history of cardiology (6). In the chapter on coronary atherosclerosis, he predicted the future of therapeutic approaches for vascular atherosclerosis. In this textbook, he wrote that "heart disease. . . is the story of a bad disease. . .the outlook for dread angina is thought to be more favorable than it was first thought. . .though the cause. . .has not been discovered, and vascular disease may never be warded off or cured, research may unearth secrets by which premature or old age may be post-poned."

Landmark studies by Otto et al. (7, 8) have described the risk factors for calcific aortic stenosis including lipids, hypertension, male gender, and increased body mass index. Emerging epidemiological studies are revealing convincing clinical development of this valvular lesion. Risk factors for calcific aortic valve disease have recently been described including male gender, hypertension, elevated levels of LDL, and smoking (6–16). Recent epidemiological studies have also defined the risk factors for the development of mitral annular calcification, which include hypertension, hypercholesterolemia, smoking, and male gender (10, 13). These risk factors are similar to those that promote the development of vascular atherosclerosis (17–19). These studies demonstrate a parallel risk factor for both of these disease processes. In 2008, we can now begin to define the cellular mechanisms important in the development of these common valve lesions and in turn think about future medical therapies for the treatment of these disease processes.

HYPERCHOLESTEROLEMIC AORTIC VALVE DISEASE

Vascular atherosclerosis has been described in the literature for hundreds of years (2). Clinically, the correlation of hypercholesterolemia and valvular disease has been well described in the patients with familial hypercholesterolemia. This patient population develops accelerated atherosclerosis within the entire vasculature and cardiac valves. Autopsy studies of these patients demonstrate a severe form of aortic stenosis associated with supravalvar narrowing in these patients (20). Familial hypercholesterolemia (FH) is characterized by raised serum LDL cholesterol levels, which result in excess deposition of cholesterol in tissues, leading to accelerated atherosclerosis and increased risk of premature coronary heart disease. FH results from defects in the hepatic uptake and degradation of LDL via the LDL-receptor pathway, commonly caused by a loss-of-function mutation in the LDL-receptor gene (LDLR) or by a mutation in the gene encoding apolipoprotein B (APOB). Recently, the proof of principle for the atherosclerotic process was demonstrated in a case report from a patient who died in 1949 (21). In this study, we reported a patient with the diagnosis of familial hypercholesterolemia IIb and prominent skin xanthomas at the time of birth. The patient died of cardiac complications at age 7 and had elevated cholesterol of over 900 mg/dl. We examined the cardiac pathology, which demonstrated coronary atherosclerosis and aortic valve atherosclerosis. Figure 4 demonstrates the development of atherosclerosis along the aortic surface of the aortic valve and in the lumen of the left circumflex (21). The arrow points to the atherosclerotic lesion along the aortic valve surface. This photo of the vasculature and the aortic valve shows that elevated lipids cause a traditional atherosclerotic lesion in the artery as well as the aortic valve surface.

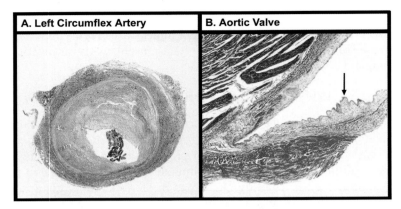

Fig. 4. Light microscopy of the aortic valve and artery from a familial hypercholesterolemia patient. Photo demonstrates the development of atherosclerosis along the aortic surface of the aortic valve and in the lumen of the left circumflex *(21)*. Used with permission.

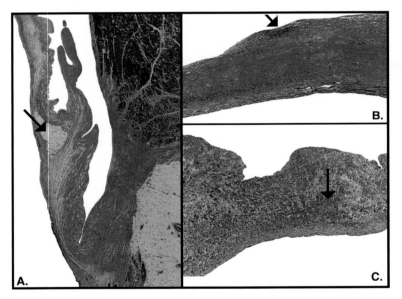

Fig. 5. Light microscopy of the mitral valve from a familial hypercholesterolemia patient. Photo demonstrates an atherosclerotic lesion developing along the atrial surface of the mitral valve from this patient.

The mitral valve from this same patient was reexamined from the autopsy heart dissection. Figure 5 demonstrates an atherosclerotic lesion developing along the atrial surface of the mitral valve from this patient. The mitral valve also demonstrates an early lipid infiltration along the surface of the valve. This report is the first to demonstrate that elevated lipids in a patient with familial hypercholesterolemia IIb-LDLR defect also induce mitral valve atherosclerosis. This study and previous studies of this patient population *(20–24)* have provided the descriptive proof of atherosclerosis involving the vascular and valvular structures. This evidence provides further proof of principle that valvular heart disease involves similar initiating events important in vascular atherosclerosis but different clinical presentations for these different valve lesions.

Another line of evidence is the work in human surgical pathological studies that demonstrate the presence of low-density lipoproteins *(25, 26)* and atherosclerosis in calcified human aortic valves. These studies indicate a similarity between the genesis of valvular and vascular disease, which suggests a common initiating cellular mechanism of atherosclerosis in these tissues *(26)*. Figure 6 demonstrates the immunohistochemistry by Olsson et al., showing the presence of oxidized LDL in cardiac valves from patients with early valvular heart disease *(25)*. This study by Olsson et al. and others *(25, 26)* proves that lipoproteins are present in the development of calcific aortic valve disease. The role of hypercholesterolemia in vascular and valvular atherosclerosis induces an inflammatory environment, which can lead to an activation of inflammatory signaling pathways in these cells that induce the initial disease pathway.

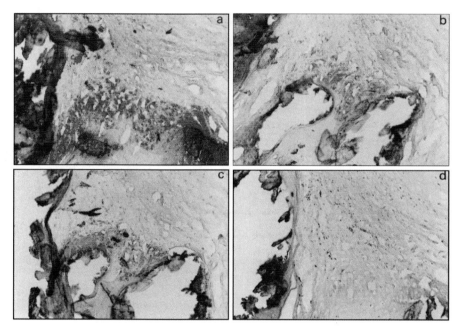

Fig. 6. Light microscopy of oxidized LDL from diseased aortic valves. Photo demonstrates the immunohisto-chemistry showing the presence of oxidized LDL in cardiac valves from patients with early valvular heart disease *(25)*.

If atherosclerotic risk factors are important in the development of left-sided degenerative valvular heart lesions, then experimental model of hypercholesterolemia provides invaluable models of cardiac valve disease. There are a growing number of experimental animal models of hypercholesterolemic valvular heart disease. These experimental in vivo models test the effects of experimental hyperc-holesterolemia on atherosclerosis in the aortic valves *(27–32)*. The rabbit model of feeding with a high-cholesterol diet has been used for years in the field of vascular atherosclerosis. Early studies demonstrate that the vascular lesion in the rabbit aorta from experimental hypercholesterolemia has a similar atherosclerotic lesion of that of the aortic valve *(28)*. After 8 weeks of 1.0% cholesterol diet, the aortic valves and aortas from these rabbits develop a similar atherosclerosis lesion *(29)*. Figure 7 shows the comparison of the vascular aorta to the aortic valve from this rabbit model.

Figure 7, Panel A1 is the normal aorta and the aortic valve demonstrating a clear aortic valve leaflet and normal appearing aorta *(32, 33)*. Figure 7, Panel A2 is the hypercholesterolemic aorta and aortic valve-marked exudative lesions along the aortic surface of the valve and extending along the aorta. Figure 7, Panel B is the longitudinal cross section of the normal diet aortic valve attached to the aorta

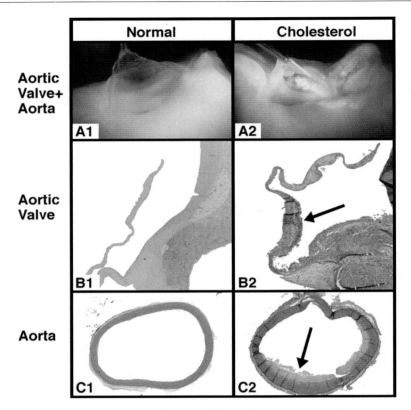

Fig. 7. Experimental hypercholesterolemia rabbit model. Photo shows the comparison of the vascular aorta to the aortic valve from this rabbit model control diet versus cholesterol diet. **(Panel A)** Gross photo of control aortic valve and aorta; **(Panel B)** light microscopy of the aortic valve attached to the aorta; **(Panel C)** cross section of thoracic aorta *(32)*. Used with permission.

with no evidence of atherosclerosis. Figure 7, Panel B2 demonstrates the fatty streak lesion along the aortic surface. The arrow points to the atherosclerotic lesion along the valve leaflet. Figure 7, Panel C1 demonstrates a cross-sectional view of the proximal thoracic aorta, which is normal in the control diet. Figure 7, Panel C2 demonstrates the atherosclerotic lesion in the vascular aorta with the arrow pointing to the fatty streak atheromatous lesion in the lumen. Further analysis of this early aortic valve lesion identified apoptosis and cellular proliferation present in the atherosclerotic valve lesion *(28)*. Drolet et al. have also tested an experimental diet including vitamin D and hypercholesterolemia in mice and found that the diet induces a hemodynamic early stenotic lesion within the aortic valve leaflets proven by echocardiography *(27)*. Figure 8 demonstrates the continuous wave Doppler waveform across the stenotic aortic valve of the rabbits treated with control in the top panel versus vitamin D and cholesterol in the bottom panel *(27)*. This is the first experimental animal model to demonstrate hemodynamic evidence of early stenosis by Doppler echocardiography.

As the experimental animal models evolved, they tested more specific cellular mechanisms important in the development of this disease process. Longer duration of cholesterol diet induces early mineralization in the valves, which is associated with abnormal endothelial nitric oxide regulation in these tissues *(34)*. This information provided the first evidence of an oxidative stress mechanism important in the activation of this disease process. A subsequent study *(35)* tested this hypothesis further in a chronic experimental model. Echocardiographic measurements and hemodynamic catheterization studies that elevated cholesterol in a genetic mouse model causes severe aortic stenosis. The study tested genetic knockout mice that lack the receptor for the low-density lipoprotein receptor and express only the

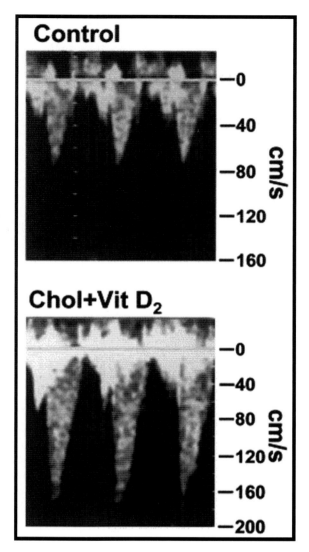

Fig. 8. Continuous wave Doppler across the aortic valve. Control versus cholesterol + vitamin D diet *(28)*. Used with permission.

receptor for the human apoB100 (LDLr$^{-/-}$apoB$^{100/100}$) in an aging genetic mouse model. This model induces mineralization as confirmed by Von Kossa staining, which stains for calcium and phosphate mineral. The study also defined the importance of an abnormal oxidation state in the diseased aortic valves from these mice. The most recent experimental cholesterol mouse model *(36)* demonstrates also the in vivo experimental evidence for multimodality imaging to diagnose aortic valve disease. These models provide critical evidence in the growing field of valvular biology that lipids play an important initiating role in the development of calcification and severe stenosis in an aging model of valvular heart disease.

AORTIC VALVE CALCIFICATION

The presence of calcification in the aortic valve is responsible for valve stenosis. Recent descriptive studies have demonstrated the critical features of aortic valve calcification, including osteoblast expression, cell proliferation, and atherosclerosis *(29, 37–39)*. These studies have shown that specific bone cell phenotypes are present in calcifying valve tissue from human specimens *(33, 40)*. The hypothesis that has been proposed by a number of laboratories is that the calcification present in aortic valve is the result of the activation of the skeleton bone phenotype. The mechanism by which bone formation develops in the valve is via the transdifferentiation of the valve interstitial cell to an osteoblast-like cell. The osteoblast cell is the main cell responsible for bone formation in skeletal bone development and repair. This cell synthesizes the proteins necessary for the mineralization and strengthening of the bone. This process is regulated at the DNA level by a number of transcription factors. Transcription factors are key proteins that are the master switch to turn on a particular gene program in the cell and therefore define the fate of the cell.

The important transcription factor in osteoblast gene differentiation is Cbfa1 *(41)*. Cbfa1 has all the attributes of a "master gene" differentiation factor for the osteoblast lineage and bone matrix gene expression. During embryonic development, Cbfa1 expression precedes osteoblast differentiation and is restricted to mesenchymal cells destined to become an osteoblast. Sox9 is important in the differentiation of mesenchymal cells to a chondrocyte lineage *(42, 43)*. Therefore, activation of these various transcription factors is important in the normal skeletal bone formation. The presence of these transcription factors in cells other than bone becomes important in defining the appearance of novel bone phenotypes.

Presence of an Osteoblast Phenotype in Aortic Valve Calcification

Mohler et al. *(38)* were the first to describe the presence of bone formation in calcifying aortic valves. Rajamannan et al. *(39)* have confirmed this finding and defined the osteoblast gene program present in calcified aortic valves. Osteoblastogenesis involves a series of complex well-orchestrated cellular pathways important in skeletal bone formation. The regulatory mechanism of osteoblast differentiation from osteoblast progenitor cells into terminally differentiated cells is via a well-orchestrated pathway. This process involves cellular proliferation and bone matrix synthesis, in response to activation of specific paracrine *(44, 45)*, and the activation of the canonical Wnt pathway *(46)*. The Wnt pathway has recently evolved in the understanding of bone formation in two different studies. Both studies were performed in independent laboratories demonstrating a high bone mass phenotype *(47, 48)* and a severe osteoporosis phenotype *(49)*.

The LDL-receptor-related protein 5 (Lrp5), a co-receptor of LDL-receptor family, has been discovered as an important receptor in the activation of skeletal bone formation via binding to the secreted glycoprotein Wnt and activating beta-catenin to induce bone formation. The canonical Wnt/Lrp5 pathway is a highly conserved pathway, which has evolved as one of the leading signaling mechanisms in early embryologic development *(50, 51)*. It is a highly conserved pathway across species *(52)*. The Wnt pathway is critical in the development of bone formation. Shao *(53)* and Rajamannan et al. *(33, 54)* have demonstrated that the Wnt pathway is a novel pathway in the reactivation of the Wnt pathway in the development of cardiovascular calcification. When Wnt binds to the Lrp5/frizzled receptor, calcification develops within the myofibroblast cell in the aortic valve *(34)*. These findings provide the evidence that the aortic valve calcification follows the spectrum of bone formation in calcifying tissues and the Wnt pathway plays an important role in the development of this disease process.

HYPERCHOLESTEROLEMIC MITRAL VALVE DISEASE

We *(55)* and others *(30)* have shown that experimental hypercholesterolemia induces an atherosclerotic lesion along the atrial surface of the mitral valve. We evaluated the mitral valves of New Zealand white rabbits assigned to 1.0% cholesterol diet for 8 weeks. The normal mitral valve as shown in Fig. 9. Panel A1 shows a thin, intact valve attached to the papillary muscle as demonstrated by the

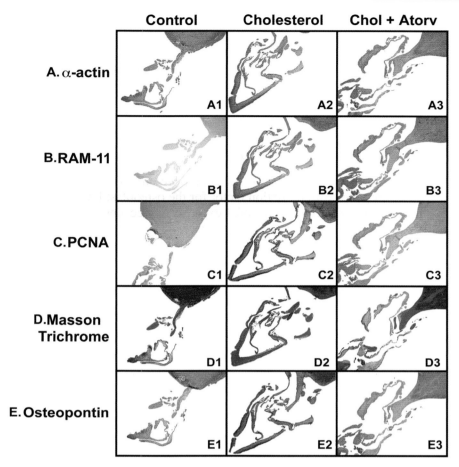

Fig. 9. Experimental hypercholesterolemia in mitral valve disease. Photo shows the control, cholesterol, and cholesterol + atorvastatin diet for 2 months. **(Panel A)** Actin immunostain; **(Panel B)** Ram-11 immunostain; **(Panel C)** proliferating nuclear antigen stain immunostain; **(Panel D)** Masson trichrome immunostain; **(Panel E)** osteopontin immunostain *(55)*. Used with permission.

α-actin immunostain. Furthermore, there was no evidence of foam cell formation (Fig. 9, Panel B1), cellular proliferation (Fig. 9, Panel C1), calcification by Masson trichrome (Fig. 9, Panel D1), and OP deposition (Fig. 9, Panel E1). Mitral valves from the hypercholesterolemic animals, on the other hand, showed considerable increase in connective tissue and collagen formation (Fig. 9, Panel D2). Likewise, there were focal areas of increased myofibroblast PCNA staining and α-actin-positive staining cells (Fig. 9, Panels A2 and C2) as well as areas staining positive for macrophages (RAM 11), suggesting foam cell infiltration (Fig. 9, Panel B2). Finally, there was significant deposition of osteopontin within the mitral valve leaflet, which is not seen in the controls (Fig. 9, Panel E2). Figure 9, Panels A3–E3 demonstrates the effects of the atorvastatin on the mitral valve for all of these treatments with marked improvement in the atherosclerotic lesion. This reduction is further demonstrated in Fig. 10 , Panel B, which shows significant decreases in the amount of all the immunohistochemical markers. We further confirmed the osteopontin RNA expression in Fig. 10, Panel A. There were significantly increased levels of osteopontin RNA gene expression in the hypercholesterolemic animals compared to either the control or atorvastatin-treated animals.

It is evident from this experimental model that the mitral valve also develops an active, complex process involving myofibroblast cellular proliferation and osteopontin expression secondary to

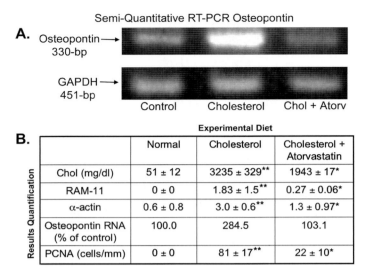

Fig. 10. Quantification of the immunohistochemistry and RT-PCR. Experimental mitral valve disease model. Used with permission.

hypercholesterolemia and that this process may be modified by atorvastatin. Osteopontin is found in active skeletal metabolism and is present in the differentiation process important in the development of valvular heart disease *(29)*. Upregulation of the protein and gene expression of these skeletal bone matrix proteins is indicative of a differentiation process that develops within the mitral valve leaflet, which is attenuated with atorvastatin therapy. The clinical significance of this finding is twofold: first is that cholesterol may be a risk factor for the development of mitral valve disease and second is the potential implications of the medical treatment of mitral regurgitation to slow the progression of this disease.

Presence of a Chondrocytic Phenotype in the Mitral Valve

We hypothesized that the underlying mechanism of degenerative valve disease may be related to the activation of the Lrp5 receptor in the spectrum of osteoblast differentiation within human diseased valve leaflets. The most common location of degenerative valves is the left side of the heart. Myxomatous mitral valve lesions causing mitral regurgitation are believed to be caused by progressive thickening due to activated myofibroblasts *(56)*. We hypothesized that the underlying mechanism of degenerative valve disease in patients who are aging, may be related to the activation of the Lrp5 receptor in the spectrum of osteoblast differentiation within human diseased valve leaflets. Young patients who present with mitral valve prolapse at a young age have a similar phenotype which is related to genetics. However, patients who develop this disease at an older age, develop a similar phenotype secondary to activation of cartilage phenotype pathways. To test this hypothesis we studied degenerative mitral valves, calcified tricuspid and bicuspid aortic valves from human surgical pathological specimens to determine if the Lrp5 signaling pathway is expressed in these diseased cardiac valves *(33)*. We found that the degenerative mitral valves in this study express a chondrocytic phenotype with the expression of chondrocyte cells in the thickened mitral valve leaflets *(33)*. Figure 11 demonstrates the immunohistochemistry stains for the osteoblast signaling markers: Lrp5, Wnt3, and PCNA. Figure 11, Panels A1, A2, B1, and B2 demonstrates a mild amount of Lrp5 and Wnt3 staining in the control valves and in the areas of hypertrophic chondrocytes in the mitral valves. Lrp5 and Wnt3 staining was increased in the calcified aortic valves (Fig. 11, Panels A3, A4, B3, and

Endochondral Bone Signaling Markers

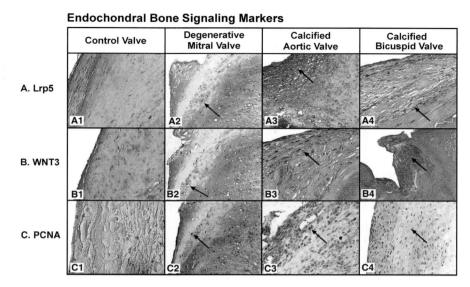

Fig. 11. Immunohistochemistry for osteoblast stains from the control, calcified tricuspid, bicuspid, and degenerative mitral valves from surgical valve. **(Panel A)** Lrp5 immunostain; **(Panel B)** Wnt3 immunostain; **(Panel C)** proliferating nuclear antigen stain *(33)*. Used with permission.

B4). Figure 11, Panels C3 and C4 demonstrates the presence of an increase in PCNA protein expression as compared to Fig. 11, Panels C1 and C2, which demonstrates a decrease in PCNA protein staining.

These data *(33)* provide the first evidence of a mechanistic pathway for the initiation of bone differentiation in degenerative valve lesions, which is expressed in the mitral valve as a cartilage phenotype and in the calcified aortic valve as a bone phenotype. These results indicate that there is a continuum of an earlier stage of osteoblast bone differentiation in the mitral valves as compared to the calcified aortic valves. This is the first study to demonstrate the presence of chondrocytes in mitral valves and osteoblasts in aortic valves, implicating this pathologic mechanism in the development of mitral regurgitation in degenerative myxomatous mitral valves and stenosis in calcific aortic valves.

EXPERIMENTAL EFFECTS OF STATINS IN ATHEROSCLEROTIC AORTIC VALVES

Our laboratory has developed models of experimental hypercholesterolemia and aortic valve atherosclerosis and valve calcification. Initially, we studied an experimental rabbit model of hypercholesterolemia for 8 weeks, which produces an atherosclerotic lesion in the aortic valve *(28)*. We then took this model to determine a number of different protocols to evaluate the development of valvular atherosclerosis and eventual mineralization in these tissues. The next level of investigation was to determine whether hypercholesterolemia induces an atherosclerotic proliferative valve lesion associated with the expression of an osteoblast-like phenotype *(29)*. During this study we also tested whether atorvastatin would inhibit this process in the aortic valve.

Figure 12 *(29)*, Panels A1 and B1 demonstrates that the normal aortic valve surface from control animals appeared thin and intact, with a smooth endothelial cell layer covering the entire surface and a thin collagen layer in the spongiosa layer of the valve, as demonstrated by hematoxylin and eosin stain and Masson trichrome stain. There were no macrophages or proliferation in the aortic valves of normal control rabbits (Fig. 12, Panels C1 and D1). In contrast, the aortic valves from the hypercholesterolemic animals demonstrated fatty plaque formation with scant accumulation of basophilic material. Foam cells converged to form a large lipid-laden lesion on the aortic endocardial surface of the valve leaflets (Fig. 12, Panel A2). There was also an increase in the blue collagen trichrome

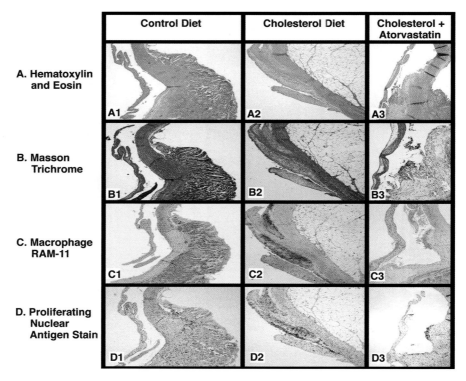

Fig. 12. Experimental hypercholesterolemia in aortic valve disease. Phcto shows the control, cholesterol, and cholesterol + atorvastatin diet for 2 months. **(Panel A)** Hematoxylin and eosin stain; **(Panel B)** Masson trichrome stain; **(Panel C)** Ram 11 immunostain; **(Panel D)** Proliferating Nuclear Antigen Stain *(29)*. Used with permission.

stain in the hypercholesterolemic aortic valves as demonstrated in Fig. 12, Panel B2. The endothelial layer on the valve surface appeared disrupted by infiltration of extracellular lipid deposits, myofibroblast cells, and foam cells that stain positive for macrophages (RAM 11), as shown in Fig. 12, Panel C2. These lesions developed primarily at the base of the leaflets and decreased in extent toward the leaflet tips. The hypercholesterolemic aortic valves also demonstrated a marked increase in myofibroblast PCNA staining along the base of the aortic valve as demonstrated in Fig. 12, Panel D2. The atorvastatin-treated rabbits demonstrated a marked decrease in the amount of atherosclerotic plaque burden, macrophage infiltration, and proliferation (Fig. 12 , Panels A3, B3, C3, D3), and these changes were most pronounced at the base of the leaflets. This study is the first experimental study to test the effect of a statin on atherosclerosis and cell proliferation on the aortic valve lesion.

Our next study was to determine if calcification was developing in the aortic valve. To test this hypothesis we tested the rabbit model for 3 months instead of 2 months to allow the valves to mineralize *(55)*. Furthermore, identification of the intermediate signaling steps between lipid accumulation, cellular proliferation, and calcification has not been clearly established. Studying the signaling pathways in disease processes helps to develop future targeted therapies for aortic stenosis. The normal aortic valve surface from control animals appeared thin and intact, with a smooth endothelial cell layer covering the entire surface and a thin collagen layer within the spongiosa. There was little to no eNOS immunostaining present in the endothelium (Fig.13, Panel A1). In contrast, the aortic valves from the hypercholesterolemic animals demonstrated an atherosclerotic lesion along the aortic surface that was identifiable by light microscopy (Fig. 13, Panel A2). Again there was no evidence of eNOS immunostaining along the surface of the aortic valve. The atorvastatin-treated rabbits demonstrated a marked decrease in the amount of atherosclerotic plaque burden (Fig. 13,

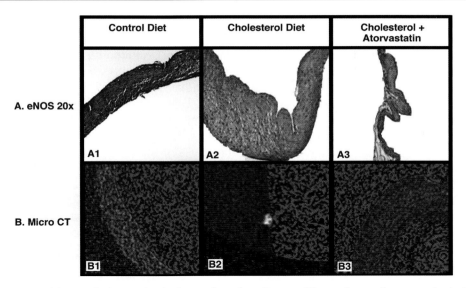

Fig. 13. Experimental hypercholesterolemia in aortic valve disease. Photo shows the control, cholesterol, and cholesterol + atorvastatin diet for 3 months. **(Panel A)** Immunohistochemistry for eNOS; **(Panel B)** MicroCT for calcification *(34)*. Used with permission.

Panel A3), with an associated positive immunostain for eNOS in the endothelial layer of the aortic valve. MicroCT was used to evaluate the development of calcification in valve leaflets and the aorta in each of the treatment groups. Control aortic valves and aortas demonstrated little to no mineralization (Fig. 13, Panel B1). The hypercholesterolemic aortic valves and aortas appeared to be in early stages of calcification (Fig. 13, Panel B2). In the group given both cholesterol and atorvastatin, the aortic valves and aortas could not be distinguished from those of the controls (Fig. 13, Panels B1 and B3).

Nitric oxide (NO) is generated in vascular endothelial cells by endothelial (eNOS) and is responsible for endothelial-dependent vasorelaxation, inhibition of smooth muscle cell proliferation, and decreased synthesis of extracellular matrix proteins. Nitric oxide (NO) is a key regulator of normal endothelial function in the vasculature. Structurally, an endothelial layer lines the aortic valve leaflet. Charest et al. *(57)* have also demonstrated that eNOS is expressed in human-calcified aortic valves indicating the first evidence in human aortic valve disease of oxidative stress. These data provide the initial evidence that endothelial nitric oxide synthase (eNOS) produced in the valve endothelium has a role in the physiologic cellular regulation of this tissue similar to its role in vascular endothelium. This inactivation of eNOS leads to a decrease in the availability of nitric oxide. This inhibitory action of hypercholesterolemia on eNOS activity may play a critical role in the development of mineralization of the atherosclerotic aortic valve over time, which can be reversed with statin therapy.

Finally,we tested the experimental hypercholesterolemic rabbit model for 6 months to determine if the valves develop extensive mineralization and if an osteoblast signaling pathway is present in the calcifying aortic valve. In this study we tested for the regulation of the Lrp5 receptor in the presence of cholesterol and statin therapy. Low-density lipoprotein receptors (LDLR) are critical in the uptake, processing, and cellular metabolism of cholesterol. In this study, the Watanabe rabbit, with a naturally occurring genetic LDLR mutation, serves as an important genetic model for the inheritable cholesterol disease familial hypercholesterolemia (FH). Studies have demonstrated that FH patients have extensive calcification in their vasculature and aortic valves *(58)*. In our most recent experimental hypercholesterolemia experiment in the naturally occurring LDL knockout Watanabe rabbit (a genetic model for FH), we demonstrated that osteoblast-like calcification develops in the rabbit aortic valves after 6 months, which is regulated by LRP5 and modified by atorvastatin treatment. These studies provide further evidence toward the multifactorial cellular pathways involved in aortic valve calcification via experimental hypercholesterolemia *(34)*.

The hematoxylin and eosin and Masson trichrome-stained hypercholesterolemic aortic valves, as shown in Fig. 14 , Panels A2, B2, and C2, demonstrate an increase in leaflet thickness, which begins at the base of the aortic valve leaflet and extends along the valve leaflet from the attachment to the aorta with an increase in the Lrp5 red-staining receptors. There is a marked increase in cellularity and collagen staining in the blue Masson trichrome throughout the leaflet lesion. The aortic valve surface from control animals appeared normal, thin, and intact, with a smooth endothelial cell layer covering the entire surface and a thin collagen layer in the spongiosa of the valve (Fig. 14, Panels A1, B1, and C1). Abnormal leaflet thicknesses did not develop when cholesterol-fed rabbits received atorvastatin with attenuation of the Lrp5 staining (Fig. 14, Panels A3, B3, and C3) *(34)*.

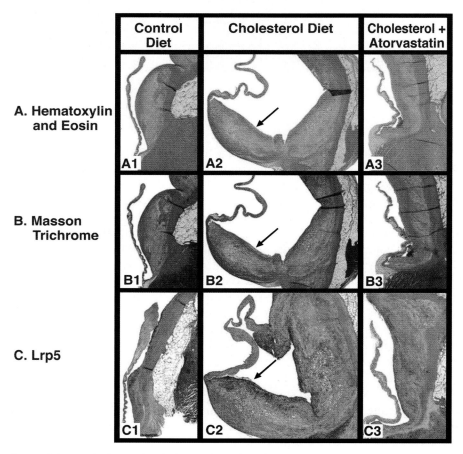

Fig. 14. Experimental hypercholesterolemia in aortic valve disease. Photo shows the control, cholesterol, and cholesterol + atorvastatin diet for 6 months. **(Panel A)** Hemotoxylin and eosin stain; **(Panel B)** Masson trichrome stain; **(Panel C)** Lrp5 stain *(54)*. Used with permission.

In this study, we demonstrate that calcification of the aortic valve leaflets develops within the valve similar to skeletal bone formation and that this mineralization occurs with the upregulation of Lrp5 receptors and bone formation in the cholesterol-treated rabbit valve and a decrease in the receptor and bone formation with the atorvastatin treatment. Lrp5 is a critical LDL co-receptor important in the differentiation of osteoblast cells in skeletal bone formation *(48, 49)*. The naturally occurring LDLR defect in Watanabe rabbits has made this species a parallel model to familial hypercholesterolemia

(FH) patients who have mutations in the LDLR *(59)*. Electron beam computed tomography studies demonstrate that FH patients have accelerated vascular and valvular atherosclerosis and calcification *(60)*. This study extends our original experimental studies demonstrating atherosclerosis and cell proliferation in a short-term cholesterol feeding in the rabbit model to demonstrate the findings in a long-term lower concentration of cholesterol feeding.

TRANSLATIONAL THERAPEUTIC IMPLICATIONS FOR AORTIC VALVE DISEASE

In summary, calcific aortic stenosis is the number one indication for valvular heart surgery in the developed world. For years this disease was thought to be due to a passive accumulation of calcium along the aortic valve surface. In the past 5 years, laboratories across the world have demonstrated that the calcification in the valve is an active biological process. There are seven retrospective studies showing that statin therapy slows the progression of stenosis especially in the earlier valve lesions. The first randomized prospective trial, SALTIRE, was a negative trial in slowing the progression of this disease. In this first randomized prospective study, testing the effects of statins in aortic valve disease was published in 2005 *(61)*. In this double-blind, placebo-controlled trial, patients with calcific aortic stenosis were randomly assigned to receive either 80 mg of atorvastatin daily or a matched placebo. Aortic valve stenosis and calcification were assessed with the use of Doppler echocardiography and helical computed tomography, respectively. The primary end points were change in aortic-jet velocity and aortic valve calcium score. However, the timing of the therapy may have had an impact on the negative outcome of this study. In the RAAVE trial *(62)* (Rosuvastatin Affecting Aortic Valve Endothelium), prospective treatment of AS with rosuvastatin targeting serum LDL slowed progression of echo hemodynamic measurements and improved inflammatory biomarkers, providing the first clinical evidence for targeted therapy in patients with asymptomatic AS. The study's aim was to assess rosuvastatin on the hemodynamic progression and inflammatory markers of AS by treating LDL in patients with AS according to the NCEP-ATPIII guidelines for 1 year. The RAAVE trial is the first prospective study to show in patients with moderate to severe stenosis that statins slow the progression of this disease. Furthermore, this study has had profound anti-inflammatory effects in improving inflammatory markers known to cause disease in the aortic valve and the vasculature. In the future, the use of statins may have a profound impact on the overall approach toward treating this disease process. The final proof of this therapeutic approach will be randomized clinical trials designed to target the disease early enough to slow the progression of calcification and delay the timing of surgical valve replacement. During a mean follow-up of 53 ± 3.2 weeks, there was decrease in aortic valve area (AVA), improvement in the peak aortic valve velocity, and slowing of the progression of the mean gradient.

SUMMARY

Recent epidemiological studies have revealed that the risk factors for arterial atherosclerosis, male gender, smoking, and elevated serum cholesterol are similar to the risk factors associated with the development of aortic valve stenosis. The growing number of models of experimental hypercholesterolemia, which produce atherosclerosis in the aortic valve and mitral valve, which are similar to the early stages of vascular atherosclerotic lesion formation. These models show that the hypercholesterolemic aortic and mitral valve develops not only an atherosclerotic lesion that is proliferative but also a lesion that expresses high levels of bone matrix proteins and osteoblast bone markers, which over time mineralize to form bone. Furthermore, if the diet is continued for a long enough time, then stenosis *(35)*develops in the aortic valve similar to that found in patients. Human mitral valve and aortic valve disease expresses a chrondrocyte and osteoblast phenotype, which parallels endochondral bone formation. Figure 15 demonstrates the cellular pathway involved in the development of aortic valve disease and Fig. 16 demonstrates the cellular pathway involved in the development of mitral valve disease.

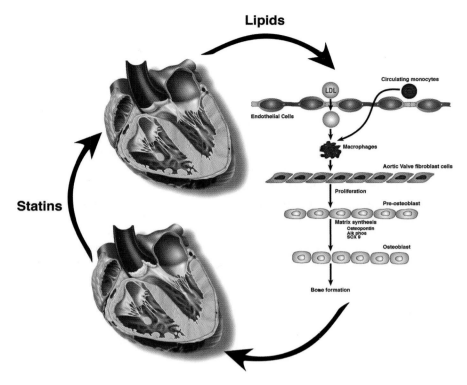

Fig. 15. The cellular pathway involved in the development of aortic valve disease*(63)*. Used with permission.

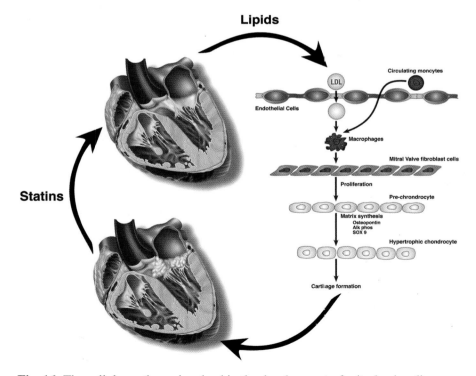

Fig. 16. The cellular pathway involved in the development of mitral valve disease.

In summary, these findings suggest that such therapy may have a potential role in patients in the early stages of this disease process to prolong the time to severe aortic stenosis and delay the time to surgical aortic valve replacement.

ACKNOWLEDGMENTS

This work was completed with the support of an American Heart Association Grant-in-Aid (0350564Z) and grants from the US National Institutes of Health (1K08HL073927-01 and 1R01HL085591-01A1). This work was completed with the support of an American Heart Association Beginning Grant-in-Aid (0060372Z). The author would like to acknowledge Mathew Holt of BodyRender.com for his artist drawings of the different valvular heart lesions. The author is the inventor on a patent for methods to slow the progression of valvular heart disease. This patent is owned by the Mayo Clinic and the author does not receive any royalties from this patent.

REFERENCES

1. Riviere L. Opera Medica Universa. Observationum medicarum, centuria IV, observatio XXI, Cordis palpitatio pulsus inaequalitas. Lugduni: Sumptibus Antoni, Cellier; 1663.
2. Stokes W. The Diseases of the Heart and Aorta. Dublin: Hodges & Smith 1845:211–2.
3. Rajamannan NM, Gersh B, Bonow RO. Calcific aortic stenosis: from bench to the bedside – emerging clinical and cellular concepts. Heart (British Cardiac Society) 2003;89(7):801–5.
4. Grande-Allen KJ, Calabro A, Gupta V, Wight TN, Hascall VC, Vesely I. Glycosaminoglycans and proteoglycans in normal mitral valve leaflets and chordae: association with regions of tensile and compressive loading. Glycobiology 2004 July;14(7): 621–33.
5. Willerson JT, Cohn JN, McAllister HA, Manabe H, Yutani C. Atlas of Valvular Heart Disease: Clinical and Pathologic Aspects. New York: Churchill Livingstone 1998.
6. Herrick JB. A short history of cardiology. Charles C Thomas, Publisher 1942:231–2.
7. Stewart BF, Siscovick D, Lind BK, et al. Clinical factors associated with calcific aortic valve disease: Cardiovascular Health Study. **J Am Coll Cardiol** 1997;29(3):630–4.
8. Otto CM, Lind BK, Kitzman DW, Gersh BJ, Siscovick DS. Association of aortic-valve sclerosis with cardiovascular mortality and morbidity in the elderly [comment]. **New Engl J Med** 1999;341(3):142–7.
9. Deutscher S, Rockette HE, Krishnaswami V. Diabetes and hypercholesterolemia among patients with calcific aortic stenosis. J Chronic Dis 1984;37(5):407–15.
10. Aronow WS, Ahn C, Kronzon I, Goldman ME. Association of coronary risk factors and use of statins with progression of mild valvular aortic stenosis in older persons. **Am J Cardiol** 2001;88(6):693–5.
11. Lindroos M, Kupari M, Valvanne J, Strandberg T, Heikkila J, Tilvis R. Factors associated with calcific aortic valve degeneration in the elderly. Eur Heart J 1994;15(7):865–70.
12. Aronow WS, Schwartz KS, Koenigsberg M. Correlation of serum lipids, calcium, and phosphorus, diabetes mellitus and history of systemic hypertension with presence or absence of calcified or thickened aortic cusps or root in elderly patients. Am J Cardiol 1987;59(9):998–9.
13. Boon A, Cheriex E, Lodder J, Kessels F. Cardiac valve calcification: characteristics of patients with calcification of the mitral annulus or aortic valve. Heart 1997;78(5):472–4.
14. Wilmshurst PT, Stevenson RN, Griffiths H, Lord JR. A case-control investigation of the relation between hyperlipidaemia and calcific aortic valve stenosis. Heart 1997;78(5):475–9.
15. Chan KL, Ghani M, Woodend K, Burwash IG. Case-controlled study to assess risk factors for aortic stenosis in congenitally bicuspid aortic valve. Am J Cardiol 2001;88(6):690–3.
16. Palta S, Pai AM, Gill KS, Pai RG. New insights into the progression of aortic stenosis: implications for secondary prevention. Circulation 2000;101(21):2497–502.
17. Whyte HM. The relative importance of the major risk factors in atherosclerotic and other diseases. Aust N Z J Med 1976;6(5):387–93.
18. Wilson PW, Castelli WP, Kannel WB. Coronary risk prediction in adults (the Framingham Heart Study). Am J Cardiol 1987;59(14):91G–4G.
19. D'Agostino RB, Kannel WB, Belanger AJ, Sytkowski PA. Trends in CHD and risk factors at age 55–64 in the Framingham Study. Int J Epidemiol 1989;18(3 Suppl 1):S67–72.
20. Sprecher DL, Schaefer EJ, Kent KM, et al. Cardiovascular features of homozygous familial hypercholesterolemia: analysis of 16 patients. **Am J Cardiol** 1984;54(1):20–30.

21. Rajamannan NM, Edwards WD, Spelsberg TC. Hypercholesterolemic aortic-valve disease. **New Engl J Med** 2003;349(7):717–8.
22. Buja LM, Kovanen PT, Bilheimer DW. Cellular pathology of homozygous familial hypercholesterolemia. **Am J Pathol** 1979 Nov; 97(2):327–57.
23. Kawaguchi A, Miyatake K, Yutani. C, et al. Characteristic cardiovascular manifestation in homozygous and heterozygous familial hypercholesterolemia. **Am Heart J** 1999 Mar; 137(3):410–8.
24. Kawaguchi A, Yutani C, Yamamoto A. Hypercholesterolemic valvulopathy: an aspect of malignant atherosclerosis. Ther Apher Dial. 2003 Aug; 7(4):439–43.
25. Olsson M, Thyberg J, Nilsson J. Presence of oxidized low density lipoprotein in nonrheumatic stenotic aortic valves. **Arterioscl Throm Vasc** 1999;19(5):1218–22.
26. O'Brien KD, Reichenbach DD, Marcovina SM, Kuusisto J, Alpers CE, Otto CM. Apolipoproteins B, (a), and E accumulate in the morphologically early lesion of 'degenerative' valvular aortic stenosis. **Arterioscl Throm Vasc** 1996;16(4):523–32.
27. Drolet MC, Arsenault M, Couet J. Experimental aortic valve stenosis in rabbits. **J Am Coll Cardiol** 2003;41(7):1211–7.
28. Rajamannan NM, Sangiorgi G, Springett M, et al. Experimental hypercholesterolemia induces apoptosis in the aortic valve. **J Heart Valve Dis** 2001;10(3):371–4.
29. Rajamannan NM, Subramaniam M, Springett M, et al. Atorvastatin inhibits hypercholesterolemia-induced cellular proliferation and bone matrix production in the rabbit aortic valve. Circulation 2002;105(22):2260–5.
30. Sarphie TG. A cytochemical study of the surface properties of aortic and mitral valve endothelium from hypercholesterolemic rabbits. **Exp Mol Pathol** 1986 Jun; 44(3):281–96.
31. Sarphie TG. Anionic surface properties of aortic and mitral valve endothelium from New Zealand white rabbits. **Am J Anat** 1985 Oct; 174(2):145–60.
32. Rajamannan NM. Role of stains in aortic valve disease. **Heart Fail Clin** 2006 Oct; 2(4):395–413. Review. No abstract available.
33. Caira FC, Stock SR, Gleason TG, et al. Human degenerative valve disease is associated with up-regulation of low-density lipoprotein receptor-related protein 5 receptor-mediated bone formation. **J Am Coll Cardiol** 2006;47(8):1707–12.
34. Rajamannan NM, Subramaniam M, Stock SR, et al. Atorvastatin inhibits calcification and enhances nitric oxide synthase production in the hypercholesterolaemic aortic valve. Heart 2005;91(6):806–10.
35. Weiss RM, Ohashi M, Miller JD, Young SG, Heistad DD. Calcific aortic valve stenosis in old hypercholesterolemic mice. Circulation 2006;114(19):2065–9.
36. Aikawa E, Nahrendorf M, Sosnovik D, et al. Multimodality molecular imaging identifies proteolytic and osteogenic activities in early aortic valve disease. Circulation 2007;115(3):377–86.
37. O'Brien KD, Kuusisto J, Reichenbach DD, et al. Osteopontin is expressed in human aortic valvular lesions [comment]. Circulation 1995;92(8):2163–8.
38. Mohler ER, 3rd, Gannon F, Reynolds C, Zimmerman R, Keane MG, Kaplan FS. Bone formation and inflammation in cardiac valves. Circulation 2001;103(11):1522–8.
39. Rajamannan NM, Subramaniam M, Rickard D, et al. Human aortic valve calcification is associated with an osteoblast phenotype. Circulation 2003;107(17):2181–4.
40. Jian B, Jones PL, Li Q, Mohler ER, 3rd, Schoen FJ, Levy RJ. Matrix metalloproteinase-2 is associated with tenascin-C in calcific aortic stenosis. **Am J Pathol** 2001;159(1):321–7.
41. Ducy P, Zhang R, Geoffroy V, Ridall AL, Karsenty G. Osf2/Cbfa1: a transcriptional activator of osteoblast differentiation [see comment]. Cell 1997;89(5):747–54.
42. Tyson KL, Reynolds JL, McNair R, Zhang Q, Weissberg PL, Shanahan CM. Osteo/chondrocytic transcription factors and their target genes exhibit distinct patterns of expression in human arterial calcification. **Arterioscl Throm Vasc** 2003;23(3):489–94.
43. Yano F, Kugimiya F, Ohba S, et al. The canonical Wnt signaling pathway promotes chondrocyte differentiation in a Sox9-dependent manner. Biochem Biophys Res Commun 2005;333(4):1300–8.
44. Jian B, Narula N, Li QY, Mohler ER, 3rd, Levy RJ. Progression of aortic valve stenosis: TGF-beta1 is present in calcified aortic valve cusps and promotes aortic valve interstitial cell calcification via apoptosis. **Ann Thorac Surg** 2003;75(2):457–65; discussion 65–6.
45. Kaden JJ, Kilic R, Sarikoc A, et al. Tumor necrosis factor alpha promotes an osteoblast-like phenotype in human aortic valve myofibroblasts: a potential regulatory mechanism of valvular calcification. Int J Mol Med 2005;16(5):869–72.
46. Aubin JE, Liu F, Malaval L, Gupta AK. Osteoblast and chondroblast differentiation. Bone 1995;17(2 Suppl):77S–83S.
47. Boyden LM, Mao J, Belsky J, et al. High bone density due to a mutation in LDL-receptor-related protein 5. N Engl J Med 2002;346(20):1513–21.
48. Little RD, Carulli JP, Del Mastro RG, et al. A mutation in the LDL receptor-related protein 5 gene results in the autosomal dominant high-bone-mass trait. **Am J Hum Genet** 2002;70(1):11–9.

49. Gong Y, Slee RB, Fukai N, et al. LDL receptor-related protein 5 (LRP5) affects bone accrual and eye development. Cell 2001;107(4):513–23.
50. Nusse R. Wnt signaling in disease and in development. Cell Res 2005;15(1):28–32.
51. Johnson ML, Rajamannan N. Diseases of Wnt signaling. Rev Endocr Metab Disord 2006;7(1–2):41–9.
52. Nusse R. Developmental biology. Making head or tail of Dickkopf. [comment]. Nature 2001;411(6835):255–6.
53. Shao JS, Cheng SL, Pingsterhaus JM, Charlton-Kachigian N, Loewy AP, Towler DA. Msx2 promotes cardiovascular calcification by activating paracrine Wnt signals. **J Clin Invest** 2005;115(5):1210–20.
54. Rajamannan NM, Subramaniam M, Caira F, Stock SR, Spelsberg TC. Atorvastatin inhibits hypercholesterolemia-induced calcification in the aortic valves via the Lrp5 receptor pathway. Circulation 2005;112(9 Suppl):I229–34.
55. Makkena B, Salti H, Subramaniam M, et al. Atorvastatin decreases cellular proliferation and bone matrix expression in the hypercholesterolemic mitral valve. **J Am Coll Cardiol** 2005;45(4):631–3.
56. Rabkin E, Aikawa M, Stone JR, Fukumoto Y, Libby P, Schoen FJ. Activated interstitial myofibroblasts express catabolic enzymes and mediate matrix remodeling in myxomatous heart valves. Circulation 2001;104(21):2525–32.
57. Charest A, Pépin A, Shetty R, et al. Distribution of SPARC during neovascularization of degenerative aortic stenosis. Heart 2006. Dec; 92(12): 1844–9. E pub 2006 May 18.
58. Pohle K, Maffert R, Ropers D, et al. Progression of aortic valve calcification: association with coronary atherosclerosis and cardiovascular risk factors. Circulation 2001;104(16):1927–32.
59. Aliev G, Burnstock G. Watanabe rabbits with heritable hypercholesterolaemia: a model of atherosclerosis. **Histol Histopathol** 1998;13(3):797–817.
60. Hoeg JM, Feuerstein IM, Tucker EE. Detection and quantitation of calcific atherosclerosis by ultrafast computed tomography in children and young adults with homozygous familial hypercholesterolemia. **Arterioscler Thromb** 1994;14(7):1066–74.
61. Cowell SJ, Newby DE, Prescott RJ, et al. A randomized trial of intensive lipid-lowering therapy in calcific aortic stenosis. N Engl J Med 2005;352(23):2389–97.
62. Moura LM, Ramos SF, Zamorano JL, et al. Rosuvastatin affecting aortic valve endothelium to slow the progression of aortic stenosis. **J Am Coll Cardiol** 2007;49(5):554–61.
63. Rajamannan NM, Calcific aortic stenosis: a disease ready for prime time. Circulation 2006 Nov 7; 114(19):2007–9.

3 Ventricular Adaptation to Valvular Heart Disease

Blase A. Carabello

CONTENTS

INTRODUCTION

Normal cardiac valves permit nearly unobstructed forward blood flow through them while preventing all but minimal backward flow. Irrespective of etiology, valvular heart disease (VHD) causes the valves to become stenotic, regurgitant, or both. In turn these lesions place pressure overload, volume overload, or both on the left and/or the right ventricles. Although molecular signaling in the heart is richly complex, ultimately the heart has only three ways for coping with hemodynamic overload. These are activation of the Frank–Starling mechanism, neurohumoral activation, and the development of hypertrophy. This chapter will focus primarily on this last aspect of the ventricular response to hemodynamic overload, the development of hypertrophy, and remodeling in response to VHD. While often used interchangeably, the two terms hypertrophy and remodeling are not entirely synonymous. Hypertrophy indicates a gain in mass. Hypertrophy can occur from an increase in ventricular wall thickness (concentric hypertrophy) or from an increase in ventricular volume (eccentric hypertrophy). In most cases of remodeling, hypertrophy has indeed occurred. However, this is not always the case. Sometimes both concentric and eccentric remodeling have occurred without hypertrophy, i.e., changes in ventricular geometry occur without an increase in mass *(1)*. This can happen only if wall thickness and radius behave discordantly, where the increase in one property is met by a decrease in the other.

Many view the processes of remodeling and hypertrophy as pathologic. However, different models of hypertrophy have found it to be either deleterious or beneficial depending upon the model investigated *(2–9)*. Most murine models create either loss or gain of function of a given signaling pathway and then focus on the amount of hypertrophy that develops and the resultant ventricular performance and mortality associated with it. There is generally implied cause and effect between the pathway studied and the hypertrophy that results. That two diametrically opposite outcomes have been observed in animals with hypertrophy suggests that the pathways for signaling hypertrophy control not only it but other cellular functions as well *(7)*. Thus one pathway leading to hypertrophy could have beneficial side effects such as also maintaining cell health, while another could create apoptosis yielding totally different outcomes unrelated to the hypertrophy. In man, although some adult myocyte replication occurs *(10)*, it is generally believed that most adult cardiac growth occurs through hypertrophy. Obviously then the very life of a growing individual is dependent on cardiac hypertrophy as the heart must grow in order to supply the body's needs. Thus some hypertrophy and remodeling are not only

From: *Contemporary Cardiology: Valvular Heart Disease*
Edited by: Andrew Wang, Thomas M. Bashore, DOI 10.1007/978-1-59745-411-7_3
© Humana Press, a part of Springer Science+Business Media, LLC 2009

not pathologic but also a prerequisite to life. Further, concentric hypertrophy develops in athletes participating in sports requiring isometric exercise such as weight lifting, while eccentric hypertrophy develops in athletes participating in isotonic exercise such as running. In both situations, muscle function is normal *(11, 12)*. Thus hypertrophy itself can be a normal and necessary process.

At issue is when in VHD are hypertrophy and remodeling compensatory and when are they dangerous, contributing to poor patient outcomes. These key questions will be addressed for each valve lesion below.

Aortic Stenosis: Concentric LV Hypertrophy, the Good, the Bad, the Ugly

Aortic stenosis (AS) is the quintessential left ventricular (LV) overload. Normally the aortic valve opens just before pressure in the LV exceeds that in the aorta and allows for equal pressure in the LV and the aorta during ejection. As the valve becomes narrowed from disease, it takes a progressively larger LV pressure to drive blood across the valve (Fig. 1) *(13)*. This extra pressure (pressure gradient between the LV and the aorta) represents the LV pressure overload. Ventricular stroke volume is determined by preload, afterload, and contractility. Afterload is often quantified as wall stress (σ), $\sigma = P \times r/2th$, where P is the LV pressure, r is the LV radius, and th is the LV thickness. As pressure increases in the numerator, it can be offset by an increased thickness (concentric hypertrophy or remodeling) in the denominator, keeping stress normal. Alternatively the radius term can decrease another mechanism by which afterload could be maintained in the normal range despite the pressure overload *(1)*.

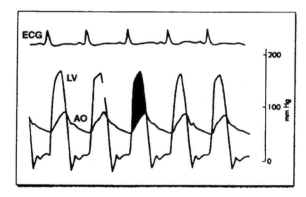

Fig. 1. The pressure gradient between the left ventricle (LV) and the aorta (Ao) in a patient with aortic stenosis is demonstrated. This pressure overload is the presumptive signal for the development of LV hypertrophy. Taken from *(13)*.

Over three decades ago, Grossman postulated that pressure overload was the mechanical signal that in some way informed the myocardium to synthesize new sarcomeres laid down in parallel, thereby increasing myocyte thickness, in turn increasing wall thickness, normalizing stress, and maintaining ventricular function *(14)*. It is likely that the mechanical signal of increased stress is transduced from the cell surface through interaction with integrins that in turn activate the various molecular pathways involved in cell growth *(15)*. The response to the initial signal is almost surely modified by the multiple signaling pathways acting in concert to yield widely disparate amounts of hypertrophy and levels of ventricular function. If the relationship between mechanical signal and compensation were perfect, then just enough hypertrophy would develop to normalize stress. However, this is not always the case *(16, 17)*. While in some patients, wall stress and ejection performance are indeed normal, in others, hypertrophy has been inadequate to normalize stress, stress is increased, and ejection fraction

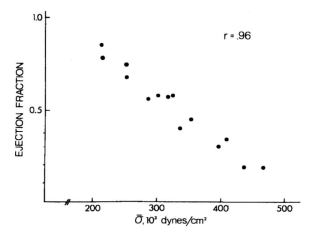

Fig. 2. Ejection fraction is plotted against mean systolic wall stress (σ, afterload) for patients with AS. Ejection performance is inversely related to afterload. Taken from *(17)*.

is reduced (Fig. 2) *(17)*. In still other patients, wall thickness is greater than is necessary to normalize stress, stress is reduced, and ejection performance is actually supernormal *(18, 19)*.

Following an increase in ventricular wall stress, the cellular machinery for causing myocardial growth is activated remarkably rapidly and within 6 hours a 35% increase in contractile protein synthesis can be detected (Fig. 3) *(20)*. This is probably too short a period of time for the transcription of new message to occur or for increase in ribosome number. Rather the acute increase in protein synthesis appears primarily due to increased efficiency of the translation of existing message by polysome formation. With systolic stress sustained over time, ribosomal number increases, adding increased capacity to increased efficiency for message translation *(21)*.

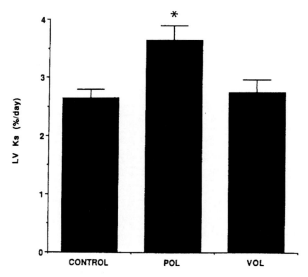

Fig. 3. The constant for myosin synthesis rate (K_s) for normal dogs and those with acute pressure overload is shown. K_s increases by 35% within 6 hours of the overload. Taken from *(20)*.

The Good. In many patients with AS, concentric left ventricular hypertrophy is present in the absence of symptoms, the key determinant of survival with the disease *(22, 23)*. In other words, asymptomatic patients have nearly normal survival irrespective of LVH. An obvious question is whether they would also be asymptomatic if no LVH developed. In some patients there is reverse remodeling where a decrease in ventricular radius allows for normal systolic wall stress without increase in thickness *(1)*. However, such patients are the minority and concentric LVH is the rule in AS. By Laplace's law, if there were no increase in wall thickness and no decrease in radius, then stress must rise as pressure rises and EF would fall. As noted above, in some animal models, LVH improves function and survival, while in other models, the absence of LVH is beneficial. This concept is amplified in Fig. 4, representing a canine model of AS, where the severity of AS was held constant yet different animals responded to the same load with vastly different amounts of hypertrophy *(24)*. In this case, reduced LVH caused

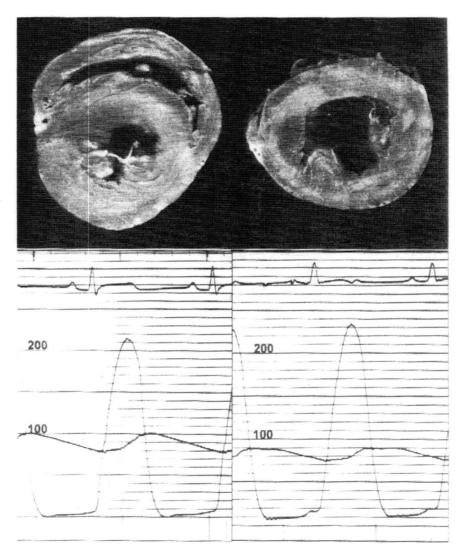

Fig. 4. Left ventricular cross sections from two dogs with similar pressure load are demonstrated. Similar load caused a vastly different amount of hypertrophy in the two dogs. Taken from *(24)*.

myocardial dysfunction at both the myocyte and the ventricular levels. Inadequate hypertrophy led to increased wall stress, in turn leading to cytoskeletal hyperpolymerization that interfered with myocyte contraction. Animals with inadequate hypertrophy had decreased LV mass despite increased load *even before* banding and never responded with enough LVH to normalize stress (Fig. 5). The differing phenotypes seen in this model suggest genetic variation among animals of the same species leading to differing outcomes. From the foregoing, it seems unlikely that hypertrophy can be viewed simplistically as positive or negative but rather it can be either according to the background in which it occurs.

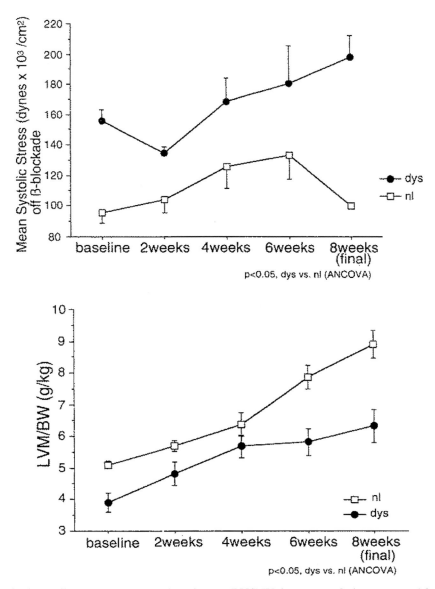

Fig. 5. Left ventricular wall stress (*upper panel*) and mass (LV/BW, *lower panel*) demonstrated for the dogs from the experiment depicted in Fig. 4 are shown. Dogs with extreme hypertrophy maintained normal function (open squares, nl), while the dogs with less hypertrophy developed dysfunction (dys). Even before banding, the dys dogs had less LV mass despite higher wall stress. Taken from *(24)*.

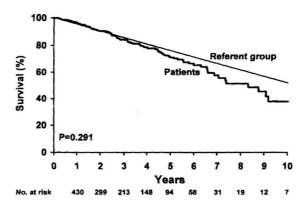

Fig. 6. Survival of asymptomatic patients with severe aortic stenosis (*thick line*) is plotted against demographic data for a matched unaffected referent population (*thin line*). While the AS group had a somewhat worse outcome, the difference was not statistically significant. Taken from *(23)*.

The Bad and the Ugly. The presence or the absence of symptoms is the key determinant of outcome in AS, as emphasized in Fig. 6 *(23)*. Survival is nearly normal in asymptomatic patients, while mortality is extreme (about 25% per year) in patients who develop angina, syncope, or the symptoms of heart failure and hypertrophy is linked to the causation of angina and heart failure. As noted above when hypertrophy fails to normalize stress, afterload increases and ejection performance falls. However, unfortunately even when hypertrophy is sufficient to maintain normal afterload, increased wall thickness may still lead to pathologic consequences. Concentric hypertrophy reduces myocardial blood flow reserve *(25, 26)*. In normal subjects, coronary blood flow can increase five- to eightfold in response to increased myocardial oxygen demand during increased workload, in turn supplying the myocardium with sufficient oxygen and nutrients to accommodate the increased metabolic demands. However, concentric hypertrophy limits flow reserve to just two- to threefold, potentially leading to exercise-induced ischemia and angina. While impaired coronary flow reserve must in part be responsible for the symptom of angina in AS patients, this alone cannot explain the onset of angina since not all patients with impaired reserve have angina and the presence of angina does not correlate well the magnitude of hypertrophy. The best correlate for the presence of angina appears to be an imbalance between the systolic ejection period (the period of oxygen consumption and oxygen debt) and the diastolic filling period (the period of coronary blood flow and oxygen debt repayment) *(27)*. Paradoxically the key determinants of myocardial oxygen consumption are systolic wall stress and heart rate. Thus on the one hand, hypertrophy helps maintain normal wall stress, thereby reducing myocardial oxygen consumption, but on the other hand, hypertrophy limits coronary blood flow and oxygen supply.

Concentric hypertrophy may also be responsible for heart failure in AS patients. While helping to maintain systolic function, increased wall thickness impairs diastolic filling so that for any given filling volume, filling pressure is increased (reduced compliance) and increased filling pressure results in pulmonary congestion. As AS progresses, myocardial fibrosis may compound diastolic dysfunction, worsening pulmonary congestion *(28, 29)*. In addition, while hypertrophy initially aids systolic performance, eventually it causes contractile dysfunction. While not entirely understood, impaired contractility appears to stem from impaired calcium handling, cytoskeletal abnormalities, ischemia (at least during exercise), and apoptosis *(30–34)*. Traditionally the view has been that there is a continuum of pressure overload hypertrophy from normal to compensated hypertrophy to heart failure. This concept has recently been challenged by findings of early divergence in gene expression between subjects that eventually did or did not demonstrate decompensation long before decompensation took place *(35)*.

These findings suggest that there may be fundamental genetic differences leading to compensation rather than a continuum that all individuals are subject to.

Thus the concentric hypertrophy of AS is a two-edged sword. It helps to compensate the pressure overload by normalizing wall stress, thereby maintaining normal ejection performance. On the other hand, hypertrophy may lead to myocardial ischemia, contractile dysfunction, and impaired diastolic filling, factors responsible for some of the symptoms of AS, portending sudden death. Hypertrophy is no doubt initiated by the hemodynamic stress of pressure overload but the results of this overload are amazingly divergent among individual subjects.

Mitral Stenosis and "Hypotrophy"

Normally in diastole there is free flow of blood from the left atrium to the left ventricle allowing for normal left ventricular filling. However, in mitral stenosis (MS), the reduced mitral orifice impairs ventricular filling, reducing cardiac output. Thus the standard view of the left ventricle in MS is that it is "protected" by the lesion and not subject to the consequences of overload. While some cases of aggressive rheumatic fever may damage the myocardium, especially in developing countries (36), in the West, myocardial contractility in MS is considered to be normal. Paradoxically, about one-third of MS patients have impaired left ventricular ejection (37). If contractility is normal in such patients, impaired ejection must be caused by either reduced preload or increased afterload and both appear to be operative. MS is not usually thought to increase left ventricular afterload, yet it in fact may. In patients with impaired ejection performance, wall thickness in MS is subnormal (Fig. 7) (37, 38). Reduced wall thickness in concert with reflexive vasoconstriction from reduced cardiac output increases wall stress impairing left ventricular ejection (36, 37). Obstruction to ventricular inflow prevents a compensatory

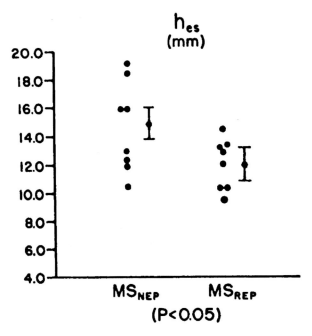

Fig. 7. Wall thickness (*h*) is demonstrated for patients with mitral stenosis and normal ejection performance (MSnep) and for MS patients with reduced ejection performance (MSrep). Thinner walls in the MSrep group led to increased wall stress. Taken from *(37)*.

increase in preload that would serve to offset the afterload excess. Following mitral balloon valvotomy, these changes are reversed *(39)*. Taken together, these findings suggest that underfilling of the left ventricle leads to remodeling such that LV wall thickness, volume, and LV mass are reduced in some MS patients.

The force required to overcome the resistance offered by the narrowed mitral valve and to fill the LV is provided by ventricular suction created by LV restoring forces and by left atrial pressure. This last component is primarily generated by the right ventricle (RV). Thus when left atrial pressure is elevated, it imparts a pressure overload on the RV. Pulmonary hypertension is further impacted by pulmonary vasoconstriction as MS worsens. Extensive animal studies of right ventricular pressure overload hypertrophy demonstrate impaired contractility even in the absence of clinical heart failure *(40)*. The predilection for myocardial dysfunction to accompany even early right ventricular pressure overload may in part be due to the odd shape of the right ventricle. This "spoon" shape may increase wall stress, leading to myocardial damage even when right ventricular pressure is only modestly elevated. Thus while the left ventricle in MS is "protected" and may even undergo a kind of atrophy, the right ventricle is exposed to pressure overload that leads to muscle dysfunction and eventually to right heart failure. In turn, pulmonary hypertension clearly worsens the prognosis for this disease *(41)*. Indeed mitral stenosis should be corrected once pulmonary hypertension is detected even if the patient is asymptomatic.

Mitral Regurgitation: A Pure Volume Overload

Most conditions that increase the demand for volume pumped by the LV are in fact a combined pressure and volume overload because in most of these disease states, the extra volume is delivered into the aorta. Increased aortic stroke volume causes widened pulse pressure and a tendency toward systolic hypertension. While this effect is most pronounced in aortic regurgitation, it is also present in hyperthyroidism, anemia, and complete heart block. However, in mitral regurgitation (MR), the excess volume pumped by the LV is ejected into the low-pressure zone of the left atrium, forward stroke volume is not increased, and systolic pressure is normal or low. Evaluation of systolic wall stress in MR finds it low in acute disease returning to normal in compensated disease *(42, 43)*. Thus MR constitutes a pure LV volume overload and is the prototype for examining the effects of pure volume overload on LV remodeling. As shown in Fig. 8 *(44)*, acute MR causes a small increase in end-diastolic volume as sarcomeres are maximally stretched by the increased volume returning from the pulmonary veins and the added regurgitant volume ejected from the LV. The extra pathway for ejection reduces afterload, decreasing end-systolic volume. Increased end-diastolic volume and decreased end-systolic volume increase total stroke volume but not enough to compensate for that lost to regurgitation. If the MR is not corrected acutely, the patient may enter the chronic compensated phase facilitated by eccentric remodeling and hypertrophy. By Grossman's hypothesis, increased end-diastolic stress initiates sarcomere addition in series, in turn elongating each myocyte, increasing total ventricular volume *(14)*. Greatly increased end-diastolic volume allows for a larger total and thus a larger forward stroke volume, returning cardiac output toward normal. Of interest is the radius to thickness ratio that develops in the process of the eccentric hypertrophy and remodeling that occurs in chronic MR. Radius increases while thickness remains static or even decreases *(42)*. This thin-walled enlarged chamber has excellent diastolic properties and actually may exhibit supernormal diastolic function, one of the few cases in all of cardiology where this occurs *(45, 46)*. Enhanced LV compliance allows the regurgitant volume to be accommodated at relatively normal filling pressure. However, the high r/th ratio is problematic for systolic function. Recall that stress = p × r/2th. Thus while MR is often thought to reduce LV afterload, the opposite may be true *(47)*. While the low-impedance pathway for LV ejection must act to reduce afterload, the remodeling that occurs works in the opposite direction to increase load. Taking a broad view of valvular heart disease and its effect on remodeling, it suggests that the pressure

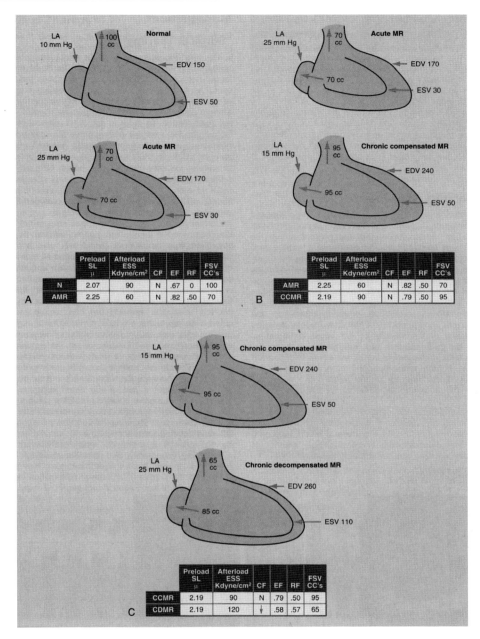

Fig. 8. The progression of ventricular remodeling in mitral regurgitation is shown. In the *upper left panel*, normal physiology is compared to that of acute MR. Acute MR facilitates ejection by decreasing afterload (end-systolic stress, ESS) and increasing preload (sarcomere length, SL). These changes increase end-diastolic volume (EDV), decrease end-systolic volume (ESV), and in the face of normal contractile function (CF), ejection fraction and total stroke volume are increased. Regurgitation of blood into the left atrium (LA) increases LA pressure while increasing regurgitant fraction (RF), in turn decreasing forward stroke volume (FSV). In the *upper right panel*, acute MR is compared to that of chronic compensated MR. Eccentric hypertrophy and remodeling have allowed EDV to increase dramatically. Ventricular dilatation increases ESS toward normal and ESV increases. However, normal CF and increased preload together with eccentric hypertrophy increase forward and total SV. Increased LA size allows LA pressure to be reduced. In the *lower panel*, compensated MR is compared to decompensated MR. Reduced contractility reduces EF (although it may remain in the "normal" range), reduces stroke volume, and increases LA pressure. Taken from *(44)*.

term in the Laplace equation is more effective than the radius term in inciting concentric hypertrophy since systolic stress increased by an increase in the Laplace radius in MR fails to cause compensatory concentric remodeling but rather leads to eccentric remodeling.

The unique mechanical signals produced by the pure volume overload of MR lead to a unique mechanism of hypertrophy. In examining myocardial protein synthesis in MR, we could never detect an increase in synthesis rate, not during acute severe MR and/or anytime during the next 3 months after MR was created *(20, 48)* (Fig. 9). Myocardial mass is held in equilibrium by balanced rates of protein synthesis and degradation. Since LV mass does increase in MR (albeit not to the degree seen in AS) and since synthesis does not increase, it appears that the eccentric hypertrophy of MR occurs by a decrease in degradation rate, an opposite mechanism from the hypertrophy of pressure overload.

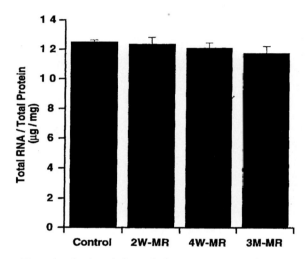

Fig. 9. Myosin synthesis rate K_s and calculated degradation rate K_d are shown at various times after creation of MR. In this model, hypertrophy appears to accrue primarily from a decrease in degradation rate. Taken from *(48)*.

While this is a surprising finding, it is corroborated by similar results from a lapine model of MR *(49)*. Further when load was imposed on contracting myocytes in systole versus diastole, different signaling pathways were activated *(50)*. Systolic load activated the MAP kinase p38 pathway, the extracellular signaling-related pathway (ERK), the JN kinase pathway (JNK), and the MEK pathway, while diastolic load activated the MAPK 38 and JNK pathways, with much less effect on the other two. Thus diastolic versus systolic loads have differential effects upon hypertrophy signaling pathways, which could form the underpinnings for differing mechanisms by which hypertrophy occurs in these two different settings.

Clinically, as with AS, remodeling has both positive and negative attributes. As noted above, if 50% of total LV stroke volume goes backward, forward stroke volume would be reduced by 50%, a reduction that cannot be well tolerated. Eccentric hypertrophy and remodeling are the key mechanisms by which total, and pari passu, forward stroke volume can be returned to normal. However, large ventricular volumes especially at end systole are associated with a poor prognosis, presumably as large end-systolic volume reflects both impaired contractility and a tendency for wall stress to become supernormal *(51, 52)*. Reduced contractility seems predicated upon a potentially reversible loss of sarcomeres and upon abnormal calcium handling *(53, 54)*.

Aortic Regurgitation: Combined Pressure and Volume Overload

In aortic regurgitation (AR), the extra volume that the LV must pump is that which leaked back into the ventricle during diastole. In systole a large stroke volume is discharged into the aorta. Because stroke volume is a key determinant of pulse pressure, pulse pressure widens as systolic pressure increases, while diastolic pressure decreases. In fact, systolic pressure in AR is about 50 mmHg than it is in MR. Thus AR represents a combined pressure and volume overload. Indeed systolic stress in AR may be as high as it is in AS, a lesion classified as pure pressure overload *(55)*. The LV responds to this dual load with dual types of hypertrophy. There is a modest increase in LV wall thickness and a greater increase in chamber radius, leading the AR left ventricle to have typically the greatest mass of all valve diseases *(42)*. Interestingly and perhaps emblematic of the dual hypertrophy that occurs, hypertrophy is initiated by an increase in protein synthesis rate but maintained by a decrease in degradation rate at least in the rabbit *(56)*. Of particular interest is how well this disease is tolerated. Despite the fact that AR produces the largest and heaviest LV in the realm of valvular heart disease, progression of the asymptomatic patient with normal LV function to either new symptoms or asymptomatic LV dysfunction occurs at the rate of only about 4% per year *(57)* (Fig. 10). Thus more than half of patients with severe disease and very large ventricles have a benign 10-year course. This observation serves to reinforce the concept that hypertrophy and remodeling cannot be viewed simplistically as either good or bad but rather must be taken in the context of adaptation versus maladaptation.

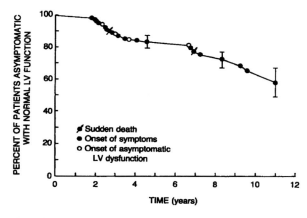

Fig. 10. The natural history of AR is demonstrated. In general, even severe AR is well tolerated for years. Taken from *(57)*.

Another provocative issue that AR raises is the effect of ACE inhibitors in treatment of the disease. ACE inhibitors are the mainstay of therapy for systolic heart failure, proven to extend life in several large clinical trials. Although the exact mechanism of benefit of these agents in heart failure is unknown, benefit is often attributed to ACE inhibitors' ability to prevent remodeling or to induce reverse remodeling. Of interest are two recent studies that suggest but do not prove that ACE inhibitors might actually be deleterious in AR patients who are not in heart failure *(58, 59)*. Because afterload is increased in patients with AR, afterload reduction seemed a reasonable therapy to forestall progression of AR. Indeed one study did demonstrate that compared to digoxin, nifedipine did slow the progression to symptom onset or LV dysfunction by about 2 years *(60)*. However, in a recent placebo-controlled trial, nifedipine failed to show benefit, and use of the ACE inhibitor enalapril tended to have deleterious effects *(58)*. In a retrospective analysis by Borer et al., ACE inhibitors also seemed delirious. Reasons for an adverse response of AR patients not in heart failure to ACE inhibitors are countless. However, one possibility is that interfering with remodeling in AR is disadvantageous.

Although marked remodeling in AR is well tolerated, tolerance is not infinite. Extreme ventricular dilatation has been associated with rare cases of sudden death, especially when end-diastolic dimension exceeds 75 mm. When end-systolic dimension exceeds 55 mm, the risk of persistent heart failure, even after successful aortic valve replacement, also increases markedly *(61)*.

Primary Tricuspid Regurgitation: Pure Right Ventricular Volume Overload

Most cases of tricuspid regurgitation (TR) result from concomitant RV pressure overloads. However, primary TR such as might occur in tricuspid endocarditis produces a pure RV volume overload. Interestingly while the volume overload of MR leads to LV dysfunction and heart failure, long-standing TR is remarkably well tolerated. Complete removal of the tricuspid valve may be tolerated for years without significant clinical sequelae. In a canine model of severe TR that caused clinical right-sided volume overload, myocytes taken from these ventricles exhibited normal contractile function *(62)*. Thus looking across the spectrum of valve disease, left-sided pressure overload and right-sided volume overload are better tolerated than left-sided volume overload and right-sided pressure overload.

SUMMARY

Valvular heart disease imparts pressure and/or volume overload on the left and/or right ventricles. These loads lead to ventricular hypertrophy and remodeling. Taking the vast amount of clinical and experimental data as whole, it seems obvious that remodeling is neither good nor bad but can be either according to the clinical situation in which it occurs. Most importantly it seems that a patient's individual genetic background is key in determining the consequences of hypertrophy and remodeling. Thus even when a given VHD seems identical in two patients, resultant LV function and mortality may be quite different.

REFERENCES

1. Kupari M, Tutro H, Lommi J. Left ventricular hypertrophy in aortic valve stenosis – preventive or promotive of systolic dysfunction and heart failure? Eur Heart J 2005;26:1790–6.
2. Meguro T, Hong C, Asai K, Takagi G, McKinsey TA, Olson EN, Vatner SF. Cyclosporine attenuates pressure-overload hypertrophy in mice while enhancing susceptibility to decompensation and heart failure. Circ Res 1999;84:735–40.
3. Rogers JH, Tamirisa P, Kovacs A, Winheimer C, Courtois M, Blumer KJ, Kelly DP, Muslin AJ. RGS4 causes increased mortality and reduced cardiac hypertrophy in response to overload. J Clin Invest 1999;104:567–76.
4. Esposito G, Rapacciuolo A, Naga Prasad SV, Takaoka H, Thomas SA, Koch WJ, Rockman HA. Genetic alterations that inhibit in vivo pressure-overload hypertrophy prevent cardiac dysfunction despite increased wall stress. Circulation 2002;105:85–92.
5. Hill JA, Karimi M, Kutschke W, Davisson RL, Zimmerman K, Wang Z, Kerber RE, Weiss RM. Cardiac hypertrophy is not a required compensatory response to short-term pressure overload. Circulation 2000;101:2863–9.
6. Levy D, Garrison RJ, Savage DD, Kannel WB, Castelli WP. Prognostic implications of echocardiographically determined left ventricular mass in the Framingham Heart Study. N Engl J Med 1990;322:1561–6.
7. Morisco C, Sadoshima J, Trimarco B, Arora R, Vatner DE, Vatner SF. Special Medical Editorial: Is treating cardiac hypertrophy salutary or detrimental: the two faces of Janus. Am J Physiol Heart Circ Physiol 2003;284:H1043–7.
8. Bueno OF, Windt LJ, Tymitz KM, Witt SA, Kimball TR, Klevitsky R, Hewett TE, Jones SP, Lefer DJ, Peng CF, Kitsis RN, Molkentin JD. The MEK1-ERK signaling pathway promotes compensated cardiac hypertrophy in transgenic mice. EMBO J 2000;19:6341–50.
9. Condorelli G, Drusco A, Stassi G, Bellacosa A, Roncarati R, Iaccarino G, Russo MA, Gu Y, Dalton N, Chung C, Latronico MV, Napoli C, Sadoshima J, Croce CM, Ross J Jr. Akt induces enhanced myocardial contractility and cell size in vivo in transgenic mice. Proc Natl Acad Sci USA 2002;99:12333–8.
10. Nadal-Ginard B, Kajstura J, Leri A, Anversa P. Myocyte death, growth, and regeneration in cardiac hypertrophy and failure. Circ Res 2003 Feb 7;92(2):139–50.
11. Hoogsteen J, Hoogeveen A, Schaffers H, Wijn PF, van der Wall EE. Left atrial and ventricular dimensions in highly trained cyclists. Int J Cardiovasc Imaging 2003 Jun;19(3):211–7.

12. D'Andrea A, Limongelli G, Caso P, Sarubbi B, Della Pietra A, Brancaccio P, Cice G, Scherillo M, Limongelli F, Calabro R. Association between left ventricular structure and cardiac performance during effort in two morphological forms of athlete's heart. Int J Cardiol 2002 Dec;86(2–3):177–84.

13. Carabello BA. Cardiovascular Diseases In Myers AR (ed) 5th ed. NMS Medicine. Lippincott, Williams & Wilkins, Philadelphia, 2004. Chapter 1: pp 1–54.

14. Grossman W, Jones D, McLaurin LP. Wall stress and patterns of hypertrophy in the human left ventricle. J Clin Invest 1975;53:332–41.

15. Lorell BH, Carabello BA. Left ventricular hypertrophy: pathogenesis, detection and prognosis. Circulation 2000 July 25;102(4):470–9.

16. Huber D, Grimm J, Koch R, Krayenbuehl HP. Determinants of ejection performance in aortic stenosis. Circulation 1981;64:126–34.

17. Gunther S, Grossman W. Determinants of ventricular function in pressure-overload hypertrophy in man. Circulation 1979;59:679–88.

18. Donner R, Carabello BA, Black I, Spann JF. Left ventricular wall stress in compensated aortic stenosis in children. Am J Cardiol 1983 Mar 15;51(6)946–51.

19. Carroll JD, Carroll EP, Feldman T, Ward DM, Lang RM, McGaughey D, Karp RB. Sex-associated differences in left ventricular function in aortic stenosis of the elderly. Circulation 1992;86:1099–107.

20. Imamura T, McDermott PJ, Kent RL, Nagatsu M, Cooper G IV, Carabello BA. Acute changes in myosin heavy chain synthesis rate in pressure versus volume overload. Circ Res 1994;75(3):418–25.

21. Nagatomo Y, Carabello BA, Hamawaki M, Nemoto S, Matsuo T, McDermott PJ. Translational mechanisms accelerate the rate of protein synthesis during canine pressure-overload hypertrophy. Am J Physiol 1999;277(6 Pt 2):H2176–84.

22. Ross J Jr., Braunwald E. Aortic stenosis. Circulation 1968;38:61–7.

23. Pellikka PA, Sarano ME, Nishimura RA, et al. Outcome of 622 adults with asymptomatic, hemodynamically significant aortic stenosis during prolonged follow-up. Circulation 2005;111:3290–5.

24. Koide M, Nagatsu M, Zile MR, Hamawaki M, Swindle MM, Keech G, DeFreyte G, Tagawa H, Cooper G IV, Carabello BA. Premorbid determinants of left ventricular dysfunction in a novel mode of gradually induced pressure overload in the adult canine. Circulation 1997;95(6):1601–10.

25. Marcus ML, Doty DB, Hiratzka LF, Wright CB, Eastham CL. Decreased coronary reserve: a mechanism for angina pectoris in patients with aortic stenosis and normal coronary arteries. N Engl J Med 1982;307:1362–6.

26. Julius BK, Spillman M, Vassali G, Villari B, Eberli FR, Hess OM. Angina pectoris in patients with aortic stenosis and normal coronary arteries: mechanisms and pathophysiological concepts. Circulation 1997;95:892–8.

27. Rajappan K, Rimoldi OE, Dutka DP, Ariff B, Pennell DJ, Sheridan DJ, Camici PG. Mechanisms of coronary micro-circulatory dysfunction in patients with aortic stenosis and angiographically normal coronary arteries. Circulation 2002;105:470–6.

28. Jalil JE, Doering CW, Janicki JS, Pick R, Clark WA, Abrahams C, Weber KT. Structural vs. contractile protein remodeling and myocardial stiffness in hypertrophied rat left ventricle. J Mol Cell Cardiol 1988;20:1179–87.

29. Peterson KL, Tsuji J, Johnson A, DiDonna J, LeWinter M. Diastolic left ventricular pressure-volume and stress-strain relations in patients with valvular aortic stenosis and left ventricular hypertrophy. Circulation 1978 July;58(1):77–89.

30. Ito K, Yan X, Feng X, Manning WJ, et al. Transgenic expression of sarcoplasmic reticulum Ca(2+) ATPase modifies the transition from hypertrophy to early heart failure. Circ Res 2001;89:422–9.

31. Nakano K, Corin WJ, Spann JF Jr, Biederman RW, Denslow S, Carabello BA. Abnormal subendocardial blood flow in pressure overload hypertrophy is associated with pacing-induced subendocardial dysfunction. Circ Res 1989 Dec;65(6):1555–64.

32. Olivetti G, Abbi R, Quaini F, et al. Apoptosis in the failing human heart. N Engl J Med 1997;336:1131.

33. Hein S, Arnon E, Kostin S, et al. Progression from compensated hypertrophy to failure in the pressure-overloaded human heart: structural deterioration and compensatory mechanisms. Circulation 2003 Feb 25;107(7):984–9.

34. Tsutsui H, Oshihara K, Cooper GT. Cytoskeletal role in the contractile dysfunction of hypertrophied myocardium. Science 1993;260(5108):682–7.

35. Buermans HPJ, Redout EM, Schiel AE, Musters RJP, Zuidwijk M, Eijk PP, van Hardeveld C, Kasanmoentalib S, Visser FC, Yistra B, Simonides WS. Micro-array analysis reveals pivotal divergent mRNA expression profiles early in the development of either compensated ventricular hypertrophy or heart failure. Physiol Genomics 2005;21:314–23.

36. Mohan JC, Khalilullah M, Arora R. Left ventricular intrinsic contractility in pure rheumatic mitral stenosis. Am J Cardiol 1989;64:240.

37. Gash AK, Carabello BA, Cepin D, et al. Left ventricular ejection performance and systolic muscle function in patients with mitral stenosis. Circulation 1983;67:148.

38. Horwitz LD, Mullins CB, Payne PM, et al. Left ventricular function in mitral stenosis. Chest 1973;64:609.

39. Fawzy Me, Choi WB, Mimish L, Sivandam V, Lingamanaicker J, Khan A, Patel A, Khan B. Immediate and long-term effect of mitral balloon valvotomy on left ventricular volume and systolic function in severe mitral stenosis. Am Heart J 1996 Aug;132(2 Pt 1):356–60.

40. Cooper G IV, Tomanek RJ, Ehrhardt JC, Marcus ML. Chronic progressive pressure overload of the cath right ventricle. Circ Res 1981;48:488–97.

41. Vincens JJ, Temizer D, Post JR, Edmunds LH, Herrmann HC. Long-term outcome of cardiac surgery in patients with mitral stenosis and severe pulmonary hypertension. Circulation 1995 Nov 1;92(9 Suppl): II137–42.

42. Carabello BA. The relationship of left ventricular geometry and hypertrophy to left ventricular function in valvular heart disease. J Heart Valve Dis 1995 Oct;4(Suppl 2):S132–8;discussion S138–9.

43. Wiensbaugh T, Spann JF, Carabllo BA. Differences in myocardial performance and load between patients with similar amounts of chronic aortic versus chronic mitral regurgitation. J Am Coll Cardiol 1984;3:916–23.

44. Carabello BA. Mitral regurgitation. Part I: basic pathophysiological principles. Mod Concepts Cardiovasc Dis 1988;57:53–8.

45. Zile MR, Tomita M, Nakano K, Mirsky I, Usher B, Lindroth J, Carabello BA. Effects of left ventricular volume overload produced by mitral regurgitation on diastolic function. Am J Physiol 1991 Nov;261(5 Pt 2):H1471–80.

46. Corin WJ, Murakami T, Monrad ES, Hess OM, Krayenbuehl HP. Left ventricular passive diastolic properties in chronic mitral regurgitation. Circulation 1991 Mar;83(3):797–807.

47. Corin WJ, Monrad ES, Murakami T, Nonogi H, Hess OM, Krayenbuehl HP. The relationship of afterload to ejection performance in chronic mitral regurgitation. Circulation 1987;76:59–67.

48. Matsuo T, Carabello BA, Nagatomo Y, Koide M, Hamawaki M, Zile MR, McDermott PJ. Mechanisms of cardiac hypertrophy in canine volume overload. Am J Physiol 1998;275(1 Pt 2):H65–74.

49. Borer JS, Carter JN, Jacobson MH, Herrold EM, Magid NM. Myofibrillar protein synthesis rates in mitral regurgitation. Circulation 1997;96(suppl 1):I–469.

50. Yamamoto K, Dang Q, Maeda Y, Huang H, Kelley R, Lee RT. Regulation of cardiomyocyte mechanotransduction by the cardiac cycle. Circulation 2001;103:1459–64.

51. Zile MR, Gaasch WH, Carroll JD, Levine HJ. Chronic mitral regurgitation: predictive value of preoperative echocardiographic indexes of left ventricular function and wall stress. J Am Coll Cardiol 1984;3:1235–42.

52. Wisenbaugh T, Skudicky D, Sareli P. Prediction of outcome after valve replacement for rheumatic mitral regurgitation in the era of chordal preservation. Circulation 1994;89:191–7.

53. Spinale FG, Ishihara K, Zile M, DeFryte G, Crawford FA, Carabello BA. Structural basis for changes in left ventricular function and geometry because of chronic mitral regurgitation and after correction of volume overload. J Thorac Cardiovasc Surg 1993 Dec;106(6):1147–57.

54. Mulieri LA, Leavitt BJ, Martin BJ, Haeberle JR, Alpert NR. Myocardial force-frequency defect in mitral regurgitation heart failure is reversed by forskolin. Circulation 1993 Dec;88(6):2700–4.

55. Sutton M, Plappert T, Spegel A, Raichlen J, Douglas P, Reichek N, Edmunds L. Early postoperative changes in left ventricular chamber size, architecture and function in aortic stenosis and aortic regurgitation and their relation to intraoperative changes in afterload: a prospective two-dimensional echocardiographic study. Circulation 1987 July;76(1):77–89.

56. Magid NM, Wallerson DC, Borer JS. Myofibrillar protein turnover in cardiac hypertrophy due to aortic regurgitation. Cardiology 1993;82(1):20–9.

57. Bonow RO, Lakatos E, Maron BJ, Epsstein SE. Serial long-term assessment of the natural history of asymptomatic patients with chronic aortic regurgitation and normal left ventricular systolic function. Circulation 1991 Oct;84(4): 1625–35.

58. Evangelista A, Tornos P, Sambola A, et al. Long-term vasodilator therapy in patients with severe aortic regurgitation. N Engl J Med 2005;353:1342–9.

59. Supino PG, Borer JS, Herrold EM, Hochreiter CA, Preibisz J, Schuleri K, Roman MJ, Kligfield P. Prognostic impact of systolic hypertension on asymptomatic patients with chronic severe aortic regurgitation and initially normal left ventricular performance at rest. Am J Cardiol 2005 Oct 1;96(7):964–70.

60. Scognamiglio R, Rahimtoola SH, Faoli G, et al. Nifedipine in asymptomatic patients with severe aortic regurgitation and normal left ventricular function. N Engl J Med 1994; 331:689–94.

61. Bonow RO, Carabello BA, Chatterjee K, de Leon AC, Faxon DP, Freed MD, Gaasch WH, Lytle BW, Nishimura RA, O'Gara PT, O'Rourke RA, Otto CM, Shah PM, Shanewise JS, Smith SC, Jacobs AK, Adams CD, Anderson JL, Antman EM, Fuster V, Halperin JL, Hiratzka LF, Hunt SA, Lytle BW, Nishimura R, Page RL, Riegel B. ACC/AHA 2006 Guidelines for the Management of Patients with Valvular Heart Disease: A Report of the American College of Cardiology/American Heart Association Task Force on Practice Guidelines (Writing Committee to Revise the 1998 Guidelines for the Management of Patients with Valvular Heart Disease). Am J Physiol Heart Circ Physiol 2001 Jan;280(1):J11–6.

62. Ishibashi Y, Rembert JC, Carabello BA, Nemoto S, Hamawaki M, Zile MR, Greenfield JC, Cooper G. Normal myocardial function in severe right ventricular volume overload hypertrophy. Am J Physiol Heart Circ Physiol 2001; 280(1):H11–6.

4

Physical Examination in Valvular Heart Disease

Carmel M. Halley and Brian P. Griffin

CONTENTS

INTRODUCTION

As the field of multimodality imaging continues to grow and build on established techniques in the assessment of valvular heart disease, it should be remembered that the cornerstone of clinical diagnosis is clinical history and physical examination. A systematic clinical examination both directs the clinician toward appropriate investigations based on clinical suspicion and aids with proper interpretation of results. The importance of clinical examination as a first step in the assessment of valvular disease is stressed by both the American Heart Association/American College Cardiology 2006 and the European Society of Cardiology 2007 guidelines *(1, 2)*. By integrating examination findings with imaging results, the clinician may improve diagnostic skills and more fully understand the underlying pathophysiology. Furthermore, employing a carefully methodical approach to physical examination provides information concerning the severity of the hemodynamic consequences of any given valvular lesion. With a clinical assessment of severity, the patient may be followed for disease progression with serial examinations. Finally, the value of time taken to perform a physical examination in establishing and continuing the rapport of the physician–patient relationship should not be underestimated. This chapter will first review a systematic approach to cardiac examination and then deal with specific valvular lesions individually.

SYSTEMATIC APPROACH

General Inspection

As with the physical examination in any disease state, the first step is general inspection of the patient, which can provide essential clues to etiology and functional status. An impression of the overall state of health and findings such as stature, nutritional status, respiratory status, and skin color may be quickly noted. Important systemic diseases and syndromes associated with valvular heart disease are outlined in Table 1.

From: *Contemporary Cardiology: Valvular Heart Disease*
Edited by: Andrew Wang, Thomas M. Bashore, DOI 10.1007/978-1-59745-411-7_4
© Humana Press, a part of Springer Science+Business Media, LLC 2009

Table 1
Physical Findings in Syndromes and Disease Associated With Valve Abnormalities

Syndrome/disease	Associated valvular abnormalities	Other physical findings	Etiology
Genetic disorders			
Marfan's syndrome	Mitral valve prolapse, aortic regurgitation	Increased height, kyphoscoliosis, high arched palate, pectus excavatum or carinatum	Autosomal dominant disorder of fibrillin gene
Down's syndrome	Endocardial cushion defects	Small head, hypertelorism, transverse palmar crease	Trisomy of chromosome 21
Turner's syndrome	Bicuspid aortic valve, pulmonic stenosis	Short stature, increased carrying angle of arms, shield-like chest with widely spaced nipples	Chromosomal disorder, 45XO
Noonan's syndrome	Pulmonic stenosis	Ptosis, low-set ears, hypertelorism, short stature	Normal genotype but Turner's-like phenotype affecting both sexes
Ehlers–Danlos syndrome	Aortic regurgitation, mitral valve prolapse	Hyperextensible joints, hyperelastic skin	Genetic disorder caused by a defect in collagen synthesis
William's syndrome	Supravalvular aortic stenosis	Elfin facies, low nasal bridge	Genetic disorder affecting chromosome 7
Systemic diseases			
Ankylosing spondylitis	Aortic regurgitation	Fixed kyphotic spine, hyperextended neck	HLA B27 association
Systemic lupus erythematosus	Libman–Sachs endocarditis and valvular regurgitation (especially if associated with anti-phospholipid syndrome)	Butterfly malar rash, vasculitis, polyarthropathy	Auto-immune condition characterized by antinuclear antibodies
Iatrogenic conditions			
Radiation heart disease	Mixed aortic valve disease, mitral and tricuspid regurgitation	Skin and sternal necrosis and scarring, recurrent pleural effusions	Calcification of valve leaflets and fibrous skeleton, typically present about 5–7 years after initial radiation
Drug-related valvular heart disease	Regurgitant lesions, carcinoid-like valvulopathy (ergotamine, pergolide)	Dependent on underlying condition, e.g., Parkinson's disease with pergolide	Ergotamine, methylsergide, anorexiant medications; pergolide

Cardiac cachexia as a result of severe heart failure manifests itself as severe weight loss and muscle wasting. Peripheral cyanosis (a bluish discoloration of exposed skin such as fingertips and earlobes) is a marker of poor peripheral perfusion. Central cyanosis (a bluish discoloration beneath the tongue due to high levels of deoxygenated hemoglobin) occurs due to intracardiac or intrapulmonary shunts. A Cheyne–Stokes pattern of breathing (periods of apnea alternating with periods of hyperpnea) can be present with low cardiac output. Peripheral stigmata of infective endocarditis include nail bed splinter hemorrhages, Osler's nodes (raised tender nodules on the pulps of fingers, toes, thenar and hypothenar eminences), and Janeway's lesions (nontender erythematous papular lesions on the palms and soles).

Pulse

The pulse should be examined with regard to rate, rhythm, volume, and character.

VOLUME

A large volume bounding pulse is typically associated with high output states such as aortic regurgitation. A small volume pulse is found with a low cardiac output and with hemodynamically significant aortic stenosis.

CHARACTER

The character or contour of the pulse is best appreciated by examining the carotid artery. With severe aortic stenosis, characteristic patterns of the pulse may include a delayed upstroke of the ascending limb (pulsus tardus), a small volume (pulsus parvus), and an anacrotic pulse (an interruption in the upstroke of the pulse due to the palpation of a prominent anacrotic notch). *In the elderly, due to changes in the peripheral vasculature, these classical contours may not be appreciable. Pulsus parvus may occur in any condition with low cardiac output (see Fig. 1).*

Pulsus bisferiens refers to a pulse pattern with two systolic peaks due to accentuated percussion and tidal waves and is present with severe aortic regurgitation and mixed aortic valve disease with predominant aortic regurgitation.

A dicrotic pulse with an accentuated upstroke and a second peak after the dicrotic notch in diastole is present in patients postaortic valve replacement with impaired left ventricular function.

Jugular Venous Pressure (JVP)

Examination of the right internal jugular venous pulse and pressure with the patient lying at an angle of 45° to the horizontal is preferable. *Features that help to differentiate the venous pulse from the carotid arterial waveform include the double undulation character (in sinus rhythm), the pattern of filling when obliterated (fills from above), the absence of pulsation on palpation, and the change in amplitude with respiration (normally decreases with inspiration).* Both the height and the character of the JVP should be assessed.

HEIGHT

The height of the JVP provides an estimate of right atrial pressure by adding 5 cm to the height of the venous impulse above the sternal angle with <9 cm water being normal. When lying at an angle of 45°, the base of the neck is in line with the sternal angle and the mid right atrium is approximately 5 cm below the sternal angle.

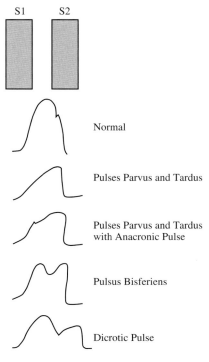

Fig. 1. The arterial pulse.

CHARACTER

The normal jugular venous pulse waveform consists of three positive and two negative waves; *a* wave represents atrial contraction just prior to left ventricular ejection and therefore just prior to the carotid artery upstroke, *c* wave represents closing of the tricuspid valve and onset of ventricular systole, *v* wave represents atrial filling with a closed tricuspid valve during ventricular systole and is coincident with the upstroke of the carotid upstroke, *x* descent represents atrial relaxation during ventricular systole, and the *y* descent is caused by the opening of the tricuspid valve and the rapid right ventricular filling from the right atrium (*see* Fig. 2).

A prominent *a* wave occurs in tricuspid stenosis, pulmonary stenosis with right ventricular hypertrophy, and pulmonary hypertension. *As patients with rheumatic tricuspid stenosis typically have other valvular lesions and are in atrial fibrillation, the finding of dominant a wave in this condition is rare and if auscultatory findings are suggestive of tricuspid stenosis, other etiologies such as right atrial myxoma obstructing the valve or carcinoid heart disease should be considered.*

A prominent *v* wave with a rapid *y* descent is classically found in tricuspid regurgitation, sometimes accompanied by systolic pulsatile motion of the earlobes in severe cases.

Precordial Motion

APICAL IMPULSE

The left ventricular apex moves toward the chest wall in early systole and the resulting apical impulse is normally brief, localized, and palpated with the examiner's fingertips in the fifth inter-

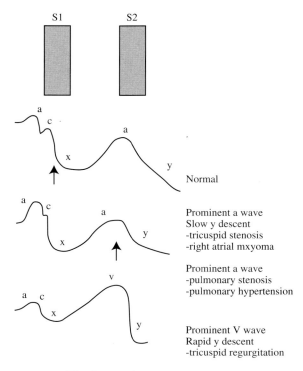

Fig. 2. Jugular venous pressure.

costal space at or just medial to the midclavicular line. The point of maximal impulse is not always the apical pulsation in disease states. For example, in severe mitral stenosis, the point of maximal impulse may be produced by the right ventricle (*see* Fig. 3).

A sustained apical impulse may result from left ventricular hypertrophy associated with aortic stenosis or with significant left ventricular dysfunction. The outward movement of the apex is prolonged and produces a diffuse heaving apical impulse that is in phase with the carotid arterial upstroke and persists during the downstroke. A palpable presystolic impulse or *a* wave may also be present; it correlates with an added fourth heart sound on auscultation.

A hyperdynamic apical impulse is felt as a thrusting impulse of increased amplitude and is found in conditions with increased stroke volume or volume overload such as mitral regurgitation or aortic regurgitation. A palpable early diastolic impulse that correlates with an added third heart sound may also be present.

A tapping (less sustained than normal) apical impulse is due to a palpable first heart sound and is associated with mitral stenosis and rarely tricuspid stenosis.

RIGHT VENTRICULAR IMPULSE

Palpation of the right ventricular impulse should be sought with the base of the hand, lifting the fingers off the chest. In health it is usually impalpable except in children or very thin adults and is a brief diastolic impulse over the left third and fourth intercostal spaces. With right ventricular hypertrophy or impairment, a prolonged left parasternal impulse may be palpable. *A similar left parasternal impulse may result from right ventricular displacement due to left atrial dilatation in severe mitral regurgitation.*

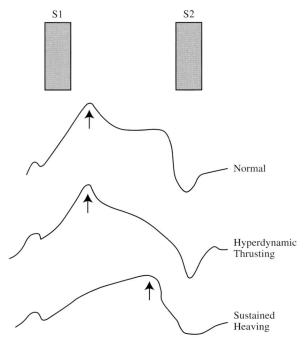

Fig. 3. The apical impulse.

THRILLS

The turbulent blood flow that produces a murmur on auscultation may be severe enough to be palpable. (A palpable murmur is classed as grade 4 or greater in intensity.) A thrill if present should be described by location (apical or basal) and by timing (systolic or diastolic). Apical thrills are palpated best with the patient in the left lateral decubitus position, while to palpate a basal thrill, the patient should be sitting up and leaning forward.

Heart Sounds

Auscultation requires a systematic approach starting with an understanding of and an ability to interpret the normal heart sounds. Abnormal heart sounds and murmurs may then be sought in specific precordial areas under varying conditions of patient position and respiration and with the addition of provocative maneuvers as needed to accentuate the findings.

FIRST HEART SOUND

The first heart sound (S1) has two components, related to mitral and tricuspid valve closure, but is usually heard as a single sound. It is best heard using the stethoscope diaphragm at the apex and the left sternal border. Its intensity is determined mainly by the mitral component. A loud S1 is audible in mitral stenosis with mobile leaflets as the valve leaflets are still separated at the end of diastole. A soft S1 may be heard in mitral stenosis when the valve leaflets are calcified and immobile. In severe aortic regurgitation, premature closure of the mitral valve due to high left ventricular filling pressure may lead to a soft S1. If the mitral valve leaflets fail to coapt fully due to prolapse or a flail segment, a soft S1 may result.

Splitting of the two components of S1 is usually due to conduction abnormalities such as right bundle branch block but may occur in Ebstein's anomaly due to delayed closure of the tricuspid valve.

Reverse splitting of the S1 may occur with severe mitral stenosis but is very difficult to appreciate clinically.

SECOND HEART SOUND

The second heart sound (S2) has two components related to the closure of the aortic (A2) and pulmonary (P2) valves with the intensity of the aortic component generally louder and heard best at the second right intercostal space. Because of lower pressure in the pulmonary circulation and a longer right ventricular ejection period compared to left ventricular ejection period, closure of the pulmonic valve occurs later than closure of the aortic. This delay is further increased during inspiration due to increased venous return, termed *physiological splitting* of the second heart sound. Therefore S2 should be examined with regard to intensity and pattern of splitting.

A loud A2 is associated with congenital aortic stenosis if the leaflets are mobile, while a soft component may occur in calcific aortic stenosis due to immobility of the leaflets. Analogously, a loud P2 is associated with pulmonary hypertension and a soft P2 is associated with pulmonic stenosis.

Persistent splitting refers to a pattern when the splitting of the two components is wider than normal and is present during both inspiration and expiration. This may occur due to a delay in P2 as in pulmonary stenosis and pulmonary hypertension. In pulmonary valve stenosis, the degree of expiratory splitting is related to the degree of the stenosis. It may also occur due to an earlier A2 such as in severe mitral regurgitation because of rapid left ventricular emptying.

Reversed or paradoxical splitting occurs when the sequence of the closure sounds is reversed with the pulmonic component first. This is audible on expiration, while a single second heart sound is heard on inspiration. When reversed splitting occurs in aortic stenosis in the absence of left bundle branch block, it indicates a hemodynamically significant lesion.

THIRD HEART SOUND

The third heart sound (S3) is a low-pitched, low-frequency early diastolic sound related to rapid early diastolic ventricular filling. It therefore correlates with the *y* descent in the jugular venous pressure and the *E* wave of transmitral inflow in Doppler echocardiography.

A left ventricular S3 (and left-sided fourth heart sound) is best heard with the bell of the stethoscope over the apex with the patient in the left lateral decubitus position. A physiological left ventricular S3 can be heard in children and adults under 40 years. A pathological left ventricular S3 is found with aortic regurgitation, mitral regurgitation, and left ventricular failure.

A right ventricular S3 (and right-sided fourth heart sound) is best heard at the left sternal border and on inspiration and is associated with tricuspid regurgitation and right ventricular failure.

FOURTH HEART SOUND

The fourth heart sound (S4) is a low-pitched, late diastolic sound related to ventricular filling during atrial systole and correlates with the *A* wave of transmitral inflow in Doppler echocardiography. An S4 is always pathological; a left-sided S4 is associated with aortic stenosis, while a right-sided S4 is found in pulmonary stenosis and pulmonary hypertension. With tachycardia, S3 and S4 if present may form a summation gallop.

ADDITIONAL SOUNDS

The opening snap is a pathological high-pitched early diastolic sound associated with mitral and tricuspid stenosis.

Systolic ejection clicks are early systolic high-pitched sounds best heard with the diaphragm of the stethoscope over the aortic or pulmonic areas in congenital aortic and pulmonic stenosis. With a bicuspid aortic valve, the click is followed by a short ejection systolic murmur with a normal S2. *In pulmonic stenosis, the systolic click can decrease or disappear with inspiration (the only right-sided auscultatory finding to do so).* Systolic ejection clicks can also be heard with a dilated aorta or a pulmonary artery.

Nonejection systolic clicks are heard most frequently in mitral valve prolapse and also in tricuspid valve prolapse and rarely in atrial septal defects and with atrial myxoma. With mitral valve prolapse, the click may be single or multiple and is a sharp, high-frequency sound heard best over the apex.

Heart Murmurs

Evaluation of a murmur involves the assessment of intensity (loudness) and pitch (frequency), configuration, area of greatest intensity, timing, and the effect of position, respiration, and dynamic maneuvers. The configuration of a murmur can be crescendo, decrescendo, crescendo–decrescendo, or plateau.

INNOCENT MURMURS

A murmur audible in the absence of any underlying cardiac structural abnormality is considered a functional or an innocent murmur, referred to as a Still's murmur in children (may be present in up to 60% of children). The mechanism is likely due to vibrations from within the aortic arch near the origins of the great vessels or from the right ventricular outflow tract and commonly relates to increased flow rate, e.g., pregnancy and anemia. The clinical ability to distinguish an innocent murmur from that which necessitates further investigation is invaluable. Innocent murmurs are usually soft and ejection systolic in nature and do not radiate widely. The hearts sounds are normal as is the apical impulse. These murmurs may change in intensity or disappear with different positions such as standing. Diastolic murmurs and most continuous murmurs are rarely, if ever, physiological. (Exceptions include the venous hum and the mammary soufflé associated with pregnancy where there are systolic and diastolic components to innocent murmurs.) The American Heart Association/American College Cardiology 2006 guidelines state that echocardiography is not recommended for asymptomatic patients with a soft midsystolic murmur identified as innocent or functional by an experienced observer.

CLASSIFICATION

Systolic murmurs are classed as holosystolic, midsystolic, early systolic, or mid–late systolic in timing. Diastolic murmurs are grouped into early, middiastolic, and presystolic murmurs.

Holosystolic murmurs occur when there is flow between two cardiac chambers with a wide pressure gradient in systole and so begin early in systole and persist until ventricular relaxation is complete, e.g., chronic mitral regurgitation.

Midsystolic murmurs are generated when blood is ejected across the semilunar valves and their configuration is crescendo–decrescendo following the pattern of increased and declining flow during ejection, e.g., aortic stenosis.

Early systolic murmurs begin with the first heart sound and end in midsystole and are heard in acute mitral regurgitation and in tricuspid regurgitation unassociated with pulmonary hypertension.

Late systolic murmurs are high pitched in quality and start after ejection and persist to S2. They occur with functional and ischemic mitral regurgitation and also in mitral valve prolapse in the presence or absence of midsystolic clicks.

Early diastolic murmurs begin at or immediately after S2 and have a decrescendo configuration, e.g., aortic regurgitation.

Middiastolic murmurs usually arise from increased flow or obstruction to flow across the mitral or tricuspid valves, so are typically heard with stenosis or severe regurgitation and also when there is increased flow across the tricuspid valve such as with an atrial septal defect.

Presystolic murmurs occur in late diastole coinciding with atrial contraction typically in mitral and tricuspid stenosis and/or more rarely as a result of functional stenosis due to an atrial myxoma.

DYNAMIC MANEUVERS

Dynamic maneuvers are very helpful in determining the etiology and significance of a murmur. Most right-sided murmurs increase with inspiration, while most left-sided murmurs increase with expiration. (Exceptions include the pulmonic ejection click associated with pulmonic stenosis, which decreases with inspiration; in the presence of right ventricular failure, the murmur of tricuspid regurgitation may not increase.)

With the Valsalva maneuver, most murmurs decrease in intensity and length; right-sided murmurs return to their baseline more quickly following release (within 2–3 beats). The two exceptions are the systolic murmurs associated with mitral valve prolapse and with hypertrophic cardiomyopathy, both of which increase in intensity. In mitral valve prolapse, the murmur also becomes longer with the Valsalva maneuver.

A similar pattern is associated with standing; most murmurs diminish with the exception of the murmurs of mitral valve prolapse (becomes louder and longer) and hypertrophic cardiomyopathy (becomes longer).

After a premature ventricular beat occurs, murmurs that are due to stenotic semilunar valves increase in intensity and murmurs due to atrioventricular valve regurgitation either do not change or become shorter (mitral valve prolapse).

After the administration of amyl nitrite, there is an initial hypotensive phase in which the murmurs of mitral regurgitation and of aortic regurgitation decrease, while those of aortic stenosis and hypertrophic cardiomyopathy increase. This is followed by a tachycardic phase in which the murmurs of mitral stenosis and right-sided lesions also increase.

Physical Examination in Pregnancy

Normal changes in the physical examination that occur in pregnancy reflect physiological changes. These decreased systemic vascular resistance and increased cardiac output with increased stroke volume and to a lesser degree, heart rate. Typical findings include a higher resting heart rate (average 10 beats/minute increase), a large volume bounding pulse, and a widened pulse pressure. The apical impulse is hyperkinetic, S1 is louder than normal, and in the later stages of pregnancy, S2 may appear widely split. A left ventricular S3 is present in most patients as is a soft midsystolic murmur at the upper left sternal border. A continuous murmur may occur due to venous hum or mammary soufflé. The mammary soufflé is typically heard in the later stages of pregnancy or the early puerperium and may be obliterated by applying firm pressure to the stethoscope or by having the patient stand. A cervical venous hum is best heard over the right supraclavicular fossa and is obliterated by digital pressure over the ipsilateral jugular vein or by turning the patient's head to the right.

In valvular lesions such as aortic stenosis and mitral stenosis, the intensity of the murmur is increased during pregnancy, while the murmurs of aortic and mitral regurgitation typically decrease in intensity.

PHYSICAL FINDINGS IN SPECIFIC VALVE LESIONS

Aortic Stenosis(AS)

GENERAL INSPECTION

The most common cause is calcific AS, which has no specific features on general inspection. AS in a younger patient is likely due to a bicuspid aortic valve. Rheumatic heart disease as a cause is increasingly rare. Supravalvular aortic stenosis may be occur as part of William's syndrome (elfin facies, small stature, multiple stenoses in the aorta, and peripheral arteries) or can be caused by lipid deposits in severe forms of familial hyperlipidemia (associated stigmata of lipid deposition such as corneal arcus, xanthelasma, and tendon xanthomata). Subvalvular AS is a congenital condition where a fibromuscular membrane is present in the left ventricular outflow tract beneath the aortic valve. It may coexist with other left-sided obstructive lesions as part of Shone's syndrome.

PULSE

There may be a plateau or an anacrotic pulse or a late peaking and small volume pulse, pulsus parvus, and tardus. The pulse pressure may be reduced. In supravalvular AS, the right brachial and carotid pulsations are of greater amplitude than the left-sided ones.

PALPATION

The apex beat is hyperdynamic and sustained due to associated left ventricular hypertrophy. A thrill in the aortic area indicates severe AS.

AUSCULTATION

S2 may become narrowly split or reversed due to delay in left ventricular ejection. The aortic component, A2, may become absent as the valve becomes more immobile (*see* Fig. 4).

In bicuspid AS, there may be an early systolic click as the relatively mobile cusps dome before coming to an abrupt halt.

The characteristic murmur is a harsh midsystolic murmur, maximal over the aortic area with radiation to the carotid arteries and sometimes to the apex. It is heard loudest with the patient upright and in full expiration. *In the elderly, the murmur can have a high-pitched musical quality, which radiates to the apex(Gallavardin phenomenon).*

In supravalvular AS, the murmur is typically best heard at the first or the second right intercostal space.

INDICATORS OF SEVERITY

Clinical signs that indicate severe AS include a plateau pulse, a palpable thrill in the aortic area, an increased duration of murmur with delayed peak, S4, paradoxical splitting of S2, absence of A2 component of S2, and signs of left heart failure. Physical findings such as timing of murmur, presence of a single second heart sound, and carotid upstroke delay have been found to correlate with stenosis as determined by peak jet velocity measured by Doppler echocardiography (*3*). The intensity of the

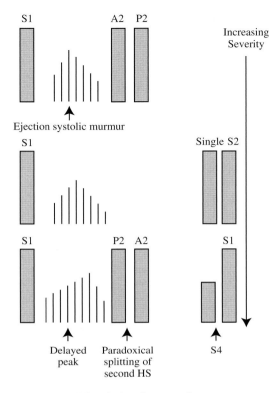

Fig. 4. Aortic stenosis.

murmur is not indicative of severity. If left ventricular systolic function is impaired, the intensity is reduced due to decreased stroke volume. No single exam finding has both high sensitivity and specificity for the presence of severe aortic stenosis; a combination of exam findings is therefore required to estimate severity.

AORTIC SCLEROSIS

Aortic sclerosis involves thickening of the valve leaflets without appreciable narrowing and is associated with a soft early peaking ejection systolic murmur localized to the aortic area with no radiation, normal heart sounds, and normal pulse character.

DYNAMIC LEFT VENTRICULAR OUTFLOW TRACT OBSTRUCTION DUE TO HYPERTROPHIC CARDIOMYOPATHY

Characteristic changes in the intensity of the murmur associated with dynamic maneuvers are helpful in differentiating the ejection systolic murmur associated with hypertrophic cardiomyopathy from that of AS. The murmur associated with hypertrophic cardiomyopathy increases with standing and decreases with sitting or squatting in contrast to the murmur of AS. The straining phase of the Valsalva maneuver increases the murmur of hypertrophic cardiomyopathy and decreases or does not change the murmur of AS. Other characteristic clinical examination findings in hypertrophic cardiomyopathy include a sharp initial upstroke of the carotid pulsation, a sustained left ventricular apical impulse that may have a bifid character, and a palpable S4.

Aortic Regurgitation (AR)

The characteristic findings are best considered in terms of onset of AR, i.e., whether acute or chronic. *In acute AR, there is sudden volume overload of a nondilated left ventricle, which results in rapid equalization of aortic and ventricular diastolic pressure. Therefore, the murmur is brief and soft with a normal pulse pressure. Elevated left ventricular end diastolic pressure leads to premature closure of the mitral valve and a soft or absent S2.*

GENERAL INSPECTION

Acute AR may be due to infective endocarditis or aortic dissection. Chronic AR may be considered as related to the valve itself (bicuspid aortic valve, rheumatic heart disease) or aortic root dilatation (Marfan's syndrome, ankylosing spondylitis, and aortitis associated with seronegative arthropathies), in which case the characteristic findings may be evident on inspection.

PULSE

The typical pulse is a collapsing, "water hammer" pulse with an associated wide pulse pressure. Many eponymous signs that relate to this characteristic pulse and pulse pressure have been described. These include Corrigan's sign (prominent carotid pulsations), De Musset's sign (nodding of the head with each heart beat), Quincke's sign (capillary pulsation in the nail bed), Mueller's sign (pulsation of the uvula with every heart beat), Duroziez's sign (systolic and diastolic murmurs in the femoral artery on gradual compression of the vessel), Hill's sign (increased blood pressure in the legs compared with the arms), and Traube's sign (double sound heard over femoral artery when the vessel is compressed distally). These signs have limited utility clinically.

PALPATION

In chronic AR, due to volume overload of the left ventricle, the apical impulse is displaced downward and laterally and is hyperkinetic.

AUSCULTATION

The characteristic murmur is a high-pitched decrescendo diastolic murmur starting immediately after S2 with a variable duration in diastole. It is maximal in intensity at the left sternal border or over the right second intercostal space and with the patient leaning forward in full expiration. An ejection systolic murmur over the aortic area and left sternal border may occur due to increased stroke volume (*see* Fig. 5).

The Austin Flint murmur is a low-pitched rumbling middiastolic murmur with a presystolic accentuation audible at the apex. The exact mechanism of this murmur is unknown but it is thought to relate to impaired opening of the anterior mitral valve leaflet due to impingement by the aortic regurgitant jet. *Unlike mitral stenosis, when the diastolic murmur is preceded by an opening snap and S1 is of increased intensity, in AR the Austin Flint murmur is preceded by an S3 and the S1 is normal or of decreased intensity. Also with the administration of amyl nitrite, the Austin Flint murmur decreases, whilst the murmur of mitral stenosis increases.*

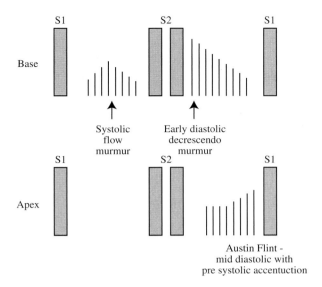

Fig. 5. Aortic regurgitation.

MIXED AORTIC AND MITRAL VALVE DISEASE

When both severe mitral stenosis and aortic regurgitation are present, the impact of aortic regurgitation on left ventricular volume is reduced as mitral stenosis restricts left ventricular filling. Therefore, the typical signs associated with a hyperdynamic circulation in isolated severe aortic regurgitation may be absent.

INDICATORS OF SEVERITY

More severe chronic aortic regurgitation is associated with a wide pulse pressure, the presence of S3, the presence of Austin Flint murmur and signs of left ventricular failure.

Mitral Regurgitation (MR)

PALPATION

With preserved left ventricular function, the apical impulse is displaced, diffuse, and hyperdynamic, reflecting volume overload of the left ventricle. With impaired left ventricular function, the apical impulse is displaced and sustained.

AUSCULTATION

S1 may be soft or absent, a left ventricular S3 may be present. The classical murmur is a blowing high-pitched, pan-systolic murmur heard maximally at the apex and in expiration with radiation to the apex. *The duration and intensity of murmur varies with loading conditions*(*see* Fig. 6).

INDICATORS OF SEVERITY

Findings suggestive of severe mitral regurgitation include low-volume pulse, S3, soft S1, signs of pulmonary hypertension, or left ventricular failure. The presence of an S3 has been correlated

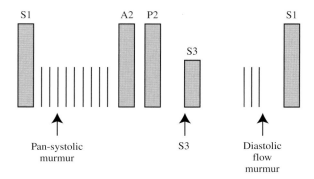

Fig. 6. Mitral regurgitation.

with severe mitral regurgitation (regurgitant fraction >40%) as measured quantitatively by Doppler echocardiography (*4*).

ACUTE MITRAL REGURGITATION

The causes of acute severe mitral regurgitation include papillary muscle rupture secondary to infarction or trauma, spontaneous chordal rupture, and infective endocarditis. *There is rapid equalization of pressure between the left ventricle and the normal-sized left atrium, so the systolic murmur may stop before S2.* The accompanying acute rise in pulmonary pressure leads to widely split S2 with a loud pulmonary component. *An added S4 often accompanies acute severe mitral regurgitation due to rigorous atrial contraction into a volume-loaded ventricle, whereas an added S3 is uncommon unlike in chronic mitral regurgitation.*

MITRAL VALVE PROLAPSE (MVP)

The classical finding is a midsystolic click generated by the tensing of the mitral apparatus as the leaflets prolapse, which is followed by a medium to high-pitched, late systolic murmur of varying duration heard maximally at the apex. Occasionally the murmur has a honking or musical quality due to high-frequency vibrations of the mitral apparatus (*see* Fig. 7).

The radiation of the regurgitant murmur typically depends on which leaflet is involved. Anterior leaflet prolapse is associated with a posteriorly directed jet and a murmur radiating to the axilla and the back. In posterior leaflet prolapse associated with an anterior regurgitant jet, the murmur can radiate to the base and the neck. *The murmur may progress to become holosystolic with progressive severity of mitral regurgitation.*

Dynamic maneuvers are used to alter the timing of the click during systole. With a decrease in preload (standing, Valsalva) or decrease in afterload (amyl nitrate administration), the click and murmur occur earlier in systole. Conversely, with an increase in LV volume (squatting) or increase in afterload (handgrip), the click and murmur occur later. Aortic or pulmonic clicks occur earlier in systole than in MVP and their timing is not affected by dynamic maneuvers.

MITRAL REGURGITATION IN HYPERTROPHIC CARDIOMYOPATHY

In obstructive hypertrophic cardiomyopathy, obstruction at the level of the left ventricular outflow precedes the onset of mitral regurgitation, which is typically a posterior jet due to systolic anterior motion of the mitral apparatus. Therefore, the typical harsh systolic murmur has an initial component

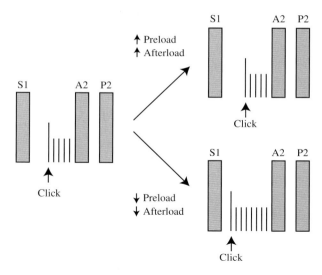

Fig. 7. Mitral valve prolapse.

related to left ventricular outflow obstruction and a later component related to mitral regurgitation. The mitral regurgitant component is heard best radiating to the axilla and the back and is mid to late systolic in timing.

Mitral Stenosis (MS)

GENERAL EXAMINATION

The mitral facies refers to the appearance of rosy coloration of the cheeks with a bluish tinge due to dilatation of the malar capillaries and it occurs in severe mitral stenosis with pulmonary hypertension. Peripheral cyanosis may also be present.

PULSE

Atrial fibrillation is common. A low-volume pulse may accompany a low cardiac output state.

JVP

The JVP may be normal; loss of *a* wave accompanies atrial fibrillation, while giant *a* waves may occur due to pulmonary hypertension.

PALPATION

The classical apical impulse is tapping in nature, which is due to a palpable S1. If pulmonary hypertension is present, a right ventricular heave and a palpable pulmonary component of S2 may be present.

AUSCULTATION

The typical murmur is low-pitched, rumbling middiastolic murmur heard best with the bell of the stethoscope over the apex with the patient in the left lateral decubitus position. An opening snap may precede the murmur if the valve leaflets are still mobile, which will also cause a loud S1 as the valve leaflets are wide apart at the onset of systole and close abruptly and loudly. *Presystolic accentuation of the murmur may occur whether or not the patient is in sinus rhythm.* The exact mechanism of this is unknown but may relate to the onset of mitral valve closure approximately 60 ms before S1. *The length of the murmur correlates with the severity of stenosis when the heart rate is normal or slow.* (Due to a shortening of diastole associated with tachycardia, the duration of the diastolic murmur is not an accurate indicator of severity.) *The intensity of the murmur, as it reflects flow across the valve, does not correlate with the severity of stenosis. The interval between A2 and the opening snap is inversely proportional to the severity of stenosis as a shorter interval will reflect higher left atrial pressure and a higher pressure gradient across the valve. An interval of 70 ms or less is consistent with severe mitral stenosis. However, this interval may not be useful in assessing the severity at fast heart rates and with other valvular lesions such as aortic stenosis, aortic regurgitation, and mitral regurgitation*(see Fig. 8).

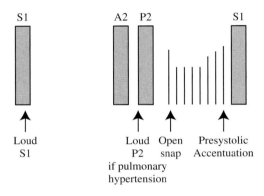

Fig. 8. Mitral stenosis.

INDICATORS OF SEVERITY

These include small pulse pressure, soft S1, short A2 opening snap interval, long diastolic murmur at normal or slow heart rate, and signs of pulmonary hypertension.

LEFT ATRIAL MYXOMA

If a left atrial myxoma prolapses across the mitral valve, the auscultatory findings may be similar to mitral stenosis with the tumor plop being similar to an opening snap and a middiastolic murmur due to obstruction. *However, the findings associated with left atrial myxoma if it is mobile will frequently vary with changes in position and from examination to examination.*

Tricuspid Regurgitation (TR)

Primary tricuspid regurgitation can occur due to rheumatic heart disease, carcinoid heart disease, Ebstein's anomaly, radiation heart disease and infective endocarditis, traumatic rupture of chordae, or right ventricular infarction. Secondary tricuspid regurgitation occurs due to pulmonary hypertension.

JVP

Characteristic findings are of *v* waves followed by a sharp *y* descent. *The liver is typically enlarged with a systolic pulsation, which correlates with systolic flow reversal in the hepatic veins as measured by pulsed wave Doppler echocardiography.* The JVP will be elevated if right ventricular failure has occurred.

PALPATION

If pulmonary hypertension is present, a palpable pulmonary component of S2 and a right ventricular heave may be detected.

AUSCULTATION

Typically the murmur of tricuspid regurgitation is pan-systolic murmur and heard maximally at the lower left sternal border on inspiration. *However, if right ventricular failure is present, the intensity of the murmur may not increase with inspiration.* It may be heard maximally near the apex due to right ventricular dilatation but will not radiate to the axilla. A right ventricular S3 can occur with severe tricuspid regurgitation.

Tricuspid Stenosis (TS)

Tricuspid stenosis is very rare and most often due to rheumatic heart disease; therefore, other valvular lesion such as mitral stenosis may also be present. Other causes include systemic lupus erythematosus, carcinoid heart disease, Fabry's disease, and Whipple's disease.

JVP

The JVP will be elevated with giant *a* waves and a slow *y* descent.

AUSCULTATION

The typical murmur is a low-pitched, middiastolic murmur with maximal intensity at left lower sternal border and during inspiration. *This increase in intensity in inspiration is known as Carvallo's sign and helps to distinguish tricuspid stenosis from mitral stenosis.* An opening snap may be present.

There may be presystolic pulsation of the liver due to forceful atrial contraction during atrial systole.

Pulmonary Regurgitation (PR)

Pulmonary regurgitation is caused by pulmonary hypertension, infective endocarditis, idiopathic dilatation of the pulmonary artery, postpulmonary valvotomy, or due to congenital absence of the pulmonary valve.

PALPATION

If pulmonary regurgitation is secondary to pulmonary hypertension, a right ventricular heave and a palpable pulmonary component of S2 may be present.

AUSCULTATION

The typical murmur known as the Graham-Steell murmur is a high-pitched, decrescendo early diastolic murmur of variable duration at the left sternal border, which is maximal with inspiration. *If pulmonary regurgitation is secondary to pulmonary hypertension, a loud pulmonary component of second heart sound and a systolic ejection murmur due to increased pulmonary blood flow may also be present. If pulmonary regurgitation is due to conditions where the pulmonary artery pressure is normal or low such as infective endocarditis or postvalvotomy, the murmur is of lower pitch. The onset of the murmur in these conditions is slightly delayed.*

Pulmonary Stenosis (PS)

As acquired pulmonary stenosis is extremely rare, almost all cases are congenital with fusion of the valve leaflets, resulting in a conical-shaped valve with restricted opening.

GENERAL INSPECTION

In cases of severe PS, peripheral cyanosis may be present. When present as part of a clinical syndrome such as Turner's syndrome or Noonan's, other phenotypical features may be present such as ptosis, low-set ears, hypertelorism, or short stature.

JVP

A giant *a* wave may occur due to increased resistance of right ventricular filling during atrial systole due to right ventricular hypertrophy. An elevated JVP indicates right ventricular failure.

PALPATION

Right ventricular hypertrophy results in a right ventricular heave; a thrill may be palpable over the pulmonic area.

AUSCULTATION

A pulmonic systolic click may be audible, which can decrease or disappear with inspiration in contrast to other right-sided lesions.

The typical murmur is a harsh ejection systolic murmur heard over the pulmonic area, which is maximal on inspiration. S2 is widely split and the degree of splitting correlates with the pressure gradient across the valve. The intensity of the pulmonary component of S2 is decreased due to a low pulmonary artery diastolic pressure. A right ventricular S4 may be present in severe PS.

SIGNS OF SEVERITY

These include late peaking murmur, presence of S4, and signs of right heart failure.

Prosthetic Heart Valves

Prosthetic heart sounds are of a higher frequency and are louder than normal heart sounds (5). The intensity of the opening and closing sounds of prosthetic heart valves varies according to the type and design of the valve and may consist of multiple clicks. *With a prosthesis in the aortic position, a diastolic murmur is abnormal. With a prosthesis in the mitral position, a pan-systolic murmur is abnormal.*

BALL–CAGE MECHANICAL VALVE

Both opening and closing clicks are loud. An ejection systolic murmur is normal in aortic and mitral positions.

BILEAFLET AND TILTING DISC MECHANICAL VALVES

A soft systolic ejection murmur can be normal when one of these prostheses is placed at the aortic position. The closing click is louder than the opening click.

BIOPROSTHETIC VALVE

A soft systolic ejection murmur is normal with aortic and mitral prostheses. A diastolic rumble can be heard in approximately 50% of mitral bioprostheses.

ROLE OF ECHOCARDIOGRAPHY

Echocardiography with spectral, color flow, and tissue Doppler provides important noninvasive information about valvular morphology, function, cardiac chamber size, ventricular function, and estimation of left ventricular filling pressure and pulmonary artery pressure.

When evaluating a patient with valvular heart disease, the role of echocardiography is to define the severity and cause of the lesion, assess hemodynamics and chamber size and function, detect coexisting abnormalities, and establish a baseline of severity. However, an echocardiogram is not required in all patients with a murmur. The American Heart Association/American College Cardiology 2006 guidelines for the management of valvular heart disease suggest that echocardiography is indicated in the assessment of asymptomatic patients with diastolic murmurs, continuous murmurs, holosystolic murmurs, murmurs that radiate to the back or the neck, late systolic murmurs with associated clicks, and loud midpeaking systolic murmurs. The guidelines also recommend echocardiography for patients with a murmur and symptoms or clinical evidence suggestive of underlying cardiac disease.

The guidelines suggest that echocardiography may be useful in asymptomatic patients with a murmur and an abnormal electrocardiogram or chest X-ray or in patients whose symptoms and/or signs are unlikely to be cardiac in origin but in whom a cardiac basis cannot be excluded by a standard evaluation.

REFERENCES

1. Bonow RO, Carabello BA, Kanu C, de Leon AC Jr., Faxon DP, Freed MD, et al. ACC/AHA 2006 guidelines for the management of patients with valvular heart disease: a report of the American College of Cardiology/American Heart Association Task Force on Practice Guidelines (writing committee to revise the 1998 Guidelines for the Management of Patients with Valvular Heart Disease): developed in collaboration with the Society of Cardiovascular Anesthesiologists: endorsed by the Society for Cardiovascular Angiography and Interventions and the Society of Thoracic Surgeons. Circulation 2006 Aug 1;114(5):e84–231.
2. Vahanian A, Baumgartner H, Bax J, Butchart E, Dion R, Filippatos G, et al. Guidelines on the management of valvular heart disease: the task force on the management of valvular heart disease of the European Society of Cardiology. Eur Heart J 2007 Jan;28(2):230–68.
3. Munt B, Legget ME, Kraft CD, Miyake-Hull CY, Fujioka M, Otto CM. Physical examination in valvular aortic stenosis: correlation with stenosis severity and prediction of clinical outcome. Am Heart J 1999 Feb;137(2):298–306.

4. Tribouilloy CM, Enriquez-Sarano M, Mohty D, Horn RA, Bailey KR, Seward JB, et al. Pathophysiologic determinants of third heart sounds: a prospective clinical and Doppler echocardiographic study. Am J Med 2001 Aug;111(2):96–102.
5. Vongpatanasin W, Hillis LD, Lange RA. Prosthetic heart valves. New Engl J Med 1996 Aug 8;335(6):407–16.

FURTHER READING

1. Braunwald E, Perloff JK. Physical Examination of the Heart and Circulation. In: Braunwald E (ed.) *Heart Disease* (7th ed.). Philadelphia: Elsevier Saunders 2005:77–106.
2. Chatterjee K. Physical Examination. In: Topol EJ (ed.) *Textbook of Cardiovascular Medicine* (3rd ed.). Philadelphia: Lippincott Williams & Wilkins 2007:193–226.
3. O'Rourke RA, Shaver JA, Silverman ME. The History, Physical Examination, and Cardiac Auscultation. In: Fuster V, Alexander RW, O'Rourke RA (eds.) *Hurst's The Heart* (10th ed.). New York: McGraw-Hill 2001:193–280.
4. Talley NJ, O'Connor S. The Cardiovascular System. In: Talley NJ, O'Connor S (eds.) *Clinical Examination, a Systematic Guide to Physical Diagnosis* (4th ed.). Oxford: Blackwell Science 2001, reprint 2003:26–29.

5 Clinical Hemodynamics in Valvular Heart Disease

Thomas M. Bashore

CONTENTS

INTRODUCTION

It is important to have a fundamental knowledge of normal hemodynamics and physiology to understand the effects of valvular heart disease on the physical examination, the noninvasive testing, the invasive evaluation, and the patient. This chapter is not meant to be comprehensive but to present the backdrop of the clinical hemodynamics that is particularly relevant to the evaluation of patients with valvular pathology. It is designed to set the stage for the more detailed hemodynamic considerations related to each of the specific valvular lesion covered in subsequent chapters.

From: *Contemporary Cardiology: Valvular Heart Disease*
Edited by: Andrew Wang, Thomas M. Bashore, DOI 10.1007/978-1-59745-411-7_5
© Humana Press, a part of Springer Science+Business Media, LLC 2009

THE CIRCULATORY SYSTEM

The heart consists of two major pumps connected in series. As shown in Fig. 1, the left ventricle (LV) pushes blood into a highly resistant system where there is elastic distension of the aorta and major branches during systole and elastic recoil of the walls of the large arteries in diastole. Histologically, the vessels become smaller, less elastic, and more muscular as the periphery is approached, and the muscular layer dominates at the arterioles. The frictional resistance is greatest in the small arteries and arterioles, and this is where the pressure drop is the greatest. In younger individuals, the wavefront travels slowly as the proximal elastic arteries and aorta dilate with systole. By the time the wavefront reaches more distal arteries, reflected waves return and boost the pulse pressure relative to the aortic pressure. As the blood advances across the arterioles and then across the capillaries to the venules, the pulsatile nature of the blood also diminishes. While it is estimated that the proximal arteries increase in size about 10% with each beat of the heart, these muscular arteries increase only about 2–3% *(1)*. Blood flow in the capillaries becomes quite slow since many capillaries arise from each arteriole. As blood returns to the heart first through the venules and then through the veins, the pressure gradually rises as the number of veins decreases in number, the thickness of the veins increases, the total cross-sectional area drops, and the velocity of blood flow in the veins increases.

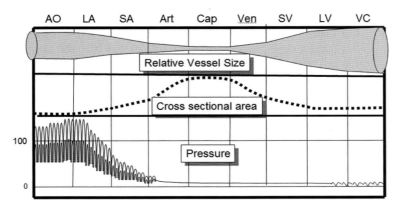

Fig. 1. Vascular flow and resistance. The relative vessel size and the area of distribution of the blood (cross-sectional area) are compared to the pressure generation observed. The pulsatile nature of the blood pressure is shown with the pulse pressure initially rising in the aorta (AO) and larger arteries (LA) then dampening and declining in the smaller arteries (SA) and arterioles (ART) and capillaries (CAP) as the vascular cross-sectional area increases. Flow in the venules (Ven), small veins (SV), large veins (LV), and vena cavae (VC) is generally nonpulsatile until the right atrial (RA) backpressure begins to be realized as the flow approaches the RA.

Blood then enters the right atrium (RA) and then the right ventricle (RV). The pulmonary bed subsequently receives the blood from the RV, but with the widespread capillary network, the pulmonary resistance is one-tenth to one-fifth of systemic resistance. On average, at any one time, two-thirds of the entire blood in the body is in the systemic veins and venules, with only 5% in the capillaries and about 11% in the aorta, arteries, and arterioles. In contrast, in the pulmonary bed, the blood volume is equally divided between the pulmonary arterial (3%), capillary (4%), and pulmonary venous vessels (5%) *(2)*. Figure 2 depicts the concept of the distribution of blood throughout the circulation. While the total blood volume is constant (an increase in one compartment must be accompanied by a decrease in another), the distribution of the circulating blood to all the different areas is determined by the output of the ventricles and the resistance of the arteriole vessels in each region of the body.

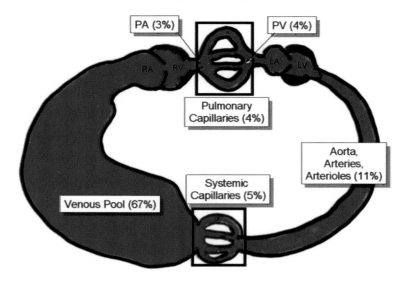

Fig. 2. Relative distribution of the blood volume within the vascular system.

NORMAL CARDIAC PRESSURE AND PRESSURE WAVEFORMS

The intracardiac pressure measurements are a reflection of not only the pressure generated within the cardiac chambers but also the pressures directly external to the heart and within the chest, including the pericardial and intrapleural pressures. This is evident by simply observing the normal pulmonary wedge tracings during respiration. The intracardiac pressures appear to swing wildly, when in fact if the intraplueral pressures are subtracted from the intracardiac recordings, there is little inherent actual pressure variation with respiration, with most of the variation due to differential filling of each of the chambers with respiration, the duration of phases in the cardiac cycle, and the compliance of the chambers.

Figure 3 schematically outlines the normal intracardiac pressure waveforms. The right atrial (RA) pressure waveforms are composed of three positive and two negative waveforms. When the atrium contracts, the chamber size is reduced in size and the RA pressure rises forming the "a" wave. Shortly afterward, ventricular contraction ensues, the tricuspid valve closes, and the RA is enlarged both by the tricuspid ring being pulled into the contracting RV and by the enlarging RA as it moves to its diastolic phase. This results in a decline in atrial pressure and an "x" descent. The positive "v" wave follows as the RA completes its diastole, the RV completes its systole, and blood returns filling the RA. The height of the "v" pressure wave is a function of both the amount of blood returning to the RA and the atrial compliance. The tricuspid valve then opens, and RA blood rushes into the right ventricle (RV), dropping the RA pressure during the rapid filling phase of the RV creating the "y" descent. The RA then slowly fills until atrial contraction occurs again, and the whole cycle repeats. The LA undergoes similar pressure changes with similar waveforms. However, because the LA must push into the less-compliant left ventricle (LV), the "a" wave is usually higher than in the RA and the "v" wave is similarly of greater magnitude due to the less-compliant and thicker-walled LA compared to the RA. In fact when the LA compliance is quite poor, giant "v" waves may occur (3). In practice, the LA pressure waveforms are assumed to be similar to the pulmonary capillary wedge waveforms, though this may not always be the case due to inherent vascular resistance in the pulmonary veins (4, 5). This difference may be particularly important when the PCW is used to track the mitral gradient; where a higher gradient may occur compared to the use of the LA pressure (6, 7). The PCW pressure is also noticeably delayed due to the longer inherent distance from the measurement to the transducer

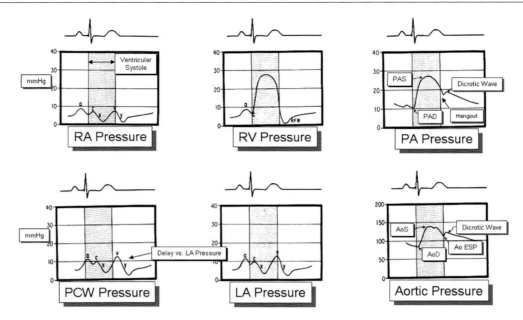

Fig. 3. Schematic representation of normal pressures and pressure waveforms. See text for definitions.

compared to direct LA pressure measurement. When tracking the gradient across the mitral valve, it becomes important to adjust for this delay.

The RV is designed as a volume pump and empties into the very compliant pulmonary circuit. RV contraction into this low-resistance system results in forward blood flow starting earlier than flow from the LV to the aorta and continuing even after the RV goes into early diastole (much like a "fall-away jump shot" in basketball). This results in the pulmonary valve closing later than the aortic valve, and this gap is referred to as "hangout." Hangout results in the familiar splitting of the second heart sound on auscultation. The increased pressure from the atrial kick creates an "a" wave just before ventricular systole. With RV systole, the RV pressure rises and the pulmonary valve opens. During RV systole, up to a 10 mmHg gradient across the RV outflow tract may be expected normally as blood is propelled forward. The RV then actively relaxes with a rapid filling wave in early diastole and then a passive filling wave in late diastole until the cycle repeats.

With inspiration the negative pleural pressures can be considered to literally draw blood from the systemic venous circulation and simultaneously pool blood in the pulmonary venous system. Inspiration therefore increases pulmonary artery blood flow and reduces blood flow to the LA. This results in an inspiratory increase in the PA pulse pressure with the increased RV stroke volume and a slight reduction in the aortic pulse pressure with the decreased LV filling. The opposite effects occur during expiration. These normal respiratory variations in stroke volume may be exaggerated by marked swings in intrapleural or intrapericardial pressures and result in the familiar *paradoxical pulse* seen in severe lung disease or pericardial tamponade where RV–LV interaction occurs and greatly reduces LV volumes with the expanding RV with inspiration.

THE IMPACT OF VASCULAR ELASTICITY AND PERIPHERAL RESISTANCE ON THE PRESSURE WAVEFORMS

Normally, despite the pulsatile nature of cardiac contraction, the flow at the capillary level continues during diastole. This is because the arteries expand during systole and store some of the ejected blood, then recoil releasing blood during diastole. From a teleological standpoint, this is good, as coronaries tend to fill in diastole. Aging results in a progressive decline in collagen and elastin in the arterial walls and an increase in vascular rigidity, though. Since the cardiac output is no longer stored in the elastic walls of the aging arterial system, the mean arterial pressure must rise to a new level so that the peripheral runoff will maintain the cardiac output.

Aging also results in arterial dilatation, and over time, while the conduit function of the arterial system is generally not affected, the cushioning function of the arterial tree is greatly affected *(8)*. The main control of the arterial pressure is not the stiffness of the large arteries, however, but the peripheral resistance and cardiac output. The pulse pressure (difference between the systolic and diastolic pressures) is a function of the stroke volume and arterial compliance. The pulse pressure is thus wider when the arterial compliance is poor.

Normally, the pressure wave travels faster than the blood itself and because of that, the arterial pressure contour becomes altered as the waveform travels down the arterial system, as shown in Fig. 4. When compared to central aortic pressure, the distal waveform becomes delayed, the incisura (the notch at aortic closure) disappears, the systolic pressure waveform elevates, and an early diastolic hump appears. These differences are much less evident in elderly patients compared to young patients with compliant aortic vasculature. The widening of the pulse pressure as the waveform approaches the periphery is primarily due to the reflected waves bouncing back from the periphery, though the tapering of the arteries, resonance, and the velocity of transmission all may contribute *(9)*. Since the pressure gradient across the aortic valve is often measured at cardiac catheterization by using the femoral arterial systolic pressure versus the LV systolic pressure, these changes are particularly relevant, especially in younger patients. An aortic pressure gradient using the LV and central aortic pressure may be quite different (larger) in a young patient than a gradient using similar sites for pressure measurement in the elderly.

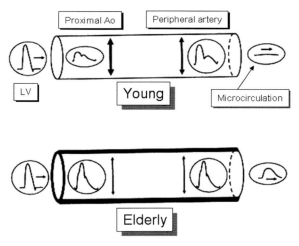

Fig. 4. Variability in the pulse pressure in the systemic circulation from the aorta to the peripheral arteries. The *upper sketch* reveals the changes from the central aorta to a peripheral artery such as the radial or the femoral artery in a young person with a compliant ascending aorta. The *lower sketch* reveals the same pressures in an elderly individual. The microcirculation is represented by the *oval* at the end of each tube. In the young, the wavefront travels slowly so that when it reflects back to the aorta, it boosts pressure in the diastole. In the elderly the wavefront travels quickly and reflects back in the systole. The cushioning effect in the young is also lost in the elderly and the microvessels are more likely to have pulsatile flow. Modified from O'Rourke MF and Hashimoto J *(8)*.

The central aortic waveform may be schematically depicted as shown in Fig. 5. In effect, the waveform is made up of a percussion wave (due to direct ejection of blood from the LV to the aorta), then tidal wave (felt to be a the forward wave in late systole merging with the reflected wave from primarily the upper extremity), and the dicrotic wave (an early diastolic wave resulting from the reflected wave primarily from the lower extremity). These waveforms have relevance in certain disease states where they are altered. For instance, in aortic stenosis there is loss of the percussion wave and an apparent "delay" in the upstroke. In hypertrophic cardiomyopathy, there is rapid early ejection of blood with about 60% before mitral–septal contact and about 40% after *(10)*. This results in the visualization of a time delay (notch) between the percussion wave and the tidal wave (spike and dome).

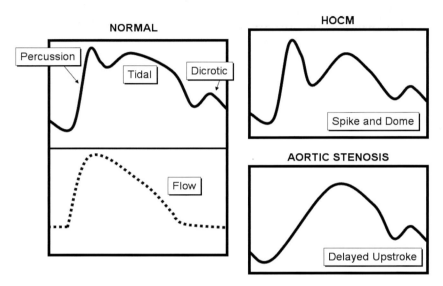

Fig. 5. Schematics of central aortic pressure and the effect of diseases on the observed waveforms. On *the left* is the normal central aortic pressure with the aortic flow depicted below it. The normal aortic waveform consists of a percussion wave that correlates with maximal forward flow, followed by a tidal wave that includes forward flow plus some reflected waveforms (mostly from the upper extremities). After aortic valve closure, there normally is a dicrotic wave primarily due to reflection from the lower extremities. On *the right* are simply exaggerated drawings of how knowledge of these components explains certain diseases. In HOCM (hypertrophic cardiomyopathy), there is rapid ejection and then reduced ejection. This often allows for separation between the percussion and tidal waves and the "spike and dome" configuration. In AS or aortic coarctation, there is loss of the percussion wave and an apparent delay in the upstroke is evident.

THE IMPACT OF A STENOSIS ON THE VASCULAR SYSTEM

In general, flow in the blood vessels is similar to flow in a pipe. As flow enters the pipe, it is considered freestream flow. Because of shear stresses between the flow and the inside surface of the pipe, the flow along the inner wall is slowed down. As flow traverses the pipe, the parallel flow profile now becomes parabolic (Fig. 6). This parabolic shape in the velocity profile is 90% evident about 10 diameters into the vessel *(11)*. Once the velocity profile is fully developed, it no longer changes. This is the point when the boundary layer thickness is midstream. At this point there is a balance between the viscous forces created by the wall and the inertial forces of the blood.

When there is a stenosis in the system, such as in a stenotic valve or coarctation or a vascular lesion, the flow is no longer laminar but distal to the stenosis. As noted in Fig. 6, the minimal area of stenosis

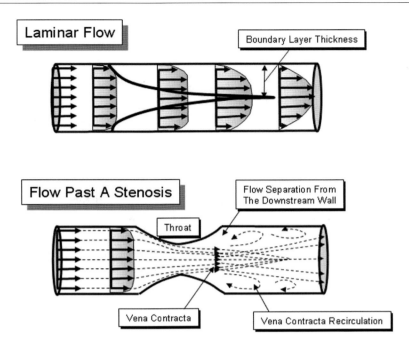

Fig. 6. Blood flow mechanics in the vascular system. Assuming a rigid straight tube, the *upper figure* depicts entrance flow and laminar flow. Freestream entry flow is altered due to the shear forces encountered between the blood and inner walls. Eventually the shape of the velocity curve is parabolic. Once a certain point is reached, the parabolic flow shape no longer changes. This is the point when there is a balance between the viscous forces by the wall and the inertial forces of the fluid and is referred to as the boundary layer thickness point and is about 10 diameters from the entry point. If a stenosis is present as depicted in the *lower figure*, flow is unable to hug the inner wall and the inertial forces continue to a point downstream (the vena contracta). Because the velocity is high, the pressure drops at this point. Eventually it will recover downstream (pressure recovery) when wall separation no longer occurs. The separation from the boundary wall results in turbulence and reversal of flow along the inner wall and vena contracta recirculation.

is referred to as the throat and this creates a flow disturbance. When the inertia forces that push the blood past this stenosis is substantial, the blood cannot turn the corner readily and flow continues past the stenosis separating from the wall. In this case, the effective minimal area is downstream from the stenosis and is referred to as the vena contracta. This inability to hug the inner walls downstream from the stenosis creates a separation of the boundary layer and a reversal of flow at the boundary surface. The flow then turns back on itself (vena contracta recirculation). As the velocity increases at the vena contracta, the pressure decreases in accordance with Bernoulli's principle. When the cross-sectional area of the vessel is restored downstream from the stenosis, the velocity recovers to what it was before the stenosis and the pressure recovers as well. This is known as pressure recovery.

Clinically, pressure recovery is primarily a concern in patients with moderate aortic stenosis (AS) and normal or only slightly dilated aortic roots (<30 mm) *(12)*. The aortic pressure at cardiac catheterization invariably will be measured after the pressure has recovered downstream. This aortic pressure will be higher than the pressure at the vena contracta, where flow velocities are maximal. The echo/Doppler utilizes these maximal flow velocities to define the aortic gradient. The result is that the gradient from the LV to this higher downstream aortic pressure will often be lower than the gradient measured by echo/Doppler from the LV to the vena contracta. This can create confusion regarding the severity of the AS as assessed by the aortic valve gradient.

SOME BASIC VENTRICULAR HEMODYNAMICS

The Pressure–Volume Relationship

Cardiac output is determined by myocardial contractility, preload, afterload, and heart rate. In 1914, Starling and colleagues showed the relationship between myocardial fiber length (sarcomere length) and developed force in diastole and systole. In the normal heart, peak force is attained at about a filling pressure of 12 mmHg or so *(13)*. This occurs when the sarcomere length is about 2.2 μm. In diastole the pressure remains low until a sharp rise occurs at the larger intracardiac volume. This increase in diastolic pressure is mostly due to noncontractile connective tissue, as the sarcomere limit is about 2.6 μm.

Clinically this concept can be translated to the intact heart by tying the pressure and volume together to form an LV pressure–volume loop (Fig. 7). The P–V loop is characterized by an isovolumic phase following mitral valve closure, an ejection phase between aortic valve opening and closure, an isovolumic relaxation phase between aortic closure and mitral opening, and early and late diastolic filling phases between mitral opening and closure. Acutely altering preload or afterload results in a series of P–V loops that represent each cardiac cycle during the intervention (Fig. 8). If done quickly, reflex

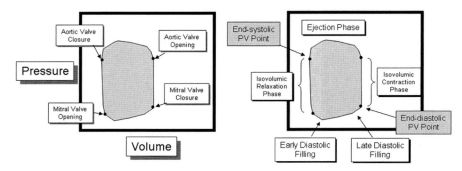

Fig. 7. The pressure–volume loop. The *left panel* defines the valvular opening and closure points. The *right panel* defines the phases of the P–V loop and points out the end-systolic and end-diastolic pressure–volume points.

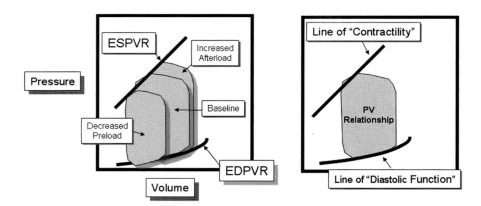

Fig. 8. Defining the end-systolic and end-diastolic pressure–volume relationships. In **Panel A**, acute changes in either preload or afterload result in a series of P–V curves being defined. *Lines* can be drawn connecting the end-systolic pressure–volume relationship (ESPVR) and the end-diastolic pressure–volume relationship (EDPVR) when these interventions are performed. The slope of the ESPVR can be used as a surrogate for the contractile function of the LV. The slope of the EDVPR can similarly be used to define diastolic function. **Panel B** then represents a single beat of the heart living within these lines of "contractile" function and "diastolic" function.

cathecholamines will not be activated. If each 10 ms point is located on each P–V loop, a linear line can be drawn among the loops, the slope of which defines *ventricular elastance*. This continues throughout the experiment and eventually a line of maximal elastance is reached (Emax). For practical purposes this slope can be defined as representing the contractile state of the ventricle and is relatively load independent *(14)*. This line is similar to the end-systolic pressure–volume points on each of the P–V loops (the ESPVR) *(15)* and can be used as a surrogate for "contractility." The linearity of this ESPVR does not tend to hold at lower ventricular volumes *(16)*.

A curvilinear line can also be drawn connecting the end-diastolic pressure–volume points from the series of P–V loops. This line can be used to represent diastolic function. The slope of the line at any given volume is often referred to as ventricular "stiffness." The inverse of stiffness is often referred to as "compliance." For the sake of simplicity, one may call this a line of "diastolic function."

Every beat of the heart, therefore, lives within this line of contractile function and diastolic performance. Clinically this concept can be used to understand how valvular disease affects this system and can be utilized to better understand the criteria used to decide when an intervention is necessary for the various valvular diseases states.

COUPLING THE HEART TO THE VENOUS SYSTEM (THE CLINICAL ISSUE OF PRELOAD)

Preload is generally defined by the amount of volume within the heart. It is a surrogate for sarcomere stretch at the onset of ventricular contraction. Measures include ventricular end-diastolic volumes, dimensions, and pressure. Recall that most of the blood volume is stored in the systemic venous system. Figure 9 relates the central venous pressure to the cardiac output. As the cardiac output increases, blood is pulled from the central venous system and the venous pressure falls. When the ventricular function curve is plotted against the venous pressure, note that it is necessary to flip the axes of the venous return curve (sometimes also called the vascular function curve). The heart operates at the intersection of the venous return curve and the cardiac function curve. At any one particular central venous pressure, one can therefore expect a certain cardiac output for that particular level of contractility. This

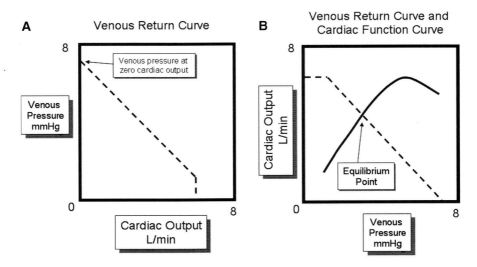

Fig. 9. The venous return curve (**Panel A**) and the cardiac function curve (**Panel B**). The heart operates at the equilibrium between the venous return curve and the cardiac function curve.

reinforces the concept that the circulatory system is a closed loop and the heart will pump what is delivered to it at the equilibrium point shown.

Adding or removing the blood volume from the venous pool creates parallel shifts in the venous return curve, assuming no change in contractility. Changes in venomotor tone do the same thing. Changes in arteriolar tone have somewhat much less effect on cardiac output (recall that the arterial system holds only about 11% of the blood volume in its entirety). The venous return curve in this situation moves counterclockwise down (arteriolar constriction) or clockwise up (arteriolar dilatation). A higher cardiac output is thus attainable when there is arteriolar vasodilation. And finally, increasing cardiac output pulls blood from the venous pool and the heart operates at a lower diastolic pressure with a lower venous pressure evident (Fig. 10).

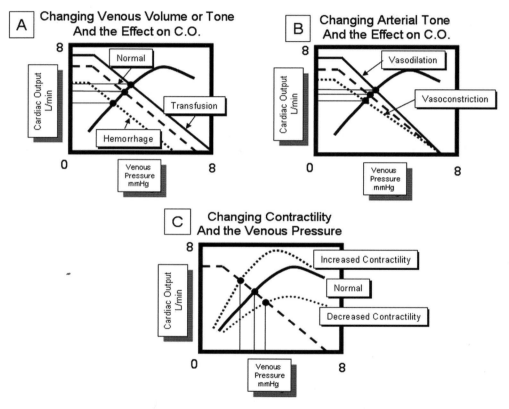

Fig. 10. The relationship between cardiac output and venous pressure when venous tone or volume is altered (**Panel A**), when arterial tone is altered (**Panel B**), or when contractility is changed (**Panel C**).

The situation described assumes only one pump (LV) and one circulation (systemic). The actual physiology involves the right ventricle and the pulmonary circuit as well. If RV function deteriorates and/or pulmonary resistance suddenly increases, systemic blood pressure, output, and pulmonary venous pressure may decline and right heart and systemic venous pressure rise. The LV is adequate to carry out the output function without the RV (witness patients with tricuspid atresia and Fontan physiology *(17)*), though the absence of an RV does have long-term impact on LV function. The sensitivity of the RV to afterload *(18)* and an understanding of its importance in maintaining adequate hemostasis continues to grow *(19, 20)*.

COUPLING THE HEART TO THE ARTERIAL SYSTEM
(THE CLINICAL ISSUE OF AFTERLOAD)

Afterload, in its strictest definition, is the force against which the heart contracts. Clinically, it is more difficult to define and two methods are often used. One method alludes to the peripheral resistance or the pulsatile input arterial impedance. The second utilizes the wall tension derived from the Law of Laplace. $\left(\text{Tension } \alpha \; \frac{\text{Pressure} \times \text{Radius}}{\text{Wall Thickness}}\right)$ Via the Law of Laplace, when the pressure within the heart increases or the heart becomes distended, then hypertrophy is stimulated to reduce wall tension. The Laplace relationship actually applies to infinitely thin walls but can be applied to the heart if corrected for wall thickness. It states that tension in the wall equals the transmural pressure across the wall times the radius of the chamber divided by wall thickness. If an increase in afterload is applied to the ventricles, then a compensatory increase in wall thickness will reduce wall stress. Pressure overload results in ventricular remodeling wherein sarcomeres are increased in parallel and wall thickness is markedly increased (concentric hypertrophy). Volume overload results in sarcomeres increasing in series (eccentric hypertrophy). This remodeling effort triggers an ever increasing sequence of events besides myocyte hypertrophy that includes altered interstitial matrix, fetal gene expression, altered calcium handling proteins, and eventually myocyte death *(21)*.

One of the definitions for afterload that is clinically applicable to the pressure–volume relationship is shown in Fig. 11 and couples the P–V loop to the arterial system. If one draws a line from the EDV point to the end-systolic pressure–volume point, the slope of that line is referred to as *arterial elastance (Ea)*.It is the ratio of the end-systolic pressure to the width of the P–V loop (stroke volume). An increase in the afterload increases the height of the P–V loop and decreases the width (increases the slope). A decrease in afterload decreases the height and increases the width of the P–V loop (decreases the slope). Variations in afterload and how they affect the P–V relationship are shown.

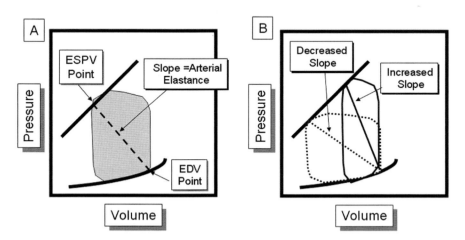

Fig. 11. The effect of afterload changes on the pressure–volume loop. **Panel A** reveals the pressure–volume relationship and the end-systolic and end-diastolic pressure–volume lines. The ESPV (end-systolic pressure–volume point on the P–V loop) and the EDV (end-diastolic volume) points are emphasized. The slope of a *line* drawn between these two points is referred to as arterial elastance and can be used as a measure of afterload in the intact heart. **Panel B** demonstrates the effects of an increase in afterload (increased slope) and a decrease in afterload (decreased slope) on the P–V loop.

THE MEASUREMENT OF THE EJECTION FRACTION

As mentioned, conceptually each beat of the heart can be thought of as living within the confines of a line of "contraction" and a line of "diastolic function." The area of the P–V loop is referred to as stroke work. The width of the P–V loop is the stroke volume (LV end-diastolic volume minus LV end-systolic volume). The ejection fraction (EF) is simply a mathematical term that relates the width of the P–V loop (the stroke volume) to the end-diastolic volume (Fig. 12A). The more narrow the loop at any particular LVEDV, the lower the EF. The wider the loop at any particular LVEDV, the higher the EF. Clinically the EF is used to define the contractile state of the LV, but clearly it is only a surrogate for the line of contractility. This becomes an even greater issue in valvular heart disease where the loading conditions vary widely.

Both the P–V relationship and the EF are profoundly affected by changes in afterload. As noted in Fig. 12B, an increase in afterload (Ea slope) without a change in the end-diastolic volume or contractility is appreciated clinically by an increase in systolic pressure and a narrowing of the

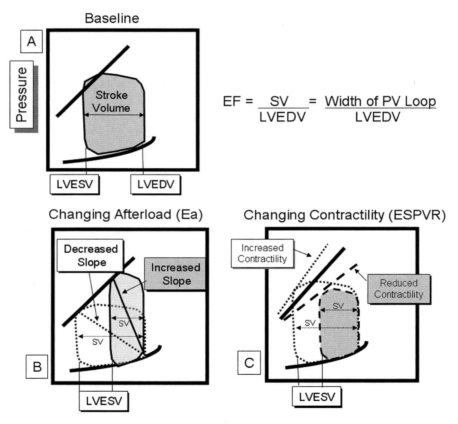

Fig. 12. The measurement of the ejection fraction (EF) and the effect of changing afterload and contractility. In **Panel A**, the EF is defined as the width of the P–V loop divided by the LV end-diastolic pressure (LVEDV). The stroke volume is the P–V loop width and is determined by simply subtracting the LV end-systolic volume (LVESV) from the LVEDV. **Panel B** examines the effect of changes in afterload, as defined by the slope of the arterial elastance (Ea). A reduced afterload and a reduced slope increase the width of the P–V loop, decrease the LVESV, and increase the EF. Increased afterload results in the opposite effect. **Panel C** examines the effects of changes in contractility as defined by the ESPVR on the EF. An increase in contractility increases the width of the P–V loop and reduces the LVESV. A reduction in contractility does just the opposite.

width of the P–V loop decreasing the measured EF. Conversely, a decrease in afterload (reduced Ea slope) with no change in contractility or end-diastolic volume widens the P–V loop and increases the measured EF.

EF is also quite sensitive to contractility changes. As shown in Fig. 12C, when there is an increase in contractility, the slope of the line of "contractility" increases, resulting in the widening of the P–V loop and a higher value for the EF. Conversely, when there is a loss of contractility, the slope of the line of contractility declines, and the EF similarly is reduced. Importantly, also observe that whenever slope of the line of contractility increases, the end-systolic volume must decrease and, conversely, when the slope of the line of contractility worsens, the end-systolic volume must increase. This additional relationship is what is used clinically to help determine the ventricular contractile function in the face of the afterload challenges presented by valvular heart disease.

USING THE EF AND END-SYSTOLIC VOLUMES FOR DECISION MAKING IN VALVULAR HEART DISEASE

Using the above concepts, the rationale for determining when there is loss of ventricular contractile function can be understood. The dependence of EF on loading conditions, particularly afterload, severely compromises its sole use in assessing patients with valvular heart disease.

The problem of using EF to define the contractile state in valvular disease is therefore complex and complicates decision making especially in patients with regurgitant valve disease. Mitral regurgitation (MR) results in an afterload decrease on the one hand and a preload increase on the other. The expected P–V loop in MR is shown in Fig. 13. The effect of MR on the P–V loop results in less isovolumic contraction, a much wider loop with a larger end-diastolic volume, and, due to the afterload reduction, a smaller end-systolic volume than normal. The P–V loop may be quite wide compared to normal, and the calculated EF is high due to what is commonly referred to clinically as the "pop-off" effect of the regurgitation. Since the decision to replace or repair a regurgitant mitral valve should be made when

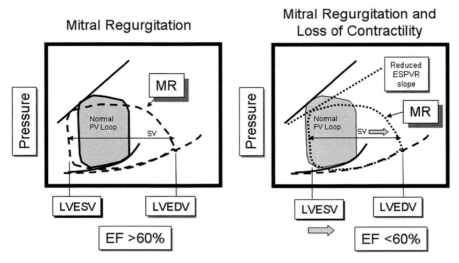

Fig. 13. Effect of MR on P–V loop and the ejection fraction (EF). In the *left panel*, the effect of MR on the P–V loop is noted. The reduced afterload results in the end-systolic volume (LVEDSV) decreasing and the increased preload results in the end-diastolic volume increasing. The width of the P–V loop is thus increased and the EF is high due to the high stroke volume (SV) relative to the LV end-diastolic volume (LVEDV). In the *right panel*, when the contractility slope declines, there is a reduction in the EF (decreased width of the P–V loop) and an increase in the LVESV.

there is any evidence for loss of contractile function, using the EF alone is clearly difficult. If the EF is abnormally high to begin with due to MR, there can be considerable loss of contractility before the EF falls into what would be considered an "abnormal" range (<55−60%). So when is contractility impaired?

The resolution to this dilemma is not only to observe what happens to the EF over time in patients with MR but also to monitor the end-systolic volume. As shown in Fig. 13, Right Panel B, when there is loss of contractility (a reduction in the end-systolic pressure–volume relationship slope), there is not only a reduction in the EF but also an increase in the end-systolic volume. These hemodynamic changes are the basis behind the valvular guidelines suggesting the use of the EF and the end-systolic dimensions as the keys to deciding on when to intervene in MR. The guidelines suggest that whenever the EF is <60% or whenever the echocardiographic LV end-systolic dimension is >4.0 cm, then that is enough to assume loss of LV contractility and enough to warrant mitral valve intervention (22) even in the absence of symptoms.

These similar concepts can be applied to the evaluation of patients with aortic regurgitation (AR). As opposed to MR patients, both afterload and preload are increased in patients with AR. When the EF is calculated using the higher LVEDV and the higher stroke volume (width of the P–V loop), the result is that the EF is often within the normal range or slightly increased (Fig. 14). With loss of contractility though, the EF falls and the end-systolic dimension increases. These concepts are the underpinning for the guideline recommendations to intervene whenever the EF falls below 55% or the end-systolic dimension by echo is >5.0 cm (22). The guidelines also suggest that an exceptionally large ventricle is also at risk, and echo dimensions >7.0 cm should be considered abnormal enough to warrant intervention.

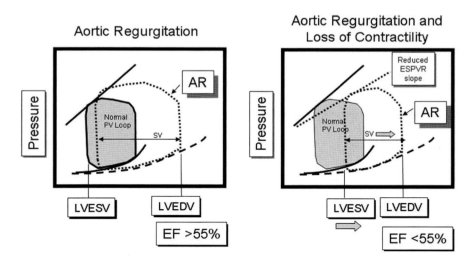

Fig. 14. Effect of aortic regurgitation on P–V loop. In the *left panel*, the pressure–volume (P–V) loop in aortic regurgitation (AR) is contrasted with that of the normal heart. AR presents both an afterload and a preload increase on the heart. The stroke volume (SV) is wide and the LV end-diastolic volume (LVEDV) is high. The resultant EF is normal or modestly elevated. In the *right panel*, when the contractile function declines, the EF drops and the LVESV increases as shown.

OTHER MEASURES OF SYSTOLIC PERFORMANCE

The EF is the only consistently derived clinical measure of ventricular systolic performance despite the problems in its use outlined above. There have been a myriad of other indices evaluated, though none have caught on in the routine clinical setting. At catheterization much effort has been made to utilize the first derivative of LV pressure (peak positive dP/dt), but it is preload, afterload, and heart rate sensitive *(23)*. It can be normalized by measuring the value at a specific isovolumic pressure, i.e., 40 mmHg. Its derivation requires high-fidelity catheter measurement and is not used clinically for decision making.

As described above, a series of P–V loops can be derived in man by acutely altering preload (usually IVC occlusion) or afterload *(24)*. This allows for the derivation of the end-systolic pressure–volume relationship or Emax [despite there being subtle differences between the two *(25)*]. The linear relationship between stroke work and the LV end-diastolic volume (preload-recruitable stroke work) *(26)* can also be determined, as it may be less sensitive to loading conditions than is the ESPVR. These types of studies are very difficult to perform, however, and require simultaneous pressure and volume measurements. This can be done with imaging modalities, such as contrast angiography or radionuclide angiography and high-fidelity catheters *(27)* or by the use of the conductance catheter and high-fidelity pressure *(28)*. The use of these parameters is confined to research applications due to the complexity and time-consuming nature of the procedures.

Most efforts outside of the measurement of EF seek to provide a noninvasive index of contractility. One index is the VCF or velocity of circumferential fiber shortening. It basically assumes that there is an endocardial or mid-wall hoop around the ventricle and the value defines the rate at which this hoop shortens. While it is preload insensitive, it is afterload sensitive *(29)*. It has been normalized for heart rate and end-systolic wall stress to address these issues (VCFc) *(30)*. The latter has also been criticized since endocardial fibers shorten more than epicardial and an end-systolic measure of wall stress ignores radial forces *(31)*.

Using echo/Doppler, the acceleration of blood into the aorta has also been proposed as an index of contractility, and while it is preload insensitive, it is also quite afterload sensitive *(32)*. The LV dP/dt from the continuous wave Doppler of the mitral regurgitation spectral signal has also been promoted but suffers from the same issues as the invasive dP/dt *(33)*.

The amount of myocardial annular or wall motion has been semiquantitated with the use of tissue Doppler methods to help understand contractile function. From an apical four-chamber view, the maximal isovolumic velocity (IVV) and its first derivative, isovolumic acceleration (IVA), have been compared favorably with invasive measurements *(34)*. Doppler tissue imaging (DTI) relies on altering receiver gains and frequency filters, so slow-moving targets, such as the myocardium or the valve annulus, can be interrogated for rate of motion. DTI can be displayed as a color map overlying the echocardiographic image as well. The rate of change across the myocardial wall, as well as the mitral annular motion, has correlated reasonably well with EF and other contractile indices *(35)*.

Since the DTI includes velocity and direction of wall motion changes, it can define displacement in millimeters. Strain rate imaging is therefore derived by simultaneously determining both velocity in two adjacent points in the myocardium and displacement between these two points. The strain rate is the instantaneous rate of change in the two velocities divided by the instantaneous distance between the two points *(35)*. Systolic strain rates are positive values and diastolic strain rates are negative values. An angle-independent method of measuring myocardial strain has also been proposed using speckle-tracking echo/Doppler imaging *(36)*, though there are little clinical data on its value at this time.

Finally, many years ago, systolic time intervals from phonocardiography were used to assess ventricular function *(37)*. These fell out of favor with the decline in phonocardiography, but a surrogate method is now available using echo/Doppler methods. As shown in Fig. 15, the index is derived by defining a total systolic time from mitral closure to mitral opening and subtracting the ejection time derived from the LV or the RV outflow jet. This difference is then divided by the ejection time to obtain a ratio called the myocardial performance index or Tei index *(38)*. A normal value is <40 ms, and the ratio worsens with ventricular dysfunction. Its time interval spans both systole and diastole. Systolic time intervals were ultimately found to be sensitive not only to contractility but also to both preload

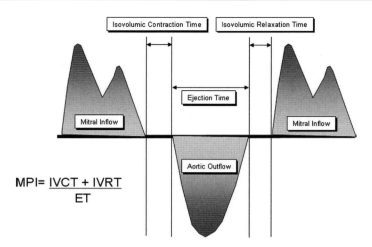

Fig. 15. The myocardial performance index. Using the mitral inflow Doppler pattern and the aortic ejection Doppler pattern, the intervals from mitral valve closure to aortic valve opening (isovolumic contraction time) and from aortic valve closure to mitral valve opening (isovolumic relaxation time) can be determined from the echo/Doppler. Often the total time from mitral closure to mitral opening is determined and the ejection time is subtracted from that to obtain the total IVCT + IVRT interval. This interval, representing both ejection and relaxation, is then divided by the ejection time (ET).

and afterload. It seems likely that this parameter will suffer a similar fate, though studies continue to suggest favorable correlations with invasive measures *(39)*.

DIASTOLIC FUNCTION AND DYSFUNCTION

Often symptoms in valvular heart disease are directly related to abnormalities in the diastolic properties of the ventricles. In simplest terms, diastole can be thought of as possessing an early active relaxation phase followed by a "passive" filling phase. At the start of diastole, myofilaments cease to generate contractile tension, and active relaxation occurs due to an energy-consuming process. Regional areas of dysfunction may affect this global process. Rapid diastolic filling is dependent upon the rate of ventricular relaxation, the elastic recoil of the ventricle, the gradient between the atrium and the ventricle, and the passive elastic properties of both the atrium and the ventricle *(23)*. "Passive" ventricular filling depends more on elastic recoil or restoring forces after systolic deformation of the ventricle, the strength of atrial contraction, and the diastolic stiffness of the ventricle. It includes a period of diastasis (slow ventricular filling) after the rapid filling of the ventricle and finally a filling boost from atrial systole. Diastolic performance is also affected by interactions due to the adjacent ventricle (LV–RV interaction), the pericardial constraint, and the duration of diastole.

Clinically, diastolic functional measurements have included evidence for *diastolic abnormalities* with no symptoms (often defined by abnormal filling patterns on echocardiography), true *diastolic dysfunction* that results in high filling pressures and symptoms of dyspnea particularly with exertion, and frank *diastolic heart failure*.

Active relaxation is affected by the systolic loading conditions (peak systolic pressure and end-systolic fiber stretch), coronary flow (referred to as the "erectile effect" early in diastole), and elastic recoil. The measurement of the active relaxation portion is difficult at best. The maximal rate of pressure decline (peak negative dP/dt) is one of the simplest measures, but it is only one point in time (about the time of aortic valve closure) and is very load and heart rate dependent. At times the isovolumic relaxation time (IVRT) has been used as a surrogate, but this is obviously affected by the end-systolic pressure as well as the atrial pressure at the cross-over when the ventricular pressure falls below the atrial pressure (mitral opening). The IVRT time would be expected to be lengthened when early active relaxation is impaired.

Probably the most effective measure, the time constant of isovolumic relaxation (often referred to as "tau") has been used invasively to describe this active relaxation interval. This is generally measured from the time of peak negative LV dP/dt (about the time of aortic valve closure) to the peak negative pressure in the LV in early LV filling. The measure is described as the time interval in milliseconds for LV pressure to decrease by about two-thirds of its initial value. The pressure decline over this brief period is fitted with various exponential mathematical decay curves (40, 41) to determine the precise interval. It is minimally affected by loading conditions. The interval increases with slower ventricular relaxation and decreases with more rapid relaxation.

The rate of rapid LV filling following the isovolumic relaxation time period has also been used as a measure of active diastolic relaxation. This can be accomplished by assessing the peak filling rate or time to peak filling rate from gated radionuclide studies (27) or by the use of echo/Doppler indices such as the peak transmitral velocity in early diastole (E wave) and tissue Doppler velocities (42). Late systolic loading may have a major impact on all these indices.

Figure 16 schematically outlines the mitral inflow velocities derived from echo/Doppler, and compares the normal and abnormal flow patterns with varying degrees of diastolic dysfunction. In healthy individuals, the mitral inflow wave (E wave) exceeds the atrial systolic wave (A wave). With age there

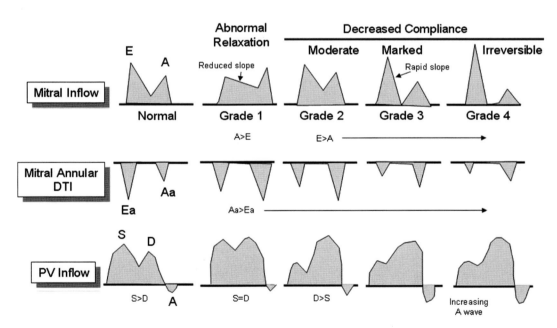

Fig. 16. Mitral valve velocities and definitions. The normal mitral Doppler inflow velocities are shown on the *left* along with normal mitral annular Doppler tissue imaging (DTI) and pulmonary vein (PV) flow. Abnormal relaxation patterns reflect slow initial filling with an increased A wave velocity compared to the early filling E wave. As the grade worsens, more and more filling occurs only in the early diastole and the associated high atrial pressure increases the velocity of the early E wave. The annulus moves more and more poorly as diastolic dysfunction ensues, though. The PV velocities reflect more filling during atrial diastole (ventricular systole – S wave) than in diastole or retrograde during atrial contraction. In abnormal relaxation, the S and D waves are similar. As compliance worsens, less filling occurs during atrial diastole and more during ventricular diastole (D > S) and more retrograde filling is noted with the atrial kick (increasing A wave). Modified from (83, p. 170).

is a loss of LV compliance and a progressive decrease in the E wave height with increase in the A wave height, so the E/A ratio may change from 2.0 or greater to less than 1.0. With increasing ventricular stiffness, it takes longer to fill the LV from the LA, and the E wave slope also declines (prolonged deceleration time). As compliance of the LV further decreases, the LV diastolic pressures rise more rapidly during diastole, and the flow from the LA to the LV completes earlier and earlier. This increases the E wave height, reduces its duration, and the flow velocity during atrial systole becomes diminished. These changes define greater grades of diastolic dysfunction. It is difficult to distinguish the moderate diastolic dysfunction pattern from the normal based on the mitral inflow pattern. By repeating the measure during Valsalva, LV filling and preload are reduced and the abnormal pattern may become evident. In restrictive cardiomyopathy, almost all filling of the LV occurs in early diastole and the E wave is very prominent and tapers off quickly. These patterns require the patient be in sinus rhythm and have a relatively normal heart rate, since high heart rates tend to merge the E and A waves.

The mitral annular DTI can be used in concert with the mitral inflow velocity waves to further characterize diastolic function. By itself, the mitral annular DTI is less subject to high heart rates or atrial fibrillation. In normal sinus rhythm, the two annular motions (Ea and Aa) parallel the transmitral flow. Normally Ea > Aa, just as in the mitral inflow pattern. The annular motion, though, is not volume dependent, and depression of mitral annular motion evident in pseudo-normal or in restrictive cardiomyopathy helps distinguish these conditions.

Of clinical importance, numerous studies have suggested a relationship between the rate of early LV filling (mitral inflow E) divided by the rate of mitral annular motion (Ea) and the pulmonary capillary wedge. In simple terms, if there is concordance between the LA pressure and how rapidly you are pulling blood into the LV in early diastole, the E/Ea ratio will be low. If there is discordance, it implies that the LV is not pulling blood from the LA, but rather there is high LA pressure pushing it forward, thus a high E/Ea ratio. Invasively, the LV end-diastolic pressure or the pulmonary capillary wedge pressure (PCWP) is used clinically to define LV diastolic dysfunction. The relationship between E/Ea ratio and pulmonary capillary wedge pressure is shown in a representative study in Fig. 17 *(43)*. There have been a variety of cutoffs of the E/Ea ratio used to define a high PCWP, ranging from 10 to 15. As

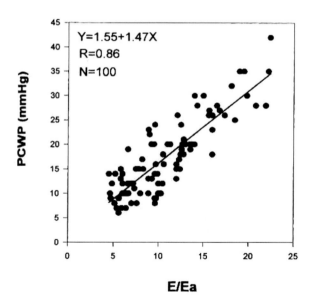

Fig. 17. The E/Ea ratio and the pulmonary capillary wedge (PCW) relationship. As noted, most patients with an E/Ea ratio <10 have a normal PCW pressure. Patients with PCW >20 usually have an E/Ea ratio >15. From Nagueh SF et al. *(84)*.

noted in the figure, the relationship is a continuous one. Many laboratories use a ratio of 15 to suggest an elevated PCWP.

The pulmonary vein (PV) velocity pattern also represents the rate of flow from the PV to the LA and provides some further diastolic functional information (Fig. 15). Recall that the atrium is in its diastole when the ventricle is in systole and during ventricular diastole, the atrium functions as a diastolic conduit to the LV until atrial systole. During atrial systole, there is a slight reversal of flow into the PV (PV "A" wave). During ventricular systole and atrial diastole, flow occurs into the LA (PV "S" wave) and this velocity is usually a little greater than in ventricular diastole (PV "D" wave). When there is decreased LV compliance, there is also decreased LA compliance and the LA pressures and volumes are elevated. There is progressively less flow through the pulmonary veins during atrial diastole, therefore, and the PV "S" wave becomes diminished. As diastolic dysfunction worsens, most of the PV flow occurs when both the atrium and the ventricle are in common diastole, and PV "D" wave dominates. Not only does the height of the PV "D" wave increase, but so does its duration. Because of the elevated LA pressure, atrial systole may also result in an increase in the retrograde PV "A" wave. Because of the difficulty in measuring PV velocities, its assessment is not always available in many laboratories.

Measurement of the "passive" filling characteristics of the diastolic ventricle is equally as difficult as the active-phase assessment. Recall from the P–V relationship that the line fitting the end-diastolic pressure–volume points is curvilinear (Fig. 8). If one takes the slope of the line at any particular point (dP/dV), the result is referred to as the ventricular diastolic elastance or stiffness at that point (Fig. 18). The reciprocal of that value at that point is called the compliance or distensibility. Note that as the volume in the chamber increases, the slope of this line eventually increases. A shift in this curve to the right implies increased chamber stiffness, while a shift to the left implies less stiffness (better compliance).

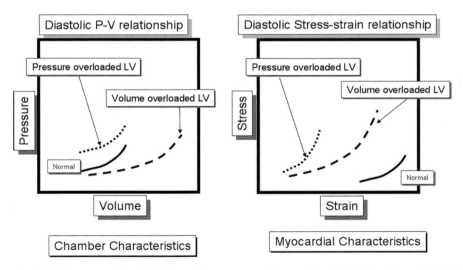

Fig. 18. Diastolic P–V loops on *the left*. Diastolic stress–strain on *the right*. The diastolic P–V relationship represents intact chamber dynamics. In the pressure-overloaded state, the sarcomeres are laid down on top of each other, the walls are thick, and the diastolic pressure is high at any given volume compared to normal. In the volume-overloaded state, the sarcomeres are laid down end-to-end, the volumes are very large, and the diastolic pressure may not be increased until the volumes get quite excessive. This clinical situation differs from the actual myocardial characteristics of the muscle itself shown on the *right* where the stress–strain relationships in both the pressure and volume overload states are abnormal.

To describe the characteristics of the ventricular myocardium rather than the intact chamber, measures of myocardial stiffness are also available. Valvular heart disease often results in myocardial hypertrophy to compensate for abnormal wall stress. This hypertrophy at times may be "inadequate" and lead to systolic dysfunction and myocardial apoptosis, which result in abnormal myocardial plasticity *(44)* and an increase in myocardial stiffness. Determining myocardial stiffness requires calculating myocardial stress–strain relationships. Stress is simply the force applied per area, and strain defines how much change in length has occurred between two points expressed as a percent of the initial length between the points. The diastolic stress–strain curves are curvilinear and they can be compared to the diastolic pressure–volume curves shown in Fig. 18 (Right panel).

Just as the slope of the diastolic P–V relationship is defined as "chamber stiffness," the slope of the myocardial stress–strain relationship is defined as "myocardial stiffness." Recent novel echocardiographic tissue Doppler *(45)* and MRI methods *(46, 47)* allow for the determination of strain rate images and provide further visual data regarding regional myocardial differences. The strain rate determined by these methods is defined as the instantaneous change in the velocities at these two points divided by the instantaneous distance between the points. Both systolic (a positive number) and diastolic (a negative number) strain rate can be determined for active contraction or relaxation (lengthening) between the two points. Color images of strain and strain rates can be overlapped with the echocardiographic images to localize regional areas of diastolic abnormalities within the myocardium. This method has been primarily applied to the identification of regional ischemic changes *(48)* and not valvular disease.

RV Function and Dysfunction Compared to the LV

RV function is important in patients with tricuspid and pulmonary valve disease and pulmonary hypertension. RV dysfunction may also occur in patients with left heart disease. RV–LV interaction is commonplace in patients with valvular heart disease. In utero the RV is the dominant ventricle, but soon after birth the pulmonary pressures fall, afterload to the RV is dramatically reduced, and the RV becomes a volume pump that is thin-walled and quite compliant. The RV has an inflow portion, an apical portion, and an outflow portion. Overall the shape is pyramidal or triangular with a crescentic appearing cross section. A variety of models have been utilized to define its geometry and none are very satisfactory *(49)*. The apical portion is heavily trabeculated compared to the LV, and that plus septal chordae to the tricuspid valve and the presence of the moderator band containing the right bundle help distinguish it from the LV. As opposed to the LV where coronary perfusion occurs mostly in early diastole, coronary flow occurs in both systole and diastole to the RV.

With RV contraction, the spiral muscles contract and then the free wall virtually milks the RV from the inferior wall and apex toward the RV outflow tract while pushing against the septum. The septum generally "belongs" to the LV but common fibers between the two chambers result in a wringing action on the RV when the LV contracts. RV dysfunction may occur from left heart disease due to the shared septum (Bernheim effect), just as LV function may be affected by RV dilatation (reversed Bernheim effect) pushing on the LV chamber. RV volume overload often results in bowing of the septum toward the LV. RV pressure overload results in flattening of the interventricular septum. RV dilatation is limited by the pericardial constraint and sudden increases in RV dilatation often result in marked increases in diastolic pressures with a rapid filling wave and "square root" sign, much as one might see in constrictive pericarditis. This is classically seen in acute RV infarction for instance.

The RV begins its ejection earlier than the LV and ends later. Because it normally pushes into a low-resistance pulmonary circuit, there is little isovolumic contraction time. Similarly ejection continues after peak RV systole, with fully 60% of ejection occurring after peak pressure *(50)*. A schematic RV P–V curve is shown in Fig. 19. The P–V loop of the RV resembles a triangle shape, reflecting the fact there is little isovolumic contraction period before the pulmonary valve opens and little isovolumic

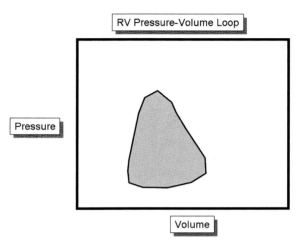

Fig. 19. Right ventricular pressure–volume loop. Note that the pulmonary valve opens and closes at a relatively low ventricular pressure, resulting in little isovolumic contraction or relaxation period.

relaxation period for the same reason. The RV end-diastolic volume is larger than the LV, therefore the EF tends to be less (normally >45%).

The thin-walled RV is felt to be at least twice as sensitive to an afterload increase as the LV *(51)*. This is particularly an issue in patients with pulmonary hypertension and those placed on mechanical ventilation. Respiration also has a more profound effect on the RV than the LV. With inspiration, the blood is literally pulled through the RV into the pulmonary circuit, resulting in an increase in RV preload and contractility and an increase in the stroke volume and ejection time. Patients on mechanical ventilation present a particular problem for the RV due to altered afterload, preload, and septal motion *(19)*. Chronic changes in RV volume overload are much better tolerated than acute changes as the pericardium and LV will accommodate the enlarging RV over time.

Measurement of RV systolic function is difficult at best. Timing intervals are dissimilar to the LV since the ejection period is longer. Due to "hangout," the pulmonary valve may even close after the tricuspid valve, allowing for no measurable isovolumic relaxation time. Cardiac MRI and computed tomography are emerging as superior to contrast angiography, echocardiography, and first-pass and gated blood pool radionuclide angiography for the determination of global RV function and volumes. CT and MRI provide information without the geometric assumptions by the use of Simpson's rule, and the RV volume, ejection fraction, wall thickness, and regional strain patterns can all be better assessed by MRI than by using echocardiographic methods *(46, 52, 53)*.

Echo/Doppler does provide a simple means of estimating peak RV systolic pressure (RVSP) by interrogating the tricuspid regurgitation (TR) velocity (RVSP = 4[TR velocity]^2 + estimated RA pressure). Visualization of the inferior vena cava (IVC) may also provide indirect information regarding RA pressure. If the IVC is normal in size and collapses with a brisk "sniff," then the RA pressure is assumed to be less than 10 mmHg. Mild elevation in the RA pressure (10–15 mmHg) is associated with normal or mildly dilated IVC and no change with sniffing, while an IVC > 2.5 mm and no change is associated with an RA pressure >15 mmHg. *(54)*. Many of the same parameters used to assess LV systolic and diastolic function have been applied to the RV with variable results including RV strain and tissue-imaging Doppler methods *(55)*. Three-dimensional echocardiography also holds promise in improving measurements of RV volume measurements *(56)*.

THE MEASUREMENT OF VALVULAR STENOSIS

Cardiac Catheterization Measurements of Valvular Stenosis Severity

The normal cardiac valves are thin and pliable, offering little resistance to blood flow. Valvular stenosis results in a progressive pressure gradient across the valve. In 1951, the Gorlins *(57, 58)* introduced an invasive method to calculate the effective orifice area of a stenotic valve using fundamental hydraulics. To calculate the stenotic valve area, the output in liters per minute that flows across the valve needs to be determined. For the mitral and tricuspid valves that means the flow in diastole only. For the aortic and pulmonary valves that means the flow in systole only. For the mitral and tricuspid valves, the flow in diastole can be determined by multiplying the diastolic filling period (DFP) (seconds per beat) and the heart rate (beats per minute) and dividing the result by the cardiac output (CO) (milliliters per minute). Similarly the flow in systole is determined by multiplying the systolic ejection period (SEP) and the heart rate and dividing the result by the measured cardiac output. The derived formula was thus the following:

$$\text{Area} = \frac{\text{Flow}}{\text{Constant} \times 44.3 \times \sqrt{\text{Mean gradient}}} \text{ or } \frac{\text{CO}/(\text{DFP or SEP})(\text{HR})}{\text{Constant} \times 44.3 \times \sqrt{\text{Mean gradient}}}$$

The SEP is the LV ejection time from the onset of the aortic pressure to the dicrotic notch, while the DFP is the time from the crossover of the LA (or PCWP) and LV pressure and the beginning of LV systole. For the aortic valve, the constant was determined to be 1.0, while the mitral valve constant (originally 0.7) was later changed to 0.85. The constants for pulmonary and tricuspid valve areas were never derived, but 1.0 is generally used. In children the cardiac index (CO/BSA) is used in place of the CO value.

The valve area measured by the Gorlin formula is subject to multiple potentials errors. Foremost is the difficulty in determining the cardiac output accurately. In low output states the effective orifice area is often calculated to be smaller than actual *(59)*. One study using TEE and simultaneous pressure measures suggested that at progressively higher outputs the Gorlin formula defined a larger valve area despite no anatomic change observed in the valve *(60)*. In addition, the pressure drop across the valve in aortic stenosis, for instance, is actually the difference in the LV pressure and the pressure at the vena contracta as measured by echo/Doppler. Pressure recovery may affect this difference as described earlier.

Since the pressure drop or gradient is a square root function, doubling the cardiac output results in a quadrupling of the gradient. The result of this is shown in Fig. 20. Note that at any particular cardiac output the valve gradient increases exponentially as the valve area drops from 1.0 cm^2 to 0.8 cm^2 to 0.6 cm^2, etc. This latter has particular relevance when an intervention such as valvuloplasty is performed. There is a marked difference in the valve gradient increasing the valve area from 0.6 to 0.8 cm^2 compared to increasing the valve area the same 0.2 cm^2 increment, from 0.8 to 1.0 cm^2, for instance. Using the incremental change in valve area to define success may be misleading as far as the impact the change makes on systolic loading of the ventricle.

When measuring gradients across each valve, it is important to obtain the pressure directly on either side of the valve. In most invasive laboratories, though, the PCWP substitutes for the LA pressure and the femoral artery pressure may substitute for the aortic pressure. With the advent of small-caliber, double-lumen pigtail catheters, the latter should be used less often. Whenever the PCWP or the femoral artery pressure is used, it is important to realign them as if they were obtained simultaneously. In addition, the differences in the femoral artery pressure and aortic pressure have been described earlier and can result in an underestimation of the aortic gradient. Similarly the differences in the PCWP and LA pressure may result in an overestimation of the mitral gradient.

An alternative to the Gorlin formula is the simplified Hakki method *(61)*. It is based on the fact that the SEP or the DFP times the heart rate produced a number about the same as the Gorlin formula

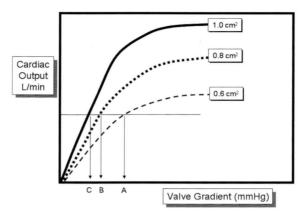

Fig. 20. Relationship of valve area, cardiac output, and valve gradient. There is a curvilinear relationship between the cardiac output and the valvular gradient at each defined valve area. When the valve area increases from 0.6 to 0.8 cm^2, the effect on the gradient is demonstrated by the change from A to B. When the valve area increases the same increment from 0.8 to 1.0 cm^2, there is much less change in the valve gradient.

constant. The formula is thus as follows:

$$\text{Valve area} = \frac{\text{Cardiac output (liters/minute)}}{\sqrt{\text{Mean pressure gradient}}}$$

As changes in diastolic time become greater than changes in systolic time at slower heart rates, it is a little unclear how heart rate affects this. Its simplicity is convenient, though, and since intervention in stenotic valve disease is primarily based on symptoms, clinically there is less importance on the derivation of a highly accurate estimated valve area.

Another alternative to the valve area measurement is the use of valve resistance. Its use has primarily been applied in aortic stenosis *(62)*. It is basically defined as the mean pressure gradient across the aortic valve divided by the cardiac output during the systolic ejection period. The formula and its correction factor are shown as follows:

$$\text{Aortic valve resistance} = \frac{\text{Mean gradient} \times (\text{SEP} \times \text{HR}) \times 1.33}{\text{Cardiac output (l/min)}}$$

The use of valvular resistance has primarily been in attempts at better definition of the valve stenosis in patients with low cardiac output, where the Gorlin formula tends to overestimate valvular stenosis severity *(63)*.

Noninvasive Measures of Valvular Stenosis Severity

Valvular stenosis can also be measured noninvasively. Most commonly this is done using echo/Doppler techniques, but both CT *(64, 65)* and MRI *(66, 67)* planimetry measures and estimated valve areas from flow characteristics continue to evolve. Besides actual planimetry *(68)*, one common concept is based on the law of conservation wherein the total amount of energy in a closed system must remain constant. The principal equation is a modified Bernoulli equation that states the pressure gradient is a function of the convective acceleration plus the flow acceleration plus the viscous friction. Its derivation is not important, as clinically what is used to measure the pressure gradient is:

$$\text{Pressure gradient} = 4 \times (\text{Maximal Doppler velocity})^2$$

Note that the peak instantaneous gradient is used and not the mean gradient, though the latter can be derived from the velocity envelope or time–velocity interval. Because the flow rate or the volume of blood passing any given point over time must be the same for all points in a closed circuit (Newton's second law of thermodynamics), a continuity equation has been derived that allows for the estimation of aortic valve area. Stated simply, the flow proximal to the aortic valve must be the same as the flow in the valve orifice (at the vena contracta). Using echo/Doppler the flow at any one point is a function of the area times the time–velocity interval. Thus, the equation is as follows:

$$\text{Area} \times \text{TVI below the valve} = \text{Area} \times \text{TVI at the vena contracta}$$

or

$$\text{Aortic valve area} = \frac{\text{Area} \times \text{TVI below the valve}}{\text{TVI at the vena contracta}}$$

The advantage of the continuity equation is that the valve area can be estimated even at low output or in the face of aortic regurgitation. The disadvantage is that minor errors in the measured radius below the valve are compounded due to the fact that area $= \pi r^2$. Thus any minor error in measuring the radius is squared.

The continuity equation can be applied to any valve, but it is most often used to define the severity of aortic stenosis. In mitral stenosis, the pressure halftime is preferred, though other methods such as planimetry with 3D echo (69) or the area determined from the proximal isovelocity surface area (70) have also been described. The pressure halftime method is derived from the mitral Doppler flow pattern in mitral stenosis. It is the time required for the maximal pressure gradient to be reduced in half. Recall from the modified Bernoulli equation that pressure is a function of velocity squared. The pressure halftime is therefore the time it takes for the peak velocity to decrease to a value of peak velocity divided by the $\sqrt{2}$. Since the $\sqrt{2}$ is about 1.4, the halftime is the time it takes for the peak velocity to reach a value of peak velocity/1.4, or stated another way, it is the time it takes for the peak velocity to reach about 0.7 times the peak velocity. The mitral valve area is then estimated by dividing the pressure halftime value in milliseconds by 220 (71).

THE MEASUREMENT OF VALVULAR REGURGITATION SEVERITY

Cardiac Catheterization Estimates of Regurgitation Severity

The measurement of the degree of valvular regurgitation is actually quite difficult by any modality. Angiography at cardiac catheterization utilizes a visual semiquantitative method (72) that describes the relative X-ray videodensity of contrast in the chamber being injected compared to the chamber receiving the regurgitant flow. In this system, 3+ regurgitation is present when there is equal contrast opacity in both chambers at some point during the injection. If the receiving chamber becomes denser than the chamber being injected, then it is considered 4+ regurgitation. If there is a minor amount of regurgitation, it is called 1+, with 2+ regurgitation defined somewhere between 1+ and 3+. This method is universally accepted, but obviously the amount of opacity of contrast seen is a function of not only the amount of regurgitation but also the size of the chamber, the rate of injection, and the presence of arrhythmia.

Angiographically a more quantitative method requires calculation of angiographic cardiac output and another measure of forward cardiac output (such as thermodilution or Fick output). Angiographic cardiac outputs require the measurement of angiographic volumes, something lost in most cardiac catheterization laboratories nowadays. If there is regurgitation, the angiographic stroke volume will be greater than the forward stroke volume. With this in mind, a representative regurgitant fraction can be calculated as follows:

$$\text{Regurgitant fraction} = \frac{\text{Angiographic SV} - \text{Forward SV}}{\text{Angiographic SV}}$$

An RF of 20% is considered mild, 20–40% moderate, 40–60% moderately severe, and >60% severe *(73)*.

Noninvasive Estimation of Regurgitant Severity

Radionuclide angiography can provide some estimate of regurgitant severity by comparing the stroke volume from the RV with the LV *(74)*. In this instance the presumption is that the RV stroke volume is similar to the forward SV, while the LV stroke volume is similar to the angiographic stroke volume. Knowing these data, a regurgitant fraction can be determined much as at cardiac catheterization.

Echo/Doppler is the most frequently used modality to estimate the severity of valvular regurgitation. There are many options. In the absence of valvular regurgitation, the stroke volume across all four valves should be equal. Using the time–velocity interval times the cross-sectional area, the stroke volume can be calculated for any valve. The amount of regurgitant volume in aortic regurgitation (AR), for instance, can then be determined by noting the difference between mitral flow and aortic flow. The regurgitant fraction in AR is thus the regurgitant volume/aortic flow × 100%. In AR, a regurgitant fraction >50% or a regurgitant volume >60 ml is considered severe regurgitation.

Regurgitant jets can be recorded using pulsed, continuous wave, or color flow Doppler imaging. Pulsed Doppler can map the regurgitant velocities, but the method requires multiple views and careful interrogation to find the maximal velocities. Pulsed Doppler of the descending aorta may also reveal diastolic flow reversal in significant AR.

Continuous wave Doppler is useful in both aortic and mitral regurgitation, though many criteria have been derived. In AR an estimate of severity can be derived from the contour of the regurgitant jet pressure halftime. As the LV diastolic pressure increases in AR, the instantaneous gradient between the aorta and the LV decreases. This results in a steeper slope to the AR Doppler velocity tracing. A pressure halftime of less than 250 ms or a slope >400 cm/sec^2 suggests severe aortic regurgitation. Many factors affect this besides the severity though, including aortic compliance, aortic pressure, LV size and compliance, and the acuity of the regurgitation *(75)*. Other methods to assess aortic regurgitation severity include the following: by color flow Doppler: (1) jet color height/left ventricular outflow tract height in parasternal long-axis view and (2) jet color area/left ventricular outflow tract area in short-axis view; by continuous Doppler: (3) regurgitant flow time–velocity integral (in centimeters) and (4) regurgitant flow time–velocity integral (in centimeters)/diastolic period (in milliseconds); by pulsed Doppler in thoracic and abdominal aorta: (5) time–velocity integral of diastolic reverse flow (in centimeters), (6) time–velocity integral of systolic anterograde flow/integral of diastolic reverse flow, (7) (time–velocity integral of diastolic reverse flow/diastolic period) × 100, and (8) diastolic reverse flow duration/diastolic period (as a percentage) *(76)*. In chronic AR, the indication for intervention requires significant AR to be present, but the effects on the LV chamber dimensions are generally more important than any of these *(22)*.

Continuous Doppler in concert with the continuity equation principle can also estimate an effective regurgitant orifice (ERO) *(77)*. As shown in Fig. 21, this is accomplished by determining the proximal isovelocity surface area (PISA). While this method is usually applied only to MR, its use has been applied to MS *(78, 79)* and AR *(80)*also. In this concept, as the blood accelerates to the regurgitant orifice, velocity aliasing occurs as a hemispheric shell forms just outside the regurgitant

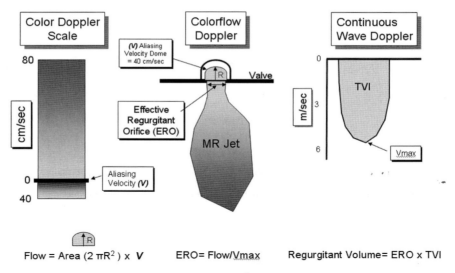

Flow = Area (2 πR²) x **V**   ERO= Flow/Vmax   Regurgitant Volume= ERO x TVI

Fig. 21. Determining the effective regurgitant orifice (ERO) and regurgitant volume using the proximal isoveloc-ity surface area (PISA) method. To *the left* is the color Doppler scale, in *the middle* the color flow Doppler image, and to *the right* the continuous wave Doppler through the orifice of the regurgitant valve. A velocity dome is found by shifting the color Doppler scale until the velocities exceed the Nyquist limit and start aliasing (40 cm/s here). Assuming a hemispheric shape, the flow of the dome at the orifice can be determined by multiplying the hemispheric area at the orifice times the aliasing velocity. If the flow at the orifice is known and the maximal velocity through the orifice is known, the area of the orifice (ERO) can be determined (*middle equation*). Deter-mining the total flow through the orifice (regurgitant volume) then requires only the area of the orifice times the time–velocity integral (TVI).

orifice. By adjusting the Nyquist limit, the size of this shell at the orifice can be maximized, allowing the hemispheric surface area to be measured. By the continuity equation, the rate of flow through the hemispheric shell at the orifice is the product of the hemispheric area ($2\pi R^2$) and the flow velocity, in this case the aliasing velocity (Va). Similar to the use of the continuity equation to determine the aortic valve area, if you know the velocity and area just prior to the orifice, it has to be the same as the velocity and the area at the orifice. The hemispheric dome area and flow velocity just before orifice is therefore equal to the effective orifice area (ERO) times the maximal flow velocity through the orifice (Vmax). The Vmax is obtained from the continuous wave Doppler.

Thus

Flow just outside the orifice = $2\pi r^2$ (Hemispheric dome area) × Aliasing velocity
Flow through the orifice = Effective orifice area × Vmax
Effective orifice area = Flow/Vmax

Once the effective orifice area is determined, the regurgitant volume can be determined by the following equation:

$$\text{Regurgitant volume} = \text{ERO} \times \text{TVI (Time–velocity interval)}$$

The routine use of proximal isovelocity surface area (PISA) is limited clinically primarily due to the difficulty in identifying the radius of the isovelocity shells and the center of the regurgitant orifice. There are other theoretic concerns as well, especially if an eccentric jet is present. In general, an ERO of >40 mm² is considered severe mitral regurgitation *(81)*. A similar method has been applied to the quantitation of tricuspid regurgitation *(82)*. Because of the difficulty in visualizing isovelocity shells that converge on the AR orifice, its use is limited in quantifying AR. Further discussions on the use of the various echo/Doppler methods can be found in the respective valvular disease chapters.

SUMMARY

A fundamental understanding of some of the basic hemodynamics allows for interpretation of the various diagnostic studies used to assess the severity of valvular lesions and provides the basis for the clinical decision making regarding when to intervene.

REFERENCES

1. Bourouyrie P, Laurent S, Benetos A. Opposing effects of aging on distal and proximal large arteries in hypertensives. J Hypertens 1992;10(Suppl 6):S87–91.
2. Levy M, Pappano A. Overview of the Circulation, Blood and Hemostasis. In: Levy M, Pappano A, editors. Philadelphia: Mosby Elsevier, 2007:1–11.
3. Fuchs RM, Heuser RR, Yin FC, Brinker JA. Limitations of pulmonary wedge V waves in diagnosing mitral regurgitation. Am J Cardiol 1982;49:849–54.
4. Mammana RB, Hiro S, Levitsky S, Thomas PA, Plachetka J. Inaccuracy of pulmonary capillary wedge pressure when compared to left atrial pressure in the early postsurgical period. J Thorac Cardiovasc Surg 1982;84:420–5.
5. Nishimura RA, Rihal CS, Tajik AJ, Holmes DR, Jr. Accurate measurement of the transmitral gradient in patients with mitral stenosis: a simultaneous catheterization and Doppler echocardiographic study. J Am Coll Cardiol 1994;24:152–8.
6. Mammana RB, Hiro S, Levitsky S, Thomas PA, Plachetka J. Inaccuracy of pulmonary capillary wedge pressure when compared to left atrial pressure in the early postsurgical period. J Thorac Cardiovasc Surg 1982;84:420–5.
7. Lappas D, Lell WA, Gabel JC, Civetta JM, Lowenstein E. Indirect measurement of left-atrial pressure in surgical patients – pulmonary-capillary wedge and pulmonary-artery diastolic pressures compared with left-atrial pressure. Anesthesiology 1973;38:394–7.
8. O'Rourke M, Hashimoto J. Mechanical factors in arterial aging. J Am Coll Cardiol 2007;50:1–13.
9. Remington JW, O'Brien LJ. Construction of aortic flow pulse from pressure pulse. Am J Physiol 1970;218:437–47.
10. Maron BJ, Gottdiener JS, Arce J, Rosing DR, Wesley YE, Epstein SE. Dynamic subaortic obstruction in hypertrophic cardiomyopathy: analysis by pulsed Doppler echocardiography. J Am Coll Cardiol 1985;6:1–18.
11. Kitajima H, Yognathan AP. Blood Flow – The Basics of the Discipline. In: Fogel MA, editor. Ventricular Function and Blood Flow in Congenital Heart Disease. Malden: Blackwell Futura Publishing, 2005:38–54.
12. Niederberger J, Schima H, Maurer G, Baumgartner H. Importance of pressure recovery for the assessment of aortic stenosis by Doppler ultrasound: role of aortic size, aortic valve area, and direction of the stenotic jet in vitro. Circulation 1996;94:1934–40.
13. Levy M, Pappano A. The Cardiac Pump. In: Levy M, Pappano A, editors. Cardiovascular Physiology. Philadelphia: Mosby Elsevier, 2007:55–79.
14. Suga H, Sagawa K, Shoukas AA. Load independence of the instantaneous pressure-volume ratio of the canine left ventricle and effects of epinephrine and heart rate on the ratio. Circ Res 1973;32:314–22.
15. Suga H. End-systolic pressure-volume relations. Circulation 1979;59:419–20.
16. Kass DA, Maughan WL. From 'Emax' to pressure-volume relations: a broader view. Circulation 1988;77:1203–12.
17. Kiani A, Shakibi JG. Fontan physiology. Circulation 1995;92:3148–50.
18. Senzaki H, Masutani S, Ishido H, et al. Cardiac rest and reserve function in patients with Fontan circulation. J Am Coll Cardiol 2006;47:2528–35.
19. Redington AN. Right ventricular function. Cardiol Clin 2002;20:341–9.
20. Redington AN. Physiopathology of right ventricular failure. Semin Thorac Cardiovasc Surg Pediatr Card Surg Annu 2006;9:3–10.
21. Sawyer DB, Colucci WS. Molecular and Cellular Events in Myocardial Hypertrophy and Failure. In: Colucci WS, Braunwald E, editors. Atlas of Heart Failure. Philadelphia: Blackwell Science, 1999:4.1–4.20.
22. Bonow RO, Carabello BA, Kanu C, et al. ACC/AHA 2006 guidelines for the management of patients with valvular heart disease: a report of the American College of Cardiology/American Heart Association Task Force on Practice Guidelines (writing committee to revise the 1998 Guidelines for the Management of Patients with Valvular Heart Disease): developed in collaboration with the Society of Cardiovascular Anesthesiologists: endorsed by the Society for Cardiovascular Angiography and Interventions and the Society of Thoracic Surgeons. Circulation 2006;114:e84–231.
23. Carroll JD, Hess OM. Assessment of Normal and Abnormal Cardiac Function. In: Zipes DP, Libby P, Bonow RO, Braunwald E, editors. Braunwald's Heart Disease. Philadelphia: Elsevier Saunders, 2005:491–507.

24. Kass DA, Midei M, Graves W, Brinker JA, Maughan WL. Use of a conductance (volume) catheter and transient inferior vena caval occlusion for rapid determination of pressure-volume relationships in man. Cathet Cardiovasc Diagn 1988;15:192–202.
25. Suga H, Nishiura N. Dissociation of end ejection from end systole of ventricle. Jpn Heart J 1981;22:117–25.
26. Feneley MP, Skelton TN, Kisslo KB, Davis JW, Bashore TM, Rankin JS. Comparison of preload recruitable stroke work, end-systolic pressure-volume and dP/dtmax-end-diastolic volume relations as indexes of left ventricular contractile performance in patients undergoing routine cardiac catheterization. J Am Coll Cardiol 1992;19: 1522–30.
27. Magorien DJ, Shaffer P, Bush CA, et al. Assessment of left ventricular pressure-volume relations using gated radionuclide angiography, echocardiography, and micromanometer pressure recordings. A new method for serial measurements of systolic and diastolic function in man. Circulation 1983;67:844–53.
28. Kass DA, Yamazaki T, Burkhoff D, Maughan WL, Sagawa K. Determination of left ventricular end-systolic pressure-volume relationships by the conductance (volume) catheter technique. Circulation 1986;73:586–95.
29. Mahler F, Ross J, Jr., O'Rourke RA, Covell JW. Effects of changes in preload, afterload and inotropic state on ejection and isovolumic phase measures of contractility in the conscious dog. Am J Cardiol 1975;35:626–34.
30. Colan SD, Borow KM, Neumann A. Left ventricular end-systolic wall stress-velocity of fiber shortening relation: a load-independent index of myocardial contractility. J Am Coll Cardiol 1984;4:715–24.
31. Gentles TL, Colan SD. Wall stress misrepresents afterload in children and young adults with abnormal left ventricular geometry. J Appl Physiol 2002;92:1053–7.
32. Peterson KL, Skloven D, Ludbrook P, Uther JB, Ross J, Jr. Comparison of isovolumic and ejection phase indices of myocardial performance in man. Circulation 1974;49:1088–101.
33. Chen C, Rodriguez L, Lethor JP, et al. Continuous wave Doppler echocardiography for noninvasive assessment of left ventricular dP/dt and relaxation time constant from mitral regurgitant spectra in patients. J Am Coll Cardiol 1994;23:970–6.
34. Vogel M, Schmidt MR, Kristiansen SB, et al. Validation of myocardial acceleration during isovolumic contraction as a novel noninvasive index of right ventricular contractility: comparison with ventricular pressure-volume relations in an animal model. Circulation 2002;105:1693–9.
35. Feigenbaum H, Armstrong WF, Ryan T. Evaluating Systolic and Diastolic Function. In: Feigenbaum H, Armstrong WF, Ryan T, editors. Feigenbaum's Echocardiography. Philadelphia: Lippincott Williams and Wilkins, 2005:138–79.
36. Amundsen BH, Helle-Valle T, Edvardsen T, et al. Noninvasive myocardial strain measurement by speckle tracking echocardiography: validation against sonomicrometry and tagged magnetic resonance imaging. J Am Coll Cardiol 2006;47:789–93.
37. Lewis RP, Rittgers SE, Froester WF, Boudoulas H. A critical review of the systolic time intervals. Circulation 1977;56:146–58.
38. Tei C, Nishimura RA, Seward JB, Tajik AJ. Noninvasive Doppler-derived myocardial performance index: correlation with simultaneous measurements of cardiac catheterization measurements. J Am Soc Echocardiogr 1997;10: 169–78.
39. Su HM, Lin TH, Voon WC, et al. Correlation of Tei index obtained from tissue Doppler echocardiography with invasive measurements of left ventricular performance. Echocardiography 2007;24:252–7.
40. Chung CS, Kovacs SJ. Physical determinants of left ventricular isovolumic pressure decline: model prediction with in vivo validation. Am J Physiol Heart Circ Physiol 2008;294:H1589–96.
41. Fogel MA. Ventricular Function – The Basics of the Discipline. In: Fogel MA, editor. Ventricular Function and Blood Flow in Congenital Heart Disease. Philadelphia: Blackwell Futura, 2005:11–37.
42. Isaaz K. Tissue Doppler imaging for the assessment of left ventricular systolic and diastolic functions. Curr Opin Cardiol 2002;17:431–42.
43. Nagueh SF, Mikati I, Kopelen HA, Middleton KJ, Quinones MA, Zoghbi WA. Doppler estimation of left ventricular filling pressure in sinus tachycardia. A new application of tissue Doppler imaging. Circulation 1998;98:1644–50.
44. Hill JA, Olson EN. Cardiac plasticity. N Engl J Med 2008;358:1370–80.
45. Baur LH. Strain and strain rate imaging: a promising tool for evaluation of ventricular function. Int J Cardiovasc Imaging 2008;24:493–4.
46. Qian Z, Lee WN, Konofagou EE, Metaxas DN, Axel L. Ultrasound myocardial elastography and registered 3D tagged MRI: quantitative strain comparison. Med Image Comput Comput Assist Interv Int Conf Med Image Comput Comput Assist Interv 2007;10:800–8.
47. Veress AI, Gullberg GT, Weiss JA. Measurement of strain in the left ventricle during diastole with cine-MRI and deformable image registration. J Biomech Eng 2005;127:1195–207.
48. Garra BS. Imaging and estimation of tissue elasticity by ultrasound. Ultrasound Q 2007;23:255–68.
49. Bashore TM. Right ventricular volumes are rarely right and are right hard to do. Catheter Cardiovasc Interv 2004;62: 52–5.

50. Redington AN, Gray HH, Hodson ME, Rigby ML, Oldershaw PJ. Characterisation of the normal right ventricular pressure-volume relation by biplane angiography and simultaneous micromanometer pressure measurements. Br Heart J 1988;59:23–30.

51. Slesnick TS, Chang AC. Right Ventricular Dysfunction in Congenital Heart Disease. In: Chang AC, Towbin JA, editors. Heart Failure in Children and Young Adults. Philadelphia: Saunders-Elsevier, 2006:218–47.

52. Catalano O, Antonaci S, Opasich C, et al. Intra-observer and interobserver reproducibility of right ventricle volumes, function and mass by cardiac magnetic resonance. J Cardiovasc Med (Hagerstown) 2007;8:807–14.

53. Catalano O, Antonaci S, Opasich C, et al. Intra-observer and interobserver reproducibility of right ventricle volumes, function and mass by cardiac magnetic resonance. J Cardiovasc Med (Hagerstown) 2007;8:807–14.

54. Feigenbaum H, Armstrong WF, Ryan T. Hemodynamics. In: Feigenbaum H, Armstrong WF, Ryan T, editors. Feigenbaum's Echocardiography. Philadelphia: Lippincott Williams and Wilkins, 2005:214–46.

55. Gondi S, Dokainish H. Right ventricular tissue Doppler and strain imaging: ready for clinical use? Echocardiography 2007;24:522–32.

56. Li J, Sanders SP. Three-dimensional echocardiography in congenital heart disease. Curr Opin Cardiol 1999;14:53–9.

57. Gorlin R, Gorlin SG. Hydraulic formula for calculation of the area of the stenotic mitral valve, other cardiac valves, and central circulatory shunts. I. Am Heart J 1951;41:1–29.

58. Gorlin WB, Gorlin R. A generalized formulation of the Gorlin formula for calculating the area of the stenotic mitral valve and other stenotic cardiac valves. J Am Coll Cardiol 1990;15:246–7.

59. Cannon JD, Jr., Zile MR, Crawford FA, Jr., Carabello BA. Aortic valve resistance as an adjunct to the Gorlin formula in assessing the severity of aortic stenosis in symptomatic patients. J Am Coll Cardiol 1992;20:1517–23.

60. Tardif JC, Rodrigues AG, Hardy JF, et al. Simultaneous determination of aortic valve area by the Gorlin formula and by transesophageal echocardiography under different transvalvular flow conditions. Evidence that anatomic aortic valve area does not change with variations in flow in aortic stenosis. J Am Coll Cardiol 1997;29:1296–302.

61. Hakki AH, Iskandrian AS, Bemis CE, et al. A simplified valve formula for the calculation of stenotic cardiac valve areas. Circulation 1981;63:1050–5.

62. Ford LE, Feldman T, Chiu YC, Carroll JD. Hemodynamic resistance as a measure of functional impairment in aortic valvular stenosis. Circ Res 1990;66:1–7.

63. Cannon JD, Jr, Zile MR, Crawford FA, Jr., Carabello BA. Aortic valve resistance as an adjunct to the Gorlin formula in assessing the severity of aortic stenosis in symptomatic patients. J Am Coll Cardiol 1992;20:1517–23.

64. Messika-Zeitoun D, Serfaty JM, Laissy JP, et al. Assessment of the mitral valve area in patients with mitral stenosis by multislice computed tomography. J Am Coll Cardiol 2006;48:411–3.

65. Piers LH, Dikkers R, Tio RA, et al. A comparison of echocardiographic and electron beam computed tomographic assessment of aortic valve area in patients with valvular aortic stenosis. Int J Cardiovasc Imaging 2007;23:781–8.

66. Friedrich M, Schulz-Menger J, Dietz R. Magnetic resonance to assess the aortic valve area in aortic stenosis. J Am Coll Cardiol 2004;43:2148–9.

67. Djavidani B, Debl K, Lenhart M, et al. Planimetry of mitral valve stenosis by magnetic resonance imaging. J Am Coll Cardiol 2005;45:2048–53.

68. Nichol PM, Gilbert BW, Kisslo JA. Two-dimensional echocardiographic assessment of mitral stenosis. Circulation 1977;55:120–8.

69. Chu JW, Levine RA, Chua S, et al. Assessing mitral valve area and orifice geometry in calcific mitral stenosis: a new solution by real-time three-dimensional echocardiography. J Am Soc Echocardiogr 2008;21:1006–9.

70. Uzun M, Baysan O, Genc C, Yokusoglu M, Karaeren H, Isik E. A nomogram for measurement of mitral valve area by proximal isovelocity surface area method. Echocardiography 2007;24:783–8.

71. Hatle L, Angelsen B, Tromsdal A. Noninvasive assessment of atrioventricular pressure half-time by Doppler ultrasound. Circulation 1979;60:1096–104.

72. Sandler H, Dodge HT, Hay RE, Rackley CE. Quantitation of valvular insufficiency in man by angiocardiography. Am Heart J 1963;65:501–13.

73. Harshaw CW, Grossman W, Munro AB, McLaurin LP. Reduced systemic vascular resistance as therapy for severe mitral regurgitation of valvular origin. Ann Intern Med 1975;83:312–6.

74. Daniel GB, Kerstetter KK, Sackman JE, Bright JM, Schmidt D. Quantitative assessment of surgically induced mitral regurgitation using radionuclide ventriculography and first pass radionuclide angiography. Vet Radiol Ultrasound 1998;39:459–69.

75. Chen M, Luo H, Miyamoto T, et al. Correlation of echo-Doppler aortic valve regurgitation index with angiographic aortic regurgitation severity. Am J Cardiol 2003;92:634–5.

76. Zarauza J, Ares M, Vilchez FG, et al. An integrated approach to the quantification of aortic regurgitation by Doppler echocardiography. Am Heart J 1998;136:1030–41.

77. Enriquez-Sarano M, Miller FA, Jr, Hayes SN, Bailey KR, Tajik AJ, Seward JB. Effective mitral regurgitant orifice area: clinical use and pitfalls of the proximal isovelocity surface area method. J Am Coll Cardiol 1995;25:703–9.

78. Rifkin RD, Harper K, Tighe D. Comparison of proximal isovelocity surface area method with pressure half-time and planimetry in evaluation of mitral stenosis. J Am Coll Cardiol 1995;26:458–65.
79. Uzun M, Baysan O, Erinc K, et al. A simple different method to use proximal isovelocity surface area (PISA) for measuring mitral valve area. Int J Cardiovasc Imaging 2005;21:633–40.
80. Tribouilloy CM, Enriquez-Sarano M, Fett SL, Bailey KR, Seward JB, Tajik AJ. Application of the proximal flow convergence method to calculate the effective regurgitant orifice area in aortic regurgitation. J Am Coll Cardiol 1998;32: 1032–9.
81. Enriquez-Sarano M, Avierinos JF, Messika-Zeitoun D, et al. Quantitative determinants of the outcome of asymptomatic mitral regurgitation. N Engl J Med 2005;352:875–83.
82. Tribouilloy CM, Enriquez-Sarano M, Capps MA, Bailey KR, Tajik AJ. Contrasting effect of similar effective regurgitant orifice area in mitral and tricuspid regurgitation: a quantitative Doppler echocardiographic study. J Am Soc Echocardiogr 2002;15:958–65.
83. Feigenbaum H, Armstrong WF, Ryan T. Evaluation of Systolic and Diastolic Function of the Left Ventricle. In: Feigenbaum H, Armstrong WF, Ryan T, editors. Feigenbaum's Echocardiography. Philadelphia: Lippincott Williams and Wilkins, 2005:138–80.
84. Nagueh SF, Middleton KJ, Kopelen HA, Zoghbi WA, Quinones MA. Doppler tissue imaging: a noninvasive technique for evaluation of left ventricular relaxation and estimation of filling pressures. J Am Coll Cardiol 1997;30:1527–33.

6 Echocardiographic Assessment of Native Valve Function

Gail E. Peterson and Lisa Forbess

CONTENTS

INTRODUCTION

Echocardiography with Doppler imaging is an essential tool in the evaluation and management of valvular heart disease. With the use of appropriate echocardiographic techniques, one can assess the etiology, severity, hemodynamic consequences, and ventricular response to valvular abnormalities. Echocardiography provides prognostic information and plays an important role in therapeutic decision making. It remains the principal modality for the diagnosis and follow-up of patients with valvular heart disease.

ECHOCARDIOGRAPHIC MODALITIES FOR THE DIAGNOSIS AND EVALUATION OF VALVULAR DISEASE

Two-Dimensional Echocardiography

A comprehensive echocardiographic evaluation of valvular disease includes two-dimensional (2-D) imaging and color-flow, pulsed, and continuous wave Doppler. Two-dimensional echocardiography can identify abnormalities in the valves and supporting structures, thus providing a mechanism for the regurgitation and/or stenosis. Measurement of chamber dimensions and ventricular function allows for an assessment of the impact of the pressure or the volume load on the heart. For example, chronic severe valvular regurgitation is almost always associated with chamber enlargement and hypertrophy; the absence of chamber remodeling in the presence of chronic regurgitation implies milder degrees of regurgitation.

From: *Contemporary Cardiology: Valvular Heart Disease*
Edited by: Andrew Wang, Thomas M. Bashore, DOI 10.1007/978-1-59745-411-7_6
© Humana Press, a part of Springer Science+Business Media, LLC 2009

Role of Color-Flow Doppler

Color-flow Doppler is an indispensable tool for the evaluation of valvular regurgitation, allowing for rapid screening for the presence and direction of the regurgitant jet and providing both qualitative and quantitative data. The regurgitant color-flow jet has three components: the flow convergence region, the vena contracta through the regurgitant orifice, and the downstream expansion of the jet in the receiving chamber (Fig. 1). Each component provides complimentary information on regurgitation severity. Knowledge of the different methods of color-flow imaging and their pitfalls is essential for accurate interpretation of valvular regurgitation.

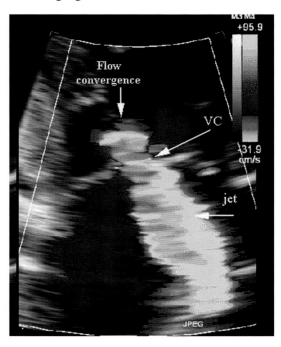

Fig. 1. Color flow of a mitral regurgitant jet showing the three components of the regurgitant jet: flow convergence, vena contracta (VC), and the downstream expansion of the jet into the left atrium.

Downstream Jet Expansion

Multiple imaging planes should be integrated during the assessment of valvular regurgitation using color-flow Doppler. The jet size or the extent of the regurgitant jet in the receiving chamber (defined by the length and width of the jet and most importantly visual assessment of the size of the regurgitant orifice) allows for quick differentiation between mild and more significant regurgitation but is less reliable for more specific quantification. The jet area is often indexed to the area of the receiving chamber, and in the case of aortic and pulmonic regurgitation, the ratio of the jet height to outflow area can provide further quantitative information (Fig. 2). However, sole reliance on color-flow Doppler can be misleading. The jet size can be affected by numerous technical, physiological, and anatomic factors *(1)*. Instrument settings such as changes in gain, pulsed repetition frequency (PRF), color scale, frequency, and wall filters can affect the size of the regurgitant jet. To optimize frame rates, the width and depth of the color Doppler sector should be minimized. An aliasing velocity of 50–60 cm/s is optimal *(2)*, since lower velocities will make the jet area larger. Color gain should be set such that random color speckle is eliminated from nonmoving areas; gain set too high leads to the appearance of larger jets. Color-flow area can also be directly influenced by the driving pressure across the valve.

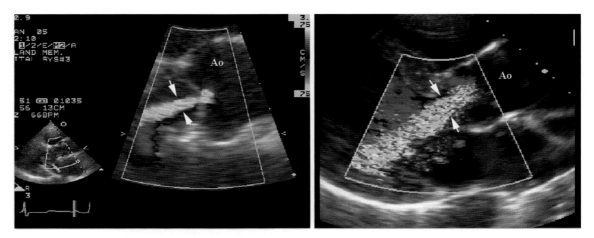

Fig. 2. Color-flow images of aortic regurgitation in the parasternal long-axis view. In the image on the left, a narrow jet is evident, comprising less than 30% of the left ventricular outflow dimension. More severe regurgitation is present in the image on the right where the regurgitant jet fills the majority of the left ventricular outflow tract.

In mitral regurgitation (MR), higher systolic blood pressure results in a larger driving force across the mitral valve, resulting in a larger jet area of MR by color flow. Jet direction is also important as it provides information about valve pathology; however, eccentric "wall-hugging" jets can lead to underestimation of regurgitant severity. A centrally directed jet may penetrate deeply into the receiving chamber even if the regurgitation is relatively mild, while an eccentric jet will appear much smaller even for more significant regurgitation.

Vena Contracta

The vena contracta is the narrowest portion of a central jet and occurs at or just downstream from the regurgitant orifice. To appropriately measure the vena contracta, it is necessary to see all three components of the color-flow jet (proximal flow acceleration, the vena contracta, and the downstream jet expansion). The cross-sectional area of the vena contracta is slightly smaller than the anatomic regurgitant orifice due to boundary effects, and it represents the effective regurgitant orifice area. Unlike the jet area, the size of the vena contracta is independent of the flow rate and driving pressure for a fixed orifice. Because it is characterized by high velocities, the vena contracta is less sensitive to technical factors such as PRF. To optimize the image for the measurement of the vena contracta, the jet size should be enlarged using the zoom view (Fig. 3), and the color sector should be sized appropriately for maximum lateral and temporal resolution. The imaging plane should be as perpendicular as possible to the commissure (e.g., the parasternal long-axis view for mitral regurgitation) and the width of the narrowest portion of the jet (the neck) is then measured.

There are many advantages to using the vena contracta for quantification of regurgitation: vena contracta is a simple measure of orifice size, it is good at identifying mild or severe regurgitation, it is not influenced by other regurgitant valves, and it does not require correction for convergence angle or adjacent walls. The vena contracta method works well for both central and eccentric jets (3). While it is not clear how to handle multiple jets, some investigators advocate adding the cross-sectional areas of the respective vena contracta (4). A disadvantage of the vena contracta method is that the range of values is small, so that small errors in measurement can result in significantly different interpretations. A 1 mm error can lead to a diagnosis of moderate rather than severe regurgitation. The vena contracta is a single temporal measurement and may not represent the overall regurgitant volume when the regurgitation occurs during only a part of systole or diastole.

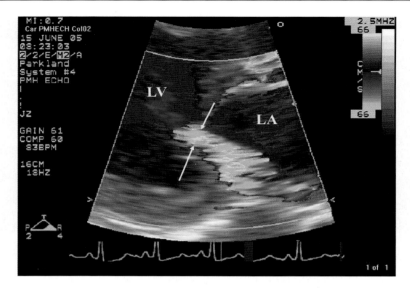

Fig. 3. Vena contracta. Parasternal long-axis view of a patient with moderate mitral regurgitation. The vena contracta (VC) is shown.

Proximal Isovelocity Surface Area

The proximal isovelocity surface area (PISA) method is based on the principle of conservation of mass: flow occurring at different locations proximal to the regurgitant orifice is equal to the flow through the regurgitant orifice. As blood approaches the regurgitant orifice, the flow accelerates. Using color-flow Doppler, roughly concentric hemispheric shells can be demonstrated, with decreasing surface area and increasing velocity as the orifice is approached (Fig. 4). To accurately calculate the PISA,

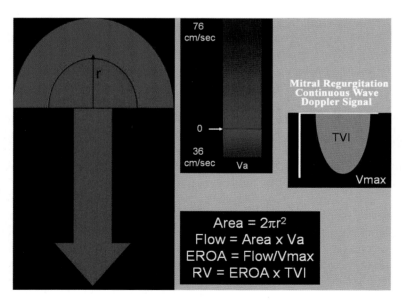

Fig. 4. Schematic representation of proximal flow acceleration. Hemispheric shells of decreasing surface area and increasing velocity can be demonstrated using color-flow Doppler. The radius (r) where the distinct *red–blue* aliasing interface to the regurgitant orifice can be measured. At this interface, the velocity is the same as the Nyquist limit identified on the velocity color scale (Va).

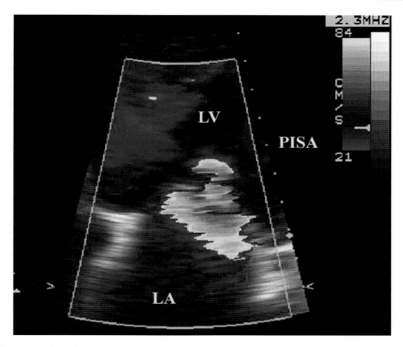

Fig. 5. Proximal flow acceleration of mitral regurgitation jet. The proximal isovolumic surface area (PISA) should be determined from a view parallel to the flow direction (e.g., apical four-chamber view for MR as shown in this figure), with a narrow sector and a zoom mode. The aliasing velocity can be decreased or the velocity baseline can be shifted toward the direction of the regurgitation to provide optimal visualization of the *red–blue* interface and to maximize the size of the radius.

the aliasing velocity needs to be adjusted so that a well-defined hemisphere is visualized (Fig. 5). The dimension of the proximal velocity hemisphere can be maximized by shifting the color Doppler Nyquist limit baseline toward the direction of regurgitation. Assuming a hemispherical shape to the isovelocity shells, the PISA can be calculated using the distance (r) from the red–blue interface to the regurgitant orifice with the formula below:

$$PISA = 2\pi r^2$$

Flow rate (ml/s) across the valve is determined by the product of the surface area of the hemispheric shell and the corresponding aliasing velocity (or the velocity at the aliasing boundary)

$$Flow\ rate\,(ml/s) = PISA\,(cm^2) \times aliasing\ velocity\,(cm/s)$$

The PISA method assumes that the maximal radius occurs at the time of the peak regurgitant flow and peak regurgitant velocity *(5)*. Based on this assumption, the maximal effective regurgitant orifice area (EROA) is derived as

$$EROA_{max}\,(cm^2) = flow\ rate\,(cm^3/s)\,/peak\ V_{reg}\,(cm/s)$$

Peak V_{reg} is the peak velocity of the regurgitant jet assessed by continuous wave Doppler. EROA determined by PISA may be slightly larger than that calculated by other means. Because PISA provides an instantaneous peak flow rate, the calculated EROA is the maximal EROA. The regurgitant volume can be calculated as the product of EROA and the time velocity integral of the regurgitant jet (VTI_{reg})

$$\text{Regurgitant volume (ml)} = \text{EROA} \left(\text{cm}^2\right) \times \text{VTI}_{\text{reg}} \text{(cm)}$$

The PISA method provides a quantitative measurement of not only lesion severity (EROA) but also volume overload (regurgitant volume). Unfortunately, the PISA method has limitations. There is less experience using PISA with lesions other than mitral regurgitation (MR). PISA measures only a single point in time and is less reliable for jets occurring in late systole (such as in mitral valve prolapse or hypertrophic cardiomyopathy). It is also invalid in the presence of multiple jets. It can be difficult to identify the precise regurgitant orifice, and any errors in measurement are squared. In eccentric jets, flow toward the regurgitant orifice is rarely hemispherical, making PISA less accurate *(6)*.

Pulsed Wave Doppler

The pulsed wave Doppler quantitative flow method is based on the principle of conservation of flow. This method allows for the calculation of regurgitant volume, regurgitant fraction, and effective regurgitant orifice area (EROA). To determine flow rate, pulsed wave Doppler is combined with 2-D imaging to calculate flow rate at a valve annulus. The annulus is the least variable anatomic area of the valvular structure, and a circular area can be assumed for all except the tricuspid valve *(2)*.

$$\text{Stroke volume (SV)} = \text{cross} - \text{sectional area (CSA)} \times \text{velocity time integral (VTI)}$$
$$\text{SV} = \pi r^2 \text{VTI}$$

In the absence of valvular regurgitation, the stroke volume at multiple valve sites is equal. However, in the setting of valvular regurgitation, stroke volume across a regurgitant valve ($\text{SV}_{\text{regvalv}}$) is larger than competent valves ($\text{SV}_{\text{compvalve}}$). An alternate method of measuring total stroke volume ($\text{SV}_{\text{regvalv}}$) is by determining LV volumes in diastole and systole with Simpson's apical method of discs. Regurgitant volume and regurgitant fraction can be calculated using the following formulas:

$$\text{Regurgitant volume (RV)} = \text{SV}_{\text{regvalv}} - \text{SV}_{\text{compvalve}}$$
$$\text{Regurgitant fraction (RF)} = \text{RV}/\text{SV}_{\text{regvalv}}$$
$$\text{Effective regurgitant orifice area (EROA)} = \text{RV}/\text{VTI}_{\text{regjet}}$$

Pitfalls of the pulsed Doppler quantitative method include errors in measurement of the valve annulus (which are then squared), failure to trace the modal velocity of the pulsed wave VTI, improper positioning of the sample volume of the pulsed wave, and improper angulation when sampling pulsed or continuous wave Doppler. Moreover, a large number of measurements must be made, with the possibility of each measurement introducing error into the calculation.

Qualitative Doppler Methods

The continuous wave (CW) Doppler spectral display can provide additional information about the severity of regurgitation *(7)*. The intensity of the Doppler signal is proportional to the number of red blood cells sampled in the regurgitant jet and typically increases with increasing regurgitant volume. The shape and the magnitude of the CW Doppler regurgitant signal provide both hemodynamic and semiquantitative assessment of regurgitant severity and are reviewed under individual valve lesions.

Acute Valvular Regurgitation

In contrast to chronic valvular regurgitation, the evaluation of acute valvular regurgitation can be limited by the appearance of small jet size by color Doppler. In part, small jet size may be related to insufficient temporal resolution in the setting of tachycardia *(8)*. Rapid equalization of pressure between the two chambers decreases orifice velocity, jet momentum, and jet area. In this setting, it can be difficult to identify the regurgitant jet by color flow, leading to a greater reliance on the accompanying 2-D abnormalities (such as papillary muscle rupture or valve perforation) and the overall clinical picture. In acute regurgitation, the vena contracta and pulsed Doppler quantitative methods remain accurate and should be included in the overall analysis.

Bernoulli Equation for Assessment of Pressure Gradients

Doppler evaluation is instrumental in the assessment of stenotic valvular disease. The pressure gradient across a valve may be calculated using the Bernoulli equation

$$\Delta P = {}^1\!/_2\rho \left(v_2^2 - v_1^2\right) + \rho \left(dv/dt\right) dx + R\left(v\right)$$

where ΔP is the pressure gradient across the valve (mmHg), ρ is the mass density of blood (1.06×10^3 kg/m^3), v_2 is the maximum velocity within the stenotic jet, v_1 is the velocity proximal to the stenosis, $(dv/dt)/dx$ is the time-varying velocity at each distance along the flowstream (local acceleration), and R is a constant describing the viscous losses. Because the values for acceleration and viscous resistance are small, they are typically eliminated. Applying a conversion factor to measure the velocity in meters per second (m/s) and pressure gradient in mmHg, the Bernoulli equation can be simplified to

$$\Delta P = 4\left(v_2^2 - v_1^2\right)$$

When the proximal velocity is <1 m/s, it can also be eliminated from the equation for further simplification

$$\Delta P = 4v_2^2$$

The modified Bernoulli equation is accurate in estimating the pressure gradient across a stenotic orifice under most conditions *(9, 10)*. The equation is less accurate when subvalve and valvular stenosis exist in tandem. When the proximal velocity is greater than 1.5 m/s, v_1 should be included in the analysis. Technical considerations are important as a significant intercept angle between the jet direction and the ultrasound beam will underestimate the degree of stenosis. Beat-to-beat variability in the presence of arrhythmias such as atrial fibrillation requires evaluation of numerous velocity profiles.

Continuity Equation

The continuity equation states that flow through a stenotic orifice is equal to flow proximal to the stenosis. Since flow equals the product of velocity and cross-sectional area of the orifice, the stenotic area can be defined as

$$\text{Stenotic area} = \text{flow/velocity across stenosis}$$

The continuity equation can be applied for pulmonary and mitral valve stenosis but is most commonly used for calculating aortic valve area *(11, 12)*.

General and Hemodynamic Considerations in Valvular Assessment

Recording the patient's blood pressure at the time of the echocardiographic examination allows for the calculation of hemodynamic data and can help put into context the degree of regurgitation (i.e., greater degrees of MR occur with higher systolic systemic blood pressure). An assessment of the right ventricular (RV) systolic pressure should be performed in all cases where an adequate tricuspid regurgitation spectral Doppler signal is present. By measuring the TR peak velocity and using the simplified Bernoulli equation, the gradient between the right ventricle and the right atrium is estimated. The change in pressure is added to an estimate of right atrial (RA) pressure to calculate RV systolic pressure. The RA pressure can be estimated using the inferior vena cava (IVC) size and response to inspiration. With RA pressure <10 mmHg, the IVC diameter is <1.7 cm and demonstrates ≥50% collapse with inspiration. A dilated IVC that does not demonstrate >50% reduction in size with inspiration indicates RA pressure >15 mmHg (Fig. 6). Pulsed wave Doppler of the pulmonary valve provides information about hemodynamics of the pulmonary vasculature. Pulmonary artery acceleration time from the onset to the peak velocity is normally greater than 140 ms and progressively shortens with increasing pulmonary hypertension. An acceleration time of <70–90 ms suggests significant pulmonary hypertension.

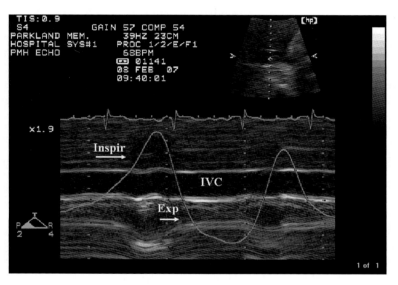

Fig. 6. M-mode of the inferior vena cava (IVC) with respiration recorded. There is no change in the dimension of the IVC during inspiration, consistent with increased right atrial pressure. Inspiration (inspir), expiration (exp), inferior vena cava (IVC).

CLINICAL APPLICATION OF ECHOCARDIOGRAPHY FOR SPECIFIC VALVULAR ABNORMALITIES

Aortic Regurgitation

Aortic regurgitation (AR) is uncommon in young otherwise healthy subjects *(13)*; however, the incidence of trivial or more AR increases with age, with an overall prevalence of 13% in men and 8.5% in women *(14)*. AR is assessed by a combination of methods that can be integrated to determine the severity (Table 1).

Echocardiographic 2-D imaging is important in determining the etiology of AR and the ventricular response to the volume load (Table 2). While mild AR may be associated with near-normal appearing valves, more significant AR is associated with abnormalities of the aortic root or the leaflets themselves (Fig. 7). Some causes of AR, such as infective endocarditis and aortic dissection, can produce acute severe AR resulting in a dramatic increase in LV filling pressure, a reduction in cardiac output, and

Table 1
Quantitative Parameters for Evaluation of Aortic Regurgitation

	Mild	Moderate	Severe
Regurgitant volume (ml/beat)	<30	30–59	≥60
Regurgitant fraction (%)	<30	30–49	≥50
EROA (cm^2)	<0.1	0.1–0.29	≥0.30
Vena contracta width (cm)	<0.3	0.3–0.6	>0.6
Jet width/LVOT width (%)	<25	25–64	≥65
Jet CSA/LVOT CSA (%)	<5	5–59	≥60

Adapted from Tables 4 and 6 of Zoghbi WA et al. *(2)*.

Table 2
Causes of Aortic Regurgitation

1. Cusp abnormalities
   a. Congenital (bicuspid, unicuspid)
   b. Calcific degeneration
   c. Myxomatous proliferation
   d. Rheumatic disease
   e. Infective endocarditis
   f. Anorectic drugs
   g. Discrete subaortic stenosis

2. Root abnormalities
   a. Idiopathic dilation of the aorta
   b. Systemic hypertension
   c. Marfan syndrome
   d. Trauma
   e. Ankylosing spondylitis
   f. Syphilitic aortitis
   g. Giant cell aortitis
   h. Ehlers-Danlos syndrome
   i. Reiter's syndrome

3. Loss of cusp support
   a. VSD with prolapse of the aortic cusp
   b. Dissection of the ascending aorta

severe pulmonary edema. Most cases of AR progress slowly over a number of years, with a prolonged asymptomatic phase. As the LV is exposed to a significant volume overload, it adapts over time by increasing LV mass in an eccentric pattern, leading to progressive chamber dilatation. Ultimately, systolic dysfunction occurs and may be irreversible.

Color-flow Doppler allows for both qualitative and quantitative assessment of AR. The maximal length of the jet penetration is not accurate in determining AR severity *(15)*. A more accurate assessment of AR is based on the jet height or the cross-sectional area of the color jet proximal to the aortic valve in the parasternal views and comparing it to the LVOT width or area just below the valve (Fig. 2) *(15, 16)*. This method has been validated angiographically *(15)*. The jet height is measured in the LVOT and must be distinguished from the vena contracta, which is measured immediately proximal to the flow convergence region.

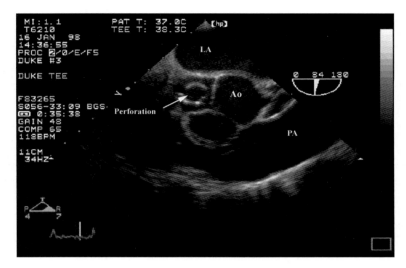

Fig. 7. Transesophageal image of a perforated aortic valve (AV perf) due to infective endocarditis. Using 2-D imaging alone, the etiology of the aortic regurgitation is determined.

Eccentric jets can be entrained along the LV wall, occupying a smaller portion of the outflow tract, and may result in underestimation of severity. Diffuse jets arising from the entire coaptation line of the aortic valve can result in overestimation of regurgitation. The aortic regurgitant orifice is dynamic during diastole, resulting in temporal variation of AR jet size.

If there is more than mild regurgitation based on qualitative color Doppler, the vena contracta can usually be measured from the parasternal long-axis view. Apical views should not be used due to splay of the color jet, which results in gross overestimation of the vena contracta. In the setting of eccentric jets, the vena contracta diameter should be measured perpendicular to the long axis of the jet rather than the long axis of the outflow tract. The vena contracta has been shown to be a reliable measurement of the severity of aortic regurgitation when compared with other methods and is more robust than the jet height and area for AR severity *(17)*. A vena contracta greater than 0.6 cm suggests severe aortic regurgitation *(see* Table 1).

There is limited experience using PISA for quantification of AR *(18)*, and there are unique technical challenges in measuring the isovelocity shells that converge on the aortic regurgitant orifice. The measurement of the flow convergence in AR should be in early diastole, closest to the peak regurgitant CW Doppler velocity. Using the flow convergence method, a calculated EROA ≥ 0.3 cm^2 is consistent with severe AR *(see* Table 1). Aortic valve calcification is common in adults with AR and can limit the ability to obtain high-quality images of the proximal convergence area. The presence of an ascending aortic aneurysm may lead to underestimation of AR by this method *(18)*.

Pulsed wave Doppler can be used in conjunction with 2-D imaging to calculate aortic regurgitant volume as the difference between transaortic and transmitral volume flow, provided there is not more than mild MR. This method has been shown to correlate well with angiographic and thermodilution methods *(19, 20)*. Pulsed wave Doppler can also be used at a single site in the proximal descending thoracic aorta to calculate forward and total stroke volume in AR *(21)*. The antegrade flow velocity integral is multiplied by the systolic cross-sectional aortic area. The flow velocity integral of the flow reversal in diastole is then multiplied by diastolic cross-sectional area. Either 2-D or M-mode imaging of the aortic arch can be used to determine both systolic and diastolic areas. A regurgitant volume ≥ 60 ml/beat and a regurgitant fraction $\geq 50\%$ suggest severe AR *(2)*.

The slope of deceleration of the CW Doppler signal provides a semiquantitative assessment of AR *(22, 23)*. The CW Doppler signal represents the pressure difference between the aorta and the LV during diastole. The pressure difference is highest at the beginning of diastole, with peak velocities of 4−6 m/s (corresponding to peak gradients of 64−144 mmHg). In mild AR there is a modest increase in LV pressure as diastole progresses, and the slope of the CW signal is relatively flat. In severe and particularly acute AR, the aortic pressure is lower in diastole and the LVEDP increases sharply during diastole, resulting in a steeper deceleration slope. The rate of change of this index is defined as the pressure half-time, the time taken for the initial pressure gradient to decrease by half (or the velocity to decrease to 70% of its peak value). A flat slope (pressure half-time >500 ms) is consistent with mild AR, while a steep slope (pressure half-time <200 ms) is consistent with severe or acute, decompensated AR *(2)*. In extreme cases, the aortic and LV pressures equalize before the end of diastole, resulting in a deceleration signal that reaches the baseline (Fig. 8). The shape of the AR signal may be affected by anything that affects LV or aortic diastolic pressure (such as systolic dysfunction, a patent ductus, or sepsis) and LV or aortic compliance. For example, a noncompliant LV develops higher pressure during diastole, resulting in a steeper slope of deceleration in the AR CW signal, not necessarily indicating severe aortic regurgitation. In the presence of tachycardia, the diastolic filling period shortens and only a few diastolic frames are displayed, limiting detection of AR by color-flow Doppler. However, in this setting, the higher sampling of CW Doppler may identify aortic regurgitation missed by color-flow Doppler.

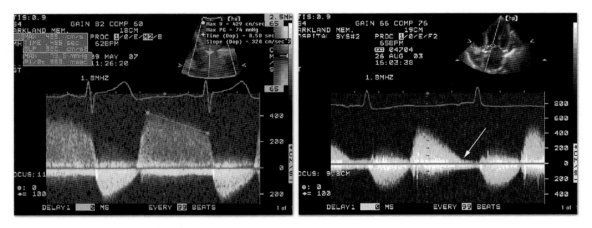

Fig. 8. Continuous wave Doppler of aortic regurgitation. The signal on the left was obtained in a patient with moderate aortic regurgitation. The pressure half-time is 393 ms, and there is a clear pressure gradient at end-diastole. The signal on the right was obtained from a patient with severe decompensated aortic regurgitation. The signal reaches the baseline before the end of diastole, demonstrating no difference in the pressures between the aorta and the left ventricle at the end-diastole.

Holodiastolic flow reversal can be demonstrated in the abdominal aorta and is highly sensitive to the presence of severe AR (Fig. 9). Holodiastolic flow reversal in the descending thoracic aorta is also sensitive to severe AR but is less specific, as it can also be present in moderate AR *(21, 24)*. Reduced compliance of the aorta, as occurs with aging, may prolong the diastolic flow reversal.

Other echocardiographic findings can provide clues regarding the presence and severity of AR. When the aortic regurgitant jet impinges on the anterior mitral leaflet, high-frequency fluttering of the leaflet can be appreciated on M-mode imaging, even in the setting of mild AR. Impaired anterior mitral leaflet opening can also occur, demonstrated by an increased distance between the "maximal anterior motion of the mitral valve E point and the most posterior motion of the ventricular septum" termed increased E-point septal separation or EPSS. In the setting of severe, decompensated AR, there is a rapid increase in LV diastolic pressure and the mitral valve closes before the onset of the QRS complex. This finding, termed systolic mitral preclosure, is best appreciated by M-mode imaging

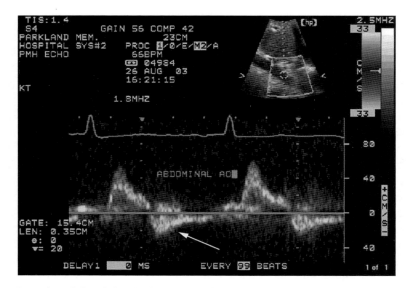

Fig. 9. Pulsed wave Doppler of the abdominal aorta obtained from the subcostal view. Diastolic flow reversal is demonstrated (*arrow*), consistent with severe aortic valve regurgitation.

(Fig. 10). Diastolic MR suggests severe acute elevation of LV end-diastolic pressures and can be seen in severe and/or acute AR (Fig. 11).

Chronic AR is typically slowly progressive, and evaluation should focus on the response of the LV to volume overload. In asymptomatic patients with chronic AR, echocardiography is instrumental in the timing of surgical intervention. Many patients with AR will develop systolic dysfunction prior to the development of symptoms, and serial monitoring is required in asymptomatic patients with severe AR who do not meet criteria for surgical management (Table 3) *(25, 26)*. Recent series involving large

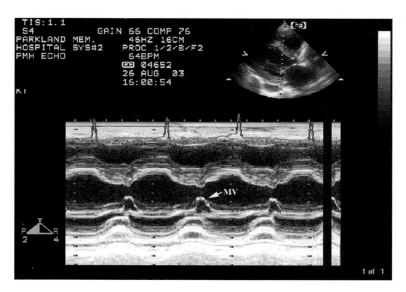

Fig. 10. M-mode parasternal long-axis view demonstrating closure of the mitral valve (MV) in diastole. This finding is related to elevated left ventricular diastolic pressure and is consistent with severe decompensated aortic regurgitation.

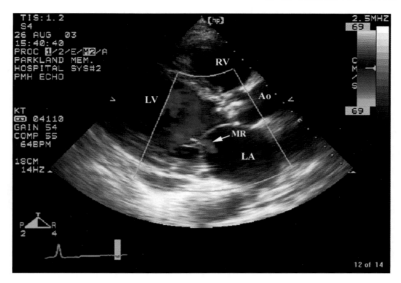

Fig. 11. Parasternal long-axis view demonstrating diastolic mitral regurgitation, seen in the setting of elevated left ventricular end-diastolic pressure in severe aortic regurgitation.

Table 3
Indications for Echocardiography in Valvular Heart Disease

Murmur: diagnosis and evaluation
Initial evaluation of a murmur when valvular or structural heart disease is suspected (diastolic, continuous, holosystolic, late systolic murmurs, and murmurs associated with ejection clicks or radiate to the neck or back or grade 3 or louder midpeaking systolic murmurs) (I)
Murmur and signs or symptoms of cardiovascular disease (CHF, ischemia, syncope or other evidence of structural heart disease) (I)

MVP: diagnosis and evaluation
Initial evaluation of patient with suspected MVP and for diagnosis of MR (I) in asymptomatic patients with physical signs of MVP (I)
To exclude MVP in patients who have been given the diagnosis but who have no clinical evidence to support the diagnosis (IIa)
For risk stratification in asymptomatic patients with physical signs of MVP or known MVP (IIa)

MVP: serial echocardiographic evaluation
Serial echo every year in patients with high-risk characteristics on initial echo or moderate-to-severe MR
Echo in patients with MVP who develop cardiovascular symptoms or exam, suggesting new significant MR

AS: diagnosis and evaluation
For diagnosis and evaluation of AS severity, and assessment of LV wall thickness, size, and function (I)

AS: serial echocardiographic evaluation
For reevaluation of patients with known AS and changes in symptoms or signs (I)
For assessment of changes in hemodynamic severity and LV function in AS during pregnancy (I)
Reevaluation of asymptomatic patients every year for severe AS, every 1–2 years for moderate AS, and 3–5years for mild AS (I)
Dobutamine stress echo to evaluate patients with low-flow/low-gradient AS and LV dysfunction (IIa)

Table 3
(Continued)

MS: diagnosis and evaluation
Diagnosis of MS, assessment of hemodynamic severity including PAP, and associated valvular disease (I)
Assessment of suitability of valve anatomy for PBMC (I)
TEE to assess for LA thrombus and degree of MR prior to PMBC (I)
TEE to assess MS when TTE is suboptimal (I)
Exercise echo in patients with MS and discordance of symptoms and MS severity by resting echo (I)

MS: serial echocardiographic evaluation
Reevaluation of known MS with change in signs or symptoms (I)
Reevaluation of patients with no symptoms and severe MS (every year), moderate MS (every 1–2 years 0),
    and mild MS (every 3–5 years) to assess PAP, hemodynamics (IIa)
Reevaluation of MV after PMBC (after minimum of 72 h after PMBC)

AR: diagnosis and evaluation
Confirm presence and severity of AR (acute or chronic) (I)
To determine etiology of AR, assessment of valve morphology, LVH, LV dimension, and EF (I)
To assess aortic root size in patients with AR and enlarged aortic root (I)

AR: serial echocardiographic evaluation
With significant AR repeat echo 2–3 months after initial evaluation to establish chronicity and stability
Mild AR: every 2–3 years
If ESD <45 mm or EDD <60 mm and stable dimensions, echo every 12 mo; if progressive dilatation, echo
    in 3 months
If ESD 45–50 mm or EDD 60–70 mm and stable dimensions, echo every 12 mo; if progressive dilatation,
    echo in 3 months
If ESD 50–55 mm or EDD 70–75 mm, echo every 4–6 months; if progressive dilatation, echo in 3 months
To reevaluate mild, moderate, or severe AR with new or changing symptoms (I)

MR: diagnosis and evaluation
Baseline evaluation of LV size, function, RV and LA size, PAP, and MR severity in any patient
    suspected of MR (I)
To determine mechanism of MR
Exercise Doppler in asx patients with severe MR to assess exercise tolerance, exercise PAP, and MR severity
    (IIa), especially when a patient's exercise tolerance is uncertain based on history
Preoperative or intraoperative TEE to establish mitral valve anatomy to assess feasibility of and to guide valve
    repair (I)
TEE indicated when TTE provides nondiagnostic information of MR severity or etiology (I)
TEE in asymptomatic patients with severe MR to determine feasibility of repair (IIa)

MR: serial echocardiographic evaluation
If moderate MR, yearly echocardiographic evaluation
Asymptomatic severe MR – echocardiogram every 6–12 months to assess LVEF, LVESD, and hemodynamics
Mild-to-moderate regurgitation and new or changing symptoms

Adapted from Refs. *(35, 155, 156)*.

numbers of patients have demonstrated preoperative LV ejection fraction (LVEF) and end-systolic (LVESD) and end-diastolic (LVEDD) dimensions predict survival and/or LV systolic function following valve replacement *(27–30)*. The development of symptoms is predicted by LVESD and LVEDD *(31–33)*, LV mass *(32)* and LVEF *(33)*. LVESD is a relatively load-independent measure of LV systolic function. Severe LV dilation is associated with increased incidence of adverse outcomes without surgical correction *(34)*. Echocardiographic indications for surgical referral are LVEF <50% or LV end-systolic dimension >55 mm *(35)*. All patients with symptomatic severe AR should be considered for valve surgery.

Transesophageal echocardiography (TEE) seldom provides additional information on transthoracic imaging, unless acoustic windows from the chest wall are poor. Color Doppler and other criteria for the assessment of AR are the same as for chest wall imaging. Because of greater difficulty in aligning Doppler signals with aortic flow, pulsed and continuous wave Doppler methods may be less accurate with TEE.

Mitral Regurgitation

The mitral valve apparatus includes the annulus, valve leaflets, chordae tendinae, papillary muscles, and the LV myocardial wall. An abnormality in one or more of these structures may result in MR, although a mild amount of regurgitation is present in 19–45% of normal mitral valves *(13, 14)*. Two-dimensional imaging should include a careful assessment of these structures to determine the etiology of regurgitation (Table 4). A flail mitral leaflet or a ruptured papillary muscle noted on 2-D imaging is specific for severe MR (Fig. 12). Evaluation of LV and LA dimensions provides clues about the chronicity and severity of regurgitation and guides appropriate timing of surgery. Chamber enlargement is not specific, as LA and LV size may be normal in acute MR. Two-dimensional evaluation is critical in determining whether the MR is functional, related to dilation of the LV or segmental wall motion abnormalities, or due to primary structural abnormalities. LV dilatation may lead to apical displacement of the papillary muscles, resulting in tethering of the mitral leaflets apically and an abnormal coaptation zone with functional MR.

Because of the increased gradient between the left ventricle and the left atrium during systole, the velocity of MR always exceeds the Nyquist limit, resulting in an aliasing pattern with a red–blue–green mosaic of color flow. Spurious signals can be mistaken for MR and include the normal posterior motion of blood in the LA from MV closure and the normal systolic inflow from the pulmonary veins. In general, large jets correspond to more regurgitation than do smaller jets. Planimetry of the jet area is not recommended as a sole means of quantification of MR. With central jets of MR, the area of the regurgitant jet indexed to LA size correlates better with the severity of regurgitation *(36)*. An indexed jet area >40% suggests severe MR. However, when MR is limited to late systole (as in mitral valve prolapse or hypertrophic cardiomyopathy), indexed jet area alone will overestimate the severity of the

Table 4
Causes of Mitral Regurgitation

1. Leaflet abnormalities
   a. Degenerative valvular disease
   b. Rheumatic heart disease
   c. Infective endocarditis, Libman-Sachs endocarditis, Marantic endocarditis
   d. Congenital cleft mitral valve
   e. Infiltrative valvular disease
   f. Diet drug valvulopathy
   g. Carcinoid (in the presence of pulmonary mets or a right-to-left cardiac shunt)

2. Abnormalities of supporting structures
   a. Dilated cardiomyopathy
   b. Left ventricular ischemia or infarction
   c. HOCM
   d. Mitral annular calcification

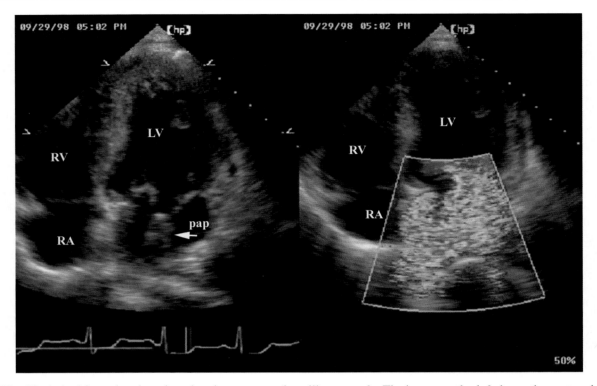

Fig. 12. Apical four-chamber view showing a ruptured papillary muscle. The image on the *left* shows the ruptured papillary muscle prolapsing into the left atrium during systole, and the color-flow Doppler image on the *right* demonstrates the severe mitral regurgitation.

MR. In acute severe MR, which is associated with elevated LA pressure and low systolic arterial blood pressure, the jet area may be small, while in patients with high systolic blood pressure and mild MR, jet area may be significant. Jet direction provides clues about the etiology of MR, as flail or prolapsing leaflets result in regurgitation directed away from the leaflet pathology (Fig. 13). Eccentric jets do not entrain blood on both sides and therefore appear smaller than central jets of similar size *(37, 38)*.

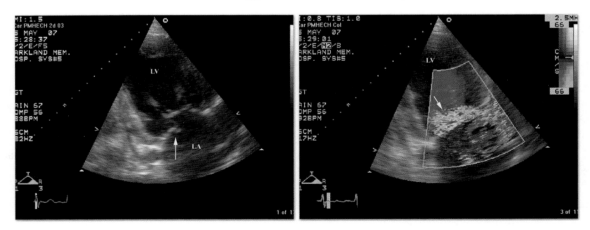

Fig. 13. Apical two-chamber view with color Doppler of a patient with a flail posterior mitral leaflet (*upward arrow in the left image*). The mitral regurgitant jet is directed anteriorly, in the opposite direction of the leaflet pathology (*downward arrow in the right image*).

Table 5
Quantitative Parameters for Evaluation of Mitral Regurgitation

	Mild	Moderate	Severe
Regurgitant volume (ml/beat)	<30	30–59	≥ 60
Regurgitant fraction (%)	<30	30–49	≥50
EROA (cm^2)	<0.2	0.2–0.39	≥0.4
Vena contracta width (cm)	<0.3	0.3–0.69	≥0.7
Jet area/LA area (%)	<20	20–40	>40
Jet area (cm^2)	<4	4–9.9	>10

Adapted from Tables 1 and 3 of Zoghbi WA et al. *(2)*.

The vena contracta method has been well validated for the assessment of MR *(39, 40)*. Because the MR jet is not usually circular and may be elongated along the zone of leaflet coaptation, vena contracta should not be measured in the apical two-chamber view, which can show a wide vena contracta even in mild MR. Vena contracta is best measured in the parasternal long-axis view on transthoracic imaging, using a zoom view of the mitral valve leaflets to improve accuracy of measurements. Often slight angulation is necessary to adequately view the proximal acceleration and the flow of convergence. A vena contracta ≥0.7 cm suggests severe MR (Table 5). Although the vena contracta is independent of driving pressure and flow for a fixed orifice *(41)*, the mitral regurgitant orifice can be dynamic, and the vena contracta may be affected by this dynamic change or by changes in hemodynamics *(42)*.

The presence of proximal flow acceleration on the LV side of the mitral valve at the usual Nyquist limit of 50–60 cm/s indicates significant MR. The PISA method has been validated in several clinical studies for measurement of regurgitant flow and EROA *(6, 43, 44)*. An EROA of ≥0.4 cm^2 is consistent with severe MR (Table 5). PISA is best measured from the apical views *(4, 45)*, and, in most cases, a single measurement in the apical four-chamber view is sufficient. However, in the setting of a noncircular orifice, PISA can be measured in both apical four and two chambers for greater accuracy *(45)*. The PISA method is less reliable for measuring flow when there is calcification of the MV leaflets or annulus. In mitral valve prolapse or hypertrophic obstructive cardiomyopathy, MR may occur only during a portion of systole, and the regurgitant volume obtained by PISA calculations will be overestimated unless adjusted by the fraction of systole during which regurgitation occurs. The PISA method tends to overestimate the regurgitant flow and orifice area in patients with eccentric jets because the flow does not approach the regurgitant orifice as a hemisphere but rather as smaller segments of a sphere. Using a radius during an earlier time in systole may help correct for overestimation of MR in the setting of eccentric jets *(46)*.

Pulsed Doppler quantitative flow has been validated for the quantitation of MR in several studies *(47–49)*. Quantitative pulsed wave Doppler provides regurgitant volume, regurgitant fraction, and orifice size. The echocardiographic measurements needed to make these calculations are shown in Fig. 14. It is accurate for multiple jets and eccentric jets and evaluates MR during the entire duration of systole. The method is not valid with combined MR and AR unless pulmonary annular data are used. A regurgitant volume of 60 ml/beat and a regurgitant fraction of 50% suggest severe MR (Table 5).

Pulsed wave Doppler also provides qualitative data regarding mitral regurgitant severity. A dominant early mitral inflow velocity is typical in severe MR due to increased diastolic flow across the MV *(50)* (Fig. 15). In the setting of severe MR, the peak E velocity is usually greater than 1.2 m/s and higher than the mitral A velocity. An increased peak mitral E wave velocity is not specific for MR, as E wave velocities are also influenced by LA pressure, LV compliance, MV stenosis, and heart rhythm abnormalities. However, a dominant A wave in the mitral filling pattern virtually excludes severe MR.

Normal pulmonary vein inflow in an adult is characterized by a systolic velocity higher than the diastolic velocity. As the severity of MR increases, the velocity of forward systolic flow in the pul-

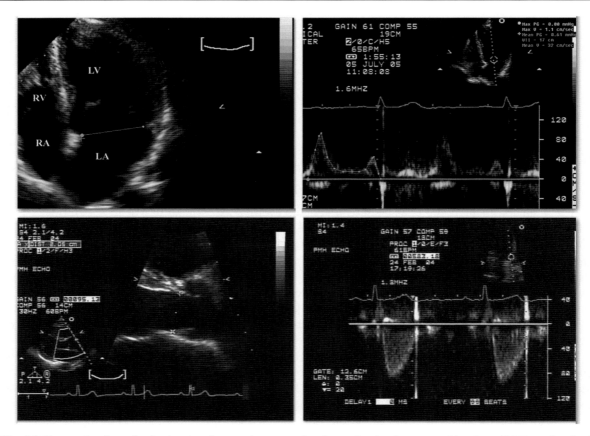

Fig. 14. Determination of mitral regurgitant volume can be determined using a combination of 2-D and pulsed wave Doppler. The mitral annulus is measured in its greatest dimension in diastole and the radius is used in the calculation of the mitral annular area (*upper left*). This is multiplied by the time–velocity integral of the mitral inflow obtained by pulsed wave Doppler at the level of the mitral annulus (*upper right*) to determine the stroke volume across the mitral valve. The LVOT area is then calculated by measuring the LVOT dimension in the parasternal long-axis view (*lower left*) and multiplied by the LVOT time–velocity integral, obtained from pulsed wave Doppler sampled just proximal to the aortic valve in the apical view, to determine the stroke volume across the aortic valve. The flow through the mitral valve is larger than that through the aortic valve, and the difference between the two represents the regurgitant volume.

monary vein decreases and eventually may be reversed (Fig. 16) (*51, 52*). Elevated LA pressure and atrial fibrillation may also result in blunting of forward pulmonary vein systolic flow (*52, 53*).

Comparison of the intensity of the MR signal to the intensity of inflow signal can provide a rapid semiquantitative assessment of MR (*7*). A faint and sometimes incomplete signal represents mild regurgitation, while a signal that is equivalent in intensity to the antegrade flow across the valve is supportive of severe regurgitation. Another approach uses the power of CW Doppler backscatter signals from the aortic outflow and mitral inflow to estimate the regurgitant fraction (*54*). The complexity of signal processing and the rather wide confidence limits, however, preclude the routine clinical use of this method.

The magnitude and shape of the MR CW Doppler signal represents the pressure gradient across the regurgitant valve over time. The mitral regurgitant peak velocity is normally 5−6 m/s, with a rapid acceleration in early systole, a rapid deceleration prior to diastole, and a mid-to-late peak of the

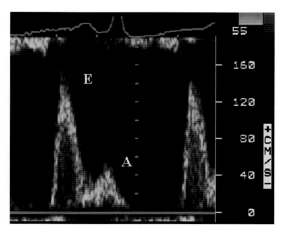

Fig. 15. Pulsed wave Doppler of mitral valve inflow in a patient with severe mitral regurgitation. The early mitral inflow velocity (E) is dominant compared to the late mitral inflow velocity (A), and E velocity is elevated at 150 cm/s.

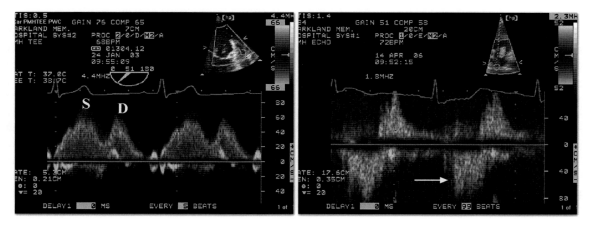

Fig. 16. Pulmonary vein Doppler pattern of a patient with mild mitral regurgitation (*left image*) shows the pulmonary vein systolic inflow velocity higher than the diastolic inflow velocity. The *right image* shows systolic flow reversal in the pulmonary vein (*arrow*) and is consistent with severe mitral regurgitation. Pulmonary vein signals are not accurate if the mitral regurgitant jet is directed into the sampled vein. Likewise, the absence of pulmonary vein flow reversal should not preclude the diagnosis of severe MR.

velocity. With severe MR, an early rise in left atrial pressure leads to a truncated, triangular, early peaking contour of the MR signal and often to a lower peak velocity.

Echocardiography plays an important role in the management of MR and provides prognostic information. Organic MR tends to be progressive, and the LV responds to this volume load by developing eccentric hypertrophy and diastolic enlargement. Over time, LV contractile dysfunction occurs and is evident by increases in systolic dimensions. Survival following mitral valve replacement is predicted by the preoperative LVEF *(55–57)* and postoperative LV systolic dysfunction is predicted by preoperative LVEF and LV end-systolic dimension *(56, 58)*. A flail mitral leaflet is associated with adverse outcomes in nonsurgically treated patients, although the risk of death is lower in the segment of patients who were asymptomatic and had normal LVEF *(59)*. Indications for surgery include LVEF <60%, LV end-systolic dimension >45 mm, or symptoms *(35)*. Asymptomatic patients not meeting these echocardiographic criteria should be followed with noninvasive studies (Table 3). Exercise echocardiography can be used in the setting of symptoms out of proportion to the MR severity and to assess functional status and hemodynamic changes in patients who are apparently asymptomatic *(60)*. In patients with PA systolic pressures >60 mmHg with exercise, mitral valve surgery should be considered *(2)*.

The feasibility of mitral valve repair, which is preferred over replacement *(61)*, can be assessed echocardiographically. Repair is more likely when there is limited calcification of the leaflets or annulus, when prolapse of only one leaflet is present, and when valve perforation or annular dilatation is the mechanism of MR.

TEE has played an important role in determining candidates for mitral valve repair and guiding valve surgery. TEE is superior to chest wall echocardiography in detailing the mitral valve anatomy and in determining MR severity *(62, 63)*. Hemodynamics are different in an anesthetized patient and can lead to the appearance of less-severe regurgitation compared with an awake or mildly sedated patient The goal of repair is a reduction of MR to mild or less, without creating significant valvular stenosis. A mean transmitral diastolic gradient of 2−4 mmHg is generally acceptable following repair.

Mitral Valve Prolapse

Echocardiographic evaluation of mitral valve prolapse provides both diagnostic and prognostic information. Mitral valve prolapse is present in 2−3% of the population *(64)*. Major echocardiographic criteria for the diagnosis include superior systolic displacement of a valve leaflet >2 mm above the annulus, coaptation of the leaflets at or superior to the annular plane, or mild to moderate superior systolic displacement of the leaflets associated with chordal rupture, MR, or annular dilatation *(65)*. Redundancy or thickening of the leaflets greater than 5 mm supports the diagnosis and may be associated with adverse outcomes *(66–68)*. Typical M-mode findings of prolapse include thickening of the mitral leaflets and posterior bowing of the mitral valve during systole (Fig. 17). The apical four-chamber view is less specific for the diagnosis of mitral valve prolapse due to the nonplanar structure of the annulus and leads to the appearance of prolapse of normal leaflets in this view. Therefore, in the assessment of mitral prolapse, the leaflets should be assessed in multiple views to document that one or both leaflets break the plane of the annulus. In approximately 20% of these patients, there is also prolapse of the tricuspid or aortic valves.

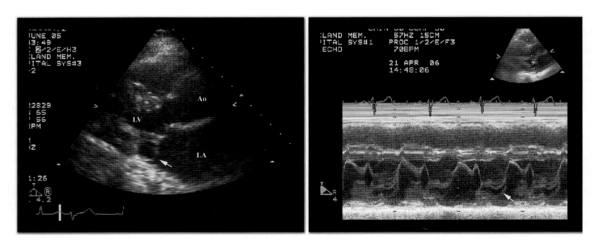

Fig. 17. Two-dimensional and M-mode images of a patient with posterior mitral leaflet prolapse. The posterior leaflet bows superior to the mitral annulus during systole (*arrow*).

Tricuspid Regurgitation

The standards for determining the severity of TR are not as robust as those for MR. Echocardiographically evident tricuspid regurgitation (TR) is present in the setting of many structurally normal valves. Mild TR is present in 15–77% of normal individuals (13, 14, 69). As is the case with other valves, the assessment of the severity of TR is dependent on integration of multiple methods of evaluation (Table 6).

Table 6
Assessment of Tricuspid Regurgitation

	Mild	Moderate	Severe
Tricuspid leaflets	Usually normal	Normal or abnormal	Abnormal/flail, lack of coaptation
RV and RA size	Normal		Moderate or greater enlargement
Vena contracta width (cm)	Absent vena contracta		>0.7
Jet area (cm^2)	<5	5–10	>10
PISA radius (cm)	≤0.5	0.6–0.9	>0.9
Jet density – CW	Faint, parabolic	Dense	Dense, early peaking triangular
Hepatic vein	Systolic dominant flow	Blunting of systolic flow	Systolic flow reversal

Adapted from Tables 8 and 9 of Zoghbi WA et al. (2).

Two-dimensional imaging helps identify the etiology of the TR. TR can be related to structural abnormalities but is most commonly secondary to annular dilation from RV enlargement, termed "functional TR." Pressure or volume loading of the right ventricle from pulmonary disease, left-to-right shunts, left heart disease, or a combination of factors can cause functional (or secondary) TR. Primary TR may be acquired or congenital. Acquired TR may result from infective endocarditis, rheumatic disease (Fig. 18), or carcinoid disease. TR is also associated with serial RV biopsies in cardiac transplant patients, presumed secondary to biotome trauma to the chordae or valve itself.

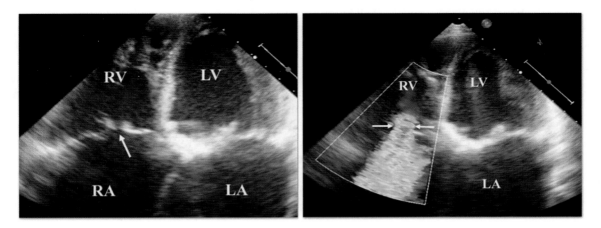

Fig. 18. Two-dimensional (*left image*) and color Doppler imaging (*right*) in rheumatic tricuspid valve disease. The leaflets are thickened and domed, and there is failure of leaflet coaptation in systole. Significant tricuspid regurgitation is evident by color Doppler (*right image*).

Indwelling RV leads may be associated with TR, either due to interference with normal leaflet coaptation or secondary fibrosis of the leaflet from physical contact with the lead. Chordal rupture from trauma or myxomatous valve disease can also occur. The most common congenital cause of TR is Ebstein's anomaly (Fig. 19). In this condition there is apical displacement of the septal and posterior leaflets with an enlarged anterior leaflet variably tethered to the RV free wall. The leaflets are redundant, elongated, and have abnormal chordal connections. If the anterior leaflet is highly redundant, RV outflow tract obstruction may result. The orifice of the TV is apically displaced relative to the anatomic annulus and is typically more than 20 mm lower than the anterior mitral valve insertion, resulting in atrialization of part of the RV. The true RV is often hypoplastic or functionally abnormal. The degree of RV atrialization, the amount of displacement of the valve insertion, and the degree of leaflet tethering are important in determining surgical approach and success of repair (70). A poor prognosis is associated with the functional RV being less than one-third of the total RV area (70).

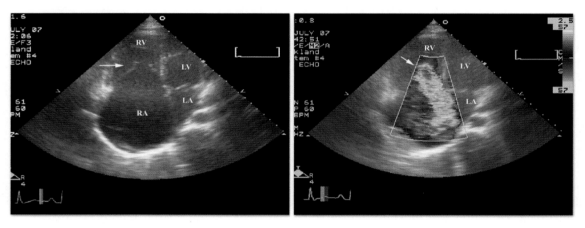

Fig. 19. Apical four-chamber view of a patient with Ebstein's anomaly with apical displacement of the tricuspid leaflets in comparison to the anterior mitral leaflet insertion.

Right atrial and right ventricular enlargement are not specific for severe TR, but their absence suggests the TR is not severe. Quantitative analysis of RV volume and function is limited by the non-geometric shape and the technical difficulties in visualizing the entire chamber. In the clinical setting, a semiquantitative analysis of RV enlargement is typical and describes mild, moderate, or severe enlargement based on RV size relative to the left ventricle. RV systolic function is generally estimated qualitatively and most easily assessed by displacement of the tricuspid valve annulus. Displacement of the tricuspid valve annulus less than 1.5 cm is associated with a poor prognosis (71). The hemodynamic response to severe low-pressure TR may be manifested by an RV volume overload pattern, demonstrated by flattening of the ventricular septum toward the LV during diastole but not systole. In high-pressure TR, the ventricular septum will be flattened throughout the cardiac cycle.

Color-flow Doppler imaging should be performed in several views to assess the size and direction of regurgitation. Color-flow mapping of TR correlates well with angiographic assessment (72, 73), and the jet area of TR is often indexed to the area of the RA (Fig. 20). The PISA method has been validated in small studies but is rarely used clinically (72, 74). The vena contracta can be used for assessment of TR severity (75) and correlates well with EROA, especially with greater degrees of TR (76, 77). Both PISA and vena contracta methods are less accurate in eccentric jets. Underestimation of severe TR has been demonstrated in up to 20–30% of patients using PISA or jet area (72).

The density and the contour of the CW Doppler signal provide qualitative data on the severity of TR. Severe regurgitation is associated with a dense signal with triangular early peaking because of the

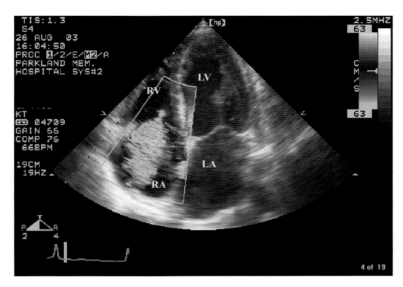

Fig. 20. Apical four-chamber view of a patient with tricuspid regurgitation. The area of the tricuspid regurgitation jet by color flow can be indexed to the area of the right atrium.

rapid rise in RA pressure (Fig. 21). Estimation of the pulmonary artery systolic pressure is a critical element in evaluating patients with cardiac and pulmonary disease, making interrogation of the TR part of the routine echocardiographic examination. In low-pressure TR, such as Ebstein's anomaly, the antegrade and the retrograde CW flow appear as near mirror images of each other, related to the high-velocity forward and low-velocity retrograde flow across a severely incompetent TV *(78)*.

Pulsed wave Doppler cannot be used to accurately calculate tricuspid regurgitant volume because of complex structure of the annulus and significant respiratory variation in tricuspid inflow. Values of early diastolic TV velocity greater than 1.0 m/s are typical in patients with severe regurgitation. With

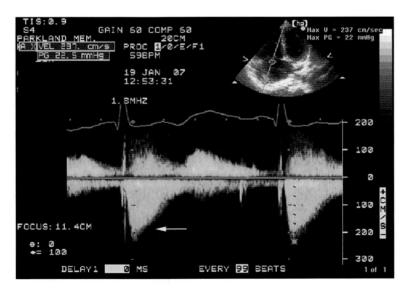

Fig. 21. Continuous wave Doppler of severe low-pressure tricuspid regurgitation. The early rise in RA pressure and a large regurgitant v-wave lead to the velocity peaking early and declining rapidly.

increasing TR severity, the hepatic vein inflow is blunted in systole, with the development of systolic flow reversal in severe TR. The sensitivity of systolic flow reversal for identifying severe TR is as high as 80% *(73)*. Hepatic vein flow patterns can also be affected by abnormal RA and RV compliance, atrial fibrillation, phase of respiratory cycle, and preload.

Pulmonary Regurgitation

A minor amount of pulmonary regurgitation (PR) may be present in 28—88% of normal individuals *(13)*. This PR is usually seen as a small, spindle-shaped jet and often central in location. Causes of pathologic PR include dilation of the pulmonary annulus (from pulmonary hypertension, left-to-right shunt, congenital absence of the pulmonary cusps, or idiopathic dilatation), rheumatic heart disease, and pulmonary hypertension. PR can also occur following percutaneous or surgical pulmonary valvuloplasty. Other abnormalities of the pulmonary valve include rare malignant tumors, endocarditis, or benign tumors such as fibroma or papilloma. Visualization of all three leaflets of the pulmonary valve can be difficult, but leaflet doming or thickening or dilatation of the pulmonary artery can help define the etiology.

Quantitation of PR is not as well validated as other regurgitant lesions, in part due to the lack of reliable standards for comparison. Color Doppler plays a major role in the assessment of PR. Jet size, the penetration depth into the RV, the vena contracta width, and the ratio of jet width to RVOT area are all used in assessing PR severity. Since jet penetration is dependent on the driving force between the pulmonary artery (PA) and RV, it is not reliable in the setting of pulmonary hypertension. In cases of severe PR, the rapidly dissipating diastolic gradient between the PA and the RV results in a brief period of color flow, and the PR severity may be underappreciated (Fig. 22). However, the vena contracta width will still be large, and the CW Doppler signal will be dense with a steep deceleration typical of hemodynamically significant PR (Fig. 23). A steep deceleration time may also occur in the setting of a noncompliant RV and is not specific for severe PR. When the clinical situation is uncertain, pulsed wave Doppler combined with 2-D measurements can be used to determine regurgitant fraction and regurgitant volume *(79)*. Because of significant overlap, standards for PR regurgitant fractions are not available. Direct evidence for hemodynamically significant PR includes RV dilation and RV volume overload pattern. Hemodynamically significant PR will lead to RV dilation and eventually to RV dysfunction. Although echocardiographic assessment of RV volume and function is semiquantitative,

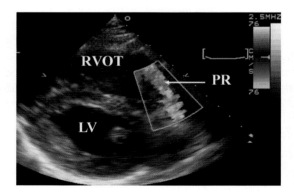

Fig. 22. Color-flow Doppler imaging of the pulmonary valve in a patient with prior surgical commissurotomy and severe pulmonary regurgitation. Spectral Doppler demonstrates a brief low-velocity regurgitant jet related to the rapid equalization of pressures in the pulmonary artery and the right ventricle. With free pulmonary regurgitation, the severity can be underappreciated, particularly in the setting of tachycardia or low frame rates; however, the vena contracta will remain large.

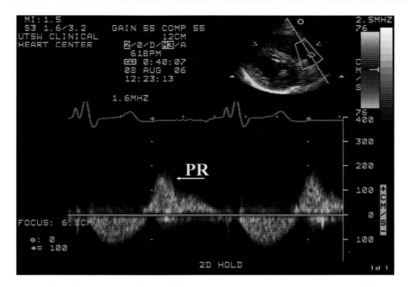

Fig. 23. Continuous wave Doppler in a patient with severe pulmonary regurgitation. The regurgitant signal has a density similar to the inflow signal, and the deceleration time is steep consistent with significant pulmonary regurgitation.

serial evaluations are essential in the clinical setting. At present, magnetic resonance imaging provides the most accurate measurement of RV volume and ejection fraction.

Aortic Stenosis

Aortic stenosis is a chronic pressure load on the heart, which results in concentric left ventricular hypertrophy and a high afterload state. Therefore, echocardiographic evaluation of aortic stenosis focuses not only on the quantitation of the severity of the valve stenosis but also on the response of the left ventricle to the pressure overload. A significant pressure load on the ventricle results in concentric left ventricular hypertrophy and subsequent diastolic dysfunction. Systolic function is preserved until late in the disease unless concomitant coronary artery disease, intrinsic myocardial disease, or other valvular or congenital heart disease is present. Full evaluation of mitral, tricuspid, and pulmonary valve function and estimation of the pulmonary artery pressure are also important elements of the echocardiographic evaluation. Details of the anatomy of the left ventricular outflow tract, valve morphology, and aortic root are essential. The most common etiology of valvular aortic stenosis is degenerative calcific disease in an apparently normal trileaflet valve. Congenital aortic valve disease is common and may be associated with a host of other anomalies. Patients with unicuspid or bicuspid valves may present with stenosis, regurgitation, or mixed stenosis and regurgitation. Serial left-sided obstructive lesions of Shone's complex can include mitral valve stenosis, tunnel subaortic stenosis from a small left ventricular outflow tract, discrete subaortic stenosis from a subaortic membrane, aortic valve stenosis, and coarctation of the aorta. Two-dimensional and Doppler imaging of the descending thoracic and abdominal aorta are necessary to rule out aortic coarctation. Supravalvular aortic stenosis is rare and may be isolated or seen with supravalvular pulmonic stenosis in patients with Williams Syndrome, a rare genetic disorder characterized by a mild-to-moderate mental retardation or learning difficulties, a distinctive facial appearance, and a unique overfriendly personality. Two-dimensional imaging in the parasternal short-axis view can provide important anatomic detail and a visual assessment of the severity of stenosis. However, reduced systolic excursion of the valve leaflets does not always mean severe stenosis. Aortic valve leaflet excursion will be reduced in low cardiac output states, such as arrhythmias or ischemia. Poor acoustic windows and heavy aortic valve calcification can limit visualization of valve opening. Direct measurement of aortic valve area by planimetry has been validated using TEE but is more difficult with chest wall imaging *(80–83)*. This approach is rarely necessary, given the reliability of Doppler methods.

Echocardiographic measures of the severity of aortic stenosis have been well validated and have become the gold standard method for grading aortic stenosis (Table 7). Catheterization is rarely needed today to assess the severity of aortic valve stenosis but may be used to assess coronary artery anatomy and hemodynamics.

Table 7

Classification of Severity of Stenotic Valve Disease

	Mild	Moderate	Severe
Aortic stenosis measurement			
Peak velocity (m/s)	<3.0	3.0–4.0	>4.0
Mean gradient (mmHg)	<25	25–40	>40
Valve area (cm^2) (valve index, cm^2/m^2)	>1.5	1–1.5	<1.0 (<0.6)
Doppler velocity index			<0.20
Mitral stenosis measurement			
Mean gradient (mmHg)	<5	5–10	>10
Valve area (cm^2)	>1.5	1.0–1.5	<1.0
Tricuspid stenosis measurement			
Mean gradient (mmHg)	<2	2–6	>6
Valve area (cm^2)			<1.0
Pulmonary stenosis measurement			
Peak velocity (m/s)			>4
Peak gradient (mmHg)	<40	40–70	>70

Adapted from Bonow RO et al. *(35)*.

The pressure gradient across a stenotic aortic valve is related to the velocity of blood flow across the stenotic orifice, as described by the modified Bernoulli equation $\Delta P = 4v^2$ and has been shown to correlate well with simultaneous pressure measurements made in the cardiac catheterization laboratory. Echocardiography utilizes the continuous wave Doppler shift to measure the maximum velocity of blood across the stenotic valve orifice. The relationship between Doppler velocity and manometric pressure measurements in the assessment of aortic valve stenosis has been well validated in in vitro models, animal models, and in patients with clinical disease *(10, 84–94)*. These studies demonstrate a close correlation between simultaneous echo and catheterization-derived mean gradients over a wide range of stenosis severity, from mild to critical aortic valve stenosis. Nonsimultaneous measurements do not correlate as well. It is important to point out a few differences between echo- and cath-derived gradients. The Doppler-derived maximum gradient is a peak instantaneous pressure gradient, which occurs at one point in time and is not the same as the "peak-to-peak gradient" often reported in a cardiac catheterization report. The peak-to-peak cath gradient refers to the pressure difference between peak LV pressure and peak aortic pressure, which are NOT simultaneous and not measured by continuous wave Doppler. Therefore, it should be no surprise that peak-to-peak cath gradients are smaller and do not correlate well with peak Doppler instantaneous pressure gradients. Doppler mean gradients are more comparable to catheterization-derived mean gradients.

Peak and mean transaortic pressure gradients are linearly related when measured by either Doppler or manometric methods. The regression equation describing this relationship is mean $\Delta P = (\text{max } \Delta P/1.45) - 2.2$ mmHg and mean $\Delta P = 2.4\ V_{\text{max}2}$ (applies only to native valves) *(95, 96)*. The linear relationship between maximum aortic velocity and mean pressure gradient is important and suggests that maximum jet velocity alone is very useful in following patients with valvular aortic stenosis. When the AS jet velocity is >4 m/s, the aortic stenosis is severe unless there is moderate regurgitation. However, high cardiac output states such as fever, anemia, arteriovenous fistula, and aortic regurgitation will increase the peak aortic velocity but not the degree of stenosis. Conversely, when low cardiac output states exist, peak aortic velocity may be modestly elevated despite critical valve stenosis.

Accurate measurement of maximum aortic jet velocity is paramount ; proper alignment of the continuous wave Doppler with the aortic stenosis jet is critical to minimize errors. The direction of the aortic jet is often eccentric and requires assessment from multiple acoustic windows, including apical five chamber, apical long axis, right parasternal, and suprasternal notch. A small dedicated continuous wave Doppler transducer is also helpful in trying to obtain the maximum aortic jet velocity. The goal is to detect the highest velocity signal with a full-spectral Doppler pattern, which can be used for measuring the peak velocity and tracing the area under the curve (Fig. 24). Measurement of peak aortic velocity is highly reproducible, with the coefficient of variability for measuring aortic jet velocity reported at 3% (97), indicating a change in peak velocity >0.2 m/s significant. Another major technical issue in recording the aortic stenosis Doppler velocity profile is insuring measurement of the AS jet as opposed to an MR signal. The AS Doppler signal will start later than the MR signal due to isovolumic

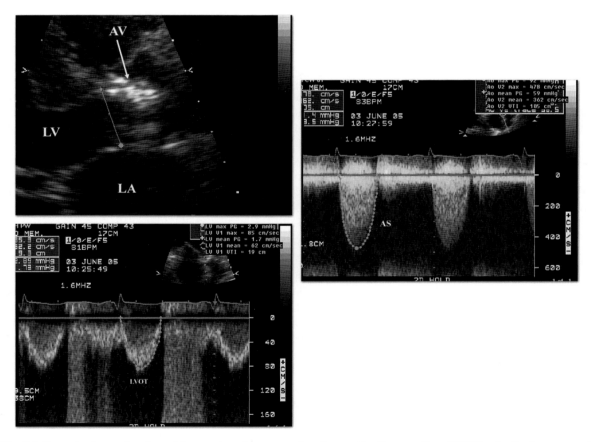

Fig. 24. Steps in the evaluation of the aortic valve area using the continuity equation. LVOT velocity is measured from an apical five-chamber view using pulse Doppler with the sample volume approximately 1 cm proximal to the aortic valve in the LVOT. LVOT diameter is measured from a 2-D parasternal long-axis view, in a high-resolution zoom view in midsystole. The LVOT diameter is measured from the inner edge of the septal endocardial echo to the leading edge of the base of the anterior mitral leaflet. The maximal peak velocity across the stenotic aortic valve is obtained by interrogating from multiple windows.

contraction and will have a shorter ejection time. The presence of AR in the spectral display diastolic flow signal may also be helpful in distinguishing AS from MR.

The phenomenon of distal pressure recovery is an important issue to keep in mind when considering the Doppler assessment of AS. Hydraulic principles demonstrate that the narrowest segment of the flow stream, the vena contracta, is actually distal to the anatomic valve orifice *(98)*. As the jet expands and decelerates distal to the vena contracta, there is an increase in aortic pressure which is termed pressure recovery. The observed magnitude of pressure recovery in native aortic valves is 5−10 mmHg, unlikely to have a major impact on clinical decision making *(99)*. Therefore, if a manometric pressure is measured in the distal aorta, the pressure difference will be less than one measured in the vena contracta. Continuous wave Doppler detects the maximum velocity and therefore reflects the pressure difference between the left ventricle and the vena contracta.

The Doppler-derived continuity equation for calculation of aortic valve area avoids an invasive procedure and avoids the use of an empirical correction factor *(11, 85, 87, 100–102)*. The principle of conservation of flow dictates that the stroke volume just proximal to the aortic valve is equal to the stroke volume (SV) in the stenotic valve orifice. For laminar flow with a spatially flat velocity profile, $SV = CSA \times VTI$, where CSA in the cross-sectional area of flow (cm^2) and the VTI is the velocity–time integral (cm). The aortic valve area (AVA) can then be calculated by the equation

$$AVA = (V_{LVOT} \times CSA_{LVOT}) / V_{ASJET}$$

V_{LVOT} is the velocity–time integral in the LVOT, measured from an apical five-chamber view using pulse Doppler, with the sample volume approximately 1 cm proximal to the aortic valve. V_{ASJET} is the velocity–time integral of the AS jet. CSA_{LVOT} is the cross-sectional area of the LVOT. In a given patient the outflow tract diameter remains relatively constant over time except when a low-flow/low cardiac output state exists and reduces the diameter. LVOT diameter is measured from a 2-D parasternal long-axis view in a high-resolution zoom view in midsystole. The LVOT diameter is measured from the inner edge of the septal endocardial echo to the leading edge of the base of the anterior mitral leaflet (Fig. 24) The largest source of variability in valve area calculation by the continuity equation lies in the measurement of the left ventricular outflow tract diameter, which is divided by two and then squared. Accurate measurement of the LVOT may not be possible in patients with poor acoustic windows and/or those with heavily calcified valves. The mean coefficient of intraobserver and interobserver measurement variability has been reported at 5.1 and 7.9%, resulting in a valve area variability of $0.15\ cm^2$ for a valve area of $1.0\ cm^2$ *(99)*. Patients with poor acoustic windows and those with heavy aortic valve and annular calcification may prove too difficult to accurately measure the LVOT diameter. For these reasons, the velocity ratio between the AS jet and the LVOT jet is also useful. The velocity ratio V_{LVOT}/V_{AS} less than 0.2 suggests severe aortic stenosis. Many patients with significant AS also have AR, usually mild to moderate in severity. Coexistent AR results in increased transaortic flow and an increase in mean gradient; however, the valve area calculation by the continuity equation remains accurate.

Serial echocardiography is used to follow disease progression in asymptomatic adults with aortic valve stenosis *(see* Table 3). Clinical symptoms predict prognosis not gradients or calculated valve areas. While the rate of hemodynamic progression is highly variable, studies reveal an increase in peak aortic jet velocity from 0.2–0.4 m/s/year, an increase in mean pressure gradient of 6−7 mmHg/year, and a decrease in aortic valve area of 0−0.3.1 cm^2/year *(103–110)*.

In patients with significant left ventricular systolic dysfunction and aortic valve stenosis, determining the severity of the AS can be problematic. Some patients with isolated severe aortic stenosis do not develop adequate hypertrophy to normalize wall stress and present with severe systolic dysfunction due to afterload mismatch. In such patients, a high transvalvular gradient is frequently present, but in rare cases only a modest gradient is seen. More commonly, patients with coexisting aortic valve disease and ischemic heart disease present with ventricular dysfunction and apparent severe AS. In both groups of patients, pressure gradients may be low due to low transaortic volume flow rates, and the calculated valve area may be <1 cm^2 even if the aortic stenosis is not really severe. One approach to this problem is to assess the degree of change in valve area with increasing transaortic flow rates. Dobutamine stress echo (DSE) has been used to distinguish severe from nonsevere valvular aortic stenosis in patients with depressed left ventricular function and low transvalvular gradients *(111)*. Dobutamine is infused in a graded fashion to a maximum dose of 20 mcg/kg/min. At each stage, ventricular function is assessed by 2-D imaging and Doppler data are obtained to reassess mean gradient and to calculate aortic valve area. The three theoretical responses to dobutamine are as follows: (1) transvalvular flow increases significantly, mean gradient increases to >40 mmHg, and valve area remains fixed at <1 cm^2; (2) transvalvular flow increases, mean gradient increases modestly but remains <40 mmHg, and valve area increases to >1 cm^2; (3) no significant change in transaortic flow, mean gradient, or valve area with dobutamine. The patients demonstrating the second type of response have been termed pseudo-severe AS. For those patients unable to augment stroke volume 20% (as assessed by velocity–time integral in the LVOT), prognosis is poor regardless of the severity of the aortic valve stenosis and suggests poor contractile reserve *(111–114)*. In patients with severe AS and a low transvaluvar pressure gradient, does the presence or the absence of LV contractile reserve help to predict operative mortality? Recent studies suggest that those without LV contractile reserve by DSE have a high operative mortality, as high as 33% *(112, 113)*. However, without surgery survival, these patients do very poorly, with survival reported as less than 15% at 3 years *(115)*. In this context, it is important to know whether the presence or the absence of contractile reserve on DSE predicts postoperative functional class, long-term survival, and postoperative ejection fraction. Quere et al. demonstrated that both patients with and without contractile reserve demonstrated a substantial improvement in functional class and ejection fraction, with survival at 2 years 92 and 90%, respectively *(114)*. At our institution, DSE is rarely used in these patients since valve replacement remains the best option for most of the patients despite the high surgical risk.

Mitral Stenosis

In adults the vast majority of mitral stenosis (MS) is due to rheumatic heart disease. Rheumatic MS is characterized echocardiographically by doming of the anterior mitral leaflet, fusion of the valve commissures and varying degrees of leaflet thickening, calcification, and chordal involvement. Instead of the normal tubular orifice, the mitral orifice appears funnel shaped. The leaflets may become thickened and calcified, particularly at the tips. If the mid and base of the leaflets are not involved, the leaflet mobility may be relatively normal apart from the fused commissures. The degree of chordal thickening, shortening, and calcification is variable (Fig. 25). Rheumatic mitral disease is often (but not always) accompanied by rheumatic involvement of the aortic, tricuspid, and rarely pulmonary valves.

Less common causes of MS include mitral annular calcification and congenital causes. Mitral annular calcification is more frequent in elderly patients and those with renal disease. Because it results in rigidity of the annulus, it more commonly results in MR. Infrequently the calcification may involve the leaflets themselves, resulting in MS. A parachute mitral valve is a congenital cause of MS characterized by insertion of all the chordae into a single papillary muscle and can be identified by 2-D parasternal views. This finding often occurs in association with serial left-sided obstructive lesions (Shone's complex), including supramitral ring, subvalvular and valvular AS, and coarctation of the aorta. A double-orifice mitral valve (Fig. 26) is another uncommon congenital condition that can result in either MS or MR *(116)* and is frequently associated with Ebstein's anomaly, coarctation of the aorta, and an atrial septal defect.

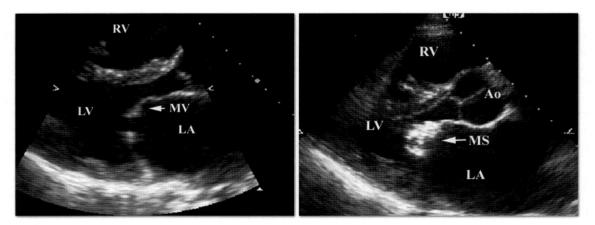

Fig. 25. Two-dimensional imaging in rheumatic mitral stenosis. The *left image* shows mildly thickened valve leaflets that are mobile and no significant calcification of the leaflets or subvalvular apparatus. The *right image* shows heavily thickened and calcified leaflets. Right ventricular dilatation and bowing of the ventricular septum is evident in the *image on the right*, consistent with right ventricular pressure overload.

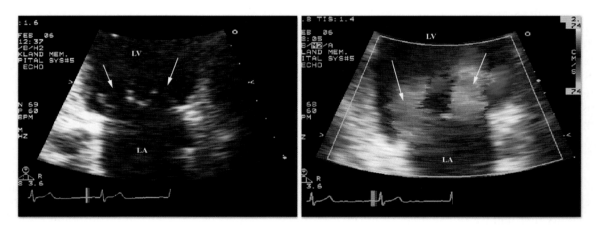

Fig. 26. Apical view of a patient with a double-orifice mitral valve; *arrows* show each orifice. Developmental fusion of the leaflets can lead to an accessory orifice, producing mitral stenosis and/or regurgitation. In up to half of cases the valve remains functionally normal, as in this patient.

The chronic pressure load of mitral stenosis has several consequences, which can be assessed echocardiographically. Over time, increased left atrial pressure results in LA enlargement, a reduction of LA contraction, atrial arrhythmias, and stasis of blood and thrombus formation within the left atrium and the left atrial appendage (Fig. 27). Increased left atrial pressure also leads to pulmonary venous and subsequently pulmonary arterial hypertension. With the advent of pulmonary hypertension, RV dilatation and pressure overload pattern may occur, along with functional TR.

With advances in 2-D echocardiography, M-mode is less routinely used in the evaluation of MS. M-mode findings characteristic of MS include increased echogenicity of the leaflets, reduced separation of the anterior and posterior leaflets, and a decreased E–F slope of mitral valve closure. The decreased E–F slope is nonspecific, however, and may also be present in the setting of impaired LV filling due to diastolic dysfunction.

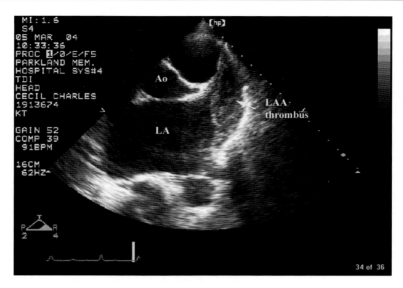

Fig. 27. Transthoracic image of a left atrial appendage thrombus (*arrow*) evident in a modified parasternal short-axis view. Transesophageal imaging should be performed to definitely exclude a thrombus.

Two-dimensional imaging of the diastolic orifice allows for planimetry of the valve area and has been validated with surgical and catheterization-determined valve areas *(117–119)*. Imaging is best performed in the parasternal short-axis view at the level of the mitral valve (Fig. 28). Instrument factors such as gain and transmission power can affect the image; higher gain can result in overstating of the leaflet boundaries and leads to the false appearance of a smaller orifice size.

The transmitral gradient can be determined by CW Doppler of the mitral inflow during diastole (Fig. 29) *(120)*. The magnitude of the pressure gradient depends not only on valve obstruction but also on volume flow rate. For example, an increase in cardiac output, tachycardia, and coexistent MR can all increase the gradient across the mitral valve.

The rate of the pressure gradient decline also provides important information about the severity of stenosis. The pressure half-time, obtained from the CW Doppler inflow signal, measures this rate of decay and is defined as the time (in milliseconds) that the initial pressure gradient decreases to half its maximum value *(121)* (Fig. 30). Studies comparing Doppler half-time data with catheterization-derived Gorlin valve areas found a linear relationship, with a half-time of 220 ms corresponding to a valve area of 1 cm^2, and have subsequently been shown to correlate well with invasive measurements of valve areas *(119, 122, 123)*.

$$\text{MVA} = 220 / PT_{1/2}$$

The mitral pressure half-time is affected by anything that changes left ventricular or atrial compliance or the driving pressure across the LA. Valve area calculation by pressure half-time is generally accurate in the setting of MR, although the early flow volume is dependent on cardiac output and MR. In this setting, the slope more distal to this initial peak velocity should be used in the calculation of pressure half-time. The ability to calculate MVA by pressure half-time is limited by significant coexistent AR. In this situation, if there is a more rapid rise in LV diastolic pressure, a shorter pressure half-time results. Conversely, if severe AR impairs mitral leaflet opening, functional MS may occur in conjunction with anatomical MS, resulting in a longer pressure half-time. However, mild-to-moderate

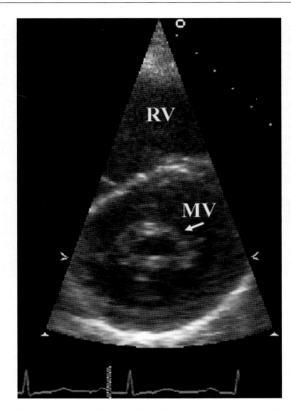

Fig. 28. Parasternal short axis of a rheumatic mitral valve. The commissures are fused, and the leaflets thickened. Careful scanning from the base toward the mitral leaflet tips helps ensure that the smallest orifice is used for planimetry.

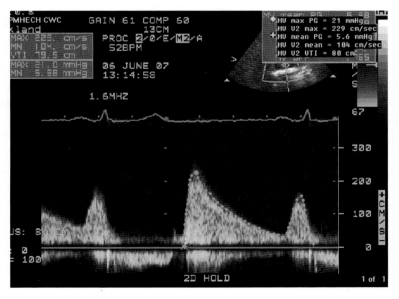

Fig. 29. Continuous wave Doppler of a mildly stenotic mitral valve. An apical approach is best for determining the transmitral gradient of the mitral valve.

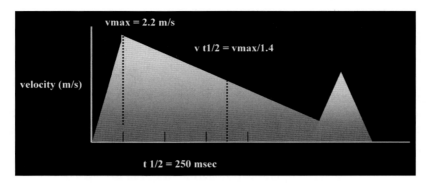

Fig. 30. Schematic representation of the pressure half-time method of calculating the mitral valve area. Using the continuous wave Doppler mitral inflow signal, the pressure half-time is defined as the time in milliseconds that the initial pressure gradient decreases to half its maximum value. The mitral valve area is obtained by dividing the pressure half-time by the constant 220.

AR does not significantly influence the pressure half-time measurement *(124)*. Pressure half-time is not accurate immediately after percutaneous mitral commissurotomy, due to opposing changes in left atrial and left ventricular compliance immediately after the procedure *(125)*. After a period of 72 h, the compliance of each chamber stabilizes and the pressure half-time can again be used for the calculation of mitral valve area.

The continuity equation may also be used for the calculation of the mitral valve area, provided there is no significant MR. Mitral valve area is equal to the transmitral valve stroke volume divided by the velocity–time integral of the MS jet. Mitral valve area calculated by the continuity equation may be less reliable than planimetry, pressure half-time, and PISA methods *(117)*. If MR is present, the transmitral volume flow rate can theoretically be calculated using the proximal isovelocity surface area method (PISA) *(126)*. The product of the cross-sectional area of the aliased boundary and the aliasing velocity equals the volume flow rate. Volumetric flow is then used with the transmitral velocity–time interval in the continuity equation *(127–129)*. The PISA method is rarely used in MS, in part because the single-color image uses the volume flow rate at only one point in diastole rather than integrated over the entire diastolic filling period.

Morphologic assessment of the mitral valve with 2-D imaging provides important information that guides therapy. Valves with significant calcification, chordal shortening, and subvalvular stenosis are not good candidates for percutaneous or surgical commissurotomy. The Wilkins score *(130)* takes into account leaflet thickening, mobility, calcification, and the extent of subvalvular involvement, each graded on a scale of 1 (minimal involvement) to 4 (severe extensive involvement). The Wilkins score has been shown to be predictive of results with mitral commissurotomy *(131)*. The degree of commissural calcification, not incorporated in the Wilkins score, is also very useful in determining appropriate candidates for percutaneous therapy *(132, 133)*. Percutaneous balloon mitral commissurotomy is contraindicated in the presence of moderate or greater MR and when a left atrial thrombus is visualized. Complications of percutaneous balloon mitral commissurotomy identified with echo include worsening of MR, a persistent atrial septal defect at the transseptal site, and cardiac perforation and development of tamponade.

The average reduction in mitral valve area in the setting of rheumatic MS is $0.09 + 0.21$ cm^2/year *(134)*. Predictors of more rapid progression include an echo score >8 and a greater initial gradient. The average reduction in mitral valve area after PBMC is 0.08 cm^2/year by planimetry and 0.06 cm^2/year by pressure half-time. The echo morphology score is the strongest predictor of restenosis *(131)*.

TEE is useful for the assessment of left atrial or left atrial appendage thrombus, particularly before percutaneous mitral commissurotomy. Thrombus within the atrium is considered a contraindication to placement of a transseptal needle and a guidewire into the left atrium. TEE can also be helpful for more definitive quantification of MR, particularly in the setting of heavy calcification when the degree of MR may be underestimated in transthoracic apical views because of acoustic shadowing. A limitation of TEE is underestimation of the degree of chordal involvement in the esophageal views because of masking by the stenotic mitral valve; transgastric views allow better visualization of the subvalvular apparatus. Transesophageal or intracardiac echo can be used during percutaneous balloon mitral commissurotomy to help guide proper position of the transseptal needle and placement of the balloon across the mitral valve. Following inflation, Doppler can be used to assess the presence and severity of MR.

Exercise echocardiography can be useful when a patient's symptoms are out of proportion to the severity of stenosis *(135)*. The restriction in LV diastolic filling in severe MS may result in low stroke volume and relatively low mean pressure gradients. With increases in volume flow rate during exercise, a significant increase in mean transmitral pressure over 15 mmHg or an increase in pulmonary systolic pressure >60 mmHg suggests hemodynamically significant MS, regardless of the resting gradient.

Tricuspid Stenosis

Tricuspid stenosis (TS) is infrequent in adults. Rheumatic disease is the most common etiology and is usually accompanied by mitral valve involvement. Echocardiographically, the rheumatic tricuspid valve appears similar to the rheumatic mitral valve, with diastolic doming of the leaflets (particularly the anterior) commissural fusion and thickening of the leaflet tips and chordae (Fig. 31). The mid portion of the leaflets typically has preserved mobility. Other causes of TS include rare congenital causes and carcinoid. In carcinoid, there is marked thickening and shortening of the TV leaflets involving the entire leaflet length. Two-dimensional imaging demonstrates leaflet immobility during diastole and failure of complete coaptation. In severe cases, the valve may appear in a fixed open position. Because of the large tricuspid valve area, a mean diastolic gradient of 2 mmHg obtained by CW Doppler can establish the diagnosis of TS. A mean gradients as low as 5 mmHg can result in congestive symptoms (Fig. 32). Spectral Doppler shows a prolonged deceleration slope of antegrade flow. Doppler quantification of TS compares well with cardiac catheterization *(136)*.

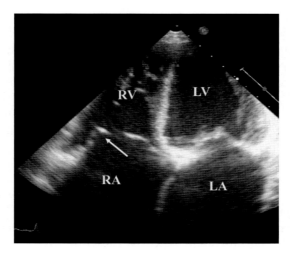

Fig. 31. Apical four-chamber image of a patient with rheumatic tricuspid stenosis. Leaflet thickening and doming, particularly of the anterior leaflet, are evident. The mitral valve is also thickened with reduced excursion. The right ventricle and both atrial are enlarged.

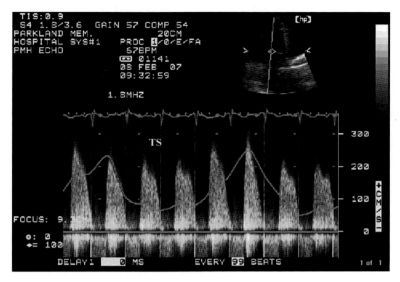

Fig. 32. Continuous wave Doppler across a stenotic tricuspid valve documenting increased velocity. Significant respiratory variation of tricuspid inflow velocities is normal.

Pulmonary Stenosis

Primary pathology of the pulmonary valve is uncommon in the adult population. The most common cause of pulmonary valvular stenosis (PS) is congenital. The leaflets may be thickened and partially fused at the commisures, two cusps may be fused, or there may be a single cone-shaped valve. In congenital PS, the commissures are fused, restricting the orifice distally. On 2-D imaging, the valve cusps appear thickened and dome during systole; valve calcification may be present in adults. Two-dimensional imaging distal to the pulmonary valve is important. Isolated supravalvular or peripheral PS is rare; however, proximal branch pulmonary artery stenosis is common in tetralogy of Fallot and after previous congenital heart surgery. Hemodynamic effects of PS are reflected in RV volume and function. RV enlargement and pressure overload pattern correspond with PS severity. Poststenotic pulmonary artery dilatation may be present but does not appear to correspond with the severity of the PS. Other causes of pulmonary stenosis include rheumatic heart disease, carcinoid and obstructing tumors. When assessing PS, it is important to identify the precise location of the increase in velocity. Using pulsed and continuous wave Doppler allows complete interrogation of the right ventricular outflow tract (RVOT), pulmonary valve, and main and proximal branch pulmonary arteries. RVOT obstruction can occur as a primary abnormality or more commonly due to physiologic hypertrophy, which can be dynamic.

There is good correlation between Doppler and catheter-derived gradients in PS. If the PA is dilated, the PV may be displaced anteriorly, making proper alignment of the Doppler signal difficult. In this setting, the subcostal or suprasternal views can be used for interrogation of the valve gradient.

NEWER TECHNOLOGIES: THREE-DIMENSIONAL ECHOCARDIOGRAPHY

Recent advances in three-dimensional (3-D) echocardiography include the availability of real-time imaging. The potential does exist for the routine use of this technique in the diagnostic evaluation of valvular heart disease *(137)*. Three-dimensional imaging can be performed with both transesophageal and transthoracic probes and has been used in the operating room and during percutaneous balloon mitral commissurotomy *(138)*. It has led to improved insight into the complex geometry of the mitral valve *(139)*, the mechanisms of functional and ischemic MR *(140)*, and the abnormalities in mitral valve prolapse *(141)*, and infective endocarditis *(142)*. Three-dimensional echo can also help guide surgical repair *(143, 144)*. Three-dimensional color-flow imaging of the proximal flow convergence region has been shown to be accurate in quantifying MR and has the theoretical advantages of not relying on the assumption of a hemispheric proximal convergence shape *(145)*. Real-time 3-D echo correlates well with 2-D and Doppler measurements of MS and with invasive measurements during percutaneous balloon mitral commissurotomy *(138, 146–148)*. Three-dimensional determination of aortic valve area in aortic stenosis compares favorably with planimetry by TEE and invasive measurements *(149, 150)*. AR has been less well studied, although 3-D calculation of aortic regurgitant volumes has been validated using an electromagnetic probe in an animal model *(151)*. Descriptions of tricuspid valve morphology by 3-D echocardiography have been reported *(152, 153)*. There is little information on the use of 3-D echo in the evaluation of the pulmonary valve *(154)*. Although 3-D echo has promise in the assessment of valvular heart disease and planning surgical strategies, clinical benefits have not yet been demonstrated in prospective studies.

CONCLUSION

The echocardiographic evaluation for valvular heart disease should be interpreted with knowledge of the clinical context and data at the time of examination. Valve function can be influenced by hemodynamic conditions. Accurate assessment of disease severity requires a comprehensive and an integrative approach of the various parameters by 2-D and Doppler methods to arrive at a coherent assessment. The more concordant the findings are as to severity of the lesion, the more accurate and conclusive is the evaluation.

REFERENCES

1. Sashn DJ. Instrumentation and physical factors related to visualization of stenotic and regurgitant jets by Doppler color flow mapping. J Am Coll Cardiol 1988;12:1354–65.
2. Zoghbi WA, Enriquez-Sarano M, Foster E, et al. Recommendations for evaluation of the severity of native valvular regurgitation with two-dimensional and Doppler echocardiography. J Am Soc Echocardiogr 2003;16:777–802.
3. Zhou X, Jones M, Shiota T, Yamada I, Teien D, Sahn DJ. Vena contracta imaged by Doppler color flow mapping predicts the severity of eccentric mitral regurgitation better than color jet area: a chronic animal study. J Am Coll Cardiol 1997;30:1393–8.
4. Tribouilloy C, Shen WF, Quere JP, et al. Assessment of severity of mitral regurgitation by measuring regurgitant jet width at its origin with transesophageal Doppler color flow imaging. Circulation 1992;85:1248–53.
5. Bargiggia GS, Tronconi L, Sahn DJ, et al. A new method for quantitation of mitral regurgitation based on color flow Doppler imaging of flow convergence proximal to regurgitant orifice. Circulation 1991;84:1481–9.
6. Enriquez-Sarano M, Miller FA, Jr, Hayes SN, Bailey KR, Tajik AJ, Seward JB. Effective mitral regurgitant orifice area: clinical use and pitfalls of the proximal isovelocity surface area method. J Am Coll Cardiol 1995;25:703–9.
7. Utsunomiya T, Patel D, Doshi R, Quan M, Gardin JM. Can signal intensity of the continuous wave Doppler regurgitant jet estimate severity of mitral regurgitation? Am Heart J 1992;123:166–71.
8. Cape EG, Yoganathan AP, Levine RA. Increased heart rate can cause underestimation of regurgitant jet size by Doppler color flow mapping. J Am Coll Cardiol 1993;21:1029–37.
9. Currie PJ, Hagler DJ, Seward JB, et al. Instantaneous pressure gradient: a simultaneous Doppler and dual catheter correlative study. J Am Coll Cardiol 1986;7:800–6.
10. Currie PJ, Seward JB, Reeder GS, et al. Continuous-wave Doppler echocardiographic assessment of severity of calcific aortic stenosis: a simultaneous Doppler-catheter correlative study in 100 adult patients. Circulation 1985;71:1162–9.
11. Zoghbi WA, Farmer KL, Soto JG, Nelson JG, Quinones MA. Accurate noninvasive quantification of stenotic aortic valve area by Doppler echocardiography. Circulation 1986;73:452–9.
12. Skjaerpe T, Hegrenaes L, Hatle L. Noninvasive estimation of valve area in patients with aortic stenosis by Doppler ultrasound and two-dimensional echocardiography. Circulation 1985;72:810–18.
13. Yoshida K, Yoshikawa J, Shakudo M, et al. Color Doppler evaluation of valvular regurgitation in normal subjects. Circulation 1988;78:840–7.
14. Singh JP, Evans JC, Levy D, et al. Prevalence and clinical determinants of mitral, tricuspid, and aortic regurgitation (the Framingham Heart Study). Am J Cardiol 1999;83:897–902.

15. Perry GJ, Helmcke F, Nanda NC, Byard C, Soto B. Evaluation of aortic insufficiency by Doppler color flow mapping. J Am Coll Cardiol 1987;9:952–9.

16. Reynolds T, Abate J, Tenney A, Warner MG. The JH/LVOH method in the quantification of aortic regurgitation: how the cardiac sonographer may avoid an important potential pitfall. J Am Soc Echocardiogr 1991;4:105–8.

17. Tribouilloy CM, Enriquez-Sarano M, Bailey KR, Seward JB, Tajik AJ. Assessment of severity of aortic regurgitation using the width of the vena contracta: a clinical color Doppler imaging study. Circulation 2000;102:558–64.

18. Tribouilloy CM, Enriquez-Sarano M, Fett SL, Bailey KR, Seward JB, Tajik AJ. Application of the proximal flow convergence method to calculate the effective regurgitant orifice area in aortic regurgitation. J Am Coll Cardiol 1998;32:1032–9.

19. Ciobanu M, Abbasi AS, Allen M, Hermer A, Spellberg R. Pulsed Doppler echocardiography in the diagnosis and estimation of severity of aortic insufficiency. Am J Cardiol 1982;49:339–43.

20. Rokey R, Sterling LL, Zoghbi WA, et al. Determination of regurgitant fraction in isolated mitral or aortic regurgitation by pulsed Doppler two-dimensional echocardiography. J Am Coll Cardiol 1986;7:1273–8.

21. Touche T, Prasquier R, Nitenberg A, de Zuttere D, Gourgon R. Assessment and follow-up of patients with aortic regurgitation by an updated Doppler echocardiographic measurement of the regurgitant fraction in the aortic arch. Circulation 1985;72:819–24.

22. Teague SM, Heinsimer JA, Anderson JL, et al. Quantification of aortic regurgitation utilizing continuous wave Doppler ultrasound. J Am Coll Cardiol 1986;8:592–9.

23. Labovitz AJ, Ferrara RP, Kern MJ, Bryg RJ, Mrosek DG, Williams GA. Quantitative evaluation of aortic insufficiency by continuous wave Doppler echocardiography. J Am Coll Cardiol 1986;8:1341–7.

24. Tribouilloy C, Avinee P, Shen WF, Rey JL, Slama M, Lesbre JP. End diastolic flow velocity just beneath the aortic isthmus assessed by pulsed Doppler echocardiography: a new predictor of the aortic regurgitant fraction. Br Heart J 1991;65:37–40.

25. Borer JS, Bonow RO. Contemporary approach to aortic and mitral regurgitation. Circulation 2003;108:2432–8.

26. Bonow RO, Lakatos E, Maron BJ, Epstein SE. Serial long-term assessment of the natural history of asymptomatic patients with chronic aortic regurgitation and normal left ventricular systolic function. Circulation 1991;84:1625–35.

27. Klodas E, Enriquez-Sarano M, Tajik AJ, Mullany CJ, Bailey KR, Seward JB. Aortic regurgitation complicated by extreme left ventricular dilation: long-term outcome after surgical correction. J Am Coll Cardiol 1996;27:670–7.

28. Turina J, Milincic J, Seifert B, Turina M. Valve replacement in chronic aortic regurgitation. True predictors of survival after extended follow-up. Circulation 1998;98:II100–6; discussion II6–7.

29. Tornos P, Sambola A, Permanyer-Miralda G, Evangelista A, Gomez Z, Soler-Soler J. Long-term outcome of surgically treated aortic regurgitation: influence of guideline adherence toward early surgery. J Am Coll Cardiol 2006;47:1012–17.

30. Michel PL, Iung B, Abou Jaoude S, et al. The effect of left ventricular systolic function on long term survival in mitral and aortic regurgitation. J Heart Valve Dis 1995;4(Suppl 2):S160–8; discussion S8–9.

31. Tarasoutchi F, Grinberg M, Spina GS, et al. Ten-year clinical laboratory follow-up after application of a symptom-based therapeutic strategy to patients with severe chronic aortic regurgitation of predominant rheumatic etiology. J Am Coll Cardiol 2003;41:1316–24.

32. Ishii K, Hirota Y, Suwa M, Kita Y, Onaka H, Kawamura K. Natural history and left ventricular response in chronic aortic regurgitation. Am J Cardiol 1996;78:357–61.

33. Tornos MP, Olona M, Permanyer-Miralda G, et al. Clinical outcome of severe asymptomatic chronic aortic regurgitation: a long-term prospective follow-up study. Am Heart J 1995;130:333–9.

34. Bonow RO, Carabello B, de Leon AC, Jr, et al. Guidelines for the management of patients with valvular heart disease: executive summary. A report of the American College of Cardiology/American Heart Association Task Force on Practice Guidelines (Committee on Management of Patients with Valvular Heart Disease). Circulation 1998;98:1949–84.

35. Bonow RO, Carabello BA, Kanu C, et al. ACC/AHA 2006 guidelines for the management of patients with valvular heart disease: a report of the American College of Cardiology/American Heart Association Task Force on Practice Guidelines (writing committee to revise the 1998 guidelines for the management of patients with valvular heart disease): developed in collaboration with the Society of Cardiovascular Anesthesiologists: endorsed by the Society for Cardiovascular Angiography and Interventions and the Society of Thoracic Surgeons. Circulation 2006;114:e84–231.

36. Helmcke F, Nanda NC, Hsiung MC, et al. Color Doppler assessment of mitral regurgitation with orthogonal planes. Circulation 1987;75:175–83.

37. Chen CG, Thomas JD, Anconina J, et al. Impact of impinging wall jet on color Doppler quantification of mitral regurgitation. Circulation 1991;84:712–20.

38. Enriquez-Sarano M, Tajik AJ, Bailey KR, Seward JB. Color flow imaging compared with quantitative Doppler assessment of severity of mitral regurgitation: influence of eccentricity of jet and mechanism of regurgitation. J Am Coll Cardiol 1993;21:1211–19.

39. Hall SA, Brickner ME, Willett DL, Irani WN, Afridi I, Grayburn PA. Assessment of mitral regurgitation severity by Doppler color flow mapping of the vena contracta. Circulation 1997;95:636–42.

40. Heinle SK, Hall SA, Brickner ME, Willett DL, Grayburn PA. Comparison of vena contracta width by multi-plane transesophageal echocardiography with quantitative Doppler assessment of mitral regurgitation. Am J Cardiol 1998;81:175–9.

41. Baumgartner H, Schima H, Kuhn P. Value and limitations of proximal jet dimensions for the quantitation of valvular regurgitation: an in vitro study using Doppler flow imaging. J Am Soc Echocardiogr 1991;4:57–66.

42. Kizilbash AM, Willett DL, Brickner ME, Heinle SK, Grayburn PA. Effects of afterload reduction on vena contracta width in mitral regurgitation. J Am Coll Cardiol 1998;32:427–31.

43. Schwammenthal E, Chen C, Benning F, Block M, Breithardt G, Levine RA. Dynamics of mitral regurgitant flow and orifice area. Physiologic application of the proximal flow convergence method: clinical data and experimental testing. Circulation 1994;90:307–22.

44. Pu M, Prior DL, Fan X, et al. Calculation of mitral regurgitant orifice area with use of a simplified proximal convergence method: initial clinical application. J Am Soc Echocardiogr 2001;14:180–5.

45. Utsunomiya T, Doshi R, Patel D, et al. Calculation of volume flow rate by the proximal isovelocity surface area method: simplified approach using color Doppler zero baseline shift. J Am Coll Cardiol 1993;22:277–82.

46. Enriquez-Sarano M, Sinak LJ, Tajik AJ, Bailey KR, Seward JB. Changes in effective regurgitant orifice throughout systole in patients with mitral valve prolapse. A clinical study using the proximal isovelocity surface area method. Circulation 1995;92:2951–8.

47. Enriquez-Sarano M, Seward JB, Bailey KR, Tajik AJ. Effective regurgitant orifice area: a noninvasive Doppler development of an old hemodynamic concept. J Am Coll Cardiol 1994;23:443–51.

48. Kizilbash AM, Hundley WG, Willett DL, Franco F, Peshock RM, Grayburn PA. Comparison of quantitative Doppler with magnetic resonance imaging for assessment of the severity of mitral regurgitation. Am J Cardiol 1998;81:792–5.

49. Dujardin KS, Enriquez-Sarano M, Bailey KR, Nishimura RA, Seward JB, Tajik AJ. Grading of mitral regurgitation by quantitative Doppler echocardiography: calibration by left ventricular angiography in routine clinical practice. Circulation 1997;96:3409–15.

50. Thomas L, Foster E, Schiller NB. Peak mitral inflow velocity predicts mitral regurgitation severity. J Am Coll Cardiol 1998;31:174–9.

51. Klein AL, Obarski TP, Stewart WJ, et al. Transesophageal Doppler echocardiography of pulmonary venous flow: a new marker of mitral regurgitation severity. J Am Coll Cardiol 1991;18:518–26.

52. Pu M, Griffin BP, Vandervoort PM, et al. The value of assessing pulmonary venous flow velocity for predicting severity of mitral regurgitation: a quantitative assessment integrating left ventricular function. J Am Soc Echocardiogr 1999;12:736–43.

53. Tice FD, Heinle SK, Harrison JK, et al. Transesophageal echocardiographic assessment of reversal of systolic pulmonary venous flow in mitral stenosis. Am J Cardiol 1995;75:58–60.

54. MacIsaac AI, McDonald IG, Kirsner KL, Graham SA, Gill RW. Quantification of mitral regurgitation by integrated Doppler backscatter power. J Am Coll Cardiol 1994;24:690–5.

55. Enriquez-Sarano M, Tajik AJ, Schaff HV, Orszulak TA, Bailey KR, Frye RL. Echocardiographic prediction of survival after surgical correction of organic mitral regurgitation. Circulation 1994;90:830–7.

56. Crawford MH, Souchek J, Oprian CA, et al. Determinants of survival and left ventricular performance after mitral valve replacement. Department of Veterans Affairs Cooperative Study on Valvular Heart Disease. Circulation 1990;81:1173–81.

57. Phillips HR, Levine FH, Carter JE, et al. Mitral valve replacement for isolated mitral regurgitation: analysis of clinical course and late postoperative left ventricular ejection fraction. Am J Cardiol 1981;48:647–54.

58. Enriquez-Sarano M, Tajik AJ, Schaff HV, et al. Echocardiographic prediction of left ventricular function after correction of mitral regurgitation: results and clinical implications. J Am Coll Cardiol 1994;24:1536–43.

59. Ling LH, Enriquez-Sarano M, Seward JB, et al. Clinical outcome of mitral regurgitation due to flail leaflet. N Engl J Med 1996;335:1417–23.

60. Armstrong GP, Griffin BP. Exercise echocardiographic assessment in severe mitral regurgitation. Coron Artery Dis 2000;11:23–30.

61. Enriquez-Sarano M, Schaff HV, Orszulak TA, Tajik AJ, Bailey KR, Frye RL. Valve repair improves the outcome of surgery for mitral regurgitation. A multivariate analysis. Circulation 1995;91:1022–8.

62. Lambert AS, Miller JP, Merrick SH, et al. Improved evaluation of the location and mechanism of mitral valve regurgitation with a systematic transesophageal echocardiography examination. Anesth Analg 1999;88:1205–12.

63. Enriquez-Sarano M, Freeman WK, Tribouilloy CM, et al. Functional anatomy of mitral regurgitation: accuracy and outcome implications of transesophageal echocardiography. J Am Coll Cardiol 1999;34:1129–36.

64. Freed LA, Levy D, Levine RA, et al. Prevalence and clinical outcome of mitral-valve prolapse. N Engl J Med 1999;341:1–7.

65. Perloff JK, Child JS, Edwards JE. New guidelines for the clinical diagnosis of mitral valve prolapse. Am J Cardiol 1986;57:1124–9.

66. Nishimura RA, McGoon MD, Shub C, Miller FA, Jr, Ilstrup DM, Tajik AJ. Echocardiographically documented mitral-valve prolapse. Long-term follow-up of 237 patients. N Engl J Med 1985;313:1305–9.

67. Marks AR, Choong CY, Sanfilippo AJ, Ferre M, Weyman AE. Identification of high-risk and low-risk subgroups of patients with mitral-valve prolapse. N Engl J Med 1989;320:1031–6.

68. Zuppiroli A, Mori F, Favilli S, et al. Arrhythmias in mitral valve prolapse: relation to anterior mitral leaflet thickening, clinical variables, and color Doppler echocardiographic parameters. Am Heart J 1994;128:919–27.

69. Klein AL, Burstow DJ, Tajik AJ, et al. Age-related prevalence of valvular regurgitation in normal subjects: a comprehensive color flow examination of 118 volunteers. J Am Soc Echocardiogr 1990;3:54–63.

70. Feigenbaum H, Armstrong WF, Ryan T. Feigenbaum's Echocardiography (6th ed.). Philadelphia: Lippincott Williams and Wilkins; 2005.

71. Lang RM, Bierig M, Devereux RB, et al. Recommendations for chamber quantification: a report from the American Society of Echocardiography's Guidelines and Standards Committee and the Chamber Quantification Writing Group, developed in conjunction with the European Association of Echocardiography, a branch of the European Society of Cardiology. J Am Soc Echocardiogr 2005;18:1440–63.

72. Grossmann G, Stein M, Kochs M, et al. Comparison of the proximal flow convergence method and the jet area method for the assessment of the severity of tricuspid regurgitation. Eur Heart J 1998;19:652–9.

73. Gonzalez-Vilchez F, Zarauza J, Vazquez de Prada JA, et al. Assessment of tricuspid regurgitation by Doppler color flow imaging: angiographic correlation. Int J Cardiol 1994;44:275–83.

74. Yamachika S, Reid CL, Savani D, et al. Usefulness of color Doppler proximal isovelocity surface area method in quantitating valvular regurgitation. J Am Soc Echocardiogr 1997;10:159–68.

75. Shapira Y, Porter A, Wurzel M, Vaturi M, Sagie A. Evaluation of tricuspid regurgitation severity: echocardiographic and clinical correlation. J Am Soc Echocardiogr 1998;11:652–9.

76. Rivera JM, Vandervoort P, Mele D, Weyman A, Thomas JD. Value of proximal regurgitant jet size in tricuspid regurgitation. Am Heart J 1996;131:742–7.

77. Tribouilloy CM, Enriquez-Sarano M, Bailey KR, Tajik AJ, Seward JB. Quantification of tricuspid regurgitation by measuring the width of the vena contracta with Doppler color flow imaging: a clinical study. J Am Coll Cardiol 2000;36:472–8.

78. Minagoe S, Rahimtoola SH, Chandraratna PA. Significance of laminar systolic regurgitant flow in patients with tricuspid regurgitation: a combined pulsed-wave, continuous-wave Doppler and two-dimensional echocardiographic study. Am Heart J 1990;119:627–35.

79. Goldberg SJ, Allen HD. Quantitative assessment by Doppler echocardiography of pulmonary or aortic regurgitation. Am J Cardiol 1985;56:131–5.

80. Dittrich HC, McCann HA, Walsh TP, et al. Transesophageal echocardiography in the evaluation of prosthetic and native aortic valves. Am J Cardiol 1990;66:758–61.

81. Hoffmann R, Flachskampf FA, Hanrath P. Planimetry of orifice area in aortic stenosis using multiplane transesophageal echocardiography. J Am Coll Cardiol 1993;22:529–34.

82. Tribouilloy C, Shen WF, Peltier M, Mirode A, Rey JL, Lesbre JP. Quantitation of aortic valve area in aortic stenosis with multiplane transesophageal echocardiography: comparison with monoplane transesophageal approach. Am Heart J 1994;128:526–32.

83. Stoddard MF, Arce J, Liddell NE, Peters G, Dillon S, Kupersmith J. Two-dimensional transesophageal echocardiographic determination of aortic valve area in adults with aortic stenosis. Am Heart J 1991;122:1415–22.

84. Hegrenaes L, Hatle L. Aortic stenosis in adults. Non-invasive estimation of pressure differences by continuous wave Doppler echocardiography. Br Heart J 1985;54:396–404.

85. Galan A, Zoghbi WA, Quinones MA. Determination of severity of valvular aortic stenosis by Doppler echocardiography and relation of findings to clinical outcome and agreement with hemodynamic measurements determined at cardiac catheterization. Am J Cardiol 1991;67:1007–12.

86. Yeager M, Yock PG, Popp RL. Comparison of Doppler-derived pressure gradient to that determined at cardiac catheterization in adults with aortic valve stenosis: implications for management. Am J Cardiol 1986;57:644–8.

87. Otto CM, Pearlman AS, Gardner CL, et al. Experimental validation of Doppler echocardiographic measurement of volume flow through the stenotic aortic valve. Circulation 1988;78:435–41.

88. Harrison MR, Gurley JC, Smith MD, Grayburn PA, DeMaria AN. A practical application of Doppler echocardiography for the assessment of severity of aortic stenosis. Am Heart J 1988;115:622–8.

89. Simpson IA, Houston AB, Sheldon CD, Hutton I, Lawrie TD. Clinical value of Doppler echocardiography in the assessment of adults with aortic stenosis. Br Heart J 1985;53:636–9.

90. Stamm RB, Martin RP. Quantification of pressure gradients across stenotic valves by Doppler ultrasound. J Am Coll Cardiol 1983;2:707–18.

91. Yoganathan AP, Valdes-Cruz LM, Schmidt-Dohna J, et al. Continuous-wave Doppler velocities and gradients across fixed tunnel obstructions: studies in vitro and in vivo. Circulation 1987;76:657–66.

92. Hatle L, Angelsen BA, Tromsdal A. Non-invasive assessment of aortic stenosis by Doppler ultrasound. Br Heart J 1980;43:284–92.

93. Callahan MJ, Tajik AJ, Su-Fan Q, Bove AA. Validation of instantaneous pressure gradients measured by continuous-wave Doppler in experimentally induced aortic stenosis. Am J Cardiol 1985;56:989–93.

94. Smith MD, Dawson PL, Elion JL, et al. Correlation of continuous wave Doppler velocities with cardiac catheterization gradients: an experimental model of aortic stenosis. J Am Coll Cardiol 1985;6:1306–14.

95. Otto CM, Pearlman AS. Doppler echocardiography in adults with symptomatic aortic stenosis. Diagnostic utility and cost-effectiveness. Arch Intern Med 1988;148:2553–60.

96. Otto CM, Davis KB, Holmes DR, Jr, et al. Methodologic issues in clinical evaluation of stenosis severity in adults undergoing aortic or mitral balloon valvuloplasty. The NHLBI Balloon Valvuloplasty Registry. Am J Cardiol 1992;69:1607–16.

97. Otto CM, Pearlman AS, Comess KA, Reamer RP, Janko CL, Huntsman LL. Determination of the stenotic aortic valve area in adults using Doppler echocardiography. J Am Coll Cardiol 1986;7:509–17.

98. Yoganathan AP. Fluid mechanics of aortic stenosis. Eur Heart J 1988;9(Suppl E):13–17.

99. Otto CM. The Practice of Clinical Echocardiography (2nd ed.). Philadelphia: WB Saunders; 2002.

100. Grayburn PA, Smith MD, Harrison MR, Gurley JC, DeMaria AN. Pivotal role of aortic valve area calculation by the continuity equation for Doppler assessment of aortic stenosis in patients with combined aortic stenosis and regurgitation. Am J Cardiol 1988;61:376–81.

101. Teirstein P, Yeager M, Yock PG, Popp RL. Doppler echocardiographic measurement of aortic valve area in aortic stenosis: a noninvasive application of the Gorlin formula. J Am Coll Cardiol 1986;8:1059–65.

102. Otto CM. The difficulties in assessing patients with moderate aortic stenosis. Heart 1999;82:5–6.

103. Lester SJ, McElhinney DB, Miller JP, Lutz JT, Otto CM, Redberg RF. Rate of change in aortic valve area during a cardiac cycle can predict the rate of hemodynamic progression of aortic stenosis. Circulation 2000;101: 1947–52.

104. Bahler RC, Desser DR, Finkelhor RS, Brener SJ, Youssefi M. Factors leading to progression of valvular aortic stenosis. Am J Cardiol 1999;84:1044–8.

105. Rosenhek R, Binder T, Porenta G, et al. Predictors of outcome in severe, asymptomatic aortic stenosis. N Engl J Med 2000;343:611–17.

106. Otto CM, Pearlman AS, Gardner CL. Hemodynamic progression of aortic stenosis in adults assessed by Doppler echocardiography. J Am Coll Cardiol 1989;13:545–50.

107. Roger VL, Tajik AJ, Bailey KR, Oh JK, Taylor CL, Seward JB. Progression of aortic stenosis in adults: new appraisal using Doppler echocardiography. Am Heart J 1990;119:331–8.

108. Faggiano P, Ghizzoni G, Sorgato A, et al. Rate of progression of valvular aortic stenosis in adults. Am J Cardiol 1992;70:229–33.

109. Peter M, Hoffmann A, Parker C, Luscher T, Burckhardt D. Progression of aortic stenosis. Role of age and concomitant coronary artery disease. Chest 1993;103:1715–19.

110. Palta S, Pai AM, Gill KS, Pai RG. New insights into the progression of aortic stenosis: implications for secondary prevention. Circulation 2000;101:2497–502.

111. deFilippi CR, Willett DL, Brickner ME, et al. Usefulness of dobutamine echocardiography in distinguishing severe from nonsevere valvular aortic stenosis in patients with depressed left ventricular function and low transvalvular gradients. Am J Cardiol 1995;75:191–4.

112. Nishimura RA, Grantham JA, Connolly HM, Schaff HV, Higano ST, Holmes DR, Jr. Low-output, low-gradient aortic stenosis in patients with depressed left ventricular systolic function: the clinical utility of the dobutamine challenge in the catheterization laboratory. Circulation 2002;106:809–13.

113. Monin JL, Monchi M, Gest V, Duval-Moulin AM, Dubois-Rande JL, Gueret P. Aortic stenosis with severe left ventricular dysfunction and low transvalvular pressure gradients: risk stratification by low-dose dobutamine echocardiography. J Am Coll Cardiol 2001;37:2101–7.

114. Quere JP, Monin JL, Levy F, et al. Influence of preoperative left ventricular contractile reserve on postoperative ejection fraction in low-gradient aortic stenosis. Circulation 2006;113:1738–44.

115. Monin JL, Quere JP, Monchi M, et al. Low-gradient aortic stenosis: operative risk stratification and predictors for long-term outcome: a multicenter study using dobutamine stress hemodynamics. Circulation 2003;108:319–24.

116. Trowitzsch E, Bano-Rodrigo A, Burger BM, Colan SD, Sanders SP. Two-dimensional echocardiographic findings in double orifice mitral valve. J Am Coll Cardiol 1985;6:383–7.

117. Faletra F, Pezzano A, Jr, Fusco R, et al. Measurement of mitral valve area in mitral stenosis: four echocardiographic methods compared with direct measurement of anatomic orifices. J Am Coll Cardiol 1996;28:1190–7.

118. Henry WL, Griffith JM, Michaelis LL, McIntosh CL, Morrow AG, Epstein SE. Measurement of mitral orifice area in patients with mitral valve disease by real-time, two-dimensional echocardiography. Circulation 1975; 51:827–31.

119. Smith MD, Handshoe R, Handshoe S, Kwan OL, DeMaria AN. Comparative accuracy of two-dimensional echocardiography and Doppler pressure half-time methods in assessing severity of mitral stenosis in patients with and without prior commissurotomy. Circulation 1986;73:100–7.

120. Holen J, Simonsen S. Determination of pressure gradient in mitral stenosis with Doppler echocardiography. Br Heart J 1979;41:529–35.

121. Hatle L, Angelsen B, Tromsdal A. Noninvasive assessment of atrioventricular pressure half-time by Doppler ultrasound. Circulation 1979;60:1096–104.

122. Come PC, Riley MF, Diver DJ, Morgan JP, Safian RD, McKay RG. Noninvasive assessment of mitral stenosis before and after percutaneous balloon mitral valvuloplasty. Am J Cardiol 1988;61:817–25.

123. Chen CG, Wang YP, Guo BL, Lin YS. Reliability of the Doppler pressure half-time method for assessing effects of percutaneous mitral balloon valvuloplasty. J Am Coll Cardiol 1989;13:1309–13.

124. Robiolio PA, Rigolin VH, Harrison JK, Kisslo KB, Bashore TM. Doppler pressure half-time method of assessing mitral valve area: aortic insufficiency does not adversely affect validity. Am Heart J 1998;136:718–23.

125. Thomas JD, Wilkins GT, Choong CY, et al. Inaccuracy of mitral pressure half-time immediately after percutaneous mitral valvotomy. Dependence on transmitral gradient and left atrial and ventricular compliance. Circulation 1988;78:980–93.

126. Bennis A, Drighil A, Tribouilloy C, Drighil A, Chraibi N. Clinical application in routine practice of the proximal flow convergence method to calculate the mitral surface area in mitral valve stenosis. Int J Cardiovasc Imaging 2002;18:443–51.

127. Rifkin RD, Harper K, Tighe D. Comparison of proximal isovelocity surface area method with pressure half-time and planimetry in evaluation of mitral stenosis. J Am Coll Cardiol 1995;26:458–65.

128. Oku K, Utsunomiya T, Mori H, Yamachika S, Yano K. Calculation of mitral valve area in mitral stenosis using the proximal isovelocity surface area method. Comparison with two-dimensional planimetry and Doppler pressure half time method. Jpn Heart J 1997;38:811–19.

129. Centamore G, Galassi AR, Evola R, Lupo L, Galassi A. The "proximal isovelocity surface area" method in assessing mitral valve area in patients with mitral stenosis and associated aortic regurgitation. G Ital Cardiol 1997;27:133–40.

130. Wilkins GT, Weyman AE, Abascal VM, Block PC, Palacios IF. Percutaneous balloon dilatation of the mitral valve: an analysis of echocardiographic variables related to outcome and the mechanism of dilatation. Br Heart J 1988;60:299–308.

131. Wang A, Krasuski RA, Warner JJ, et al. Serial echocardiographic evaluation of restenosis after successful percutaneous mitral commissurotomy. J Am Coll Cardiol 2002;39:328–34.

132. Sutaria N, Northridge DB, Shaw TR. Significance of commissural calcification on outcome of mitral balloon valvotomy. Heart 2000;84:398–402.

133. Cannan CR, Nishimura RA, Reeder GS, et al. Echocardiographic assessment of commissural calcium: a simple predictor of outcome after percutaneous mitral balloon valvotomy. J Am Coll Cardiol 1997;29:175–80.

134. Gordon SP, Douglas PS, Come PC, Manning WJ. Two-dimensional and Doppler echocardiographic determinants of the natural history of mitral valve narrowing in patients with rheumatic mitral stenosis: implications for follow-up. J Am Coll Cardiol 1992;19:968–73.

135. Cheriex EC, Pieters FA, Janssen JH, de Swart H, Palmans-Meulemans A. Value of exercise Doppler-echocardiography in patients with mitral stenosis. Int J Cardiol 1994;45:219–26.

136. Ha JW, Chung N, Jang Y, Rim SJ. Tricuspid stenosis and regurgitation: Doppler and color flow echocardiography and cardiac catheterization findings. Clin Cardiol 2000;23:51–2.

137. Mumm B, Baumann R, Hyca M. Three-dimensional echo for the assessment of valvular heart disease. Cardiol Clin 2007;25:283–95.

138. Zamorano J, Perez de Isla L, Sugeng L, et al. Non-invasive assessment of mitral valve area during percutaneous balloon mitral valvuloplasty: role of real-time 3D echocardiography. Eur Heart J 2004;25:2086–91.

139. Sugeng L, Coon P, Weinert L, et al. Use of real-time 3-dimensional transthoracic echocardiography in the evaluation of mitral valve disease. J Am Soc Echocardiogr 2006;19:413–21.

140. Kwan J, Shiota T, Agler DA, et al. Geometric differences of the mitral apparatus between ischemic and dilated cardiomyopathy with significant mitral regurgitation: real-time three-dimensional echocardiography study. Circulation 2003;107:1135–40.

141. Ahmed S, Nanda NC, Miller AP, et al. Usefulness of transesophageal three-dimensional echocardiography in the identification of individual segment/scallop prolapse of the mitral valve. Echocardiography 2003;20:203–9.

142. Schwalm SA, Sugeng L, Raman J, Jeevanandum V, Lang RM. Assessment of mitral valve leaflet perforation as a result of infective endocarditis by 3-dimensional real-time echocardiography. J Am Soc Echocardiogr 2004;17:919–22.

143. Delabays A, Jeanrenaud X, Chassot PG, Von Segesser LK, Kappenberger L. Localization and quantification of mitral valve prolapse using three-dimensional echocardiography. Eur J Echocardiogr 2004;5:422–9.

144. Macnab A, Jenkins NP, Bridgewater BJ, et al. Three-dimensional echocardiography is superior to multiplane transesophageal echo in the assessment of regurgitant mitral valve morphology. Eur J Echocardiogr 2004;5:212–22.

145. Iwakura K, Ito H, Kawano S, et al. Comparison of orifice area by transthoracic three-dimensional Doppler echocardiography versus proximal isovelocity surface area (PISA) method for assessment of mitral regurgitation. Am J Cardiol 2006;97:1630–7.

146. Zamorano J, Cordeiro P, Sugeng L, et al. Real-time three-dimensional echocardiography for rheumatic mitral valve stenosis evaluation: an accurate and novel approach. J Am Coll Cardiol 2004;43:2091–6.

147. Xie MX, Wang XF, Cheng TO, Wang J, Lu Q. Comparison of accuracy of mitral valve area in mitral stenosis by real-time, three-dimensional echocardiography versus two-dimensional echocardiography versus Doppler pressure half-time. Am J Cardiol 2005;95:1496–9.

148. Sugeng L, Weinert L, Lammertin G, et al. Accuracy of mitral valve area measurements using transthoracic rapid freehand 3-dimensional scanning: comparison with noninvasive and invasive methods. J Am Soc Echocardiogr 2003;16:1292–300.

149. Ge S, Warner JG, Jr, Abraham TP, et al. Three-dimensional surface area of the aortic valve orifice by three-dimensional echocardiography: clinical validation of a novel index for assessment of aortic stenosis. Am Heart J 1998;136:1042–50.

150. Menzel T, Mohr-Kahaly S, Kolsch B, et al. Quantitative assessment of aortic stenosis by three-dimensional echocardiography. J Am Soc Echocardiogr 1997;10:215–23.

151. Shiota T, Jones M, Tsujino H, et al. Quantitative analysis of aortic regurgitation: real-time 3-dimensional and 2-dimensional color Doppler echocardiographic method – a clinical and a chronic animal study. J Am Soc Echocardiogr 2002;15:966–71.

152. Faletra F, La Marchesina U, Bragato R, De Chiara F. Three dimensional transthoracic echocardiography images of tricuspid stenosis. Heart 2005;91:499.

153. Schnabel R, Khaw AV, von Bardeleben RS, et al. Assessment of the tricuspid valve morphology by transthoracic real-time-3D-echocardiography. Echocardiography 2005;22:15–23.

154. Citro R, Salustri A, Gregorio G. Images in cardiovascular medicine. Three-dimensional reconstruction of pulmonary valve endocarditis. Ital Heart J 2001;2:938–9.

155. Douglas PS, Khandheria B, Stainback RF, et al. ACCF/ASE/ACEP/ASNC/SCAI/SCCT/SCMR 2007 appropriateness criteria for transthoracic and transesophageal echocardiography: a report of the American College of Cardiology Foundation Quality Strategic Directions Committee Appropriateness Criteria Working Group, American Society of Echocardiography, American College of Emergency Physicians, American Society of Nuclear Cardiology, Society for Cardiovascular Angiography and Interventions, Society of Cardiovascular Computed Tomography, and the Society for Cardiovascular Magnetic Resonance endorsed by the American College of Chest Physicians and the Society of Critical Care Medicine. *J Am Coll Cardiol* 2007;50:187–204.

156. Cheitlin MD, Armstrong WF, Aurigemma GP, et al. ACC/AHA/ASE 2003 guideline update for the Clinical Application of Echocardiography: summary article. A report of the American College of Cardiology/American Heart Association Task Force on Practice Guidelines (ACC/AHA/ASE Committee to Update the 1997 Guidelines for the Clinical Application of Echocardiography). *J Am Soc Echocardiogr* 2003;16:1091–110.

7   Aortic Stenosis

Paul Sorajja and Rick A. Nishimura

ETIOLOGY

Aortic stenosis is a hereditary or acquired disease in which there is progressive obstruction to left ventricular outflow. The long-standing increased afterload results in pressure hypertrophy of the left ventricle, leading to symptoms of angina, dyspnea, and syncope. It is important to diagnose and assess the severity of aortic stenosis, for severe symptomatic aortic stenosis left untreated has a poor prognosis *(1)* . Proper diagnosis and treatment of aortic stenosis results in improvement of symptoms and prolongation of life.

The most common cause of aortic obstruction is valvular stenosis. However, supravalvular and discrete subvalvular aortic stenosis may occur and need to be differentiated from intrinsic valve disease, since the timing and the type of treatment differ for these less-common causes of outflow obstruction.

Supravalvular Aortic Stenosis

Supravalvular aortic stenosis is a congenital abnormality consisting of narrowing of the ascending aorta immediately superior to the aortic valve (Fig. 1). This narrowing may consist of a single discrete stenosis or a long tubular lesion of the entire ascending aorta. Supravalvular aortic stenosis is uncommon, accounting for less than 1% of patients with aortic stenosis. Supravalvular stenosis may be associated with other congenital abnormalities such as coronary dysplasia, elfin facies, mental retardation, coarctation of the aorta, hypercalcemia, and peripheral pulmonic stenosis. There is a high prevalence of supravalvular aortic stenosis in Williams Syndrome, which is due to an autosomal dominant mutation in the elastin gene. The diagnosis of supravalvular aortic stenosis should be suspected clinically when there is a thrill felt in the right carotid artery but not in the left carotid artery, due to the high-velocity jet of blood directed toward the innominate artery. Imaging of the entire

From: *Contemporary Cardiology: Valvular Heart Disease*
Edited by: Andrew Wang, Thomas M. Bashore, DOI 10.1007/978-1-59745-411-7_7
© Humana Press, a part of Springer Science+Business Media, LLC 2009

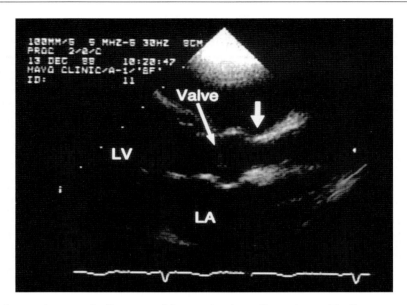

Fig. 1. Supravalvular aortic stenosis. Parasternal long-axis view of a patient with discrete supravalvular aortic stenosis (*thick arrow*). LA, left atrium; LV, left ventricle.

ascending aorta, either by magnetic resonance or computed tomographic angiography, confirms the diagnosis. Operation usually consists of replacement of the ascending aorta, depending on the extent of narrowing.

Subvalvular Aortic Stenosis

Subvalvular aortic stenosis occurs in less than 10% of all patients presenting with aortic stenosis. It can be due to a discrete subvalvular ridge or diffuse tunnel-like narrowing of the entire outflow tract (Fig. 2). In the presence of severe hypertrophy of the left ventricle, additional dynamic outflow

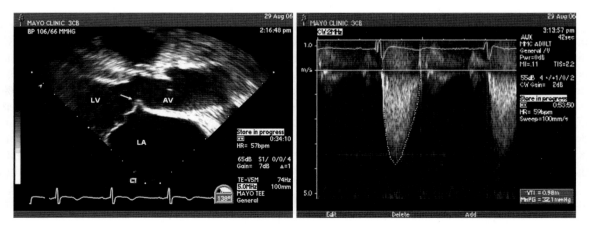

Fig. 2. Subaortic stenosis. *Left,* Transesophageal echocardiogram showing a discrete subaortic membrane (*arrow*) below the aortic valve (AV). LA, left atrium; LV, left ventricle. *Right,* Subaortic gradient from the same patient (mean, 32 mmHg).

obstruction from systolic anterior motion of the mitral valve may occur. Aortic regurgitation frequently accompanies subvalvular aortic stenosis due to valve damage from the high-velocity jet emanating from the subvalvular stenosis. Subvalvular aortic stenosis should be suspected on echocardiography when there is a high velocity across the left ventricular outflow tract in the absence of immobile aortic valve cusps. Treatment is surgical myectomy and direct resection of the subvalvular ridge. Operation should be performed for severe obstruction associated with symptoms. However, operation may also be reasonable for the asymptomatic patient, as resection may be "curative" and prevent progressive aortic valve regurgitation.

Valvular Aortic Stenosis

The most common location of aortic stenosis is obstruction at the level of the valve. The etiology of valvular aortic stenosis depends upon the age at which the patient presents. Patients with symptomatic aortic stenosis in their teens or early twenties usually have a congenital abnormality, such as a unicuspid or a fused bicuspid valve. Middle-aged patients in their forties to sixties who present with symptomatic valvular aortic stenosis usually have a calcified bicuspid valve or a valve previously damaged by rheumatic heart disease (Fig. 3).

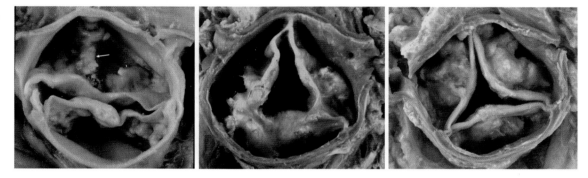

Fig. 3. Gross pathological specimens from patients with aortic stenosis of three different etiologies. *Left*, Bicuspid aortic stenosis. Two cusps (anterior and posterior) are present. *Arrow* indicates a calcified raphe. *Middle*, Rheumatic aortic stenosis. Two commissures are fused, in addition to prominent fibrosis and calcification. *Right*, Degenerative aortic stenosis. Extensive calcification is present in the valve pockets, with preservation of the commissures. Courtesy, Dr. William D. Edwards, Mayo Clinic.

Bicuspid aortic valve is the most common congenital heart disease, occurring in approximately 2% of the population *(2)*. It can lead to stenosis or regurgitation over time but may remain with minimal hemodynamic effects for decades. Bicuspid aortic stenosis is the most common reason for aortic valve replacement in patients aged <70 years. Importantly, bicuspid aortic stenosis is associated with a generalized aortopathy due to fragmentation of the fibers of the elastic media. This aortopathy can present as coarctation, aortic dilation, or dissection.

In older patients, the most common cause of aortic stenosis is senile degenerative aortic stenosis. These patients commonly present with symptoms in their seventies or eighties, due to progressive degenerative changes with calcific deposits at the base of the aortic valve cusps (Fig. 3). Calcific valvular aortic stenosis is now thought to be a part of a generalized atherosclerotic process and is frequently found in conjunction with coronary artery and cerebrovascular disease. It is an active disease process characterized by lipid accumulation, inflammation, and calcification *(3–6)*.

PATHOPHYSIOLOGY

The pathophysiology of valvular aortic stenosis is one of progressive obstruction and the resultant compensatory changes. With increasing left ventricular outflow tract obstruction, there is pressure hypertrophy of the left ventricle (7). Left ventricular cavity size and systolic function is initially maintained, as the increase in left ventricular wall thickness acts as a compensatory mechanism to normalize wall stress (Fig. 4). The development of pressure hypertrophy is initially a beneficial adaptation. However, this hypertrophy may result in reduced coronary flow reserve and oxygen supply–demand mismatch (8). These hypertrophied hearts are also more sensitive to diffuse subendocardial ischemic injury, which may result in both systolic and diastolic dysfunction. In elderly women, there may be an inappropriate degree of myocardial hypertrophy, which leads to a high perioperative morbidity and mortality (9).

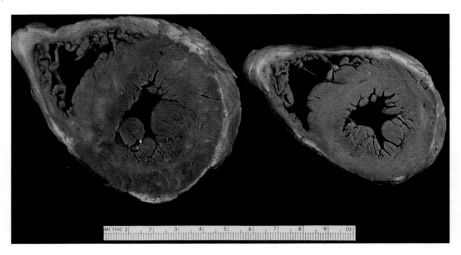

Fig. 4. Pressure hypertrophy of the left ventricle due to aortic valvular stenosis. *Left,* Severe concentric hypertrophy in a patient who had severe aortic stenosis. Patchy subendocardial fibrosis is also present. *Right,* Normal heart, for comparison. Courtesy, Dr. William D. Edwards, Mayo Clinic.

As the obstruction progresses to a critical level, the high afterload "overwhelms" the left ventricle and systolic function begins to decrease. With continued severe afterload excess, myocyte degeneration and fibrosis occurs and produces irreversible left ventricular systolic dysfunction. In these patients, both the high afterload and the intrinsic myocardial disease significantly increase wall stress and a vicious cycle of deterioration in ventricular function ensues.

Many patients with aortic stenosis will remain asymptomatic for years, even with severe obstruction. Symptoms of angina, dyspnea, and syncope occur after a long latent period and are due to multiple mechanisms. Angina pectoris may occur due to diffuse subendocardial ischemia from abnormalities of coronary flow and flow reserve, progressive hypertrophy resulting in myocardial oxygen supply–demand mismatch, and severe abnormalities of diastolic dysfunction (8). Diastolic dysfunction occurs from prolonged ventricular relaxation caused by myocyte hypertrophy and afterload excess, as well as an increase in myocardial stiffness from hypertrophied myocytes and interstitial fibrosis (10, 11). Dyspnea results from the high left atrial pressure generated by the diastolic filling abnormalities. Syncope is usually due to abnormal vasodepressor reflexes caused by the high left ventricular intracavitary pressures. Once systolic dysfunction is present, severe heart failure symptoms occur. Secondary pulmonary hypertension may subsequently lead to signs and symptoms of right-sided heart failure.

It is important to determine the severity of aortic stenosis based upon hemodynamic measurements. The outcome of these patients is related to the severity of the lesion at diagnosis, indicating that aortic stenosis does represent a disease continuum. The following criteria have been defined by the ACC/AHA Valvular Heart Disease guidelines committee and are based upon outcome data from natural history studies *(12)* :

Severity of aortic stenosis	Aortic valve area (cm^2)	Mean gradient (mmHg)	Peak velocity (m/s)
Mild	>1.5	<25	<3.0
Moderate	1–1.5	25–40	3.0–4.0
Severe	<1.0	>40	>4.0
Critical	<0.6	>60	>5.0

*In very small or large patients, it may be necessary to use a valve area indexed to body surface area. Severe aortic stenosis is defined in this manner as <0.5 cm^2/m^2.

Although there are now well-defined categories of hemodynamic severity, therapeutic decisions should not be based upon a single hemodynamic value. It is always necessary to take into consideration the patient's presenting symptoms and concomitant factors such as the status of the left ventricle when deciding upon timing of operation.

CLINICAL MANIFESTATIONS

Clinical Presentation

Many patients with aortic stenosis will remain asymptomatic for decades. The diagnosis of aortic stenosis is usually made in the asymptomatic patient on the basis of a systolic murmur on auscultation and confirmed by echocardiography. Symptoms, when they occur, usually consist of one or more of the classic triad of exertional dyspnea, angina, and syncope. Following symptom onset, there is a high mortality rate with an average survival of 2–3 years. The development of symptoms therefore is a critical point in the natural history of patients with aortic stenosis. Sudden death rarely is the initial manifestation of severe aortic stenosis, occurring at a rate of less than 1% per year in asymptomatic patients.

Patients with aortic stenosis may undergo sudden hemodynamic deterioration. This can occur from the onset of rapid atrial fibrillation, with loss of atrial contraction and abbreviated diastolic filling times. Hypotension and pulmonary edema may result and emergency cardioversion is required. Other patients may deteriorate due to hypotension from vasodilators, anesthetic agents, blood loss, or even vagal reactions. In patients with severe aortic stenosis, any element of systemic hypotension can lead to decrease in perfusion of the coronary arteries, myocardial ischemia, further reduction in cardiac output, and further decreases in aortic diastolic pressures. Rapid reversal of this "death spiral" is essential and should be done with vasoconstrictors that raise systemic pressure and restore coronary perfusion.

Physical Examination

The physical examination is important for diagnosis and estimation of severity of aortic stenosis. The contour of the carotid upstroke is a reliable indicator of the severity of aortic stenosis in most patients. There will be both *parvus* (small pulse) and *tardus* (slow upstroke) in patients with severe aortic stenosis. In older patients with a noncompliant vasculature, there may not be the typical findings on carotid palpation. The jugular venous pressure will usually be normal in the absence of end-stage left ventricular systolic dysfunction. A sustained bifid left ventricular impulse indicates concomitant left ventricular hypertrophy. A systolic thrill, if present, indicates the presence of severe aortic stenosis, usually with a mean gradient >50 mmHg.

Accurate auscultation is an essential component of evaluating patients with aortic stenosis. An absent aortic component of the second heart sound indicates severe calcification of the aortic valve. A fourth heart sound is frequently audible, indicating the increased workload in the left atrium imposed by the diagnostic filling abnormalities of the left ventricle. The turbulence across the aortic valve always produces a systolic ejection murmur. It is not necessarily the intensity but the timing of the murmur that determines the severity of aortic stenosis. In those patients with mild aortic stenosis, the murmur has an early peak and the duration ends before the second heart sound. As aortic stenosis becomes more severe, the peak intensity of the murmur occurs in mid-to-late systole, and the murmur extends into the second heart sound.

CLINICAL ASSESSMENT

Electrocardiography and Chest Radiography

The electrocardiographic findings in patients with aortic stenosis are usually that of left ventricular hypertrophy and left atrial enlargement. If atrial fibrillation is present, concomitant mitral valve disease or thyroid disease should be considered. The chest X-ray may demonstrate enlargement of the ascending aorta and a left ventricular predominance. The lateral view is essential to look for calcification of the ascending aorta (i.e., porcelain aorta), which poses high risk for operation *(13)* .

Echocardiography

Two-dimensional and Doppler echocardiography is the imaging modality of choice for the diagnosis and quantification of aortic stenosis. Two-dimensional echocardiography allows the determination of the location of the obstruction (supravalvular, valvular, or subvalvular). In some patients with discrete subvalvular aortic stenosis, transesophageal echocardiography may be required for further definition. Short-axis images from two-dimensional echocardiography demonstrate the number of aortic cusps and the degree of cusp fusion or restricted cusp opening in valvular aortic stenosis. Overall, a heavily calcified aortic valve with restricted opening is usually seen with severe stenosis (Fig. 5). However, the visual appearance and motion of the aortic valve does not always correlate with severity. A noncalcified severely stenotic bicuspid valve may appear to open fully on short-axis view due to the "doming" that occurs (Fig. 6). A heavily calcified aortic valve may have only mild stenosis.

Two-dimensional echocardiography is also useful for determining the status of the left ventricle and the degree of hypertrophy. Left atrial enlargement indicates concomitant diastolic dysfunction. The

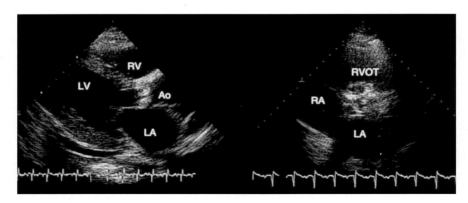

Fig. 5. Senile degenerative aortic stenosis on echocardiography. *Left,* Parasternal long-axis view. *Right,* Parasternal short-axis view. AV, aortic valve; LA, left atrium; LV, left ventricle.

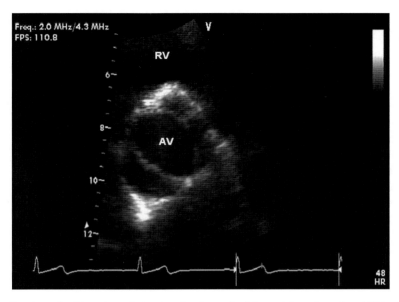

Fig. 6. Bicuspid aortic stenosis. Parasternal short-axis view of a bicuspid aortic valve (AV) showing the typical bowing aortic cusps. RV, right ventricle.

presence of other valvular abnormalities (aortic regurgitation or mitral/tricuspid valve disease) can also be determined by echocardiography. Patients with a bicuspid valve frequently have an associated aortopathy, manifested by aortic dilatation, aortic dissection, or coarctation of the aorta. Thus, visualization and Doppler interrogation of the ascending and descending aorta is an important part of the echocardiographic examination.

Although the presence of aortic stenosis can be reliably made by two-dimensional echocardiography, the severity of aortic stenosis cannot be determined by visualization of valve motion alone. Therefore, Doppler echocardiography must be used to further assess the severity of aortic stenosis. The velocity obtained by continuous wave Doppler across the aortic valve provides an accurate and reproducible measurement of valve gradient by application of the modified Bernoulli equation

$$\text{Pressure gradient (mmHg)} = 4v^2$$

where v is the peak Doppler velocity (m/s).

Both the maximal instantaneous gradient and the mean aortic valve gradient can be derived from continuous wave Doppler velocity. However, this does require a detailed meticulous study using multiple sites of interrogation in order to ensure that the Doppler beam is parallel to the stenotic jet. One of the major pitfalls of Doppler echocardiography is underestimation of the gradient when the Doppler beam is not parallel to the aortic velocity jet.

Using the continuity equation, the aortic valve area can be calculated noninvasively by Doppler echocardiography. The left ventricular outflow tract (LVOT) diameter is measured from the parasternal long-axis view and converted to the LVOT area. From an apical approach with pulsed-wave Doppler, the LVOT velocity is obtained and traced to derive the time–velocity integral (TVI). The following formula is then used for calculation of aortic valve area:

Continuity equation

$$\text{Aortic valve area} = \frac{(\text{LVOT}_{\text{TVI}}) \times (\text{LVOT}_{\text{area}})}{(\text{AV}_{\text{TVI}})}$$

Calculation of aortic valve area does require a skilled echocardiographer to ensure accurate measurement of the LVOT diameter and proper positioning of the same volume in the outflow tract. Small errors in diameter measurement result in significant errors in the calculation of area. In each patient, there needs to be a correlation between the valve gradient, the valve area, and the stroke volume.

Cardiac Catheterization

The principal indication for invasive assessment is when there is a discrepancy in the severity of aortic stenosis between the clinical and echocardiographic findings. Proper performance of right heart catheterization for cardiac output determination is essential for the assessment of aortic stenosis in the cardiac laboratory. The assessment of the severity of aortic stenosis requires accurate measurement of the left ventricular and ascending aortic pressures and of cardiac output. Indicator dilution and the Fick method constitute the main techniques for measurement of cardiac output in the catheterization laboratory.

FORMULA FOR CARDIAC OUTPUT BY FICK

$$\text{Cardiac output } (1/\text{min}) = \frac{\text{Oxygen consumption(ml/min)}}{(A - VO_2) \bullet 1.34 \text{ ml/g} \bullet \text{Hgb (g/dl)} \bullet 10 \text{ (dl/l)}}$$

where $A - V\ O_2$ is the difference in oxygen saturation between the arterial and the venous circulation.

Cardiac output using the indicator dilution method is inaccurate in the presence of significant bradycardia or tachycardia, significant valvular regurgitation, and irregular rhythms. The Fick method overcomes these limitations, but its accuracy requires a steady state and thus it cannot be used for the measurement of acute changes (e.g., during pharmacologic interventions or exercise). The Fick method requires measurement of myocardial oxygen consumption. When possible, both methods should be performed in an individual study to identify outlier results.

The left ventricular and ascending aortic pressures should be measured simultaneously, either via two arterial accesses or via a single arterial access and a transseptal puncture for left ventricular pressure (Fig. 7). The left ventricular pressure should be obtained with an end-hole catheter with only two side holes such as a multipurpose or Rodriguez catheter. A Judkins coronary catheter should not be used. Without side holes, catheter entrapment may occur. Erroneous measurements also may arise if there are multiple side holes more proximally, particularly in the presence of intraventricular pressure gradients. The mean aortic valve gradient alone can be used to help define the severity of aortic valvular stenosis in patients with a normal cardiac output in the absence of significant aortic regurgitation (mild, <25 mmHg; moderate, 25–40 mmHg; severe, >40 mmHg).

The pullback of a single catheter from the left ventricle to the aorta may sometimes be performed to determine the peak-to-peak systolic gradient. However, the peak-to-peak gradient is not physiologic as it is derived from nonsimultaneous recordings (Fig. 7). The peak-to-peak gradient may approximate the true mean aortic valve gradient in some circumstances, particularly at high-pressure gradients (>50 mmHg). However, the peak-to-peak gradient does not accurately reflect lower aortic valve gradients and may be erroneous in patients with irregular arrhythmia or low cardiac output. In some laboratories, the femoral artery pressure obtained from the sidearm of the sheath is substituted for the ascending aortic pressure. Errors in aortic valve assessment with this method occur because of the time delay for the pressure wave to travel from the ascending aorta to the periphery and because of the overshoot phenomenon that is characteristic of peripheral artery pressures (Fig. 8).

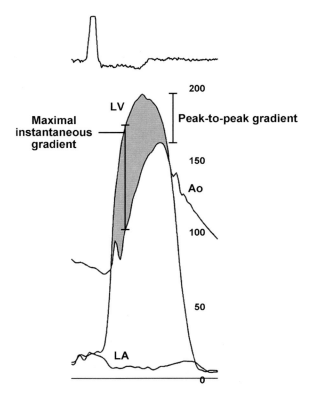

Fig. 7. Aortic valve gradients. Maximum instantaneous gradient is the maximum pressure difference at any time between the left ventricle and the aorta. "Peak-to-peak" is a nonsimultaneous measure of the aortic and left ventricular pressure difference. Shaded area is the area of planimetry for calculation of mean valvular gradient. Ao, aortic pressure; LA, left atrial pressure; LV, left ventricular pressure. Reprinted with permission from Cardiovascular Medicine, 3rd edition, Sorajja P and Nishimura RA, Assessment and therapy of valvular heart disease in the catheterization laboratory, pp. 463–486, with permission from Springer-Verlag London Limited.

Gorlin and Gorlin originally derived the formula for calculation of stenotic valve areas in 1951 *(14)*:

Gorlin equation

$$\text{Arotic valve area} \left(\text{cm}^2\right) = \frac{\text{low (ml/sec)}}{44.3 \bullet C \bullet \sqrt{\Delta P}}$$

where ΔP is the mean transvalvular pressure gradient (mmHg) and C is an empirical constant. For aortic valve area calculations, C is assumed to be 1.0. *Flow* refers to absolute forward flow across the valve expressed in millimeters per second and is derived from the cardiac output and the duration of forward flow, which is the systolic ejection period for the aortic valve. Overall, the variability in valve area calculation using the Gorlin equation is ±0.2 cm². Greater errors in using the Gorlin equation occur in patients with bradycardia or tachycardia and when there is significant regurgitation.

Hakki and coworkers derived a simplified version of the Gorlin equation *(15)*. In this derivation, they observed that the product of heart rate, forward flow, and the Gorlin constants approximated 1 for most calculations.

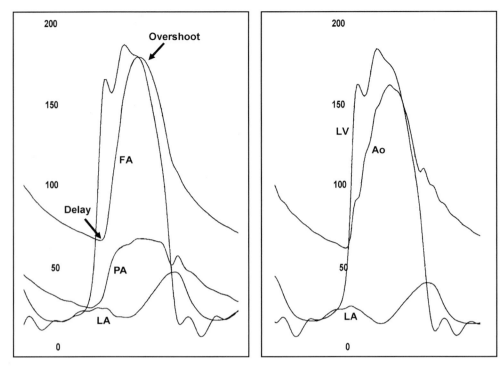

Fig. 8. Central aortic and peripheral arterial pressure tracings from one patient with aortic stenosis. *Left*, Simultaneous left ventricular (LV), left atrial (LA), pulmonary artery (PA), and femoral artery (FA) recordings. There is a temporal delay in the femoral artery tracing because of the transmission of pressure from the central aorta to the periphery. This delay can lead to under- or overestimation of the gradient and erroneous calculation of the aortic valve area. Also, due to the femoral artery overshoot, there does not appear to be a "peak-to-peak" gradient. *Right*, Simultaneous left ventricular (LV), ascending aortic (Ao), and left atrial (LA) recordings from the same patient. Note the presence of the aortic valve gradient that was not evident on the tracings on the left-hand side. Reprinted with permission from Cardiovascular Medicine, 3rd edition, Sorajja P and Nishimura RA, Assessment and therapy of valvular heart disease in the catheterization laboratory, pp. 463–486, with permission from Springer-Verlag London Limited.

Hakki equation

$$\text{Valve area}\left(\text{cm}^2\right) = \frac{\text{Cardiac output (L/min)}}{\sqrt{\Delta P}}$$

As in the Gorlin equation, the mean pressure gradient is used for the calculation of the valve area using the Hakki equation. Similar to the Gorlin equation, the major limitation of the Hakki equation occurs in patients with bradycardia, tachycardia, or coexistent regurgitation.

An Integrated Approach to Diagnosis

The evaluation of aortic stenosis is based upon the history, the physical examination, and a comprehensive echocardiography. For most patients, two-dimensional echocardiography readily identifies the calcified stenotic aortic valve, and Doppler echocardiography reliably estimates the severity of aortic stenosis in the majority of patients. However, errors may occur in the noninvasive assessment of the severity of the stenosis, mainly from poor alignment of the Doppler signal with the aortic jet, which results in underestimation of the gradient. This underestimation is the most common error in the noninvasive evaluation of aortic stenosis, especially in less-experienced laboratories. Rarely, the severity of aortic stenosis is overestimated, such as when a mitral regurgitation jet is erroneously identified as that due to aortic stenosis. In addition, the modified Bernoulli equation may not be applicable in the presence of severe anemia, a high cardiac output state, or concomitant subvalvular obstruction. In these instances, the modified Bernoulli cannot be applied as contribution from flow acceleration or viscous friction cannot be ignored.

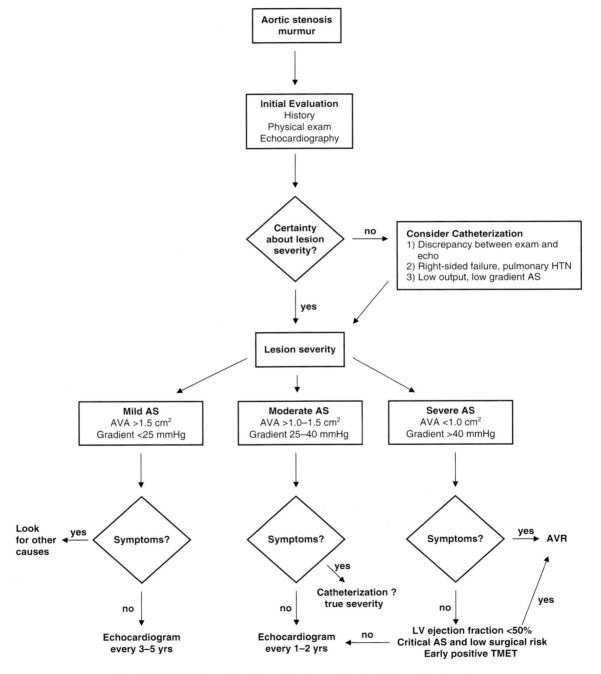

Fig. 9. Clinical algorithm for evaluating patients with aortic stenosis.

Asymptomatic patients who have findings on physical examination of mild aortic stenosis need no further testing if the aortic valve opens >10 mm on two-dimensional imaging and the mean gradient is <25 mmHg on Doppler echocardiography. Similarly, no further hemodynamic evaluation is required when there are findings of severe aortic stenosis on clinical examination and the mean gradient by echocardiography is >40 mmHg, as the degree of aortic stenosis should be severe (Fig. 9). However, when there is a significant discrepancy between the bedside findings and those found on echocardiography, cardiac catheterization may be required to complete the hemodynamic evaluation.

There may be patients who have echocardiographic findings consistent with only mild aortic stenosis but have symptoms or the physical examination would suggest more severe aortic stenosis. There may be patients who have echocardiographic features of severe aortic stenosis, yet the physical examination is not consistent with severe stenosis. In these cases, cardiac catheterization is required to further evaluate the true severity of aortic stenosis.

There are other instances in which a hemodynamic cardiac catheterization is warranted. These situations usually arise when the hemodynamics obtained by echocardiography are not congruent with the diagnosis of isolated aortic stenosis. Patients with severe pulmonary hypertension should undergo concomitant catheterization to examine other etiologies of pulmonary hypertension, such as intrinsic pulmonary vascular disease or mitral valve disease. Cardiac catheterization may also be required for patients who present with an enlarged right ventricle on echocardiography. Isolated aortic stenosis itself should not result in severe pulmonary hypertension or right heart failure unless there is severe left ventricular systolic dysfunction.

Most patients with concomitant mitral regurgitation will not require further diagnostic testing if the mitral valve morphology is normal on two-dimensional echocardiography. In these patients, the high left ventricular pressure from the outflow tract obstruction will lead to an increase in the severity of mitral regurgitation. Intraoperative transesophageal echocardiography should be performed following aortic valve replacement to determine whether residual mitral regurgitation will require additional operative intervention. Alternatively, those patients who have significant structural abnormalities of the mitral valve may require additional operative intervention on the mitral valve. A left ventriculogram should not be performed in patients with severe aortic stenosis, as this may cause acute hemodynamic compromise.

NATURAL HISTORY

The natural history of patients with aortic stenosis is dependent upon the severity of this stenosis as well as concomitant comorbid problems. Patients usually do not develop symptoms or impaired survival until the degree of aortic stenosis is at least moderately severe. Survival begins to shorten when the peak Doppler aortic valve velocity is >4 m/s, corresponding to a mean valve gradient of >40 mmHg. Once the patient becomes symptomatic with severe aortic stenosis, the outlook is poor. With the onset of heart failure, there is a 50% 2-year mortality. With the onset of angina or syncope, there is a 50% 3- to 5-year mortality (1, 16). In patients with aortic stenosis and left ventricular dysfunction, the prognosis is dismal if left untreated. Depressed ejection function from afterload excess improves after aortic valve replacement in many patients.

The prognosis of patients with *asymptomatic* severe aortic stenosis has been difficult to elucidate, resulting in more controversy regarding appropriate timing of treatment. Sudden death may occur in these patients, but the incidence is less than 1% per year. Nevertheless, aortic stenosis is a progressive disease and symptoms develop with a high frequency once the stenosis becomes severe. For asymptomatic patients with a Doppler velocity of >4 m/s, the event-free survival is only 20–33% at 3–5-year follow-up (Fig. 10) (17–19). Event-free survival is worse in patients with heavily calcified valves, documented rapid rate of progression, and older patients with concurrent coronary atherosclerosis. These observations have implications for timing of valve surgery in the asymptomatic patient.

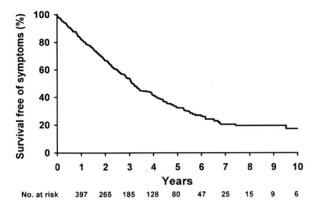

Fig. 10. Outcome of patients with asymptomatic severe aortic stenosis. Survival free of symptoms is shown with censoring at the time of aortic valve surgery. The probability of remaining free of cardiac events, including cardiac death and aortic valve surgery, was only 63% at 2 years. Reprinted with permission from Pellikka PA et al. *(19)* with permission from Lippincott Williams & Wilkins.

The rate of progression of aortic stenosis is highly variable. Once moderate aortic stenosis is present, the average increase in valve gradient is 7 mmHg per year and the average decrease in valve area is 0.1 cm^2 per year *(20)*. Progression of aortic stenosis may be dependent upon underlying atherosclerotic processes and can be more rapid in senile calcific valve disease than in congenital or rheumatic disease *(18)*.

MANAGEMENT

The management of patients with aortic stenosis depends upon the severity of aortic stenosis and the presence or absence of symptoms (Fig. 11). In patients with only mild stenosis and no symptoms, management is continued observation. Serial echocardiography should be performed every 3–5 years in

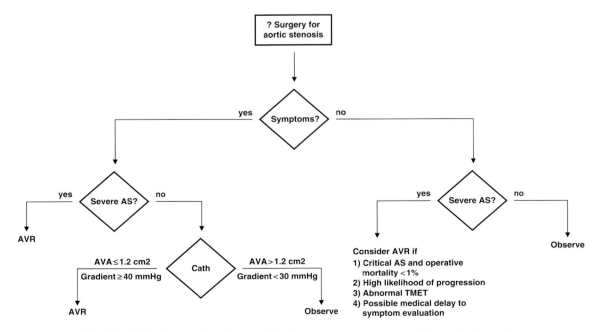

Fig. 11. Clinical algorithm for considering surgery in patients with aortic stenosis.

patients with mild aortic stenosis and every 1–2 years in those with moderate stenosis. Prompt echocardiography should be performed anytime there is new symptom onset. Infective endocarditis prophylaxis should be followed. Patients with moderate-to-severe aortic stenosis should avoid athletics, which require high dynamic and static muscular demands. There are no proven medical treatments to slow or prevent disease progression. However, aggressive lipid lowering therapy may be of benefit, especially in patients with less-severe valve calcification, and will ameliorate progression of vascular atherosclerosis that frequently coexists and increases their comorbidity.

Symptomatic Patient

Patients with symptoms and severe aortic stenosis should be considered for operation with aortic valve replacement. Delays to surgery have been associated with poorer outcome following operation (21). Over the past two decades, the risk of operation has decreased substantially. Isolated aortic valve replacement in a patient less than 70 years old should be able to be performed with a risk of less than 1%. The risk should be less than 2–3% among septuagenarians and even less than 5% in octogenarians in the absence of significant comorbidities. Therefore, age is not a contraindication to surgery (22). Concomitant coronary artery bypass grafting should be performed for coronary atherosclerosis when epicardial lesions are >50%.

Asymptomatic Patient

The treatment of the asymptomatic patient with severe aortic stenosis is more controversial. When there is left ventricular dysfunction, valve replacement is indicated even in asymptomatic patients. In these patients, the critical increase in afterload has started to overwhelm the compensatory mechanisms of left ventricular hypertrophy and the outcome is poor without surgical intervention.

In patients with normal systolic function, the initial ACC/AHA Guidelines for Valvular Heart Disease initially considered aortic valve replacement to be a Class III indication in asymptomatic patients. However, longitudinal studies have now shown poor event-free survival patients with severe aortic stenosis, even if asymptomatic (17–19). Importantly, aortic valve replacement can also now be done with a low operative mortality and there is enhanced durability of the new prostheses. Thus, surgery is reasonable to consider in asymptomatic patients when there is critical aortic stenosis (gradient >60 mmHg and valve area <0.6 cm^2) and the expected operative mortality is <1.0%. Aortic valve replacement may also be considered for adults with severe asymptomatic aortic stenosis if there is evidence or high likelihood of rapid progression or when there may be delayed rapid access to medical care if symptoms arose. Progression of aortic stenosis may be considered rapid when the Doppler peak velocity increases by >0.3 m/s per year or when the valve area decreases by >0.1 cm^2 per year (17, 8).

Treadmill testing may be appropriate in further risk stratifying patients with asymptomatic severe aortic stenosis. Exercise testing is relatively safe if done under strict monitored conditions and may provide incremental information to the initial history. Exercise testing should never be performed in a symptomatic patient with aortic stenosis. However, it may be beneficial in the patient who does not admit to symptoms yet has a limited exercise capacity on objective stress testing. These patients are truly symptomatic and should be considered for operation. In addition, patients who have an abnormal blood pressure response (<20 mmHg rise) or develop ST segment abnormalities with exercise are at higher risk for events (23–26). In one study, symptom-free survival at 2 years was 19% in "asymptomatic" patients with an abnormal exercise testing versus 85% in patients with normal exercise tolerance and no abnormalities (27). Thus, exercise testing can identify patients who may benefit from prophylactic aortic valve replacement.

Therapeutic Challenges

THE ELDERLY PATIENT

Octogenarians now represent the most rapidly expanding segment of the general population. In the United States, it is predicted that the number of individuals older than 80 years of age will increase from 6.9 million in 1990 to 25 million by the year 2050 *(28)*. Calcific aortic stenosis increases in prevalence with age and is extremely common in this age group. In a random population sampling in Finland, severe aortic valve calcification was present in 7% of persons aged between 55 and 71 years and in 17% of persons older than 80 years of age *(29)*. Furthermore, among persons between 75 and 86 years of age, 2.9% had severe aortic stenosis (valve area <0.8 cm^2) *(29)*.

The elderly patient with severe aortic stenosis poses a therapeutic challenge. In considering elderly patients for aortic valve replacement, important factors include the presence of symptoms, physiologic age, patient expectations, anticipated future activities, and comorbidity. Both patients and their families must have a clear understanding of not only the anticipated benefits but also the possible complications of surgery, particularly neurologic events. Cerebrovascular disease is a common comorbidity that significantly influences postoperative outcome. Approximately one-fourth of patients with aortic stenosis will have either asymptomatic or symptomatic cerebrovascular disease.

The operation itself carries a higher risk than in younger patients. Extensive calcification of the aorta and annulus as well as fragile tissue presents significant technical difficulties for the surgeon. In addition, particularly in women, the aortic root and annulus may be small and require concomitant enlargement to accommodate the valve prosthesis. Furthermore, protruding arch atheroma occurs in one-fifth of patients >65 years of age and significantly increases the risk of stroke and mortality during cardiac surgery *(30)*.

Historically, the perioperative mortality for patients older than 80 years of age undergoing aortic valve replacement ranged from 10 to 20% *(31–35)*. Over the past two decades, however, the perioperative risk has improved significantly. The current mortality for nonreoperative surgery in this age group ranges from 5 to 8% but decreases to 3% for patients with isolated aortic stenosis and no significant comorbidities *(36–39)*. Major postoperative complications, nevertheless, remain high, with the incidence of permanent stroke between 4 and 6%. Rehabilitation can also be a problem, as elderly patients take longer to recover from surgery. In one study, prolonged hospital stay (>14 days) occurred in 28% of patients >80 years of age following aortic valve replacement *(37)*.

Nonetheless, survival has clearly improved in these elderly patients with severe symptomatic aortic stenosis who undergo aortic valve replacement. Survival is 80–85% at 1 year and 60–70% at 5 years, which is similar to an age- and sex-matched population without aortic valve disease *(37, 39, 40)*. Most patients report improved functional capacity and quality of life, with more than 90% of patients feeling better after surgery *(41, 42)*. Thus, operation should not be withheld due to age. However, the risks and benefits of the operation need to be discussed in detail with the patient and family.

LOW-OUTPUT, LOW-GRADIENT AORTIC STENOSIS

Patients with aortic stenosis may present with a low cardiac output and low valvular gradient (<30 mmHg) due to concomitant left ventricular systolic dysfunction *(43–46)*. The aortic valve area measures to be in the severe range (<1.0 cm^2) and often is <0.7 cm^2. In these instances, the small aortic valve area may represent either (1) end-stage critical aortic stenosis or (2) mild aortic stenosis and cardiomyopathy due to another etiology. In the latter instance, the left ventricle does not have enough power to fully open the aortic valve, resulting in a low "calculated" valve area that erroneously suggests severe intrinsic valvular stenosis.

Importantly, it is never "too late" to operate on a patient with severe aortic stenosis even in the presence of left ventricular dysfunction. Thus, one must determine whether or not the aortic stenosis is truly severe. In these patients, dobutamine stress is performed either during echocardiography or in the cardiac catheterization laboratory (Fig. 12) *(43–45)*. The purpose of dobutamine is to attempt to normalize the cardiac output. When the cardiac output can be normalized and the mean gradient exceeds 40 mmHg, severe valvular aortic stenosis is present and the patient should undergo surgery. However, if the cardiac output is normalized and the gradient remains <30 mmHg, there is no severe intrinsic aortic stenosis and these patients would not benefit from aortic valve replacement *(44, 5)*.

There are some patients in whom the cardiac output does not increase with dobutamine infusion. These patients lack "contractile reserve," which is defined as a stroke volume rise of <20% during peak dobutamine infusion. Patients without contractile reserve have significantly increased perioperative mortality and may continue to have significant heart failure following aortic valve replacement *(45, 46)*. Nevertheless, if patients with truly severe aortic stenosis can survive operation despite the lack of contractile reserve, some will have improvement in ventricular function and symptoms *(47)*. Given these observations and the poor outlook of unoperated severe aortic stenosis, the absence of contractile reserve therefore is not a contraindication to surgery.

Noncardiac Surgery

Patients who present with severe aortic stenosis and need noncardiac surgery pose a therapeutic challenge. Severe aortic stenosis is one of the highest risk factors for complications following noncardiac surgery *(48–50)*. The indications for aortic valve replacement in these settings are largely the same as in the absence of noncardiac surgery. For all patients with symptoms and severe aortic stenosis, the ACC/AHA guidelines recommend aortic valve replacement preoperatively if the noncardiac surgery is elective and can be delayed for several months. However, a more difficult challenge arises when the patient with severe aortic stenosis is asymptomatic and needs noncardiac surgery. Although the risk of noncardiac surgery is increased, patients can undergo noncardiac surgery relatively safely if meticulous attention is given to intraoperative and postoperative hemodynamics *(51, 52)*. Monitoring of preload and delivering rapid infusions of fluid or blood are essential to prevent precipitous hypotension. In the presence of hypotension, rapid treatment with vasopressors must be performed to prevent the "death spiral" that can result from decreased perfusion of the hypertrophied myocardium. Percutaneous aortic balloon valvotomy may sometimes be used with critical aortic stenosis prior to noncardiac surgery, but there is a high rate of complications and little data supporting its efficacy in this setting *(53–55)*.

Cardiac Surgery with Concomitant Aortic Stenosis

Frequently, surgery for severe coronary disease or aortic root dilatation is required in patients with concomitant aortic stenosis. Even if there are no symptoms attributable to the aortic stenosis, aortic valve replacement is always indicated for patients with severe aortic stenosis who undergo coronary artery bypass grafting, aortic surgery, or other heart valve surgery.

Conversely, there is more controversy about aortic valve replacement in asymptomatic patients with less-severe aortic stenosis who need to undergo these other cardiac surgeries. Several studies have shown rapid subsequent progression of aortic stenosis when aortic valve replacement was not undertaken during these other cardiovascular surgeries. Rapid progression may be due to a diffuse atherosclerotic process as the etiology for both the calcific aortic stenosis and the coronary artery disease. Importantly, the risk of repeat operation is higher in these patients due to the fibrosis and scarring from the first operation as well as the frequent presence of a patent left internal mammary artery bypass graft, which could be damaged during a second sternotomy *(56)*. Therefore, it has been proposed that select patients with less-severe aortic stenosis be considered for aortic valve replacement at the time of the initial operation.

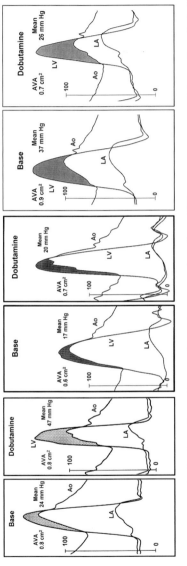

Fig. 12. Representative hemodynamic findings from three patients demonstrating three different responses to dobutamine. *Left*, There was an increase in both cardiac output and gradient in response to dobutamine. The valve area remained 0.8 cm². The patient had severe aortic stenosis at operation and was in NYHA Class I following surgery. *Middle*, There was an increase in cardiac output but only a mild change in the gradient. This represents mild aortic stenosis. *Right*, There was no change in cardiac output, a decrease in the valve gradient, and hypotension occurred during the study. Severe aortic stenosis was found at operation, but the patient died of heart failure 2 years later. Reprinted with permission from Nishimura RA et al. (*44*) with permission from Lippincott Williams & Wilkins.

Aortic valve replacement is considered reasonable for patients with moderate aortic stenosis undergoing coronary artery bypass grafting, aortic surgery, or other heart valve surgery (57). For patients with milder aortic stenosis, consideration should also be given to concomitant aortic valve replacement if the valve is found to be significantly calcified at the time of operation because of the likelihood of rapid progression in these patients.

AORTIC DILATATION

Patients with aortic stenosis may have concomitant aortic dilatation. In some patients, aortic dilatation is secondary to aortic trauma from the aortic stenosis jet. Among patients with a bicuspid aortic valve, there is frequently a concomitant aortopathy. This aortopathy results in aortic dilatation independent of the hemodynamic consequence of the aortic stenosis. Importantly, patients with aortopathy that is associated with a bicuspid aortic valve are at increased risk for rupture and dissection.

Echocardiography is the primary imaging technique for identifying patients with aortic stenosis in whom the aortic root or the ascending aorta is enlarged. In those patients with enlargement on screening, other imaging techniques such as cardiac magnetic resonance imaging or computerized tomography should be performed to look at the full extent and size of the aorta as well as to assess the transverse arch and descending aorta.

Operation to repair the aortic root or replace the ascending aorta is recommended for these patients. The type of operation is dependent upon the presence of effacement of the sinotubular junction. In patients with a dilated sinus, complete root replacement with reimplantation of both coronary arteries is necessary. For patients who have enlargement of the ascending aorta distal to the sinotubular junction, only replacement of the ascending aorta is necessary.

Overall, patients with bicuspid valves should undergo elective repair of the aortic root and replacement of the ascending aorta if the diameter of the structure exceeds 5.0 cm. Normalizing to body surface area may be indicated in a very small or large patient, with a value >2.5 cm/m^2 being the indication for operation. Among patients who undergo aortic valve replacement for severe aortic stenosis, aortic root repair or replacement of the ascending aorta is performed if the diameter is greater than 4.5 cm.

New Therapeutic Options

For young patients with congenital or rheumatic aortic stenosis, balloon valvotomy is associated with excellent acute and long-term success, with relief of stenosis and improvement in symptoms. Conversely, for patients with calcific severe aortic stenosis, surgical aortic valve replacement presently is the only effective therapy. While balloon aortic valvuloplasty leads to a ~50% reduction in the valve gradient acutely, restenosis occurs in all patients and is the major limitation of the procedure (55, 58–60). Balloon aortic valvuloplasty therefore is reserved only for patients as a bridge to valve replacement or, in very few select patients, as a means of symptom palliation.

While balloon aortic valvuloplasty failed to live up to its early promise, novel approaches for percutaneous aortic valve replacement have emerged. In the largest reported experience, Cribier and coworkers performed percutaneous aortic valve implantation in 36 nonsurgical patients (mean age, 80 years) with end-stage calcific aortic stenosis (60). This percutaneous valve prosthesis (Edwards-Lifesciences) consists of three bovine pericardial leaflets mounted on a balloon-expandable stainless steel stent and can be delivered via an antegrade or retrograde approach (Fig. 13) (61, 2). Successful delivery occurred in 75% of patients, with an increase in the effective aortic valve area from 0.60 ± 0.09 cm^2 to 1.70 ± 0.11 cm^2, a decrease in the gradient from 37 ± 13 mmHg to 9 ± 2 mmHg, and an increase in left ventricular ejection fraction from $45 \pm 18\%$ to $53 \pm 14\%$ at follow-up. Complications included two deaths, early migration of the prosthesis ($n = 2$), and moderate or severe paravalvular regurgitation ($n = 15$), but coronary artery patency was preserved in all patients. In a separate study, Grube and coworkers also have evaluated the CoreValve aortic valve prosthesis (Fig. 14) (63). Unlike the Cribier-Edwards

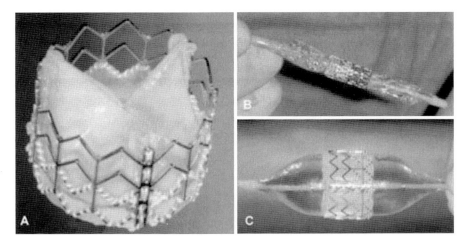

Fig. 13. The Cribier-Edwards percutaneous aortic valve. Reprinted from Cribier et al. *(61)* Copyright 2006, with permission from American College of Cardiology Foundation.

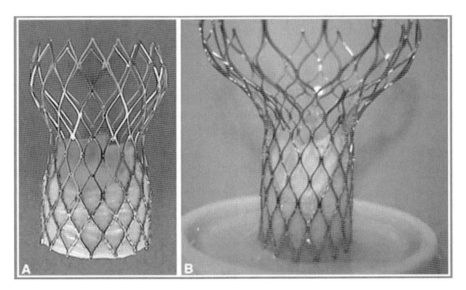

Fig. 14. The CoreValve self-expanding valve prosthesis. Reprinted from Grube E et al. *(63)* with permission from Lippincott Williams & Wilkins.

valve, the CoreValve aortic valve prosthesis is self-expanding with a broad superior segment, which facilitates positioning in the aortic root. Implant success was 84% in a study of 25 patients with only 2 cases of residual perivalvular regurgitation. Another relatively less-invasive approach being evaluated is transapical aortic valve replacement *(64, 5)*.

Technological development of suitable prostheses is ongoing, with targeting of the major obstacles to successful percutaneous treatment of aortic stenosis. These challenges include (1) accurate placement within the native valve without obstruction of the native coronary arteries; (2) minimizing the risk of embolization of the prosthesis and native valve debris; (3) retention of the prosthetic position without paravalvular regurgitation; and (4) long-term durability. Overcoming these challenges will help to address the increasing prevalence of aortic stenosis due to aging of the population, in whom management may also become more complex and require innovative therapies.

REFERENCES

1. Ross J Jr, Braunwald E. Aortic stenosis. Circulation 1968;38:(Suppl 1):61–7.
2. Roberts WC, Ko JM. Frequency by decades of unicuspid, bicuspid, and tricuspid aortic valves in adults having isolated aortic valve replacement for aortic stenosis, with or without associated aortic regurgitation. Circulation 2005;111: 920–5.
3. O'Brien KD, Reichenbach DD, Marcovina SM, Kusisto J, Alpers CE, Otto CM. Apolipoproteins B, (a), and E accumulate in the morphologically early lesion of 'degenerative' valvular aortic stenosis. Arterioscler Thromb Vasc Biol 1996;16:523–32.
4. Olsson M, Thyberg J, Nilsson J. Presence of oxidized low density lipoprotein in nonrheumatic stenotic aortic valves. Arterioscler Thromb Vasc Biol 1999;19:1218–22.
5. Rajamannan NM, Subramaniam M, Rickard D, Stock SR, Donovan J, Springett M, Orszulak T, Fullerton DA, Tajik AJ, Bonow RO, Spelsberg T. Human aortic valve calcification is associated with an osteoblast phenotype. Circulation 2003;107:2181–4.
6. Olsson M, Dalsgaard CJ, Haegerstrand A, Rosenqvist M, Ryden L, Nilsson J. Accumulation of T lymphocytes and expression of interleukin-2 receptors in nonrheumatic stenotic aortic valves. J Am Coll Cardiol 1994;23:1162–70.
7. Sasayama S, Ross J Jr, Franklin D, Bloor CM, Bishop S, Dilley RB. Adaptations of the left ventricle to chronic pressure overload. Circ Res 1976;38:172–8.
8. Julius BK, Spillmann M, Vassalli G, Villari B, Eberli FR, Hess OM. Angina pectoris in patients with aortic stenosis and normal coronary arteries. Mechanisms and pathophysiological concepts. Circulation 1997;95:892–8.
9. Orsinelli DA, Aurigemma GP, Battista S, Krendel S, Gaasch WH. Left ventricular hypertrophy and mortality after aortic valve replacement for aortic stenosis. A high risk subgroup identified by preoperative relative wall thickness. J Am Coll Cardiol 1993;22:1679–83.
10. Gaasch WH, Levine HJ, Quinones MA, Alexander JK. Left ventricular compliance: mechanisms and clinical implications. Am J Cardiol 1976;38:645–53.
11. Hess OM, Ritter M, Schneider J, Grimm J, Turina M, Krayenbuehl HP. Diastolic stiffness and myocardial structure in aortic valve disease before and after valve replacement. Circulation 1984;69:855–65.
12. Bonow RO, Carabello B, Chatterjee K, DeLeon AC, Faxon DF, Freed MD, Gaasch WH, Lytle BW, Nishimura RA, O'Gara PT, O'Rourke RA, Otto CM, Shah PM, Shanewise J. ACC/AHA 2006 Guidelines on the management of patients with valvular heart disease: a report of the ACC/AHA Task Force on Practice Guidelines (Writing Committee to Revise the 1998 Guidelines for the Management of Patients with Valvular Heart Disease). American College of Cardiology Web site. Available at: http://www.acc.org/clinical/statements.htm
13. Schreiber C, Lange R. Porcelain aorta: therapeutical options for aortic valve replacement and concomitant coronary artery bypass grafting. Ann Thorac Surg 2006;82:381.
14. Gorlin R, Gorlin G. Hydraulic formula for calculation of area of stenotic mitral valve, other cardiac values and central circulatory shunts. Am Heart J 1951;41:1–29.
15. Hakki AH, Iskandrian AS, Bemis CE, Kimbiris D, Mintz GS, Segal BL, Brice Cl. A simplified valve formula for the calculation of stenotic cardiac valve areas. Circulation 1981;63:1050–5.
16. Horstkotte D, Loogen F. The natural history of aortic valve stenosis. Eur Heart J 1988;9(Suppl E):57–64.
17. Otto CM, Burwash IG, Legget ME, Munt BI, Fujioka M, Healy NL, Kraft CD, Miyake-Hull CY, Schwaegler RG. Prospective study of asymptomatic valvular aortic stenosis. Clinical, echocardiographic, and exercise predictors of outcome. Circulation 1997;95:2262–70.
18. Rosenhek R, Binder T, Porenta G, Lang I, Christ G, Schemper M, Maurer G, Baumgartner H. Predictors of outcome in severe, asymptomatic aortic stenosis. N Engl J Med 2000;343:611–17.
19. Pellikka PA, Sarano ME, Nishimura RA, Malouf JF, Bailey KR, Scott CG, Barnes E, Tajik AJ. Outcome of 622 adults with asymptomatic, hemodynamically significant aortic stenosis during prolonged follow-up. Circulation 2005;111:3290–5.
20. Faggiano P, Aurigemma GP, Rusconi C, Gaasch WH. Progression of valvular aortic stenosis in adults: literature review and clinical implications. Am Heart J 1996;132:408–17.
21. Gjertsson P, Caidahl K, Oden A, Bech-Hanssen O. Diagnostic and referral delay in patients with aortic stenosis is common and negatively affects outcome. Scand Cardiovasc J. 2007;41:12–18.
22. Kvidal P, Bergstrom R, Horte LG, Stahle E. Observed and relative survival after aortic valve replacement. J Am Coll Cardiol 2000;35:747–56.
23. Atwood JE, Kawanishi S, Myers J, Froelicher VF. Exercise testing in patients with aortic stenosis. Chest 1988;93: 1083–7.
24. Clyne CA, Arrighi JA, Maron BJ, Dilsizian V, Bonow RO, Cannon RO, III. Systemic and left ventricular responses to exercise stress in asymptomatic patients with valvular aortic stenosis. Am J Cardiol 1991;68:1469–76.
25. Das P, Rimington H, Chambers J. Exercise testing to stratify risk in aortic stenosis. Eur Heart J 2005;26:1309–13.

26. Alborino D, Hoffman JL, Fournet PC, Bloch A. Value of exercise testing to evaluate the indication for surgery in asymptomatic patients with valvular aortic stenosis. J Heart Valve Dis 2002;11:204–9.

27. Amato MCM, Moffa PJ, Werner KE, Ramires JAF. Treatment decision in asymptomatic aortic valve stenosis: role of exercise testing. Heart 2001;86:381–6.

28. Spencer, G. US bureau of the census: Projections of the population of the United States, by age, sex and race: 1988 to 2080. Current Population 1989, Series P-25, No. 1018.

29. Lindroos M, Kupari M, Heikkila J, Tilvis R. Prevalence of aortic valve abnormalities in the elderly: an echocardiographic study of a random population sample. J Am Coll Cardiol 1993;21:1220–5.

30. Stern A, Tunick PA, Culliford AT, Lachmann J, Baumann FG, Kanchuger MS, Marschall K, Shah A, Grossi E, Kronzon I. Protruding aortic arch atheromas: risk of stroke during heart surgery with and without aortic arch endarterectomy. Am Heart J 1999;138:746–52.

31. Olsson M, Granstrom L, Lindblom D, Rosenqvist M, Ryden L. Aortic valve replacement in octogenarians with aortic stenosis: a case-control study. J Am Coll Cardiol 1992;20:1512–6.

32. Elayda MA, Hall RJ, Reul RM, Alonzo DM, Gillette N, Reul GJ Jr, Cooley DA. Aortic valve replacement in patients 80 years and older. Operative risks and long-term results. Circulation 1993;88(5 pt 2):II11–16.

33. Bessou JP, Bouchart F, Angha S, Tabley A, Dubar A, Mouton-Schleifer D, Redonnet M, Fournier JF, Arrignon J, Soyer R. Aortic valvular replacement in octogenarians. Short-term and mid-term results in 140 patients. Cardiovasc Surg 1999;7:355–62.

34. Gilbert T, Orr W, Banning AP. Surgery for aortic stenosis in severely symptomatic patients older than 80 years: experience in a single UK centre. Heart 1999;82:138–42.

35. Freeman WK, Schaff HV, O'Brien PC, Orszulak TA, Naessens JM, Tajik AJ. Cardiac surgery in the octogenarian: perioperative outcome and clinical follow-up. J Am Coll Cardiol 1991;18:29–35.

36. Edwards FH, Peterson ED, Coombs LP, DeLong ER, Jamieson WR, Shroyer ALW, Grover FL. Prediction of operative mortality after valve replacement surgery. J Am Coll Cardiol 2001;37:885–92.

37. Akins CW, Daggett WM, Vlahakes GJ, Hilgenberg AD, Torchiana DF, Madsen JC, Buckley MJ. Cardiac operations in patients 80 years old and older. Ann Thorac Surg 1997;64:606–14.

38. Society of Thoracic Surgeons National Cardiac Surgery Database. http://www.sts.org/sections/stsnationaldatabase/riskcalculator/

39. Asimakopoulos G, Edwards MB, Taylor KM. Aortic valve replacement in patients 80 years of age and older: survival and cause of death based on 1100 cases: collective results from the UK Heart Valve Registry. Circulation 1997;18:3403–8.

40. Olsson M, Granstrom L, Lindblom D, Rosenqvist M, Ryden L. Aortic valve replacement in octogenarians with aortic stenosis: a case-control study. J Am Coll Cardiol 1992;20:1512–6.

41. Olsson M, Janfjall H, Orth-Gomer K, Unden A, Rosenqvist M. Quality of life in octogenarians after valve replacement due to aortic stenosis. A prospective comparison with younger patients. Eur Heart J 1996;17:583–9.

42. Shapira OM, Kelleher RM, Zelingher J, Whalen D. Fitzgerald, C., Aldea GS, Shemin RJ. Prognosis and quality of life after valve surgery in patients older than 75 years. Chest 1997;112:885–94.

43. deFilippi CR, Willett DL, Brickner ME, Appleton CP, Yancy CW, Eichhorn EJ, Grayburn PA. Usefulness of dobutamine echocardiography in distinguishing severe from nonsevere valvular aortic stenosis in patients with depressed left ventricular function and low transvalvular gradients. Am J Cardiol 1995;75:191–4.

44. Nishimura RA, Grantham JA, Connolly HM, Schaff HV, Higano ST, Holmes DR Jr. Low-output, low-gradient aortic stenosis in patients with depressed left ventricular systolic function: the clinical utility of the dobutamine challenge in the catheterization laboratory. Circulation 2002;106:809–13.

45. Monin JL, Monchi M, Gest V, Duval-Moulin AM, Dubois-Rande JL, Gueret P. Aortic stenosis with severe left ventricular dysfunction and low transvalvular pressure gradients: risk stratification by low-dose dobutamine echocardiography. J Am Coll Cardiol 2001;37:2101–7.

46. Monin JL, Quere JP, Monchi M, Petit H, Baleynaud S, Chauvel C, Pop C, Ohlmann P, Lelguen C, Dehant P, Tribouilloy C, Gueret P. Low-gradient aortic stenosis: operative risk stratification and predictors for long-term outcome: a multicenter study using dobutamine stress hemodynamics. Circulation 2003;108:319–24.

47. Quere JP, Monin JL, Levy F, Petit H, Baleynaud S, Chauvel C, Pop C, Ohlmann P, Lelguen C, Dehant P, Gueret P, Tribouilloy C. Influence of preoperative left ventricular contractile reserve on postoperative ejection fraction in low-gradient aortic stenosis. Circulation 2006;113:1718–20.

48. Goldman, L. Aortic stenosis in noncardiac surgery: underappreciated in more ways than one?. Am J Med 2004;116:60–2.

49. Kertai MD, Bountioukos M, Boersma Eric, Bax Jeroen J, Thomson Ian, Sozzi Fabiola, Klein Jan, Roelandt Jos RTC, Poldermans Don. Aortic stenosis: an underestimated risk factor for perioperative complications in patients undergoing noncardiac surgery. Am J Med 2004;116:8–13.

50. Zahid M, Sonel AF, Saba S, Good CB. Perioperative risk of noncardiac surgery associated with aortic stenosis. Am J Cardiol 2005;96:436–8.
51. O'Keefe JH, Shub C, Rettke SR. Risk of noncardiac surgical procedures in patients with aortic stenosis. Mayo Clin Proc 1989;64:400–5.
52. Torsher LC, Shub C, Rettke SR, Brown DL. Risk of patients with severe aortic stenosis undergoing noncardiac surgery. Am J Cardiol 1998;81:448–52.
53. Levine MJ, Berman AD, Safian RD, Diver DJ, McKay RG. Palliation of valvular aortic stenosis by balloon valvuloplasty as preoperative preparation for noncardiac surgery. Am J Cardiol 1988;62:1309–10.
54. Roth RB, Palacios IF, Block PC. Percutaneous aortic balloon valvuloplasty: its role in the management of patients with aortic stenosis requiring major noncardiac surgery. J Am Coll Cardiol 1989;13:1039–41.
55. Hayes SN, Holmes DR, Nishimura RA, Reeder GS. Palliative percutaneous aortic balloon valvuloplasty before noncardiac operations and invasive diagnostic procedures. Mayo Clin Proc 1989;64:753–7.
56. Odell JA, Mullany CJ, Schaff HV, Orszulak TA, Daly RC, Morris JJ. Aortic valve replacement after previous coronary artery bypass grafting. Ann Thorac Surg 1996;62:1424–30.
57. Jeremy J, Pereira MB, Balaban K, Lauer MS, Lytle B, Thomas JD, Garcia MJ. Aortic valve replacement in patients with mild or moderate aortic stenosis and coronary bypass surgery. Am J Med 2005;118:735–42.
58. Safian RD, Berman AD, Diver DJ, McKay LL, Come PC, Riley MF, Warren SE, Cunningham MJ, Wyman RM, Weinstein JS. Balloon aortic valvuloplasty in 170 consecutive patients. N Engl J Med 1988;319:125–30.
59. Rahimtoola SH, Catheter balloon valvuloplasty for severe calcific aortic stenosis: a limited role. J Am Coll Cardiol 1994;23:1076–8.
60. Otto CM, Mickel MC, Kennedy JW, Alderman EL, Bashore TM, Block PC, Brinker JA, Diver D, Ferguson J, Holmes DR Jr. Three-year outcome after balloon aortic valvuloplasty. Insights into prognosis of valvular aortic stenosis. Circulation 1994;89:642–50.
61. Cribier A, Eltchaninoff H, Tron C, Bauer F, Agatiello C, Nercolini D, Tapiero S, Litzler P-Y, Bessou J-P, Babaliaros V. Treatment of calcific aortic stenosis with the percutaneous heart valve: mid-term follow-up from the initial feasibility studies: the French experience. J Am Coll Cardiol 2006;47:1214–23.
62. Webb JG, Chandavimol M, Thompson CR, Ricci DR, Carere RG, Munt BI, Buller CE, Pasupati S, Lichtenstein S. Percutaneous aortic valve implantation retrograde from the femoral artery. Circulation 2006;113:842–50.
63. Grube E, Laborde JC, Gerckens U, Felderhoff T, Sauren B, Buellesfeld L, Mueller R, Menichelli M, Schmidt T, Zickmann B, Iversen S, Stone GW. Percutaneous implantation of the CoreValve self-expanding valve prosthesis in high-risk patients with aortic valve disease: the Siegburg first-in-man study. Circulation 2006;114:1616–24.
64. Dewey TM, Walther T, Doss M, Brown D, Ryan WH, Svensson L, Mihaljevic T, Hambrecht R, Schuler G, Wimmer-Greinecker G, Mohr FW, Mack MJ. Transapical aortic valve implantation: an animal feasibility study. Ann Thorac Surg 2006;82:110–16.
65. Ye J, Cheung A, Lichtenstein SV, Pasupati S, Carere RG, Thompson CR, Sinhal A, Webb JG. Six-month outcome of transapical transcatheter aortic valve implantation in the initial seven patients. J Cardio Thor Surg 2007;31:16–21.

8 Aortic Regurgitation

Vera H. Rigolin and Robert O. Bonow

CONTENTS

INTRODUCTION

Aortic regurgitation (AR) is a common disorder throughout the world. This disorder may be due to a variety of diseases of the aortic valve and/or the aortic root. Patients with severe AR may remain asymptomatic for several years. However, if preload reserve or compensatory hypertrophy is insufficient, afterload mismatch will result, eventually resulting in systolic dysfunction. Surgical correction of AR is the only definitive treatment once symptoms or systolic dysfunction develop. The etiology, clinical presentation, natural history, and management strategies for patients with AR are discussed.

Aortic regurgitation (AR) is a common worldwide disorder. The prevalence of AR in the United States has been reported to be between 4.9% in Framingham cohort up to 10% in Strong Heart study. The range in disease prevalence may be due to racial differences in the study groups (whites vs. native Americans) or differences in the prevalence of rheumatic heart disease. The prevalence of AR increases with age, and severe AR is found more commonly in men compared to women *(1)*.

ETIOLOGY

AR may result from a primary valve disorder or from a disorder of the aortic root. Primary disorders of the valve include degenerative calcific aortic stenosis in which some degree of AR is present in 75%; infective endocarditis in which AR may result from poor leaflet coaptation due to the presence of a vegetation or leaflet destruction; trauma that may result in a tear in the aorta with subsequent leaflet

From: *Contemporary Cardiology: Valvular Heart Disease*
Edited by: Andrew Wang, Thomas M. Bashore, DOI 10.1007/978-1-59745-411-7_8
© Humana Press, a part of Springer Science+Business Media, LLC 2009

prolapse; congenital abnormalities of the aortic valve such as a bicuspid, unicuspid, or quadricuspid valve, or rupture of congenitally fenestrated valve; other congenital defects such as large ventricular septal defects and subaortic membranes; rheumatic heart disease with retraction of the aortic valve leaflet due to scarring and fibrosis; and myxomatous infiltration of the AV resulting in leaflet prolapse. Other systemic disorders that may affect the aortic valve include lupus erythematosus, giant cell arteritis, Takayasu's arteritis, ankylosing spondylitis, Jaccoud's arthropathy, Whipple's disease, and Crohn's disease. Prior to their removal from the market, appetite suppressant drugs were also reported to cause AR *(2)*.

Bicuspid aortic valves are of particular concern due to their unique pathology and association with aortic root enlargement. Bicuspid valves develop from abnormal cusp formation during valvulogenesis. Bicuspid valves may reflect a developmental continuum of valve disorders, ranging from unicuspid valves (the most severe abnormality) to bicuspid valves (moderate abnormality) to trileaflet valves (normal) to the more rare quadricuspid valves *(3)*. The abnormal tissue found in bicuspid valves may be related to deficient microfibrillar proteins. Inadequate production of fibrillin-1 during valvulogenesis may disrupt formation of the aortic cusps and weaken the aortic root *(3)*. Bicuspid aortic valves occur in 1−2% of the population and are more common in males. Familial clustering has been noted, so echocardiographic screening of first degree relatives is warranted. Aortic stenosis is the most common complication of bicuspid valves. AR usually results from cusp prolapse, fibrotic retraction, or dilatation of the sinotubular junction.

Patients with bicuspid aortic valves are also at risk of developing aortic aneurysms that are prone to rupture and dissection. The presence of associated vascular disease is unrelated to the severity of the valve disease itself. Progressive aortic root enlargement has also been noted following surgical aortic valve replacement. Thus, diligent routine screening of the aortic root in patients with bicuspid valves is imperative.

AR due to aortic root disease is now more common than primary valve disease. According to one study that evaluated 268 patients who underwent aortic valve replacement for pure AR, the etiology of the AR was valvular in 46% and the aortic root in 54% of patients *(4)*. The causes of root enlargement include age-related (degenerative) dilatation, degeneration of the extracellular matrix as an isolated condition or associated with Marfan syndrome or congenitally bicuspid aortic valves, aortic dissection, systemic hypertension, osteogenesis imperfecta, syphilitic aortitis, ankylosing spondylitis, giant cell arteritis, the Behçet syndrome, psoriatic arthritis, and other forms of arthritis associated with ulcerative colitis, relapsing polychondritis, and the Reiter syndrome. Aortic root enlargement causes AR due to annular dilatation. This results in leaflet separation and loss of coaptation. Tension on the leaflets from the regurgitation may also result in scarring, which in turn, interferes with coaptation by shortening the leaflets *(2)*.

The Marfan syndrome also deserves special consideration due to its unique characteristics. Marfan syndrome is an autosomal dominant disorder caused by a defect in the gene that encodes fibrillin. Similar aortic pathology occurs in genetic disorders related to transforming growth factor-β (TGF-β) receptors, such as the Loeys–Dietz syndrome *(5)*. In these conditions, aortic root aneurysmal dilatation and aortic dissection are the major causes of morbidity and mortality. Characteristic findings on echocardiography include dilatation of the aortic root and ascending aorta with loss of tapering of the sinotubular junction. AR develops due to incomplete central coaptation of the stretched leaflets due to annular dilatation and increased leaflet stress and strain. The anterior leaflet of the mitral valve is often elongated and prolapses into the left atrium. There is often some degree of mitral regurgitation *(6)*. The risk factors for aortic dissection include a family history of cardiovascular events, generalized aortic root dilatation, degree of aortic root dilatation, and the ratio of the actual sinus dimension/predicted sinus dimension. A dimension less than or equal to 1.3 is a predictor of good long-term outcome *(7)*.

PATHOPHYSIOLOGY

In patients with AR, the total left ventricular (LV) stroke volume is the sum of the forward plus the regurgitant stroke volume. Normal forward cardiac output is maintained by an increase in total stroke volume corresponding to the severity of regurgitation. The increase is achieved by progressive dilatation of the left ventricle with increased end-diastolic and end-systolic volumes. In addition, unlike mitral regurgitation, LV afterload is also increased in AR as the elevated end-diastolic volume increases LV wall stress, which represents impedance to myocardial shortening that must be overcome for ejection to occur. In addition, the increased stroke volume that is ejected into the high-impedance aorta often creates systolic hypertension (6), which further increases ventricular afterload. Thus, chronic AR represents a combination of elevated preload and elevated afterload.

Afterload is best described in terms of end-systolic wall stress, which is the product of ventricular pressure and radius divided by twice the wall thickness The volume overload associated with AR results in compensatory eccentric hypertrophy whereas the pressure overload results in superimposed concentric hypertrophy (8). Preload is normalized due to eccentric hypertrophy and the addition of new sarcomeres in series. Increased systolic wall stress and afterload are a stimulus for concentric hypertrophy as well. Therefore, as the disease progresses, the combination of preload reserve and continued compensatory hypertrophy allows the left ventricle to maintain normal wall stress and thus normal ejection performance. These compensatory mechanisms allow patients to remain asymptomatic for years. Since left atrial pressure increases late in the course of the disease, symptoms develop slowly and late when AR is chronic (1). However, if preload reserve or compensatory hypertrophy is insufficient, afterload mismatch will result, eventually resulting in systolic dysfunction (9). Initially the depressed ejection fraction is due to afterload mismatch and is therefore reversible with correction of the valve disorder. However, if left untreated, permanent contractile dysfunction may develop (8, 10). Progression of LV dysfunction may also be due in part to myocardial fibrosis. The left ventricle of patients with AR has been noted to have abnormal extracellular matrix production by cardiac fibroblasts, featuring a high proportion of noncollagen extracellular matrix, especially fibronectin with very little change in collagen synthesis (11).

CLINICAL PRESENTATION

Patients with AR usually remain asymptomatic for years. As the left ventricle decompensates, both end-diastolic volume and end-diastolic pressure increase. In later stages of dysfunction, right-sided pressures also rise. Cardiac output then fails to meet the body's demands, and symptoms of heart failure ensue. The most common initial symptom is shortness of breath which first develops with exercise, then later at rest. Patients may also be aware of a strong, pounding heart beat. Sinus tachycardia may develop with minimal exertion. Palpitations may also result from supraventricular or ventricular premature beats (12). Syncope may occur due to diminished diastolic blood pressure (9).

Anginal chest pain can also occur in the absence of coronary artery disease. Coronary blood flow in AR is affected by decreased diastolic perfusion pressure and by increased LV oxygen demands due to the increased LV wall stress and mass. There is a compensatory increase in the coronary artery dimensions in AR but, as in other forms of pathologic hypertrophy, the increase in myocardial mass decreases the capillary muscle density. Thus, in many patients with chronic severe AR, coronary blood flow reserve is reduced and is insufficient to keep up with the demands of the increased LV mass. The result is subendocardial ischemia during periods of increased oxygen demands, such as during exercise, resulting in anginal chest pain (6).

Physical examination. The findings on physical examination in patients with chronic AR are mainly related to the increased stroke volume and widened pulse pressure. The apical impulse is diffuse, laterally and inferiorly displaced due to LV enlargement. The augmented stroke volume often creates a hyperdynamic apical impulse. A rapid ventricular filling wave can often be palpated at the apex and there may also be systolic retraction of the parasternal region. A systolic thrill may be heard at the base of the heart, the suprasternal notch, and the carotid arteries. At times, a carotid shudder is palpable (2). The carotid pulse is usually bounding with a pronounced upstroke followed by a rapid runoff (waterhammer or Corrigan's pulse) and there may be a bifid systolic pulse (bisferiens pulse). The bisferiens pulse may also be appreciated in the brachial and femoral arteries.

The heart sounds are usually altered in patients with chronic AR. Although S1 is often normal, S2 is increased or decreased depending on the etiology of the AR. A loud closure sound is associated with a dilated aortic root. A soft S2 is found when the AR is due to abnormally thickened and retracted leaflets. Ejection clicks can be heard in young patients with bicuspid valves (6). The presence of an S3 may signify a failing left ventricle (2).

The classic murmur of chronic AR is that of a blowing diastolic murmur along the left sternal border. The murmur is best heard with the diaphragm of the stethoscope when the patient is sitting up and leaning forward with held exhalation. The murmur is also accentuated by maneuvers that increase blood pressure such as squatting or isometric exercise. The murmur decreases with maneuvers that decrease blood pressure such as standing, amyl nitrate inhalation, or the strain phase of the Valsalva maneuver. The murmur is loudest along the right sternal border if the AR is related to pathology of the aortic root. On the other hand, the murmur is best heard in left sternal border (3–4 intercostal spaces) if the cause of the AR is related to diseased valves. A systolic outflow murmur radiating to the carotids, resulting from the increased stroke volume, is a common finding, and this harsh systolic murmur is often more easily appreciated than the high-pitched diastolic blow (2).

Mild degrees of AR result in a murmur only in early diastole. As the severity of AR increases, the murmur becomes more holodiastolic. However, when the left ventricle decompensates, the increase in LV end-diastolic pressure and the rapid decrease in the aortic diastolic blood pressure result in a diminished gradient between the left ventricle and the aorta, which then shortens the murmur (9).

Patients with severe AR may also demonstrate a second diastolic murmur hear best at the apex (Austin-Flint murmur), which is low pitched. This diastolic rumble, similar to that of mitral stenosis in pitch and intensity, has been postulated to represent physiological mitral stenosis caused by the rapid increase in LV diastolic pressure and by the jet of AR hitting the mitral valve (9). Others have concluded that this murmur is related to the AR jet directed at the anterior leaflet of the mitral valve and the LV free wall, causing vibrations that are appreciated on auscultation as a diastolic rumble (6). Other peripheral signs of AR related to the widened pulse pressure and increased stroke volume are listed in Table 1.

Table 1
Peripheral Signs of Severe, Chronic Aortic Insufficiency

De Musset's sign	Head bobbing in synch with arterial pulse
Quinke's pulse	Pulsation of nail beds when mild pressure is placed on the nail
Duroziez's sign	Systolic and diastolic bruit heard over the femoral artery with gentle compression of the stethoscope
Traube sign (also known as "pistol shot sounds")	Booming systolic and diastolic sounds heard over the femoral artery
Müller sign	Systolic pulsations of the uvula
Hill's sign	Increase in lower extremity systolic blood pressure > 40 mm Hg compared to the brachial artery

Acute AR may be a catastrophic illness and may be difficult to diagnose. Medically treated patients have mortality up to 75%, whereas surgical therapy reduces mortality to 25% range. Diagnosis is often difficult since the ventricle has not had time to enlarge. Thus the large stroke volume and wide pulse pressure, which are responsible for the physical exam signs of AR, are not present. With the sudden decrease in forward stoke volume, the cardiac output can only be maintained by an increase in heart rate. Patients usually present with tachypnea, tachycardia, and pulmonary edema. The physical exam is of a quiet precordium, a soft first heart sound, and a short diastolic murmur. The soft S1 is related to early closure of the mitral valve. Thus only the tricuspid valve contributes to S1. Early closure of the mitral valve noted on echo is a poor prognostic sign and should prompt rapid surgical correction. The importance of rapid surgical correction for acute severe AR, even in cases of endocarditis, is imperative since medical therapy can often worsen the hemodynamics *(9)*.

CLINICAL ASSESSMENT

The progressive enlargement and hypertrophy of the left ventricle in chronic severe AR usually result in characteristic changes in most diagnostic modalities. The electrocardiogram may be normal or show LV hypertrophy with or without strain. The presence of the strain pattern correlates with ventricular dilatation and hypertrophy. Left axis deviation may also be present. With early LV volume overload, there are prominent Q waves in leads I, aVL, and V3–V6. As the disease progresses, the prominent initial forces decrease but the total QRS amplitude increases *(2)*. An example of an ECG of a patient with severe AR is shown in Fig. 1. The chest X-ray demonstrates an enlarged cardiac silhouette as well enlargement of the aorta, if present (Fig. 2).

Currently, two-dimensional (2D) echocardiography is the principal diagnostic tool for patients with AR. The echocardiogram is able to demonstrate the size and function of the left ventricle as well as the

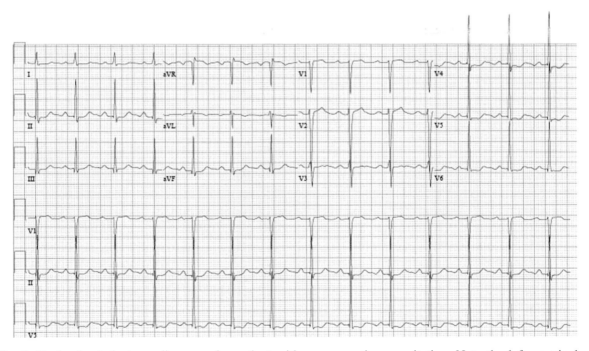

Fig. 1. Twelve-lead electrocardiogram of a patient with severe aortic regurgitation. Note the left ventricular hypertrophy and the strain pattern.

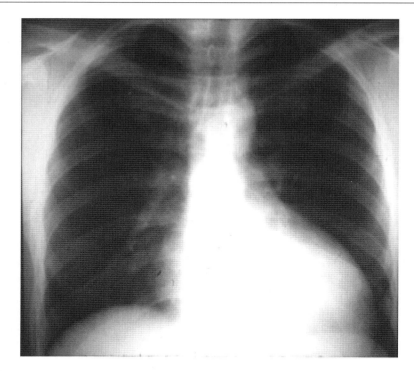

Fig. 2. Chest X-ray of a patient with severe aortic regurgitation. Note the marked cardiomegaly.

morphology of the aortic valve and ascending aorta. Color and spectral Doppler are then used to further quantify the severity of AR. Semi-quantitative echocardiographic measures of AR severity include the size of the left ventricle, the AR jet width measured by color Doppler in the LV outflow tract, measurement of the vena contracta width using color Doppler, assessment by spectral Doppler of flow reversal in the descending aorta, and measurement by spectral Doppler of pressure halftime. Quantitative measures of AR severity include proximal flow convergence (PISA) and calculation of regurgitant volume and fraction using stroke volume determinations across the mitral and aortic valves *(13)*. The specific supportive signs and quantitative parameters are shown in Table 2. The echocardiographic images of a patient with severe AR due to giant cell arteritis are shown in Fig. 3.

Cardiac catheterization is usually only needed in selected cases when noninvasive imaging is inconclusive. It is most often used to assess coronary anatomy prior to surgery in patients in whom coronary artery disease is suspected.

Radionuclide imaging is useful when echo images are technically difficult or when there is a discrepancy between clinical and echo findings. This technique is able to provide accurate ejection fraction, measurement of the LV/RV stroke volume ratio (to help quantify the AR), and the assessment of LV function before and during exercise *(2)*.

Magnetic resonance imaging is also useful to measure LV volumes and ejection fraction, particularly when echocardiography is unable to accurately provide this information. This technique is also invaluable to assess the size and structure of the aorta (Fig. 4A). Velocity-coded cine magnetic resonance imaging provides direct measurement of forward and regurgitant flow across the aortic valve (Fig. 4B).

Exercise testing may be useful to identify patients with early systolic dysfunction when such information is not readily available by history or by resting imaging of the heart. On exercise ECG, at least 0.1 mV of ST segment depression is associated with lower resting and exercise LV ejection fraction,

Table 2
Application of Specific and Supportive Signs and Quantitative Parameters in the Grading of Aortic Regurgitation

	Mild	Moderate	Severe
Specific signs for AR severity	Central jet, width < 25% of LVOT Vena contracta <0.3 cm^{2†} No or brief early diastolic flow reversal in descending aorta	Signs of AR>mild but no criteria for severe AR	Central jet, width ≥ 65% of LVOT Vena contracta >0.6 cm^{2†}
Supportive signs	Pressure halftime >500 ms Normal LV size*	Intermediate values	Pressure halftime <200 ms Holodiastolic aortic flow reversal in descending aorta Moderate or greater LV enlargement**
Quantitative parameters‡R VOl, ml/beat	< 30	30–44 45–59	≥ 60
RF, %	< 30	30–39 40–49	≥ 50
EROA, cm^2	< 0.10	0.10–0.19 0.2–0.29	≥ 0.3

*LV size applied only to chronic lesions; normal 2D measurements: LV minor axis ≤ 2.8 cm/m^2; LV end-diastolic volume ≤82 ml/m^2.

†At a nyquist limit of 50–60 cm/s.

**In the absence of other etiologies of LV dilatation

‡Quantitative parameters can help subclassify the moderate regurgitation group into mild to moderate and moderate to severe as shown.

AR, aortic regurgitation; EROA, effective regurgitant orifice area; LV, left ventricle; LVOT, left ventricular outflow tract; R Vol, regurgitant volume; RF, regurgitant fraction.

Reproduced from Zoghbi et al. *(13)* with permission.

higher wall stress, and greater end-systolic dimension. Reduced oxygen consumption and anaerobic threshold are also predictive of LV dysfunction. The change in ejection fraction with exercise reflects contractile reserve and is predictive of clinical outcome *(6)*. Rest followed by exercise ejection fraction can be measured by echocardiography or by radionuclide angiography.

NATURAL HISTORY

As noted previously, patients with chronic AR usually remain asymptomatic for many years. The morbidity and mortality of the disease are related to the severity of regurgitation, the etiology of the aortic valve disease, the presence of symptoms, and the size and function of the left ventricle. The natural history of mild AR is unknown, but it is likely that most of these patients do not progress to more severe regurgitation *(6)*. The knowledge about the natural history of severe AR is limited by studies with small sample sizes as well as inconsistent reporting of symptoms and parameters of LV function such as internal dimensions and ejection fraction. The current treatment guidelines for AR from the American Heart Association and the American College of Cardiology *(14)* are based on nine published studies with a total of 593 patients and a mean follow-up of 6.6 years *(15–23)*. The composite results of these studies are outlined in Table 3. The rate of progression to symptoms or LV dysfunction averaged 4.3% per year, the rate of sudden death was less than 0.2% per year, and the rate of development of LV dysfunction without symptoms reported in seven out of the nine studies was 1.2% per year *(14)*.

Five out of seven of the natural history studies were consistent in identifying age, end-systolic dimension (or volume), end-diastolic dimension (or volume), and exercise ejection fraction as high risk markers in patients with severe AR *(17–19, 22, 23)*. In one study, an end-systolic dimension of greater than 50 mm resulted in a risk of death, symptoms, or LV dysfunction of 19% per year. In the patients with end-systolic dimensions between 40 and 50 mm, the risk was 6% per year. No patients

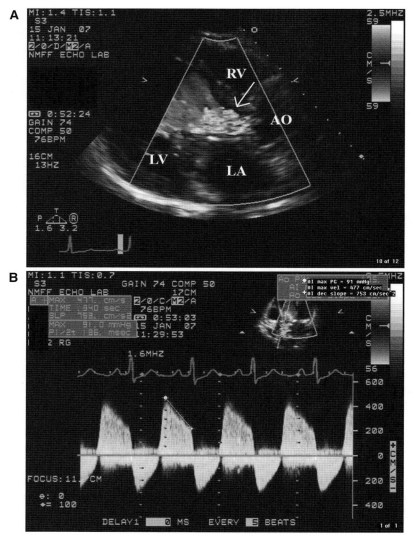

Fig. 3. Two-dimensional echocardiographic images of a patient with severe aortic regurgitation related to giant cell arteritis. In **panel A**, the parasternal long-axis view is shown. Note that the jet of aortic insufficiency (marked by the *arrow*) is as wide as the left ventricular outflow tract. In **panel B**, the pressure halftime of the aortic regurgitation jet is < 200 ms. In **panel C**, there is diastolic flow reversal noted in the descending aorta. **Panel D** shows marked thickening of the descending aorta noted on the intra-operative transesophageal echocardiogram. Biopsy during surgery showed marked inflammation of the aorta and the aortic valve. LA, left atrium; LV, left ventricle; RV, right ventricle; Ao, aorta.

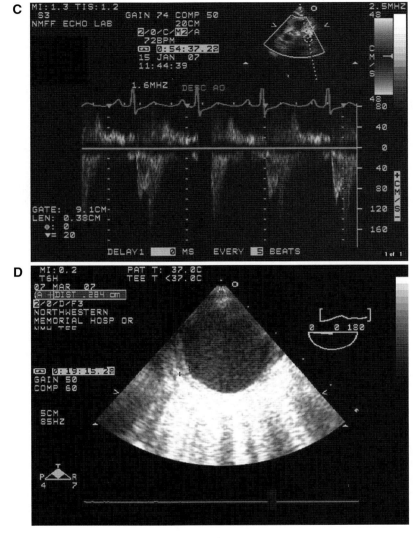

Fig. 3. *(Continued)*

with an end-systolic dimension below 40 mm developed an adverse cardiac event during the 8-year follow-up *(18)*. These findings emphasize the importance of noninvasive imaging in the assessment of these patients.

Severe symptoms, including dyspnea or angina (NYHA and Canadian class III–IV) identify a high risk population since annual mortality in this group is near 25% *(25)*. Patients with Class 2 symptoms have an annual mortality of 6.3% *(1)*. However, some patients may develop LV dysfunction in the absence of symptoms. The limited data on asymptomatic patients with LV dysfunction suggest that the majority of such patients will go on to develop symptoms requiring aortic valve replacement within 2–3 years *(26–28)*. In addition, more than 25% of patients who die or develop systolic dysfunction do so without warning signs *(16–19, 22)*. LV dysfunction that is short lived is often reversible with surgical correction of the valve disease. However, long-standing LV dysfunction reduces the chances of LV recovery following surgery *(29)* (Fig. 5). Therefore, periodic noninvasive assessment of LV function is important, even in patients with no symptoms.

A   **B**

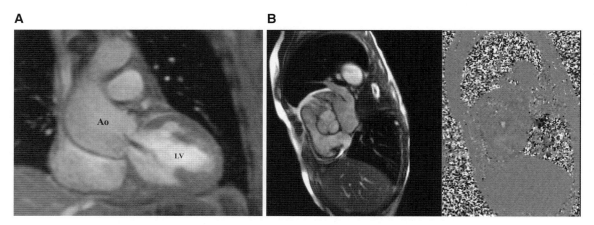

Fig. 4. Two patients who underwent magnetic resonance imaging are shown. **Panel A** demonstrates a patient with a bicuspid aortic valve, aortic regurgitation, and a dilated aortic root. **Panel B** shows a patient with a trileaflet aortic valve and aortic regurgitation. The *left image* in **panel B** is the corresponding velocity map image. Ao, aorta; LV, left ventricle.

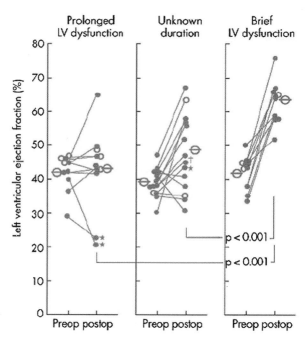

Fig. 5. Change in left ventricular (LV) ejection fraction at rest pre- and 6 months postoperatively in patients with severe aortic regurgitation and prolonged LV dysfunction (>14 months), LV dysfunction of unknown duration, and brief dysfunction (≤14 months). *Open symbols* indicate asymptomatic patients. *Asterisks* indicate patients who subsequently died from heart failure, and the *cross* identifies a patient who subsequently died suddenly. Reproduced from Bonow et al. *(29)* with permission.

Table 3
Studies of the Natural History of Asymptomatic Aortic Regurgitation

References	Number of patients	Mean follow-up, years	Progression to symptoms, death, or LV dysfunction Rate/year (%)	Progression to asymptomatic LV dysfunction (n)	Progression to asymptomatic LV dysfunction Rate/year (%)	Mortality (no. of patients)	Comments
Bonow et al. (15, 18)	104	8.0	3.8	4	0.5	2	Outcome predicted by LV ESD, EDD, change in EF with exercise, and rate of change in ESD and EF at rest with time
Scognamiglio et al. (16)*	30	4.7	2.1	3	2.1	0	Three patients developing asymptomatic LV dysfunction initially had lower PAP/ESV ratios and trend toward higher LV ESD and EDD and lower FS
Siemienczuk et al. (17)	50	3.7	4.0	1	0.5	0	Patients included those receiving placebo and medical dropouts in a randomized drug trial; included some patients with NYHA FC II symptoms; outcome predicted by LV ESV, EDV, change in EF with exercise, and end-systolic wall stress
Scognamiglio et al. (19)*	74	6.0	5.7	15	3.4	0	All patients received digoxin as part of a randomized trial
Tornos et al. (20)	101	4.6	3.0	6	1.3	0	Outcome predicted by pulse pressure, LV ESD, EDD, and EF at rest
Ishii et al. (21)	27	14.2	3.6	–	–	0	Development of symptoms predicted by systolic BP, LV ESD, EDD, mass index, and wall thickness. LV function not reported in all patients

Table 3
(Continued)

References	Number of patients	Mean follow-up, years	Progression to symptoms, death, or LV dysfunction Rate/year (%)	Progression to asymptomatic LV dysfunction (n)	Progression to asymptomatic LV dysfunction Rate/year (%)	Mortality (no. of patients)	Comments
Borer et al. (22)	104	7.3	6.2	7	0.9	4	20% of patients in NYHA FC II; outcome predicted by initial FC II symptoms, change in LV EF with exercise, LV ESD, and LV FS
Tarasoutchi et al. (23)	72	10	4.7	1	0.1	0	Development of symptoms predicted by LV ESD and EDD. LV function not reported in all patients
Evangelista et al. (24)	31	7	3.6	–	–	1	Placebo control group in 7-year vasodilator clinical trial
Average	593	6.6	4.3	37	1.2	(0.18%/year)	

*Two studies by same authors involved separate patient groups.

Abbreviations: BP, blood pressure; EDD, end-diastolic dimension; EDV, end-diastolic volume; EF, ejection fraction; ESD, end-systolic dimension; ESV, end-systolic volume; FC, functional class; FS, fractional shortening; LV, left ventricular; NYHA, New York Heart Association; PAP, pulmonary artery pressure.

Reproduced from Bonow et al. (14) with permission.

MANAGEMENT

General Principles

Echocardiography is the most widely used noninvasive tool to assess LV dimensions, volumes, and ejection fraction. In cases in which the echo is technically suboptimal, other techniques such as radionuclide angiography or cardiac magnetic resonance imaging may be useful. In general, patients with mild AR and normal LV size and function should undergo a clinical evaluation at least once per year. Routine echocardiography can be performed every 2–3 years unless there is evidence of progression of disease before that time (14). However, whether or not there is a high likelihood of progression will depend on the etiology of the disorder. Thus, careful evaluation of valve and aortic anatomy in order to determine the etiology of the AR will help determine the frequency and intensity of follow-up (6).

Asymptomatic patients with severe AR and normal LV size and function should undergo clinical exams and echocardiography yearly unless symptoms arise beforehand. Patients with significant LV dilatation (end-diastolic dimension greater than 60 mm) require clinical evaluations every 6 months and echocardiographic imaging every 6–12 months. Patients with very severe LV dilatation (end-diastolic dimension greater than 70 mm or end-systolic dimension greater than 50 mm) may require serial echoes every 4–6 months (14).

Patients with mild to moderate AR or those with severe AR and normal LV size and function may participate in aerobic exercise. However, patients with severe AR and significant LV dilatation should abstain from heavy exertion of aerobic exercise (14). Patients with systolic dysfunction and/or symptoms related to the valve disorder are candidates for surgery and need to be counseled against strenuous exertion.

Medical Therapy

Systemic arterial diastolic hypertension, if present, should be treated. Vasodilators such as nifedipine or angiotensin-converting enzyme (ACE) inhibitors are preferred, and beta-blocking agents should be used with great caution because of their negative inotropic and chronotropic effects. Atrial fibrillation and bradyarrhythmias are poorly tolerated and should be prevented if possible and aggressively treated if they develop (2). Vasodilator therapy is not recommended in patients with mild or moderate AR and normal LV function in the absence of systemic hypertension since the prognosis in this group is excellent without treatment.

The benefits of chronic vasodilator therapy in asymptomatic patients with severe AR and normal ejection fraction remain controversial. The benefits of nifedipine for such patients were initially suggested by a study by Scognamiglio et al. (19). This prospective study evaluated the use of long-acting nifedipine over a 6-year period. At the end of the study, fewer patients in the nifedipine group needed aortic valve surgery due to symptoms or LV dysfunction. However, this study enrolled a small number of patients and had few endpoints. In addition the nifedipine group was compared to a group that received digoxin rather than to a placebo control group. A second trial studied 95 patients randomly assigned to placebo, long-acting nifedipine, or enalapril in an open label fashion for 7 years (24). At the end of the study, there was no difference in mortality, rate of surgical indications, or changes in LV mass, mean wall stress, ejection fraction, or regurgitant volume. In patients who underwent surgery, the postoperative LV volumes and ejection fraction were similar in all groups. Thus, in this study long-term vasodilator therapy did not slow the progression to surgical correction nor did it alter ventricular remodeling (Fig. 6). In light of these findings, definitive recommendations for the use of chronic long-acting nifedipine or ACE inhibitors in asymptomatic patients with severe AR are not possible (14).

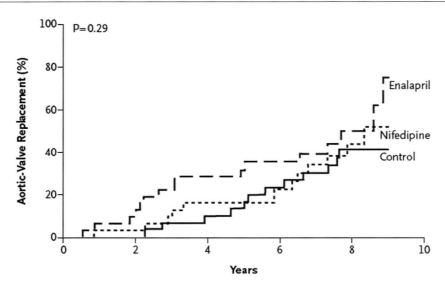

Fig. 6. Probability of aortic valve replacement in three patient groups randomized to placebo, enalapril, and nifedipine in a prospective clinical trial. Neither drug altered the natural history compared to placebo. Reproduced from Evangelista et al. *(24)* with permission.

Vasodilators may be helpful in patients who have symptoms and/or LV dysfunction but are not surgical candidates. They may also be useful short term for improving the hemodynamic profile of patients with severe heart failure prior to undergoing aortic valve surgery *(14)*.

Patients with AR are at risk for endocarditis. Therefore, meticulous dental care and routine dental exams and cleanings are imperative. However, due to the growing evidence that taking prophylactic antibiotic may cause more harm than good, there has been a recent major change in philosophy regarding the use of prophylactic antibiotics. According to the new guidelines from the American Heart Association and the American College of cardiology, only the following individuals who are at the highest risk of developing endocarditis should receive prophylactic antibiotics prior to dental and other procedures: those with artificial heart valves, a prior history of endocarditis, certain specific, serious congenital lesions (including unrepaired or incompletely repaired cyanotic congenital heart disease, including palliative shunts and conduits, a completely repaired congenital heart defect with prosthetic material or device, whether placed by surgery or by catheter interventions, during the first six months after the procedure, any repaired congenital heart defect with residual defect at the site or adjacent to the site of a prosthetic patch or prosthetic device), and those who have undergone a cardiac transplant and develop a problem in a heart valve *(30)*.

Surgical Therapy

Surgical correction of AR is indicated only for those with severe regurgitation. Patients with mild AR are not candidates for surgery due to their excellent long-term prognosis. In individuals with severe AR, surgical therapy should be considered for patients with symptoms irrespective of LV function. On the other hand, surgery is recommended when resting ejection fraction is less than 50% regardless of the presence of symptoms. Surgery is also reasonable to consider when the left ventricle is significantly dilated (end-diastolic dimension is greater than 75 mm or the end-systolic dimension is greater than 55 mm). Surgical correction may be considered in patients with moderate AR who are undergoing coronary artery bypass grafting surgery or repair of an aortic root aneurysm. Finally, surgery may also be considered in asymptomatic patients with normal ejection fraction (greater than 50%), a dilated left ventricle (end-diastolic dimension greater than 70 mm or end-systolic dimension of 50 mm) when there is evidence of progressive LV dilatation, declining exercise tolerance, or abnormal hemodynamic response to exercise *(14)*. Progressive expansion of the aortic root or the presence of an aortic aneurysm greater than 5.0 cm in diameter should undergo surgical repair despite the degree of AV disease *(14)*. A management strategy for patients with chronic severe AR is outlined in Fig. 7.

The LV dimensions used as threshold values for surgical intervention must be used cautiously in women and men of small stature. In a study by Klodas et al. *(31)*, baseline characteristics and post-

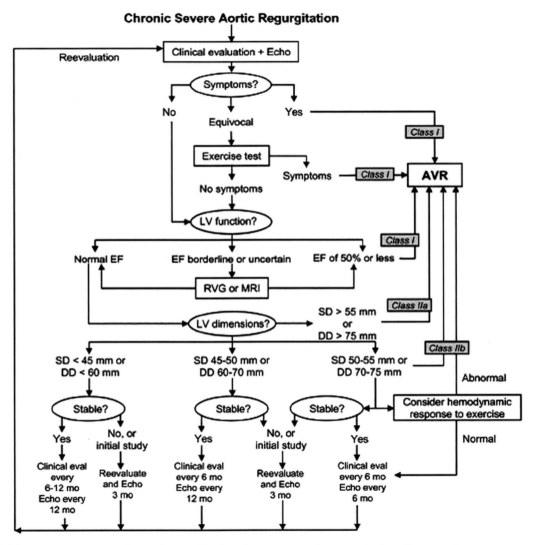

Fig. 7. Management strategy for patients with chronic, severe aortic regurgitation. Preoperative coronary angiography should be performed routinely determined by age, symptoms, and risk factors. Angiography may also be useful if echocardiography and clinical findings are discordant. "Stable" refers to stable echocardiographic measurements. In some centers, serial follow-up may be performed with radionuclide angiography (RVG) or magnetic resonance imaging (MRI) rather than echocardiography (echo) to assess left ventricular (LV) volume and systolic function. AVR, aortic valve replacement; DD, end-diastolic dimension; EF, ejection fraction; Eval, evaluation; SD, end-systolic dimension. Reproduced from Bonow et al. *(14)* with permission.

operative outcomes were compared between 51 women and 198 men undergoing surgery for isolated aortic regurgitation between 1980 and 1989. Women more often had surgery for heart failure symptoms as opposed to LV enlargement and more often for class III–IV symptoms. Operative mortalities were similar in women and men (3.9% and 4.5%, respectively). Among operative survivors, 10-year survival was worse for women than for men (39 ± 9% vs. 72 ± 4%, $P=$ 0002) and, in contrast with men, was worse than expected for women ($P<.0001$). This study implies that the unadjusted LV diameter surgical criteria established in men may not be applicable to women since the women in this study developed more severe symptoms despite similar LV dimensions as men when corrected for body surface area. The excessive late mortality noted in the women in this study suggests that surgical correction of aortic regurgitation may need to be considered at an earlier stage in women. However, the data supporting the use of cardiac dimensions corrected for body surface area are limited, thus clinical judgment is needed when treating individuals of women and men of small stature *(14)*.

Impaired LV function at rest is the basis for selecting patients for operation; normal LV function at rest with failure of the ejection fraction to rise normally with exercise is not considered an absolute indication for surgery, but may be an early indicator of impending LV dysfunction rest *(2)*. A decrease in ejection fraction with exercise should not be used as the sole indicator of surgery in asymptomatic patients with normal LV function at rest since the change in ejection fraction in these patients is complex and multifactorial. The exercise ejection fraction is a relatively nonspecific response related to the degree of volume overload as well as exercise-induced changes in preload, heart rate, and peripheral resistance *(14)*. Exercise testing may therefore be most useful to assess patients with unclear symptoms or borderline LV dysfunction.

The treatment of choice for patients with symptoms is surgery. Patients who are not candidates for surgery should receive aggressive medical therapy for heart failure, including ACE inhibitors and possibly other vasodilators, digitalis, salt restriction, diuretics. Beta blockers should be avoided *(2)*.

Emergency surgery is the preferred method of treatment for acute severe AR. Afterload reduction is appropriate while the patient is being prepared for surgery. Beta blockers are contraindicated since cardiac output is maintained through an increase in heart rate, and lowering the heart rate may acutely worsen the hemodynamic situation. Intra-aortic balloon counterpulsation is absolutely contraindicated. Antibiotics should be given if endocarditis is suspected.

Surgical correction using bioprosthetic or mechanical valves is the preferred method of correction. The use of homografts or pulmonary autografts is used less often due to concerns about durability. Valve repair is possible in experienced centers in selected cases such as bicuspid valves with prolapsing leaflets with minimal sclerosis. However, outcomes have generally been less favorable than repair of the mitral valve *(12)*. Valve-sparing surgery is being performed with increasing frequency in patients with relatively normal valves who require surgery for aortic root aneurysms. In a study by David et al. *(32)*, 167 patients underwent AV reimplantation during aortic root surgery. The mean follow-up was 5.1 ± 3.8 years. Survival at 10 years was 92%. Freedom from moderate or severe AR was 94 ± 4%; freedom from aortic valve replacement was 95 ± 4% at 10 years.

According to the Society of Thoracic Surgeons national database [www.sts.org ref], the overall risk of aortic valve replacement surgery is 4% when performed in isolation and 6.8% when performed with CABG. This risk is considerably lower in high-volume centers and in patients with no symptoms (1–2%) and in those with better preoperative LV function (8% if ejection fraction $\leq$ 35% vs. 2% for ejection fraction $\geq$ 50%). For patients with ascending aortic aneurysms, an ascending aortic graft with a prosthesis is associated with a mortality of 1–10%, depending on symptoms, LV size and function, and severity of AR *(1)*, as well as the experience of the surgical team.

The majority of patients who undergo surgery experience improvement in symptoms as well as reduction in LV size and mass. A small percentage of patients, however, do not improve. Such patients are those in Class NYHA III or IV heart failure preoperatively or those with severe LV dysfunction preoperatively. Perioperative mortality is dependent on the presence of other co-morbidities as well as the skill of the surgical team. Late mortality of 5–10% is noted in patients with severe LV enlargement or prolonged LV dysfunction prior to surgery *(2)*. Chaliki et al. *(33)* reported postoperative results in 450 patients with severe AR who underwent surgery from 1980 to 1995. Patients with very low preoperative LV ejection fraction (less than 35%) had higher operative and postoperative mortality and heart failure after surgery (Fig. 8). However, it is also noteworthy that postoperative ejection fraction improved significantly, and most patients did not have heart failure (Fig. 9). Therefore, although patients with severely depressed ejection fraction have a higher post-op mortality, many experience an improvement in ejection fraction after valve replacement and thus should not be denied surgery.

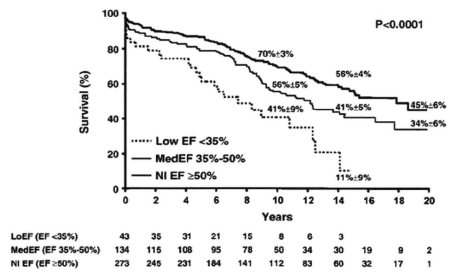

	0	2	4	6	8	10	12	14	16	18	20
LoEF (EF <35%)	43	35	31	21	15	8	6	3			
MedEF (EF 35%-50%)	134	115	108	95	78	50	34	30	19	9	2
NI EF (EF ≥50%)	273	245	231	184	141	112	83	60	32	17	1

Fig. 8. Survival after aortic valve replacement in 450 patients with aortic regurgitation subdivided on the basis of the preoperative ejection fraction (EF). Reproduced from Chaliki et al. *(33)* with permission.

Patients continue to require clinical monitoring after surgical correction. An echocardiogram should be obtained prior to hospital discharge or at the first postoperative outpatient visit in order to establish a baseline with which to compare future studies. In general, there is usually a rapid decline in LV diastolic volume following surgery, and the initial decline in LV end-diastolic dimension is predictive of long-term LV systolic function and survival *(34)*. On the other hand, the LV ejection fraction often declines immediately following valve replacement due to the reduced preload and may take several months to improve. After the initial postoperative evaluation, the patient should be seen and examined again at 6 and 12 months following surgery, then yearly thereafter. If the postoperative echocardiogram in an asymptomatic patient indicates that LV systolic function is normal and there has been a substantial reduction in LV volumes, follow-up echocardiograms are only needed if there is a new murmur, suspicion of valve dysfunction, or concerns about LV function *(14)*.

Patients with persistent LV dysfunction postoperatively should be treated with ACE inhibitors and beta blockers, according to guideline recommendations for patients with LV dysfunction from other causes. These patients should undergo repeat echocardiography at the 6- and 12-month post-op visits and then as clinically indicated thereafter *(14)*.

Patients who have undergone valve replacement surgery should continue to receive meticulous dental care and should take prophylactic antibiotics before dental and other medical procedures that may produce bacteremia *(30)*.

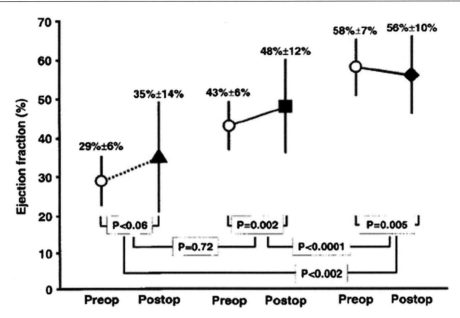

Fig. 9. Left ventricular ejection fraction (EF) before and after aortic valve replacement in patients with aortic regurgitation. Ejection fraction increased in patients with preoperative left ventricular systolic dysfunction. Reproduced from Chaliki et al. *(33)* with permission.

ACKNOWLEDGEMENT

The authors would like to thank Ms Angelene Delk for her administrative assistance.

REFERENCES

1. Enriquez-Sarano M, Tajik AJ. Clinical practice: aortic regurgitation. N Engl J Med 2004;351:1539.
2. Otto CM, Bonow RO. Valvular heart disease. In: Libby P, Bonow RO, Mann DL, Zipes DP, Eds. *Braunwald's Heart Disease: A Textbook of Cardiovascular Medicine* (8th ed). Philadelphia: Elsevier Science 2007;1625–1693.
3. Fedak PWM, Verma S, David TE, Leask RL, Weisel RD, Butany J. Clinical and pathophysiological implications of a biscuspid aortic valve. Circulation 2002;106:900–904.
4. Roberts WC, Ko JM, Moore TR, Jones, WH. Causes of pure aortic regurgitation in patients having isolated aortic valve replacement at a single US tertiary hospital (1993–2005). Circulation 2006;114:422.
5. Loeys BL, Schwarze U, Holm T, et al. Aneurysm syndromes caused by mutations in the TGF-β receptor. N Engl J Med. 2006;355:788–98.
6. Otto CM. In: Otto CM, Ed. *Valvular Heart Disease* (2nd ed). Philadelphia: WB Saunders; 2004, pp. 302–335.
7. Legget ME, Unger TA, O'Sullivan CK, et al. Aortic root complications in Marfan's syndrome: identification of a lower risk group. Heart 1996;75(4):389–95.
8. Rigolin VH, Bonow RO. Hemodynamic characteristics and progression to heart failure in regurgitant lesions. Heart Failure Clin 2007;2:453–460.
9. Carabello BA. Progress in mitral and aortic regurgitation. Prog Cardiovasc Dis 2001;43:457–75.
10. Bonow RO. Chronic aortic regurgitation. CardiolClin 1998;16(3):449–61.
11. Borer JS, Truter S, Herrold EM, et al. Myocardial fibrosis in chronic aortic regurgitation: molecular and cellular responses to volume overload. Circulation 2002;105:1837.
12. Maurer G. Aortic regurgitation. Heart 2006;92:994.
13. Zoghbi WA, Enriquez-Sarano M, Foster E, et al. Recommendations for evaluation of the severity of native valvular regurgitation with two-dimensional and Doppler echocardiography. J Am Soc Echocardiogr 2003;16:777.
14. Bonow RO, Carabello BA, Chatterjee K, et al. ACC/AHA 2006 guidelines for the management of patients with valvular heart disease: a report of the American College of Cardiology/American Heart Association Task Force on Practice

Guidelines (writing committee to revise the 1998 guidelines for the management of patients with valvular heart disease): developed in collaboration with the Society of Cardiovascular Anesthesiologists: endorsed by the Society for Cardiovascular Angiography and Interventions and the Society of Thoracic Surgeons. Circulation 2006;114:e1–148.

15. Bonow RO, Rosing DR, McIntosh CL, et al. The natural history of asymptomatic patients with aortic regurgitation and normal left ventricular function. Circulation 1983;68:509–17.

16. Scognamiglio R, Fasoli G, Dalla VS. Progression of myocardial dysfunction in asymptomatic patients with severe aortic insufficiency. Clin Cardiol 1986;9:151–6.

17. Siemienczuk D, Greenberg B, Morris C, et al. Chronic aortic insufficiency: factors associated with progression to aortic valve replacement. Ann Intern Med 1989;110:587–92.

18. Bonow RO, Lakatos E, Maron BJ, Epstein SE. Serial long term assessment of the natural history of asymptomatic patients with chronic aortic regurgitation and normal left ventricular systolic function. Circulation 1991;84:1625–35.

19. Scognamiglio R, Rahimtoola SH, Fasoli G, Nistri S, Dalla VS. Nifedipine in asymptomatic patients with severe aortic regurgitation and normal left ventricular function. N Engl J Med 1994;331:689–94.

20. Tornos MP, Olona M, Permanyer-Miralda G, et al. Clinical outcome of severe asymptomatic chronic aortic regurgitation: a long term prospective follow-up study. Am Heart J 1995;130:333–9.

21. Ishii K, Hirota Y, Suwa M, Kita Y, Onaka H, Kawamura K. Natural history and left ventricular response in chronic aortic regurgitation. Am J Cardiol 1996;78:357–61.

22. Borer JS, Hochreiter C, Herrold EM, et al. Prediction of indications for valve replacement among symptomatic patients with chronic aortic regurgitation and normal left ventricular performance. Circulation 1998;97:525–34.

23. Tarasoutchi F, Grinberg M, Spina GS, et al. Ten-year clinical laboratory follow-up after application of a symptom-based therapeutic strategy to patients with severe chronic aortic regurgitation of predominant rheumatic etiology. J Am Coll Cardiol 2003;41:1316–24.

24. Evangelista A, Tornos P, Sambola A, Permanyer-Miralda G, Soler-Soler J. Long term vasodilator therapy in patients with severe aortic regurgitation. N Eng J Med 2005;353:1342–9.

25. Dujardin KS, Enriquez-Sarano M, Schaff HV, Bailey KR, Seward JB, Tajik AJ. Mortality and morbidity of chronic aortic regurgitation in clinical practice: a long term follow-up study. Circulation 1999;99:1851–7.

26. Henry WL, Bonow RO, Rosing DR, Epstein SE. Observations n the optimum time for operative intervention for aortic regurgitation II: serial echocardiographic evaluation of asymptomatic patients. Circulation 1980;61:484–92.

27. McDonald IG, Jelinek VM. Serial M-mode echocardiography in severe chronic aortic regurgitation. Circulation 1980;62:1291–6.

28. Bonow RO. Radionuclide angiography in the management of asymptomatic aortic regurgitation. Circulation 1991;84(Suppl I):I-296–302.

29. Bonow RO, Rosing DR, Maron BJ, et al. Reversal of left ventricular dysfunction after aortic valve replacement for chronic aortic regurgitation: influence of duration of preoperative left ventricular dysfunction. Circulation 1984;70:570–9.

30. Wilson W, Taubert KA, Gewitz M, et al. Prevention of Infective Endocarditis. Guidelines From the American Heart Association. A Guideline From the American Heart Association Rheumatic Fever, Endocarditis, and Kawasaki Disease Committee, Council on Cardiovascular Disease in the Young, and the Council on Clinical Cardiology, Council on Cardiovascular Surgery and Anesthesia, and the Quality of Care and Outcomes Research Interdisciplinary Working Group. Circulation. Published on-line April 19, 2007 (www.americanheart.org).

31. Klodas E, Enriquez-Sarano M, Tajik AJ, Mullany CJ, Bailey KR, Seward JB. Surgery for aortic regurgitation in women: contrasting indications and outcomes compared with men. Circulation 1996;94:2472–8

32. David TE, Feindel CM, Webb GD, Colman JM, Armstrong S, Maganti M. Aortic valve preservation in aortic root aneurysm: results of the reimplantation technique. Ann Thorac Surg 2007;83:S732–5.

33. Chaliki HP, Mohty D, Avierinos JF, et al. Outcomes after aortic valve replacement in patients with severe aortic regurgitation and markedly reduced left ventricular function. Circulation 2002;106:2687.

34. Bonow RO, Dodd JT, Maron BJ, et al. Long-term serial changes in left ventricular function and reversal of ventricular dilatation after valve replacement for chronic aortic regurgitation. Circulation 1988;78:1108–20.

9 Mitral Stenosis

Nazanin Moghbeli and Howard C. Herrmann

CONTENTS

ETIOLOGY

The leading cause of mitral stenosis (MS) throughout the world is rheumatic carditis. Approximately 60% of patients with pure mitral stenosis have a history of rheumatic fever, although in some parts of the developing world, the initial episode of rheumatic fever may be unrecognized due to scarcity of health-care resources (1).

The diagnosis of rheumatic fever is made using the Jones criteria in a patient with a history of strep-tococcal infection. To make the diagnosis, two major criteria or one major and two minor criteria must be met. Major criteria include carditis, polyarthritis, chorea, erythema marginatum, and subcutaneous nodules. Minor criteria include arthralgias, fever, high acute phase reactants like C-reactive protein or erythrocyte sedimentation rate, and a prolonged PR interval (Table 1). In addition to the major and minor criteria listed above, there must be evidence of streptococcal infection 2–4 weeks earlier (either a positive throat culture for group A beta-hemolytic streptococci, a positive rapid streptococcal antigen test, or elevated streptococcal antibody titers) (2).

The incidence of rheumatic fever is declining in the United States, concomitant with a shift to more disadvantaged populations including children and immigrants. However, there have been several recent recurrences in the United States. In developing areas of the Indian subcontinent, Middle East, and Asia, rheumatic fever remains more frequent.

Other causes of mitral stenosis include congenital malformation of the mitral valve, as well as acquired conditions such as mitral annular calcification (3). The differential diagnosis of mitral stenosis should also include other causes of obstruction to left ventricular filling such as left atrial myxoma, cor triatriatum, and idiopathic pulmonary vein obstruction (4). In the current era of pulmonary vein isolation as treatment for atrial fibrillation, pulmonary vein stenosis should also be considered.

From: *Contemporary Cardiology: Valvular Heart Disease*
Edited by: Andrew Wang, Thomas M. Bashore, DOI 10.1007/978-1-59745-411-7_9
© Humana Press, a part of Springer Science+Business Media, LLC 2009

Table 1
**Jones Criteria for Diagnosis of Rheumatic Fever. To Make the
Diagnosis of Rheumatic Fever, Either Two Major or One Major and
Two Minor Criteria Must be Present**

Major criteria	Minor criteria
Carditis	Arthralgias
Polyarthritis	Fever
Chorea	Elevated C-reactive protein
Erythema marginatum	Elevated erythrocyte sedimentation rate
Subcutaneous nodules	Prolonged PR interval

PATHOPHYSIOLOGY

The normal mitral valve is a complex structure including the annulus, a large-diameter C-shaped anterior leaflet that divides the left ventricular inflow and outflow tracts, the posterior leaflet, the two papillary muscles, and the attaching chordae tendinae. From a hemodynamic standpoint, all of these structures contribute to the pattern of blood flow from the left atrium to the left ventricle. It is simplistic, but useful, to think of the mitral valve opening as a circular area. However, it should not be forgotten that this area is an approximation of a more complex funnel-like 3D structure.

The primary hemodynamic abnormality in mitral stenosis is obstruction of left ventricular inflow at the mitral valve level, caused by restricted mitral valve opening due to an abnormal mitral valve apparatus. The normal mitral valve area is 4−5 cm^2. When the mitral valve area is narrowed to less than 2.5 cm^2, an increased pressure gradient is needed to propel blood forward from the left atrium to the left ventricle. This leads to increased left atrial pressure, which is in turn transmitted to the pulmonary veins *(5)*. When pulmonary venous pressure is greater than plasma oncotic pressure, pulmonary edema results. Long-standing pulmonary venous hypertension can in turn cause changes in the pulmonary arterioles, including intimal hyperplasia and medial hypertrophy leading to pulmonary arterial hypertension. Chronic pulmonary arterial hypertension causes right ventricular dysfunction and congestive heart failure. When obstruction to left ventricular filling is severe enough, a reduction in stroke volume and cardiac output will result.

Abnormalities in mitral stenosis may include different parts of the mitral valve apparatus: commissures, cusps, chordae, or a combination. The rheumatic process causes thickening and fusion of the commissures, leading to limited movement of the leaflet tips. This, in turn, causes narrowing of the mitral orifice from a tubular to a funnel shape, leading to obstruction of flow from the left atrium to the left ventricle during diastole *(6)*. In cross section, the opening may resemble a "fish mouth" (Fig. 1). The subvalvular apparatus is often involved, with fusion, shortening, fibrosis, and calcification of the mitral chordae *(7)*. Shortening of the chordae can also lead to malcoaptation of the mitral valves resulting in mitral regurgitation.

The development of rheumatic carditis is thought to be due in part to molecular mimicry. Streptococcal M proteins share epitopes with myosin and with valvular endothelium. It is believed that antibodies to the M proteins cross react with myosin and proteins in the valvular endothelium, causing destruction of the valve. Further damage to the valvular structures then occurs as a result of turbulent blood flow through the stenotic valve and leads to further thickening and calcification of the valvular apparatus *(8)*.

It is important to remember that rheumatic carditis can affect other cardiac valves and the myocardium. Mitral stenosis in isolation occurs in 25−40% of patients, with an additional 40% of patients having both MS and mitral regurgitation (MR). The aortic and tricuspid valves can also be involved in up to 25% of patients with rheumatic carditis *(4)*. Left ventricular dysfunction can

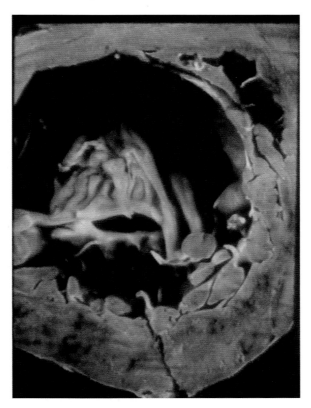

Fig. 1. Pathologic specimen of a rheumatic mitral valve. Note the thickened and fused commissures, narrow "fish-mouth" orifice, and fused and shortened chordae.

occur due to direct myocardial involvement by the rheumatic process or as a consequence of valvular dysfunction.

CLINICAL MANIFESTATIONS

History

The initial phase of mitral stenosis is often asymptomatic. In early stages of disease, symptoms occur only with exercise, anemia, atrial fibrillation, or pregnancy. These conditions all increase cardiac output and decrease diastolic filling time, which cause elevation of left atrial pressure and associated symptoms *(9)*.

The primary symptom of dyspnea results from elevated left atrial and pulmonary venous pressures *(4)*. Patients may cough, wheeze, or exhibit hemoptysis due to rupture of the thin, dilated bronchial veins from elevated left atrial pressures. Pulmonary edema and, rarely, pulmonary infarction can occur. Chest pain may be due to right ventricular hypertrophy, or rarely, embolism of a coronary artery, although often no inciting etiology is found. Atrial fibrillation with or without an embolic event can occur. The risks of embolic phenomena are highest in patients of older age, and those with dilated left atria, low cardiac output, and atrial fibrillation, but can occur even in mild mitral stenosis *(10)*. Finally, patients may describe peripheral edema and increased abdominal girth if right ventricular failure has developed from long-standing pulmonary hypertension *(4)*.

Other less commonly occurring sequela include endocarditis. Ortner's syndrome has been described due to compression of the left recurrent laryngeal nerve by a dilated left atrium or dilated pulmonary artery, resulting in hoarseness *(4)*.

Physical Exam

Palpation of the precordium will likely reveal a normal apical impulse, as the left ventricle is not affected in pure mitral stenosis. There may, however, be a right ventricular heave at the left parasternal region due to right ventricular hypertrophy.

Auscultation will reveal a diastolic murmur or "rumble" at the apex. The intensity and duration of the rumble increases with higher gradients between the left atrium and the left ventricle. There may be an opening snap (OS) as the stenotic mitral valve opens, and a loud S1 as the stenotic leaflets close. The presence of an OS usually indicates a pliable, non-calcified valve morphology. The interval between A2 and the opening snap can be suggestive of the severity of stenosis. If the A2-OS interval is shorter than 60–70 ms, severe mitral stenosis is likely present, as high left atrial pressures will lead to earlier opening of the mitral valve leaflets relative to aortic valve closure. An interval longer than 100 ms is suggestive of a milder degree of stenosis. As progressive calcification occurs and the mitral valve is more difficult to open, the OS may be harder to appreciate. P2 may be loud and high pitched if pulmonary hypertension is present.

The audibility of the mitral stenosis murmur may be improved by placing the patient in the left lateral decubitus position. Other maneuvers that increase the intensity of the murmur include sit-ups and mild exercises that increase the heart rate, decrease diastolic time, and increase the gradient *(11)*.

"Mitral facies" may be manifest as purple-pink patches on the cheeks and is a result of systemic vasoconstriction from the low cardiac output state of mitral stenosis. Pulse volumes may be diminished if cardiac output is sufficiently reduced *(4)*.

CLINICAL ASSESSMENT

The initial clinical assessment rests on obtaining a detailed history of symptoms as described above. Symptoms of dyspnea and orthopnea may first be described in the setting of exercise, fever, pregnancy, anemia, or atrial fibrillation, as these states lead to shortened diastolic filling time and increased left atrial pressures *(4)*.

The electrocardiogram may reveal atrial fibrillation or sinus rhythm with left atrial enlargement. The chest X-ray often reveals left atrial enlargement and dilated pulmonary arteries *(4)*.

Echocardiography is critical in the assessment of mitral stenosis. Two-dimensional echo will reveal the morphology of the mitral valve and allow determination of the parts of the mitral valve apparatus that are involved. For instance, thickening and fusion of the commissures is usually present and visible on echo. The leaflet tips are limited in mobility, and the anterior leaflet classically has a "hockey stick appearance" when viewed in the parasternal long axis view. In short axis, the orifice of the mitral valve appears funnel shaped as opposed to a normal tubular shape, and commissural fusion can be best appreciated in these views (Fig. 2). Left atrial enlargement is invariably present, and although better seen with transesophageal echo, left atrial thrombus is sometimes appreciated on transthoracic echo *(12)*.

Echocardiography is also critical in determining the suitability of the mitral valve for percutaneous repair. Several scoring systems have been developed to predict favorable outcome with percutaneous balloon valvotomy, the most frequently used one being the Wilkins criteria. This system assigns a score of 1–4 for each of the following factors, with 16 being the highest score and indicating the least likelihood for successful percutaneous intervention: leaflet rigidity, thickening, calcification, and subvalvular thickening and calcification *(13)*.

DETERMINATION OF SEVERITY BY ECHOCARDIOGRAPHY

To determine mitral valve severity using echo, planimetry of the mitral valve tips should be done in the parasternal short-axis view. Care should be taken to start imaging at the apex in order to obtain

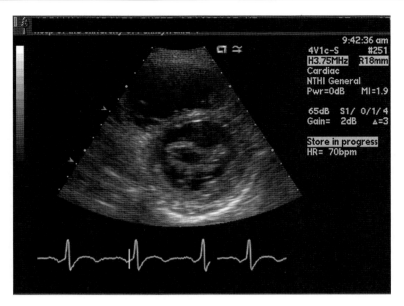

Fig. 2. Short-axis two-dimensional transthoracic echocardiographic image of a stenotic mitral valve. The commissural fusion and narrowed orifice are apparent.

the smallest orifice for planimetry *(7)*. An accurate measurement may be difficult if the mitral valve orifice is highly irregular.

Peak and mean doppler gradients across the mitral valve are obtained from the parasternal long axis and apical 4 chamber views *(12)*. A gradient of >10 mm Hg is considered severe, 5–10 mm Hg moderate, and <5 mm Hg mild mitral stenosis.

The mitral valve area (MVA) is calculated using the continuity equation as follows:

$$MVA = \frac{\text{transmitral SV}}{MV_{VTI}}$$

where SV is stroke volume defined as the product of the velocity time integral (VTI) in the left ventricular outflow tract (LVOT) and the cross-sectional area of the LVOT *(7)*. MV_{VTI} is the velocity time integral measured across the mitral valve by continuous wave Doppler.

A mitral valve area of <1 cm^2 indicates severe MS, 1–1.5 cm^2 moderate, and >1.5 cm^2 mild mitral stenosis. The calculation of the MVA using the continuity equation is only accurate when there is no significant concomitant mitral regurgitation, which can change the measurement of stroke volume and thereby lead to underestimation of MVA.

The Doppler waveform should also be examined to determine the severity of mitral stenosis. There is a characteristic Doppler flow across the normal mitral valve in sinus rhythm with an initial peak (E) corresponding to early rapid blood flow across the mitral valve in the first part of diastole. As left ventricular pressures rise with early diastolic filling, transmitral flow decreases and diastasis is achieved. This represents the time in diastole where left atrial (LA) pressures equal left ventricular (LV) pressures. As the left atrium contracts, there is a second peak in the Doppler tracing (A) reflecting late diastolic flow across the mitral valve.

In mitral stenosis, this normal Doppler pattern is altered by restriction of diastolic flow into the LV by a stenotic mitral valve. This leads to an earlier and higher initial peak as high left atrial pressure accelerates early ventricular filling. However, the slope of the descending E waveform is decreased due to restricted flow across the stenotic mitral valve. It is this slope that is used to calculate MVA by pressure halftime (Fig. 3).

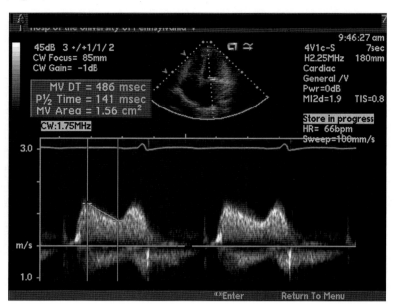

Fig. 3. The Doppler echocardiographic pattern of diastolic flow into the LV by a stenotic mitral valve is illustrated. The slope of the wave form from the initial peak of left atrial pressure is used to calculate the mitral valve area using the pressure halftime formula (*see* text for details).

Pressure halftime (PHT) represents the decay in pressure between the left atrium and the left ventricle and is a measure of the time it takes for the pressure of the early peak to decay in half. The slope of this flow is proportional to the degree of stenosis. A smaller orifice leads to a slower rate of pressure decline and therefore a longer pressure half-time. Severe MS leads to slow pressure recovery (i.e., long pressure halftime) as the diastolic pressure never declines to zero – in other words, a gradient is still present at end diastole *(12)*. PHT can be used to calculate MVA with the following relationship:

$$MVA = 220/PHT$$

Pitfalls of Using Echo

When obtaining Doppler gradients and pressure halftime, care must be taken to have the ultrasound beam parallel to the jet of flow. If this is not done, the gradients and PHT will underestimate the severity of stenosis.

Pressure halftime measurement cannot be used if there is concomitant MR or LV dysfunction. Both of these states alter the pressure gradient across the MV; MR by virtue of raising LA pressure and LV dysfunction by raising LVEDP. Therefore the pressure decay measured if one or both of these conditions are present will not reflect pure pressure decay across the MV *(16)*. Finally, aortic insufficiency may preclude accurate measurement of PHT as the regurgitant volume into the LV will lead to more rapid rate of rise of pressure in early diastole and lead to a shorter pressure halftime thereby underestimating severity. Alternatively, severe AI may lead to early closure of the mitral valve and lengthen the PHT leading to overestimation of mitral stenosis severity.

Finally, it is important to remember that pressure gradients vary with both valve area and flow rate (i.e., cardiac output). If the cardiac output is low due to restricted filling, one can underestimate the pressure gradient and the MVA, either by echo or by catheterization *(7)*. Alternatively, if the diastolic filling period is diminished due to rapid heart rate, such as in atrial fibrillation, the gradient across the mitral valve will be increased.

CATHETERIZATION

The role of cardiac catheterization is to obtain information about the hemodynamic effects of mitral stenosis, measure the mitral valve gradient, calculate cardiac output, and use this information to calculate mitral valve area. Since the apical diastolic rumble is pathognomonic and the echocardiographic features diagnostic, the role of catheterization in MS is often confirmatory. Coronary angiography can be performed if questions exist regarding the co-existence of coronary artery disease, either as an alternative explanation for symptoms or as preoperative evaluation should mitral valve surgery be considered.

The most accurate way to measure intra-cardiac pressures is to directly measure the pressure in the chamber in question. For example, left atrial pressure is most accurately measured via transseptal puncture from the right atrium into the left atrium. This direct measurement allows determination of exact left atrial pressures and simultaneous LV pressure for determining mitral valve gradients, which can be particularly important when smaller gradients exist. However, in most cases the pulmonary capillary wedge pressure (PCWP) can be used as a surrogate for left atrial tracing. The PCWP waveform will be delayed by 55–100 msec relative to the LA pressure. It is therefore important to phase shift the peak of the V wave to the downslope of the LV pressure tracing prior to determining the mean gradient by planimetry (Fig. 4). Even with adequate correction of the wedge pressure for the time delay relative to left atrial pressure, the wedge pressure falls more slowly than the true left atrial pressure and tends to overestimate the gradient (and underestimate the valve area) by a small, and not usually clinically relevant, amount. The PCWP should not be used as a surrogate for LA pressure if the patient has significant lung disease as this can falsely elevate the PCWP (14).

Large V waves are often present in severe mitral stenosis and can identify co-existing mitral regurgitation. However, this finding is not very specific as large V waves are present in any condition in which left atrial compliance is diminished.

The hemodynamic impact of MS can be determined based on right heart catheterization measurements. The right atrial pressures and right ventricular pressures should be within the normal range in mild to moderate mitral stenosis. The pulmonary artery (PA) pressure is usually normal in mild disease, but as the disease progresses, chronically elevated LA pressures will lead to elevation in PA pressures. If this is longstanding and severe, irreversible pulmonary hypertension and elevation in right ventricular end diastolic pressure (RVEDP) will result.

Pulmonary artery catheterization is also used to determine cardiac output using either the Fick or the thermodilution method. The cardiac output is then used to calculate a mitral valve gradient with Gorlin equation described as follows:

$$MVA \left(cm^2\right) = \frac{CO/(DFP \times HR)}{K\sqrt{MVG}}$$

where CO is cardiac output in mL/min, DFP is diastolic filling period in seconds, and MVG is the mean valve gradient in mm Hg. K is a constant derived by Gorlin and Gorlin and is 37.9 for the mitral valve (15). The diastolic filling period is the time of the cardiac cycle spent in diastole, which is the time where there is flow across the mitral valve. The time in seconds is measured on the pressure tracing at

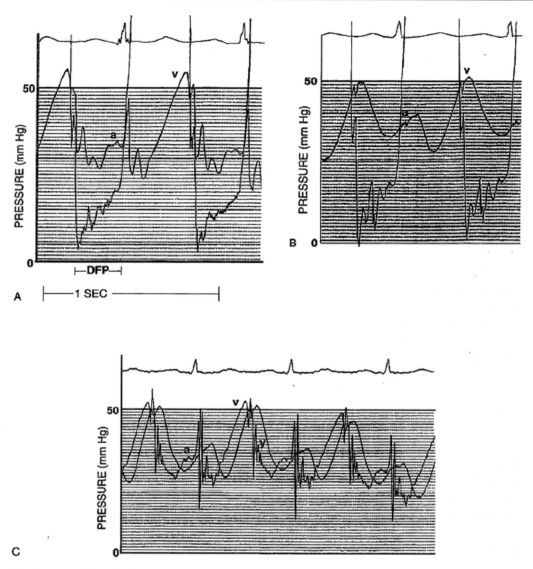

Fig. 4. Simultaneous left atrial and left ventricular pressure tracings are shown in a patient with rheumatic mitral stenosis and a mitral valve area of 1.0 cm^2 (**panel A**). The mean diastolic pressure gradient of 19 mm Hg is apparent and the diastolic filling period (DFP) is shown. **Panel B** demonstrates the rightward displacement (time delay) in the a and v waves when a simultaneous wedge pressure is recorded instead of a direct left atrial pressure measurement in the same patient. The left atrial pressure and pulmonary capillary wedge pressure were recorded simultaneously in **panel C** to demonstrate the time delay of ~75 msec and the attenuated pressure descent after the v wave on the wedge recording. Reproduced with permission from *(14)*.

fast paper speeds (100 mm/sec) from mitral valve opening to valve closure (Fig. 4). The time per beat is multiplied by the heart rate to derive the total diastolic filling period in seconds per minute *(16)*.

A quick estimation of the mitral valve area can be done using the Hakki equation described as CO/$\sqrt{}$MVG. However, this corresponds most accurately to the MVA when the heart rate is between 60 and 100 beats per minute. For a patient in sinus rhythm, the gradient should be averaged across 5 beats, while an average of 10 beats should be used for the patient in atrial fibrillation.

Pitfalls

The Gorlin equation was developed in 1951 by Gorlin and Gorlin and usually corresponds to echocardiographic measurements of MVA *(17)*. However, when co-existing mitral regurgitation is present, the Gorlin equation often underestimates the true area. This is because the cardiac output used in the Gorlin equation does not include the regurgitant fraction from MR which increases flow across the mitral valve in diastole.

It is also difficult to use the Gorlin equation in patients with low cardiac output, other valvular lesions, or atrial fibrillation. In these situations, echo information should be carefully integrated with catheterization data to determine severity of mitral stenosis.

The cardiac output determination is critical and can be obtained by the thermodilution technique in the absence of significant tricuspid regurgitation. Alternatively, the cardiac output can also be determined in the patient with multivalvular disease by the indicator dilution technique or using the Fick principle which relates the patient's oxygen consumption to the arterio-venous oxygen difference *(16)*.

In patients with a low cardiac output and/or a low gradient, the valve area calculation is highly dependent on the gradient, and extra care should be taken in its determination. The administration of saline to raise the flow and gradient if the left atrial pressure is not already too high may improve the accuracy of the calculations. Exercise can also be performed in the catheterization laboratory to help determine in a patient with a low gradient whether a patient's symptoms are due to mitral stenosis or another cause.

Heart rate also effects the measurement of mitral valve gradients. Slow heart rates (i.e., long RR intervals) allow equilibration of LA and LV pressures at end diastole while in faster HR, this equilibration never occurs. The longer the diastolic period, the more time is allowed for the pressure in the LA to decay to match LV pressures at end diastole. Therefore, higher gradients are calculated in tachycardia, which often explains the presence of symptoms during exercise, pregnancy, or atrial fibrillation.

EXERCISE TESTING

Exercise testing is indicated in the subset of patients who have symptoms that could be consistent with MS, but do not have clinical or echocardiographic evidence of moderate or severe MS. In this population, exercise can yield changes in the transmitral gradient or pulmonary artery pressures, which, if correlated with symptoms, implicate MS as the culprit in the patient's symptoms. Treadmill testing or bicycle testing with Doppler of transmitral and tricuspid velocities can be done. Alternatively, hemodynamics can be measured with a PA catheter during exercise. Patients who experience elevation of PA systolic pressure (PASP) greater than 60 mm Hg, a mean transmitral gradient of greater than 15 mm Hg, or PA pressures greater than 25 mm Hg likely have significant MS and are likely to benefit from intervention *(18, 19)*.

NATURAL HISTORY AND MANAGEMENT

Rheumatic mitral stenosis is a disease that is progressive, usually with a latent phase of 20–40 years from the initial rheumatic insult to the development of symptoms. Symptoms gradually increase in severity over several years and may take up to 10 years to become disabling. While the 10-year survival in patients with little or no symptoms is 80%, once significant symptoms do occur, the 10-year survival is a mere 0–15% (367–69) *(16)*. Importantly, in less developed countries, severe MS may develop as early as the early twenties. This may be due to repeated strep infections or due to a more virulent initial infection.

Individuals with rheumatic fever have a high risk of developing recurrences and need antimicrobial prophylaxis against future episodes of streptococcal infection. Since recurrence rates decrease with increasing age, prophylaxis is usually recommended for a limited period of time, although the exact duration is disputed *(17)*. The World Health Organization recommends antibiotic prophylaxis with penicillin for 5 years following the initial episode of rheumatic fever or up to age 18. Prophylaxis should be continued to at least 10 years if mild MR is present or until age 25, and should be continued for a lifetime if severe MS is present. Penicillin can be given in oral form as 4,000 Units twice daily or as intramuscular benzathine penicillin G 1.2 Million Units every 4 weeks *(20)*.

Although percutaneous or surgical intervention is the only definitive treatment for relief of mitral valve obstruction, there are several components of medical therapy that should be implemented to alleviate symptoms. Prompt treatment of tachycardia to prevent hemodynamic compromise is crucial. This includes treatment of tachycardia due to fever, anemia, hyperthyroidism, as well as counseling to avoid excessive physical exercise. Tachycardia increases flow across the stenotic valve and decreases diastolic filling time, both of which lead to further increase in LA pressures. The use of beta blockers and calcium channel blockers to decrease chronotropy has been shown to improve symptoms that result from tachycardia in the appropriate patient *(21)*. If pulmonary edema is present, diuretic therapy can be used to improve congestion.

Atrial fibrillation is a common occurrence in patients with MS, occurring in up to 40% of patients *(22)*. This is due to chronic LA pressure and volume overload and may also result from interatrial fibrosis caused by the rheumatic process *(19)*. For this reason, atrial fibrillation (AF) may persist or develop even after surgical treatment of MS. Treatment of atrial fibrillation involves rate control with beta blockers, digoxin, or calcium channel blockers, or cardioversion and maintenance of sinus rhythm with amiodarone in the appropriate patient. MS patients with paroxysmal or persistent AF are at increased risk for systemic emboli and therefore should be maintained on warfarin therapy.

In addition to MS patients with atrial fibrillation, any patient with MS who has a history of a prior embolic event or left atrial thrombus should be maintained on anticoagulation, regardless of underlying rhythm (Class I). Anticoagulation for patients with severe MS and left atrial dimension $\geq$ 55 mm with or without spontaneous contrast on echo is a class IIB recommendation *(23)*.

SPECIAL POPULATIONS

Pregnancy can cause severe hemodynamic stress on the heart. Plasma volume expands by 40%, which can increase left atrial pressures and increase the gradient across the mitral valve. Pregnant patients also experience an increase in heart rate, which shortens diastole and increases transmitral gradients. Finally, delivery poses major shifts in volume which can lead to a sudden increase in LA pressure and pulmonary edema.

Patients with mild to moderate MS can usually be managed with beta blockers and diuretics, although these must be used with caution so as not to lead to systemic hypotension and placental hypoperfusion. Patients with severe MS may not tolerate the hemodynamic stress of pregnancy and should be referred for intervention prior to conception or delivery.

The patient with mitral stenosis and severe pulmonary hypertension requires special consideration. These patients have an increased risk during cardiac surgery and may have a lesser risk with percutaneous balloon valvuloplasty *(24)*. The decision to perform balloon valvuloplasty in this setting requires a careful balancing of the probably lower risk of the balloon procedure with the likely greater and more sustained reduction in pulmonary artery pressure that can be achieved with the greater mitral valve area provided by a surgical prosthesis. Careful follow-up of patients after balloon valvuloplasty is essential to document the reduction in pulmonary pressure and the development of any recurrence *(25)*. Maneuvers to assess the reversibility of pulmonary hypertension, such as inhaled nitric oxide or other pulmonary vasodilators, may be useful to predict the response to treatment of mitral stenosis *(26)*.

INTERVENTIONS

Timing of Intervention

According to the 2006 ACC/AHA guidelines, intervention is recommended in symptomatic patients with moderate to severe MS. Asymptomatic patients with moderate to severe MS should be referred for intervention in the presence of pulmonary hypertension (PASP >50 mm Hg at rest or >60 mm Hg with exercise) *(24)*.

Mitral valve area should not be the sole criterion used to select patients for either percutaneous or surgical intervention. Several studies have demonstrated that symptomatic patients with mild and moderate stenosis may have substantial improvement in symptoms following successful intervention *(27)*. In this regard, the Gorlin formula may underestimate the severity of mitral stenosis in some patients due to large body size or high cardiac output.

Procedures

Given that mechanical obstruction to diastolic inflow in the left ventricle is the primary pathology in mitral stenosis, the definitive treatment of this disease is relief of the obstruction. This can be obtained by several methods, all of which will be discussed in more detail in Chapter 12, but will be briefly outlined below.

Percutaneous mitral valve balloon valvuloplasty (PMBV) is the treatment of choice in patients with moderate to severe MS who have non-calcified valves without significant subvalvular involvement, as described by the Wilkins criteria above. It is contraindicated in patients with left atrial thrombus, moderate to severe mitral regurgitation, or subvalvular involvement. The indications for PMBV are summarized in Table 2.

Table 2
Indications for Percutaneous Mitral Balloon Valvotomy (PMBV) for Mitral Stenosis

Class I
   1. PMBV is effective for symptomatic patients with moderate or severe MS and valve morphology favorable for PMBV in the absence of left atrial thrombus or moderate to severe MR.
   2. PMBV is effective for asymptomatic patients with moderate or severe MS and valve morphology favorable for PMBV who have pulmonary HTN (PASP >50 mm Hg at rest or >60 mm Hg with exercise) in the absence of LA thrombus or moderate to severe MR.

Class IIA
   1. PMBV is reasonable for patients with moderate to severe MS who have a nonpliable calcified valve, are in NYHA functional class III–IV, and are either not candidates for surgery or are at high risk for surgery.

Class IIB
   1. PMBV may be considered for asymptomatic patients with moderate or severe MS and valve morphology favorable for PMBV who have new onset atrial fibrillation in the absence of LA thrombus or moderate to severe MR.
   2. PMBV may be considered for symptomatic patients with MV area greater than 1.5 cm^2 if there is evidence of hemodynamically significant MS based on pulmonary artery systolic pressure greater than 60 mm Hg, PCWP of 25 mm Hg or more, or mean MV gradient greater than 15 mm HG during exercise.
   3. PMBV may be considered as alternative to surgery for patients with moderate or severe MS who have a nonpliable calcified valve and are in NYHA class III–IV.

CLASS III
   1. Not indicated for patients with mild MS.
   2. Should not be performed in patients with moderate to severe MR or LA thrombus.

Adapted from the ACC/AHA Guidelines *(23)*

If a patient's anatomy is not suitable for PMBV or if there is another contraindication, surgical repair is the preferred alternative. Surgical repair may involve open commissurotomy if the valve morphology is suitable. However, this operation is no more efficacious than PMBV. Mitral valve replacement is reserved for patients in whom surgical repair is not feasible.

REFERENCES

1. Wood P. An appreciation of mitral stenosis, clinical features. Br Med J 1954;4870:1051–63.
2. Guidelines for the Diagnosis of Rheumatic Fever. Jones Criteria, 1992 update. Special Writing Group Committee on Rheumatic Fever, Endocarditis, and Kawasaki Disease of the Council on Cardiovascular Disease in the Young of the American Heart Association. Jama 1992;268(15):2069–73.
3. Roberts WV, Perloff J. Mitral valvular disease: a clinicopathologic survey of the conditions causing the mitral valve to function abnormally. Ann Intern Med 1972;77:939–75.
4. Zipes DP, Libby P, Bonow RO, Braunwald EB. Heart Disease: A Textbook of Cardiovascular Medicine (7th ed). Philadelphia: Elsevier Science; 2004.
5. Braunwald E, Moscovitz HL, Mram SS, et al. The hemodynamics of the left side of the heart as studied by simultaneous left atrial, left ventricular, and aortic pressures; particular reference to mitral stenosis. Circulation 1955;12:69–81.
6. Rusted IE, Scheifley CH, Edwards JE. Studies of the mitral valve, II: certain anatomic features of the mitral valve and associated structures in mitral stenosis. Circulation 1956;14:398–406.
7. Otto CM, Pearlman AS. Textbook of Clinical Echocardiography. Philadelphia, PA: W.B Saunders Company; 1995.
8. Galvin JE, Hemric ME, Ward K, Cunningham MW. Cytotoxic MAb from rheumatic carditis recognizes heart valves and laminin. J Clin Invest 2000 Jul;106(2):217–24.
9. Hugenholtz PG, Ryan TJ, Stein SW, Belmann WH. The spectrum of pure mitral stenosis: hemodynamic studies in relation to clinical disability. Am J Cardiol 1962;10:773–84.
10. Rowe JC, Bland EF, Sprague HB, White PD. The course of mitral stenosis without surgery ten- and twenty-year perspectives. Ann Intern Med 1960;52:741–9
11. Murphy JG. Mayo Clinic Cardiology Review. Philadelphia, PA: Lippincott Williams and Wilkins; 2000, pp. 290–3.
12. Feigenbaum H. Feigenbaum's Echocardiography. Philadelphia, PA: Lippincott Williams and Wilkins; 2004.
13. Wilkins GT, Wey-man AE, Abascal VM, Block PC, Palacios IF. Percutaneous balloon dilatation of the mitral valve: an analysis of echocardiographic variables related to outcome and the mechanism of dilatation. Br Heart J 1988;60:299–308.
14. Herrmann HC. Mitral, Pulmonic, Tricuspid, and Prosthetic Valve Disease. In: Cardiac Catheterization, Uretsky BF, Eds. Malden, MA: Blackwell Science, Inc.; 1997, pp. 375–96.
15. Gorlin R, Gorlin SG. Hydraulic formula for calculation of stenotic mitral valve, other cardiac valves, and central circulatory shunts. Am Heart J 1951;41:1.
16. Selzer A, Cohn KE. Natural history of mitral stenosis: a review. Circulation 1972;45:878–90.
17. Dajani A, Taubert K, Ferrieri P, Peter G, Shulman S. Treatment of acute streptococcal pharyngitis and prevention of rheumatic fever: a statement for health professionals. Committee on rheumatic fever, endocarditis, and Kawasaki disease of the council of cardiovascular disease in the young, the American Heart Association. Pediatrics 1995 Oct;96 (4 pt 1):758–64.
18. Tamai J, Nagata S, Akaike M, et al. Improvement in mitral flow dynamics during exercise after percutaneous transvenous mitral commissurotomy: noninvasive evaluation using continuous wave Doppler technique. Circulation 1990;81:46–51.
19. Aviles RJ, Nishimura RA, Pellikka PA, Andreen KM, Holmes D. Utility of stress Doppler echocardiography in patients undergoing percutaneous mitral balloon valvotomy. J Am Soc Echocardiogr 2001;14:676–81.
20. World Health Organization. Rheumatic fever and rheumatic heart disease: a report of a WHO expert consultation. Geneva. WHO, 20 Oct to 1 Nov 2001. WHO Tech Rep Ser 2001;923.
21. Nakhjavan FK, Katz MR, Maranhao V, Goldberg H. Analysis of influence of catecholamine and tachycardia during supine exercise in patients with mitral stenosis and sinus rhythm. Br Heart J 1969;31:753–61.
22. Rowe JC, Bland EF, Sprague HB, White PD. The course of mitral stenosis without surgery ten- and twenty-year perspectives. Ann Intern Med 1960;52:741–9
23. Bonow RO, Carabello BA, Chatterjee J, et al. ACC/AHA 2006 guidelines for the management of patients with valvular heart disease. J Am Cell Cardiol 2006;48:1–148.
24. Vincens J, Temizer D, Post JR, Edmunds LH, Herrmann HC. Long-term outcome of cardiac surgery in patients with mitral stenosis and severe pulmonary hypertension. Circulation 1995;92(Suppl II):II-137–42.

25. Herrmann HC. Acute and chronic efficacy of percutaneous mitral commissurotomy: implications for patient selection. Cath and Cardiovasc Diag 1994;(Suppl 2):61–8.
26. Mahoney PD, Loh E, Blitz LR, Herrmann HC. Hemodynamic effects of inhaled nitric oxide in women with mitral stenosis and pulmonary hypertension. Am J Cardiol 2001;87:188–92.
27. Herrmann HC, Feldman T, Isner JM, et al. Comparison of results of percutaneous balloon valvuloplasty in patients with mild and moderate mitral stenosis to those with severe mitral stenosis. Am J Cardiol 1993;71:1300–3.

10 Mitral Regurgitation

*Maurice Enriquez-Sarano, Vuyisile T. Nkomo,
and Hector I. Michelena*

CONTENTS

NORMAL MITRAL STRUCTURE AND FUNCTION
ETIOLOGY AND MECHANISM OF MITRAL REGURGITATION
PATHOPHYSIOLOGY
CLINICAL MANIFESTATIONS
LABORATORY ASSESSMENT
NATURAL HISTORY
MANAGEMENT
REFERENCES

Mitral regurgitation (MR) is characterized by systolic blood flow reversal from the left ventricle (LV) to the left atrium (LA). MR etiology is predominantly degenerative in developed countries and rheumatic in developing countries. Doppler echocardiography is the noninvasive tool of choice for evaluation of MR and its consequences. Advances in MR surgery and better understanding of MR natural history have led to a more proactive surgical MR management and better outcomes.

NORMAL MITRAL STRUCTURE AND FUNCTION

The mitral valve is formed by four components: annulus, leaflets, chordae tendineae, and papillary muscles (1, 2). The annulus is asymmetrical, ellipse-shaped with an anterior fibrous portion (one-third of the annulus) shared with the aortic annulus and a posterior dynamic portion (2). The two mitral leaflets, anterior and posterior, attach at their bases to the corresponding anterior annulus and posterior annulus and are asymmetric. The anterior leaflet has a narrower base but greater leaflet length compared to the posterior leaflet (2). Leaflets are separated by commissures positioned anterolaterally and posteromedially (2). Primary chordae tendineae attach to leaflets' tips and secondary chordae tendineae attach to leaflets' body (1). The chordae attach to the two papillary muscles (anterolateral and posterolateral) affixed to the LV wall. Physiologically, pre-closure of mitral leaflets follows atrial contraction and approximates the two leaflets. Competent mitral closure during systole relies on the position of the anterior leaflet, forming a veil parallel to systolic flow in the LV outflow tract, and on the coaptation of leaflets, which creates strong shear forces. Coaptation over the rough zones on the atrial surfaces of both leaflets create high friction resistance. Finally, contraction of the posterior annulus approximates the leaflets enhancing coaptation. Disruption of any of these anatomic elements may result in coaptation loss and MR.

From: *Contemporary Cardiology: Valvular Heart Disease*
Edited by: Andrew Wang, Thomas M. Bashore, DOI 10.1007/978-1-59745-411-7_10
© Humana Press, a part of Springer Science+Business Media, LLC 2009

ETIOLOGY AND MECHANISM OF MITRAL REGURGITATION

Etiology and mechanism are not synonymous and a single cause (etiology) may generate MR by different mechanisms (Table 1). Etiology of MR is generally stratified as *ischemic* (MR due to consequences of coronary disease not fortuitous association of both) and *nonischemic* (all other causes). Mechanisms of MR are stratified as *functional* (mitral valve is structurally normal and MR is due to valve deformation caused by ventricular remodeling) or as *organic* (intrinsic valve lesions). MR mechanism is further specified by leaflet movement (Carpentier's classification): Type I (normal valve movement such as annular dilatation, perforation), Type II (excessive movement), and Type III (restrictive movement, IIIa: diastolic restriction such as rheumatic disease; IIIb: systolic restriction as in functional MR). Etiology and mechanism of MR are shown in Table 1. MR lesion localization is also defined by Carpentier description: The two commissures, anterolateral and posteromedial, separate the leaflets and opposing leaflet segments are labeled P1–A1 externally, P2–A2 centrally, and P3–A3 medially. This common framework of anatomic and echocardiographic analysis is essential in defining reparability for a specific patient and a specific surgical team. Major specific causes are as follows.

Table 1
Etiology and Mechanism of MR

| | | MR mechanism | | | | |
| | | Organic MR | | | Functional MR | |
		Type I*	Type II**	Type IIIa***	Type I*	Type IIIb***
MR etiology	Nonischemic	*Endocarditis*: perforation *Degenerative*: annular calcification *Congenital*: cleft leaflet	*Degenerative*: billowing/ flail leaflets *Endocarditis*: ruptured chordae *Traumatic*: ruptured chord/PM *Rheumatic*: acute RF	*Rheumatic*: chronic RF *Iatrogenic*: radiation/ drug *Inflammatory*: lupus/ anticardi-olipin, eosinophilic endocardial disease, endomy-ocardial fibrosis	Cardiomyopathy, myocarditis left ventricular dysfunction (any cause)	
	Ischemic		Ruptured PM		Functional ischemic MR	

*Type I: Mechanism involves normal leaflet movement
**Type II: Mechanism involves excessive valve movement
***Type III: Restricted valve movement, IIIa in diastole, IIIb in systole
MR, mitral regurgitation; PM, papillary muscle; RF, rheumatic fever.

Rheumatic Mitral Regurgitation

Rheumatic MR is usually associated with some fusion of commissures, but may be pure in young patients with active rheumatic carditis *(3)*. Severe rheumatic MR requiring surgical correction is frequent in developing countries *(4, 5)* but is rare in developed countries *(6)*. In pure active rheumatic MR, annulus dilatation and anterior leaflet prolapse from chordal elongation are noted *(3)*. In chronic rheumatic MR, retractile fibrosis of leaflets and chordae causes loss of coaptation and repair is difficult because it requires leaflet elongation *(7)*.

Degenerative Mitral Regurgitation

Degenerative MR includes myxomatous degeneration of the mitral valve with resultant mitral valve prolapse (abnormal movement of leaflet tissue beyond the annulus plane into the left atrium during systole) with or without ruptured chordae, mitral valve leaflet sclerosis or calcification, and mitral annulus calcification.

Primary mitral valve prolapse is due to diffuse or localized myxomatous degeneration of the mitral valve leaflets and or chordae, which results in leaflet thickening and redundancy and chordal elongation. Myxomatous degeneration is due to increased water content and accumulation of glycosaminoglycans *(8)*, collagen alteration *(9, 10)*, as well as dysfunctional regulation of the degradation–regeneration process of the leaflet matrix support tissue *(11)*. Diffuse myxomatous degeneration of leaflets characterizes the "floppy" mitral valve (also called Barlow's disease), with bileaflet prolapse, extensive valve hooding and chordal elongation with or without rupture, along with annular dilatation and possible dislocation. Localized myxomatous degeneration *(12)* is seen in older patients, more often in men than in women, and involves more commonly the posterior leaflet and is generally associated with chordal rupture causing a flail leaflet. Calcification of the mitral annulus and hypertension may precede occurrence of chordal rupture. Primary mitral valve prolapse is usually sporadic, but may be familial *(13–15)*. In western countries, mitral valve prolapse is the most frequent cause of severe MR requiring surgery *(6)*.

Secondary prolapse of mitral leaflets without primary myxomatous degeneration can be seen in rheumatic mitral valve disease, blunt thoracic trauma, endocarditis complicated by ruptured chordae, myocardial infarction associated with elongation or rupture of the papillary muscles, hypertrophic cardiomyopathy associated with chordal rupture and volume contraction of the LV.

Degenerative MR without mitral valve prolapse is usually due to mitral valve leaflet sclerosis or calcification with or without associated annulus calcification. The degree of mitral valve regurgitation associated with this type of degeneration of the mitral valve is usually mild.

Ischemic and Functional Mitral Regurgitation

The mechanism of ischemic and functional MR is similar, in that mitral leaflets are intrinsically normal, but their coaptation is incomplete *(16)* because of annular and left ventricular dilatation due to ischemia, previous myocardial infarction and scarring, aneurysm formation, cardiomyopathy, or myocarditis. However, myocardial infarction of a wall adjacent to the papillary muscles may be associated with incomplete or complete papillary muscle rupture (a form of organic MR). Papillary muscle rupture is associated with severe MR and hemodynamic compromise and is a surgical emergency *(17)*. It is a complication typically involving the posteromedial papillary muscle because of its single blood supply *(17)*.

Infective Endocarditis

Infective endocarditis causes MR mainly through tissue destruction causing chordal rupture or leaflet perforation. Infective endocarditis accounts for approximately 5% of cases of severe MR.

Other Causes of MR

Other causes of MR include *connective tissue diseases* such as Marfan syndrome, Ehlers–Danlos syndrome, pseudo-xanthoma elasticum, osteogenesis imperfecta, Hurler's disease, systemic lupus erythematosus and antiphospholipid antibody syndrome; *cardiac trauma*, blunt or penetrating;

myocardial diseases such as hypertrophic cardiomyopathy or sarcoidosis; *endocardial lesions*due to eosinophilic syndromes, endocardial fibroelastosis, carcinoid tumors, ergot toxicity, radiation toxicity, diet–drugs toxicity *(18)*; *congenital* lesions such as isolated cleft mitral valve or associated with persistent atrio-ventricular canal, corrected transposition with or without Ebstein abnormality of the left atrio-ventricular valve; and *(6) cardiac tumors* such as valve myxoma or fibroelastoma.

PATHOPHYSIOLOGY

Anatomic malcoaptation of mitral leaflets during systole results in a regurgitant orifice (ERO), which under the influence of the pressure gradient between LV and LA allows abnormal regurgitant flow into the LA. The sum of regurgitant flow throughout systole is the regurgitant volume (RVol) accumulated in the LA, which re-enters the LV during the next diastole so that MR results in volume overload of LA and LV.

The systolic pressure gradient between the LV and LA begins with closure of the mitral valve (S1) and persists after closure of the aortic valve (S2) up to mitral opening *(19)*. Thus, regurgitant flow lasts in systole as long as the ERO and is typically holosystolic. However, ERO can be dynamic depending on the cause of MR *(20)*. In mitral valve prolapse, the ERO appears or increases in mid-to-late systole with parallel variations in regurgitant flow *(20, 21)*. With small ERO not caused by mitral prolapse, ERO may become smaller during systole, thus limiting MR to early systole *(19)*. Determinants of RVol are the area of ERO *(22)*, the regurgitant gradient, and duration of regurgitation, so that RVol may vary with dynamic interventions. Additionally, in both organic MR *(23)* and functional MR *(24)*, ERO increases with increased afterload or ventricular volume and decreases with decreased afterload or improved contractility, but is independent of changes in heart rate *(23)*. Even vasodilators in severe MR may result in ERO changes with little change in LV–LA gradient *(25)*.

In the mitral regurgitant system, there is conservation of energy produced by the LV so that the sum of its components (kinetic and potential energies) remains constant. Kinetic energy is reflected by RVol and potential energy by LA pressure V-wave *(26)*. LA compliance is one of the major determinants of the V-wave and LA pressure *(26)*. In acute severe MR, LA is smaller and less compliant compared to chronic severe MR, so that a similar RVol will result in higher V-wave and LA pressure. Therefore, for any given ERO, acute MR translates more into higher LA pressure or potential energy and smaller RVol than in chronic MR *(22)*. In chronic MR, which progresses slowly over time, LA remodels and accommodates the RVol so that normal or near normal LA pressure is maintained despite severe MR and clinical tolerance may be excellent *(27)*.

Left ventricular dilatation is another consequence of volume overload and myocardial mass is increased proportionately to LV dilatation *(28)*. LV dilatation is typically less pronounced than in aortic regurgitation of similar degree *(29)*. LV end-diastolic volume and wall stress increase *(29)* and LV shape becomes more spherical. LV end-systolic volume is increased, but end-systolic wall stress is usually within normal limits *(30)*. LV dysfunction is a frequent and serious complication of severe MR *(31, 32)*, but is difficult to characterize because of preload and afterload changes. Those involve decrease in instantaneous impedance to ejection during systole while end-systolic wall stress (measure of afterload) is within normal limits *(30)*. However, the usual inverse relation of end-systolic wall stress to ejection fraction is maintained in MR *(33)*. LV dysfunction is associated with myocardial interstitial fibrosis, reduction in myofiber content, and decrease in myofiber contractility *(34)*. Diastolic LV dysfunction in severe MR is difficult to diagnose, but may be present in patients with severe MR and systolic dysfunction *(35)*. In patients with apparently normal systolic function, LV diastolic dysfunction is one of the mechanism explaining reduced functional capacity *(36)*.

Ischemic/Functional MR has a different physiology from organic MR as the primary disease involves LV dysfunction secondarily causing MR. The MR is due to localized LV deformation with apical and posterior displacement of the papillary muscles causing tethering and tenting of the leaflets and loss of coaptation surface *(37, 38)*. The RVol in ischemic MR is usually less than in organic MR *(39)* and the LV and LA dilatation are in excess to the degree of MR *(22)*. Despite this appearance of low-volume regurgitation, MR is associated with elevated LA pressure *(22)* and poor clinical outcome with reduced survival *(40)*, and heart failure in acute myocardial infarction *(40, 41)* and chronic ischemic heart disease *(42, 43)*.

Natriuretic peptides are elevated in clinical *(44)* and experimental *(45)* studies of organic MR. A-type natriuretic peptide elevation is related to LA pressure elevation *(44)*, but is relatively nonspecific *(46)*. B-type natriuretic peptide activation reflects hemodynamic, ventricular, and atrial consequences of MR rather than its degree *(47, 48)*. B-type natriuretic peptide activation is an independent predictor of death and heart failure in organic MR *(47)*. In dogs with organic MR, systemic activation of the renin–angiotensin system may occur *(49)*. Tissue levels of angiotensin II, however, are markedly elevated with organic MR *(50, 51)* irrespective of hemodynamic alterations. The role of the angiotensin system activation in subsequent development of LV hypertrophy and interstitial fibrosis in organic MR is not fully elucidated.

CLINICAL MANIFESTATIONS

The clinical manifestations of MR, symptoms, physical examination features, and electrocardiographic or radiographic changes are determined by the severity of MR, by the rapidity of MR development, and by the LA and LV functions and compliances. In developing countries, MR is a complication of rheumatic disease predominantly in young patients *(3, 5)*. In developed countries, rheumatic disease has decreased substantially, and MR is mostly degenerative, related to older age *(52, 53)* with patients presentation with severe MR most often in the sixth decade of life *(54)*. Overall, clinical examination is insensitive as compared to echocardiography in detecting mitral valve diseases, rheumatic *(55)*, or degenerative *(52)*.

Manifestations

Acute severe MR may be caused by spontaneous chordal rupture, papillary muscle rupture postinfarction, endocarditic perforation of mitral leaflets or chordal rupture and by leaflet rupture from trauma. It is associated with development of marked elevation of LA pressure due to a large regurgitant orifice and normal sized noncompliant LA. Acute dyspnea from pulmonary congestion is the predominant symptom. Papillary muscle rupture from myocardial infarction or blunt trauma may present with florid pulmonary edema and/or cardiogenic shock from low cardiac output. Development of acute dyspnea and atypical chest pain in a patient with MVP may signal acute chordal rupture.

Chronic severe MR is associated with LA enlargement and increased LA compliance, which tends to maintain normal or near normal LA pressure. Patients may remain asymptomatic for years despite severe MR. The typical symptoms are exertional dyspnea or fatigue relieved by resting. Severe exertional dyspnea, paroxysmal nocturnal dyspnea, frank pulmonary edema, or hemoptysis may also develop, but this is usually later in the course of MR and may be triggered by atrial fibrillation or increase in degree of MR. Sudden death as the initial presentation of MR is possible *(56)*.

Physical Examination

Mitral regurgitation is usually diagnosed because of a murmur when no or minimal symptoms are present *(54)*. Blood pressure is usually normal and carotid upstroke brisk. A palpable apical thrill is characteristic of severe MR but is rare while the apical impulse is more usually forceful and laterally displaced. A right ventricular heave may be present along the left sternal border with associated right ventricular dilatation.

The murmur of MR is systolic, heard best at the apex with the patient in the left lateral decubitus position. The murmur is often holosystolic, but is typically mid-late systolic and associated with a systolic click when caused by MVP. A MR murmur of short duration usually corresponds to mild MR, but with myocardial infarction and functional MR, severe MR may be soft or silent *(57)*. Therefore, the presence and intensity of murmur is a poor detector of ischemic or functional MR *(40, 41)*. The murmur radiates toward the axilla, but radiates posteriorly toward the spine when associated with anterior leaflet prolapse, and radiates anteriorly toward the base when associated with posterior leaflet prolapse *(58)*. When the murmur radiates to the base, it may be difficult to distinguish from that of aortic stenosis or from left ventricular outflow tract obstruction. A distinguishing feature is the lack of murmur intensity beat-to-beat variation with MR, such as with postextrasystolic beats *(59)* or atrial fibrillation while marked murmur variation would be expected with aortic stenosis or dynamic left ventricular outflow tract obstruction. Amyl nitrite reduces MR murmur intensity and increases that of obstructive lesions. MR murmur increases with isometric exercise or phenylephrine, while these maneuvers decrease obstructive murmurs. The murmur of MR also needs to be distinguished from

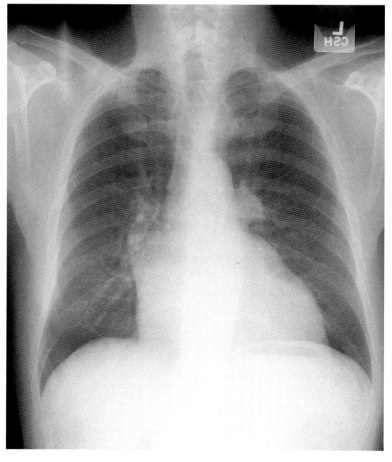

Fig. 1. Chest radiography in a patient with severe mitral regurgitation. Note the cardiomegaly, enlarged atrial appendage visible on the left contour of the heart, the enlarged left atrium and dilated pulmonary arteries.

that of ventricular septal defect since both are holosystolic. The murmur of ventricular septal defect is heard best at left sternal border instead of apex and may be associated with a parasternal thrill.

S1 intensity is usually normal, but may be decreased in chronic severe MR associated with defective leaflets or increased in rheumatic MR. Presence of S3 is directly related to MR degree in organic MR *(60)* and is often associated with a diastolic rumble which is low pitched and heard best in the left lateral decubitus position. In ischemic/functional MR, S3 reflects more restrictive LV filling than severity of MR.

Radiography

Cardiomegaly from LV enlargement and particularly LA enlargement is common in chronic severe organic MR (Fig. 1) and in ischemic/functional MR. Pulmonary edema and congestion is rare in chronic severe MR but is common in acute severe MR. A giant left atrium may signal mixed mitral valve disease. Calcification of the mitral leaflets is rarely seen but calcification of the mitral annulus is common particularly with degenerative MR and is best seen on lateral views, as a dense C-shaped opacity in the posterior cardiac silhouette.

Electrocardiogram

The electrocardiogram may be normal in patients with MR, even severe, particularly if it is acute. Sinus tachycardia may be present, particularly in the context of heart failure. The most frequent finding is LA enlargement in sinus rhythm while atrial fibrillation (Fig. 2), paroxysmal or permanent, ultimately affects 50% of patients within 10 years of diagnosis in sinus rhythm *(31)*. Left ventricular

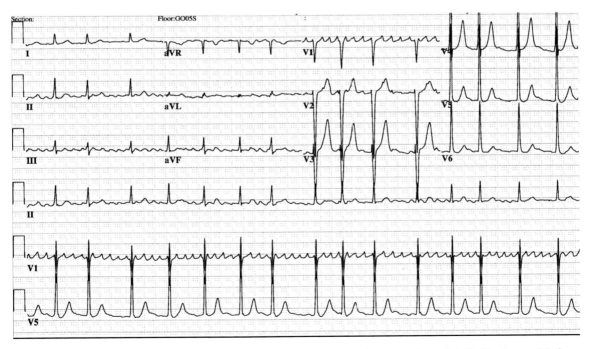

Fig. 2. Electrocardiogram in a patient with severe mitral regurgitation. Note the atrial fibrillation and left ventricular hypertrophy.

enlargement is less frequent *(61)* and right ventricular hypertrophy rare. In patients with ischemic or functional MR, Q waves and left bundle branch block may be noted.

Clinical Presentation Patterns

The clinical presentation combine various signs into suggestive patterns and are summarized in Table 2.

Table 2
Patterns of Clinical Presentations

	MVP syndrome	Chronic MR	Acute MR	Ischemic/functional MR
Symptoms	Chest pain	Fatigue	pulmonary edema	CHF
Physical examination	Mid-systolic click, murmur	Loud murmur S3	Loud murmur S4	Soft murmur S4, S3
ECG	ST-T Changes	Atrial fibrillation	Normal, sinus tachycardia	Q waves, LBBB
CXR	Pectus excavatum	Cardiomegaly	Normal heart size, pulmonary edema	Cardiomegaly, pulmonary edema

CXR, chest radiography; ECG, electrocardiogram; LBBB, left bundle branch block; MVP, mitral valve prolapse; S3 and S4, third and fourth heart sounds

LABORATORY ASSESSMENT

Doppler Echocardiography

Doppler echocardiography is the tool of choice in assessing valvular heart disease. The goals of Doppler echocardiography in MR are to assess the morphology and reparability of the mitral valve apparatus, the severity of MR, the LV and LA size and function, and the hemodynamic consequences of MR. This is achieved by use of two-dimensional echocardiography with directed M-mode measurements, color flow imaging, pulsed wave and continuous wave Doppler, and transesophageal echocardiography. The role of three-dimensional echocardiography remains undetermined.

MORPHOLOGY OF THE MITRAL VALVE APPARATUS

Rheumatic Mitral Valve Disease. Chronic rheumatic mitral valve disease is characterized by varying degrees of thickening of the leaflets and chordae, fusion of the commissures, and calcification of valvular and subvalvular components. The posterior leaflet is retracted and tethered with limited mobility (Fig. 3). The anterior leaflet may be doming in diastole from commissural fusion or be retracted limiting the length of coaptation. Similar lesions of thickened, retracted, and immobile mitral leaflets may be observed with diet-drugs or ergot toxicity. Similar leaflet thickening and retraction may result from anticardiolipin antibody syndrome with associated nonbacterial thrombotic endocarditis vegetations. Mitral valve prolapse in chronic rheumatic MR may occur after chordal rupture, while acute rheumatic valvulitis causes MR by elongation of the chordae and dilatation of the annulus and associated anterior leaflet prolapse.

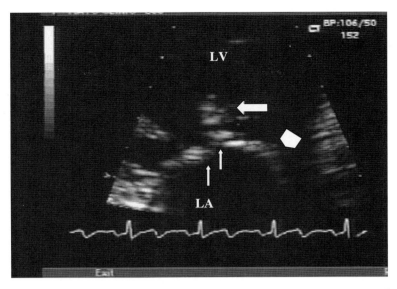

Fig. 3. Echocardiogram in a patient with rheumatic mitral regurgitation. The long *arrows* show the distal thickening of leaflets, the *arrowhead* the anterior leaflet doming, and the large *arrow* the thickening and shortening of subvalvular apparatus. LV, left ventricle; LA, left atrium.

Degenerative Mitral Regurgitation. Mitral valve prolapse from myxomatous disease is the most common form of degenerative mitral valve disease associated with clinically significant MR. It is diagnosed by passage of mitral leaflet tissue ≥2 mm beyond the annulus plane into the LA visualized from the parasternal long axis view during systole (Fig. 4). Echocardiography defines myxomatous changes of mitral leaflets, diffuse or localized (most often the posterior leaflet), with marked but pliable thickening and excessive leaflet tissue. Associated chordal ruptures *(62)* cause unsupported or flail segments which appear as complete eversion (Fig.5) with or without a floating echo density corresponding to a ruptured chordae (Fig. 6) typically seen in the left atrium during systole *(63)*. Defining the extent and localization of prolapse is essential for reparability and possible recurrence of MR postrepair and can be difficult in commissural lesion emphasizing the need for a thorough examination of the valve.

Mitral annulus calcification may accompany myxomatous mitral changes, with bright echogenic mitral annulus, typically involving the posterior annulus that may encroach on adjacent leaflet, ventricular or atrial tissue. Mild calcification is usually inconsequential, but moderate or severe annular calcification may cause loss of normal annulus contraction during systole and obstruction to diastolic flow *(64)*. The risk of developing degenerative mitral annulus and leaflet calcification is higher in patients with systemic diseases such as hypertension, end stage kidney disease, rheumatoid arthritis, or with diseases such as Marfan syndrome that affect the fibrous skeleton of the heart. Annular calcification is a limitation to valve repair when it is extensive and should be carefully delineated.

Endocarditic Mitral Regurgitation. Echocardiographic features of MR related to endocarditis include leaflet vegetations, flail segments, valve perforation, or annular abscess. Flail leaflets are easily identified by transthoracic echocardiography but ruptured chordae *(63)*, vegetations *(65)*, valvular aneurysms, and annular abscesses are detected with better sensitivity by transesophageal than transthoracic echocardiography.

Ischemic/Functional Mitral Regurgitation. Functional MR is a ventricular disease for which echocardiography may show global or regional wall motion abnormalities. The mechanism of

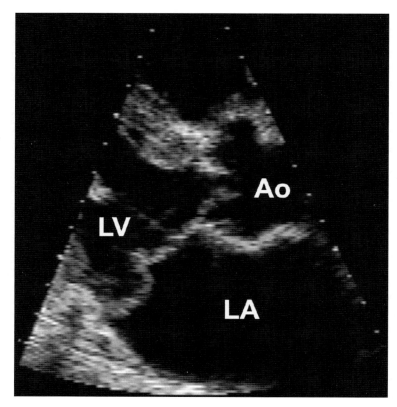

Fig. 4. Echocardiogram of a patient with mitral valve prolapse. Note the prolapse of the posterior leaflet and posterior displacement of the annulus. LV, left ventricle; LA, left atrium; Ao, aorta.

functional MR, irrespective of its etiology, is apical and posterior displacement of the papillary muscles that despite normal mitral leaflets causes tenting of leaflets due to abnormal traction by the strut (secondary) chordae (Fig. 7). Tenting combined with reduced annulus contraction during systole *(16, 66)* leads to incomplete coaptation and MR, which is in general central. Ischemic papillary muscle rupture is diagnosed based on a free floating mass (Fig. 8) attached to chordae and causing a flail leaflet in the setting of a myocardial infarction *(17)*.

Valve reparability is a function of the lesions and skills of the surgeon. Therefore, there are no uniform echocardiographic criteria for a repairable valve. However, reparability is higher with excess than retracted tissue and durability of repair is higher with posterior leaflet involvement than with anterior leaflet involvement *(67)* or valve tethering *(68)*. Thus the ideal repair case is the flail posterior leaflet due to primary ruptured chords, which in advanced repair centers can be repaired in >90% of cases *(63, 69)*.

ASSESSMENT OF MR SEVERITY

Assessment of MR severity is now conducted according to the American Society of Echocardiography guidelines *(70)*, using specific, supportive, and quantitative signs (Table 3).

Color flow imaging jet detection is highly sensitive in diagnosing MR but should be used with caution for MR severity assessment. The origin and direction of MR depend on MR etiology and mechanism. For instance, posterior mitral leaflet prolapse or flail is associated with an anteriorly directed jet

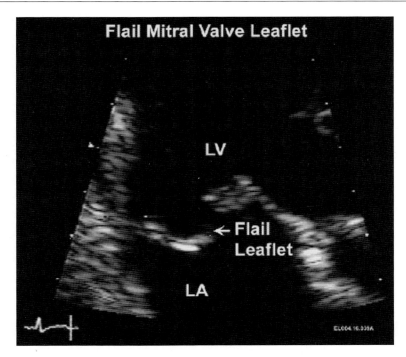

Fig. 5. Flail leaflet seen by transthoracic echocardiography.

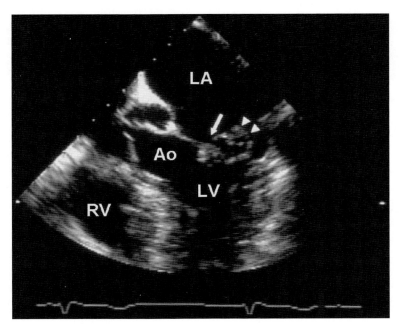

Fig. 6. Flail leaflet seen by transesophageal echocardiography. The *arrowheads* indicate the flail segment and the arrow the ruptured chordae. RV, right ventricle.

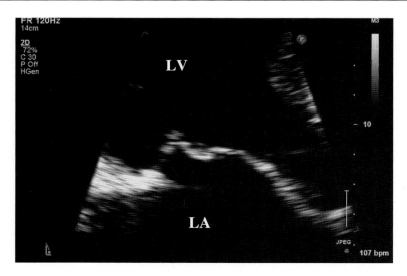

Fig. 7. Ischemic mitral regurgitation. Note the tenting of the leaflets above the mitral annulus.

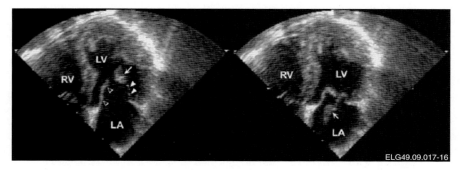

Fig. 8. Ruptured papillary muscle. The *left image* is in diastole showing (*arrow*) the ruptured papillary muscle in the left ventricle and the *right image* shows in systole the papillary muscle head in the left atrium. The *arrowheads* indicate mitral leaflets. RV, right ventricle.

whereas prolapse or flail of the anterior leaflet causes a posteriorly directed jet of MR and functional MR has usually a central jet. The extent of the jet into the LA is influenced by its momentum, and thus by its regurgitant velocity and flow. Jet length into the LA, jet to jet area ratio, or jet area can be measured *(71)*. Small MR jets correspond consistently to mild MR *(39)*. However, eccentric jets impinge on the LA wall and are constrained and MR may be underestimated *(39)*. Conversely, central jets are not constrained, expand more in large atria, and may overestimate RVol *(39)*. Therefore, for interpreting a jet as reflective of severe MR, it has to be large or reaching deep into LA and to be associated with wide vena contracta or large flow convergence. The vena contracta is the smallest neck of the regurgitant flow below the flow convergence *(72)*. Direct measurement of the width of the vena contracta provides an index of the ERO and is superior to jet area in estimating MR severity via transthoracic *(73)* or transesophageal *(72)* echocardiography. Transesophageal echocardiography does not overcome the limitations of jet expansion and may show larger jets, but can be useful in delineating extent of eccentric jets because of better resolution.

Pulmonary venous velocity profile is useful in showing flow reversal by pulsed wave Doppler, as a specific sign of severe MR *(74)*. However, systolic flow reversal in pulmonary veins is determined

Table 3
Gradation of MR by Doppler echocardiography

	Mild	Moderate		Severe
Specific signs	• Small central jet <4 cm² or <10% of LA. • Vena contracta width <0.3 cm • No or minimal flow convergence	MR more than mild, but no criteria for severe MR		• Vena contracta width ≥0.7 cm with large central MR jet (area >40% of LA) or with a wall-impinging jet of any size • Large flow convergence • Systolic reversal in pulmonary veins • Prominent flail leaflet or ruptured papillary muscle
Supportive signs	• Systolic dominant flow in pulmonary veins • A-wave dominant mitral inflow • Low density Doppler MR signal • Normal LV size	MR more than mild, but no criteria for severe MR		• Dense, triangular Doppler MR signal • E-wave dominant mitral inflow (E > 1.2 m/s) • Enlarged LV and LA size (particularly with normal LV function)
Quantitative parameters				
RVol (mL/beat)	<30	30–44	45–59	≥60
RF (%)	<30	30–39	40–49	≥50
ERO (cm²)	<0.20	0.20–0.29	0.30–0.39	≥0.40

ERO, effective regurgitant orifice area; LA, left atrium; LV, left ventricle; MR: mitral regurgitation; RF, regurgitant fraction; RVol: regurgitant volume.

Modified from Zoghbi et al. *(70)*.

not only by MR severity, but also by LA pressure and may be absent in severe MR, underscoring the insensitivity of this sign *(75)*.

Anatomic features are specific for severe MR when a flail leaflet or ruptured papillary muscle are diagnosed. However, approximately 15% of patients with flail leaflets have only moderate MR and care should be applied in using this sign.

Supportive signs include pulsed-Doppler mitral inflow patterns, which with E predominance are compatible with moderate or severe MR while A predominance suggests more mild MR. Continuous wave Doppler appearance of partial or faint density suggests mild MR. Enlarged LA and LV suggest severe MR (Fig. 9).

Quantitative methods measure volume overload as RVol, calculated as the difference between total stroke volume and forward stroke volume. In addition, quantitative echocardiography measures regurgitant lesion severity as ERO *(22, 76)* calculated as

$$ERO = \text{regurgitant flow/regurgitant velocity, or}$$
$$ERO = \text{regurgitant volume/regurgitant TVI}$$

where TVI is the time velocity integral of the regurgitant jet.

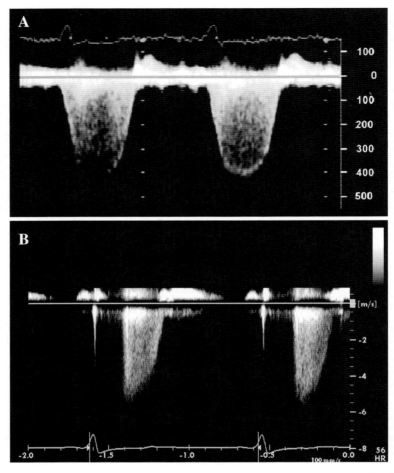

Fig. 9. Continuous wave Doppler of mitral regurgitation. In **A** is shown a dense holosystolic signal. In **B** is shown a purely end-systolic signal.

There are several methods to provide these measurements, all based on application of the conservation of mass principle. Quantitative Doppler measures mitral and aortic stroke volumes using pulsed wave Doppler (Fig. 10). Pitfalls are related to mitral stroke volume measurements, which can be technically challenging and have a significant learning curve *(77)*. Quantitative two-dimensional echocardiography uses LV volumes to calculate total stroke volume. Proximal isovelocity surface area (PISA) directly measures the regurgitant flow by analyzing the zone of flow convergence proximal to the regurgitant orifice. Color flow mapping precisely defines blood velocity at the flow convergence (Fig. 11) to calculate regurgitant flow, and combined with velocity and regurgitant TVI, measured by continuous wave Doppler, allows calculation of RVol and ERO *(76)*.

Comprehensive assessment of MR involves utilization of the entire array of available information *(70)*. Qualitative assessment is sufficient in general to diagnose mild MR but does not provide direct signs of moderate MR. For laboratories proficient in use of quantitative methods, these provide direct positive diagnosis of all grades of MR, concordant assessment using multiple methods in a single examination and superior prognostic prediction *(78)*. In general, severe MR is considered present with ERO ≥ 0.40 cm^2 or with RVol ≥ 60 mL/beat *(79)*. However, functional/ischemic MR is associated with

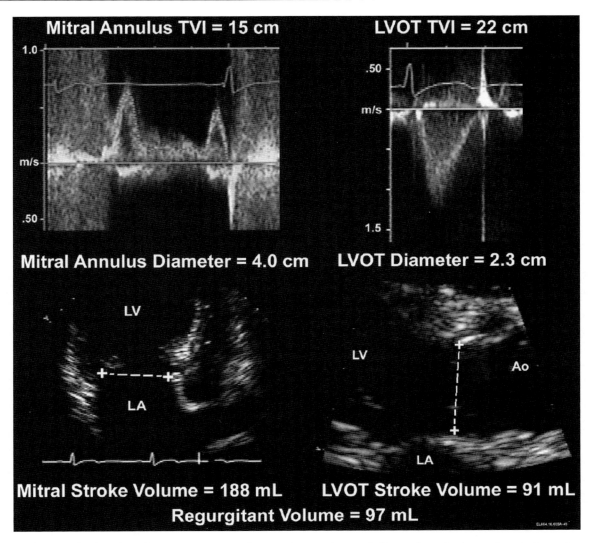

Fig. 10. Quantitative Doppler measurement of regurgitant volume. *Left* are the mitral annular stroke volume measurements and *right* the left ventricular outflow tract (LVOT) stroke volume measurements. The difference between these two stroke volumes is the regurgitant volume.

poor outcome with smaller ERO $\geq$0.20 cm^2 *(43)*, so that the interpretation of "severe MR" may be different for organic and functional MR.

ASSESSMENT OF LV AND LA SIZE AND FUNCTION

The size, mass, and wall stress of the LV and LA size can be obtained by M-mode diameters *(80–82)*, and LV volumes can be reliably measured by two-dimensional measurements *(83, 84)*. LV ejection fraction can be calculated from M-mode or two-dimensional measurements *(85)* or can be visually estimated *(86)*. These measures have shown their prognostic value for survival under medical management *(54)* and postoperatively *(80, 87)*. Ejection fraction $\leq$60% or LV end-systolic diameter $\geq$40 mm are considered reflective of overt LV dysfunction *(88)*. LA volume is simple to obtain

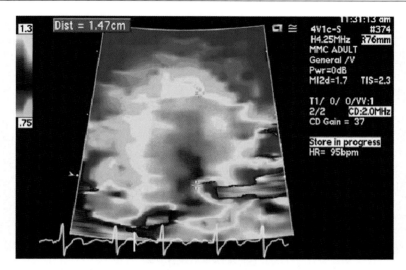

Fig. 11. Color flow imaging of the flow convergence for the PISA (proximal isovelocity surface area) measurement. Note the displacement of the color baseline allowing clear visibility of the flow convergence in *yellow*.

by two-dimensional echocardiography, reliable and predictive of the occurrence of atrial fibrillation during follow-up *(89)*.

Radionuclide and Other Noninvasive Imaging Studies

Left and right ventricular end-diastolic and end-systolic dimensions, volumes, and ejection fractions can also be assessed by ECG gated radionuclide angiography *(90)*, but arrhythmias such as atrial fibrillation and ventricular ectopy limit this technique. The mitral regurgitant fraction can be calculated by using the ratio of LV to RV stroke volume *(91)*. Magnetic resonance imaging shows the jet of MR and offers the possibility of quantitative assessment of regurgitation *(92)*. Resolution of valvular imaging is insufficient to determine reparability.

Exercise Testing

Electrocardiographic changes induced by exercise are nonspecific and in general exercise testing is performed with imaging or with cardiopulmonary metabolic assessment. Exercise-induced LV dysfunction detected by radionuclide angiography is not uncommon in patient with severe MR, but the significance of this finding on long-term prognosis is not clear. Imaging with echocardiography during exercise may be used to judge changes in LV function *(93)*, but also changes in the severity of MR *(94)*, which are associated with subsequent outcome. These techniques are relatively labor-intensive and accuracy may remain a problem. In contrast cardiopulmonary exercise testing is standardized and allows defining functional capacity (peak oxygen consumption) *(95)*, which is often markedly reduced even in asymptomatic patients *(36)*.

Cardiac Catheterization

Cardiac catheterization is rarely used for initial diagnosis of MR, but may be an important adjunct if Doppler echocardiography is poor and inadequate. Qualitative assessment of MR severity relies on degree and persistence of LA opacification during LV angiography using the Sellers criteria *(96)*.

This method has important limitations *(97)*. Cardiac catheterization can determine RVol by comparing estimated angiographic LV stroke volume to LV forward stroke volume calculated by the Fick or thermodilution methods *(98)*. Angiographic stroke volume often overestimates true stroke volume and calculations may be erroneous and difficult to verify by repeat testing. The major hemodynamic consequences of MR, decreased cardiac output, and elevated pulmonary wedge pressure can be assessed invasively. The large V-wave of the pulmonary wedge pressure is more common in acute severe MR but also occurs in cardiac condition with poor LA compliance without severe MR.

Left ventricular end-diastolic and end-systolic volumes and ejection fraction by quantitative angiography correlate with MR severity and with LV systolic impairment and are useful prognosticators of clinical outcome *(32, 99)*. More complex indices such as LV wall stress, maximum LV elastance, passive diastolic stiffness *(35)*, and LV systolic stiffness can also be measured, but incremental value of these measurements to traditional LV size and ejection fraction measures remains to be fully defined.

Cardiac catheterization defines coronary anatomy by selective coronary angiography. Coronary angiography should be performed preoperatively in patients with severe MR and older than 40–50 years since obstructive coronary artery disease continues to be frequent in patients with severe MR even in the absence of angina *(100)*.

Strategy of Utilization of Diagnostic and Laboratory Testing

Doppler echocardiography usually defines presence, etiology, and severity of MR as well as associated valve lesions and attendant adverse consequences on LV and LA. It is the test of choice for initial assessment of MR, for follow-up, as well as for pre-surgical assessment. Transesophageal echocardiography adds incremental value to transthoracic echocardiography, but only when the latter is incomplete *(63)*. Transesophageal echocardiography is used extensively intraoperatively to assess results of mitral valve surgery *(101)*. Coronary angiography is indicated preoperatively depending on the age of the patient. Left ventricular angiography need not be performed for redundant testing since it does not add materially to comprehensive noninvasive information, unless there is absolute need to corroborate echocardiography because of concern over its validity *(22, 102)*. Therefore, not all tests need to be performed in all patients with severe MR *(88)*, but testing does have to be individualized depending on patient characteristics and results of noninvasive testing.

NATURAL HISTORY

Natural history of MR has not been well defined in the pre-surgical era. This is in large part due to imprecise assessment of MR severity. In unoperated patients with clinically significant MR, survival was found to be as high as 60% at 10 years in some studies *(103)*, but as low as 46% *(104)* or lower at 27% *(105)* at 5 years. Patients with mild rheumatic MR have a good prognosis *(106)*, but those with severe MR do not *(107)*. More recent data aimed at filling these gaps of knowledge. One useful model is MR due to flail leaflets, which in the vast majority of cases is severe. Patients with this condition incur 10-year survival under medical management lower than expected survival *(54)*, underscoring the serious nature of severe organic MR despite the rarity of symptoms at diagnosis. While some studies in young patients with healthy participant bias and mostly moderate MR have observed less impressive mortality *(108)*, coherent data in mitral valve prolapse *(109)*, flail leaflets *(110)*, and any etiology of severe MR (78) show excess mortality with medical management of severe MR (Fig. 12).

Patients with severe MR also incur notable morbidity. Patients with severe MR due to MVP develop symptoms indicating surgery at a rate of 10% per year *(111)*. In patients with flail leaflets, heart failure occurs in 63% 10 years after diagnosis and 30–40% of those initially in sinus rhythm develop permanent atrial fibrillation after 10 years *(54)*, and 50% develop paroxysmal or permanent atrial fibrillation *(112)*. In addition, 90% of patients with flail mitral leaflets will either die or undergo surgery

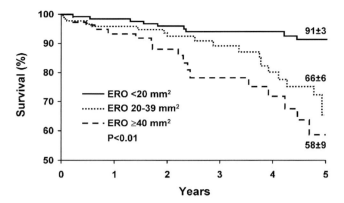

Fig. 12. Survival under medical management of patients with organic mitral regurgitation according to the effective regurgitant orifice area measurement. From Enriquez-Sarano et al. *(78)* with permission of the Massachusetts Medical Society.

after 10-year follow-up. MR progression is usually slow at 5–8 mL per year, but can be as high as 20 mL per year in those with a new flail mitral leaflet *(113)*. The mechanism of MR progression is the increase in ERO associated to increase in annular size. Regression in MR degree is infrequent but can be achieved with afterload reduction *(113)*. Progression of LV dysfunction in patients treated medically is not well defined.

Unexpected sudden death is a dreaded complication of severe MR and occurs more often when there is associated LV dysfunction *(56)*, but may occur with normal systolic function in asymptomatic patients *(107)*. Sudden death in severe MR occurs at an overall rate of 1.8% per year, more frequently in symptomatic patients or those with reduced LV systolic function *(114)*. Sudden death occurs at a rate of 0.8% per year in those asymptomatic with preserved systolic function *(114)*.

The predictors of a poor outcome in patients with severe MR treated medically are as follows:

1. NYHA class III–IV symptoms *(104)*, even if transient with diuretic therapy *(54)*;
2. pulmonary hypertension;
3. increased LV end-diastolic volume or arteriovenous difference in oxygen *(115)*;
4. reduced LV ejection fraction *(54)*;
5. marked LA enlargement *(89, 112)*;
6. B-type natriuretic peptide activation *(47)*;
7. reduced functional capacity *(36)*; and
8. large ERO ($\geq$0.40 cm^2) *(78)*.
9. Atrial Fibrillation *(112)*.

MANAGEMENT

Principles

Mitral valve surgery should be considered for patients with severe organic MR because outcome with surgical treatment is superior to medical management *(78, 110, 116)*, particularly if repair can be performed *(110)*. Comparison of prognosis in patients treated medically and surgically shows better survival with surgery *(107)*, particularly when offered early *(116)*, even in patients with reduced LV systolic function *(115)*. However, no clinical trial has yet been conducted.

In ischemic MR, many doubts remain on the best approach to treatment, so that surgical indication remains guided by symptoms.

Medical Management

Chronic afterload reduction with vasoactive drugs for management of chronic severe MR is not proven to improve outcome, and vasoactive drugs are not recommended as mainstay therapy of substitute for mitral valve surgery (88). Hydralazine has been shown acutely to lower aortic impedance and increase stroke volume while decreasing severity of MR, but this drug is not well tolerated and there are no long-term studies showing beneficial effect (25). Angiotensin converting enzyme inhibitors have been studied in small series (117–119), but their long-term efficacy is not well defined and there are discrepancies in terms of their effect of the degree of MR (120) and LV remodeling (121). Diuretic therapy is helpful in the control of symptoms of heart failure. Atrial fibrillation is rate controlled with a combination of beta blockers and digoxin and anticoagulation is indicated. Beta blockers are also particularly helpful in patients with MVP and palpitations. Long-term maintenance of sinus rhythm with cardioversion or antiarrhythmic drugs is difficult in patients with severe MR or large LA, but sinus rhythm may be restored by mitral valve repair particularly if it has been of short duration preoperatively (122).

Rheumatic fever prophylaxis should be given to patients with previous rheumatic fever and its duration is tailored according to presence and severity of rheumatic valve disease (123). The role of bacterial endocarditis prophylaxis in patients with valve diseases has been revised (124), and patients with MR from myxomatous mitral valve disease or rheumatic MR are no longer recommended to receive prophylaxis. Patients with previous mitral valve replacement should continue to receive prophylaxis (124). Good oral hygiene is emphasized to reduce the risk of infective endocarditis (124).

For patients with ischemic MR, medical therapy (vasodilators or beta blockers) may reduce MR and are warranted before a surgical decision is made. Biventricular pacing may be useful.

Surgical Management

Surgical techniques for management of severe MR are centered around valve repair. Briefly, the goal of mitral valve surgery should be to repair the valve and not replace it, unless mitral valve repair is impossible or unsuccessful. The approach is via the traditional sternotomy and more recently "minimally invasive" procedures via smaller sternotomy or thoracotomy or port access are being utilized.

Intraoperative transesophageal echocardiography does not interfere with the surgical procedure and should be performed intraoperatively to assess adequacy of mitral valve repair such as for residual regurgitation or stenosis or development of systolic anterior motion of the mitral leaflets with dynamic left ventricular outflow tract obstruction (101). If mitral valve repair is inadequate, mitral valve replacement should be performed.

Mitral valve repair or reconstruction has a lower mortality compared to mitral valve replacement (125, 126), although direct comparison is hindered by the fact that patients undergoing mitral valve repair are typically younger than those undergoing valve replacement (125). Operative mortality in earlier series of mitral valve replacement was reported to be between 5 and 12% (127) but in the more recent era is 1−2% in patients younger than 75 years with organic MR undergoing mitral valve repair or replacement (80). Although operative mortality has decreased for patients above the age of 75 years, it remains higher at around 4−5% compared to 1−2% for patients younger than 75 years (128). Age, symptoms, and coronary artery disease are the strongest predictors of operative mortality (80), but LV function in patients with organic MR is not a predictor of operative mortality and therefore even patients with reduced systolic function have a reasonable chance of surviving surgery (80). Operative mortality for ischemic MR is higher at 6−10%.

Postoperative survival is better following mitral valve repair than after mitral valve replacement and restores expected survival in those who are asymptomatic or have minimal symptoms prior to surgery. In our experience with a population with a mean age of 62 years, the overall 5- and 10-year survival is 83 and 68%, respectively, for mitral valve repair, compared to 69 and 52% for mitral valve replacement (125).

In the majority of patients undergoing mitral valve surgery there is symptomatic improvement by at least one functional class and most patients become asymptomatic. However, postoperative heart failure and reoccurrence of symptoms do occur in operative survivors due in two-thirds of cases to residual LV dysfunction *(87)*. Postoperative heart failure in a minority of cases is related to mitral prosthetic valve failure or failure of repair *(87)*. Recurrent MR requires reoperation after valve repair in 5–10% of patients within 10 years *(67)*, more frequently after repair of ischemic MR *(68)*.

Postoperative mortality after mitral valve surgery is related predominantly to residual LV dysfunction *(32, 80)*. The majority of patients demonstrate a fall in LV ejection fraction after mitral surgery *(28, 31)*. Overall, LV dysfunction following mitral valve surgery occurs in 41% of patients and in 32% of those with organic MR *(31)*. The decline in LV ejection fraction after mitral valve surgery may be explained by several factors including permanent irreversible myocardial damage, intraoperative myocardial insult, diminished preload after correction of MR, and increase in impedance to LV ejection after elimination of MR. However, LV systolic dysfunction is probably already present even before most of the patients are operated given the relationships between pre- and postoperative LV function *(28, 30–32, 99)*. and between preoperative LV function and postoperative survival *(80, 81, 129)*. In patients with MR, because of altered loading conditions, LV contractile function may be depressed while LV ejection fraction remains normal and multiple and complex indices of LV function have been proposed *(30, 33, 129)*. LV ejection fraction, however, remains a useful and powerful predictor of postoperative LV ejection fraction *(28, 31, 32)* and survival *(80)*. Generally, LV ejection fraction can be expected to decrease by 10% early following mitral valve surgery *(28, 31, 32)*, but more decline is observed in patients with marked increase in LV end-systolic diameter *(31, 81)*, volume *(32, 99)*, or wall stress *(31)* and in patients with severe symptoms or coronary artery disease *(31)*. Although surgical correction of severe MR provides better outcomes than medical therapy *(115)*, patients with LV ejection fraction <50% have a high postoperative late mortality *(80)*. Also, although patients with a "borderline" reduced LV ejection fraction between 50 and 60% have a better late postoperative outcome, they too show excess late mortality compared to patients with a preoperative LV ejection fraction of >60% *(80)*. Therefore, long-term outcome of mitral valve surgery is best in those patients with LV ejection fraction >60% and end-systolic diameter <40 mm *(80, 88)*.

Preoperative symptoms impact negatively postoperative survival after surgery for severe MR *(130)*. NYHA class III or IV symptoms are a strong and independent predictor of postoperative excess postoperative mortality *(130)*. Conversely, patients with NYHA class I or II symptoms incur very low operative mortality *(130)* and excellent long-term survival similar to expected survival *(130)*.

Atrial fibrillation, if present before mitral valve surgery, usually persists unless it was of short duration preoperatively *(122)* and the Maze procedure can be preformed for atrial fibrillation at the time of mitral valve surgery with minimal additional risk *(131)*. Postoperative atrial fibrillation requires long-term anticoagulation, but its impact on excess risk postoperatively appears only modest *(87)*. Late risk of thromboembolism favors mitral valve repair over replacement *(125, 126)* and the risk of postoperative bleeding is obviously higher in those needing anticoagulation either because of a mechanical valve or because of atrial fibrillation *(125)*.

Indications for Surgery in Organic MR

Indications for mitral valve surgery can be summarized as follows *(88)*:

TRADITIONAL INDICATIONS FOR ORGANIC MR

1. Patients with acute severe MR;
2. Patients with chronic severe MR and severe symptoms (NYHA functional class III or IV) even if they improve with medical therapy;

3. Patients with minimal symptoms (NYHA functional class II); and
4. Patents who are asymptomatic, but have signs of LV dysfunction (LV ejection fraction <60% or LV end-systolic dimension ≥40−45 mm).

ADVANCED INDICATIONS

Patients who are asymptomatic (NYHA functional class I) and have preserved LV ejection fraction >60% and LV end-systolic dimension <40 mm, but have atrial fibrillation or pulmonary hypertension.

EARLY SURGERY FOR ORGANIC MR

Patients who are asymptomatic (NYHA functional class I) and have preserved LV ejection fraction >60% and LV end-systolic dimension <40 mm and with a repairable valve. These patients can be expected to do very well with surgery and their postoperative survival is the same as expected survival *(80, 130)*. This indication is controversial, class IIa in American guidelines *(88)* and IIb in European guidelines *(132)*.

The controversy is related to exposing patients to the risk of surgery when surgery is not justified by either symptoms of LV dysfunction. Therefore, certain conditions must be met if asymptomatic patients without LV dysfunction are referred for surgery:

a. systematic quantitation of MR with multiple imaging modalities if necessary to make sure it is severe MR
b. low operative risk of 1−2%
c. high probability of valve repair which means surgery must be preformed by a surgeon experienced in this operation
d. intraoperative transesophageal echocardiogram should be available and performed to assess adequacy of repair.

Indication for Surgery in Ischemic MR

Indications are much more circumspect than in organic MR and require severe MR persistent despite full medical therapy and persistent symptoms despite treatment. The choice of repair versus replacement remains disputed *(133, 134)*, and in view of the limited survival expected (due to LV dysfunction), valve replacement with a bioprosthesis may be warranted in patients with severe and ongoing LV remodeling *(135)*.

REFERENCES

1. Lam JH, Ranganathan N, Wigle ED, Silver MD. Morphology of the human mitral valve. I. Chordae tendineae: a new classification. Circulation 1970;41:449–58.
2. Ranganathan N, Lam JH, Wigle ED, Silver MD. Morphology of the human mitral valve. II. The value leaflets. Circulation 1970;41:459–67.
3. Marcus RH, Sareli P, Pocock WA, Barlow JB. The spectrum of severe rheumatic mitral valve disease in a developing country. Correlations among clinical presentation, surgical pathologic findings, and hemodynamic sequelae. Ann Intern Med 1994;120:177–83.
4. Essop MR, Nkomo VT. Rheumatic and nonrheumatic valvular heart disease: epidemiology, management, and prevention in Africa. Circulation 2005;112:3584–91.
5. Nkomo VT. Epidemiology and prevention of valvular heart diseases and infective endocarditis in Africa. Heart 2007;93:1510–9.

6. Olson LJ, Subramanian R, Ackermann DM, Orszulak TA, Edwards WD. Surgical pathology of the mitral valve: a study of 712 cases spanning 21 years. Mayo Clin Proc 1987;62:22–34.

7. Acar C, de Ibarra JS, Lansac E. Anterior leaflet augmentation with autologous pericardium for mitral repair in rheumatic valve insufficiency. J Heart Valve Dis 2004;13:741–6.

8. Grande-Allen KJ, Griffin BP, Ratliff NB, Cosgrove DM, Vesely I. Glycosaminoglycan profiles of myxomatous mitral leaflets and chordae parallel the severity of mechanical alterations. J Am Coll Cardiol 2003;42:271–7.

9. Baker PB, Bansal G, Boudoulas H, Kolibash AJ, Kilman J, Wooley CF. Floppy mitral valve chordae tendineae: histopathologic alterations. Hum Pathol 1988;19:507–12.

10. van der Bel-Kahn J, Duren DR, Becker AE. Isolated mitral valve prolapse: chordal architecture as an anatomic basis in older patients. J Am Coll Cardiol 1985;5:1335–40.

11. Rabkin E, Aikawa M, Stone JR, Fukumoto Y, Libby P, Schoen FJ. Activated interstitial myofibroblasts express catabolic enzymes and mediate matrix remodeling in myxomatous heart valves. Circulation 2001;104:2525–32.

12. Hickey AJ, Wilcken DE, Wright JS, Warren BA. Primary (spontaneous) chordal rupture: relation to myxomatous valve disease and mitral valve prolapse. J Am Coll Cardiol 1985;5:1341–6.

13. Disse S, Abergel E, Berrebi A, et al. Mapping of a first locus for autosomal dominant myxomatous mitral-valve prolapse to chromosome 16p11.2–p12.1. Am J Hum Genet 1999;65:1242–51.

14. Trochu JN, Kyndt F, Schott JJ, et al. Clinical characteristics of a familial inherited myxomatous valvular dystrophy mapped to Xq28. J Am Coll Cardiol 2000;35:1890–7.

15. Freed LA, Acierno JS, Jr, Dai D, et al. A locus for autosomal dominant mitral valve prolapse on chromosome 11p15.4. Am J Hum Genet 2003;72:1551–9.

16. Izumi S, Miyatake K, Beppu S, et al. Mechanism of mitral regurgitation in patients with myocardial infarction: a study using real-time two-dimensional Doppler flow imaging and echocardiography. Circulation 1987;76:777–85.

17. Kishon Y, Oh JK, Schaff HV, Mullany CJ, Tajik AJ, Gersh BJ. Mitral valve operation in postinfarction rupture of a papillary muscle: immediate results and long-term follow-up of 22 patients. Mayo Clin Proc 1992;67:1023–30.

18. Connolly HM, Crary JL, McGoon MD, et al. Valvular heart disease associated with fenfluramine-phentermine. N Engl J Med 1997;337:581–8.

19. Yellin EL, Yoran C, Sonnenblick EH, Gabbay S, Frater RW. Dynamic changes in the canine mitral regurgitant orifice area during ventricular ejection. Circ Res 1979;45:677–83.

20. Schwammenthal E, Chen C, Benning F, Block M, Breithardt G, Levine RA. Dynamics of mitral regurgitant flow and orifice area. Physiologic application of the proximal flow convergence method: clinical data and experimental testing. Circulation 1994;90:307–22.

21. Enriquez-Sarano M, Miller FA, Jr, Hayes SN, Bailey KR, Tajik AJ, Seward JB. Effective mitral regurgitant orifice area: clinical use and pitfalls of the proximal isovelocity surface area method. J Am Coll Cardiol 1995;25:703–9.

22. Enriquez-Sarano M, Seward JB, Bailey KR, Tajik AJ. Effective regurgitant orifice area: a noninvasive Doppler development of an old hemodynamic concept. J Am Coll Cardiol 1994;23:443–51.

23. Yoran C, Yellin EL, Becker RM, Gabbay S, Frater RW, Sonnenblick EH. Dynamic aspects of acute mitral regurgitation: effects of ventricular volume, pressure and contractility on the effective regurgitant orifice area. Circulation 1979;60:170–6.

24. Keren G, Bier A, Strom JA, Laniado S, Sonnenblick EH, LeJemtel TH. Dynamics of mitral regurgitation during nitroglycerin therapy: a Doppler echocardiographic study. Am Heart J 1986;112:517–25.

25. Chatterjee K, Parmley WW, Swan HJ, Berman G, Forrester J, Marcus HS. Beneficial effects of vasodilator agents in severe mitral regurgitation due to dysfunction of subvalvar apparatus. Circulation 1973;48:684–90.

26. Grose R, Strain J, Cohen MV. Pulmonary arterial V waves in mitral regurgitation: clinical and experimental observations. Circulation 1984;69:214–22.

27. Braunwald E, Awe WC. The syndrome of severe mitral regurgitation with normal left atrial pressure. Circulation 1963;27:29–35.

28. Enriquez-Sarano M, Hannachi M, Jais JM, Acar J. [Hemodynamic and angiographic results following surgical correction of mitral insufficiency. Apropos of 51 repeated catheterizations]. Arch Mal Coeur Vaiss 1983;76:1194–203.

29. Wisenbaugh T, Spann JF, Carabello BA. Differences in myocardial performance and load between patients with similar amounts of chronic aortic versus chronic mitral regurgitation. J Am Coll Cardiol 1984;3:916–23.

30. Starling MR, Kirsh MM, Montgomery DG, Gross MD. Impaired left ventricular contractile function in patients with long-term mitral regurgitation and normal ejection fraction. J Am Coll Cardiol 1993;22:239–50.

31. Enriquez-Sarano M, Tajik AJ, Schaff HV, et al. Echocardiographic prediction of left ventricular function after correction of mitral regurgitation: results and clinical implications. J Am Coll Cardiol 1994;24:1536–43.

32. Crawford MH, Souchek J, Oprian CA, et al. Determinants of survival and left ventricular performance after mitral valve replacement. Department of Veterans Affairs Cooperative Study on Valvular Heart Disease. Circulation 1990;81:1173–81.

33. Corin WJ, Monrad ES, Murakami T, Nonogi H, Hess OM, Krayenbuehl HP. The relationship of afterload to ejection performance in chronic mitral regurgitation. Circulation 1987;76:59–67.

34. Urabe Y, Mann DL, Kent RL, et al. Cellular and ventricular contractile dysfunction in experimental canine mitral regurgitation. Circ Res 1992;70:131–47.

35. Corin WJ, Murakami T, Monrad ES, Hess OM, Krayenbuehl HP. Left ventricular passive diastolic properties in chronic mitral regurgitation. Circulation 1991;83:797–807.

36. Messika-Zeitoun D, Johnson BD, Nkomo V, et al. Cardiopulmonary exercise testing determination of functional capacity in mitral regurgitation: physiologic and outcome implications. J Am Coll Cardiol 2006;47:2521–7.

37. He S, Fontaine AA, Schwammenthal E, Yoganathan AP, Levine RA. Integrated mechanism for functional mitral regurgitation: leaflet restriction versus coapting force: in vitro studies. Circulation 1997;96:1826–34.

38. Otsuji Y, Handschumacher MD, Schwammenthal E, et al. Insights from three-dimensional echocardiography into the mechanism of functional mitral regurgitation: direct in vivo demonstration of altered leaflet tethering geometry. Circulation 1997;96:1999–2008.

39. Enriquez-Sarano M, Tajik AJ, Bailey KR, Seward JB. Color flow imaging compared with quantitative Doppler assessment of severity of mitral regurgitation: influence of eccentricity of jet and mechanism of regurgitation. J Am Coll Cardiol 1993;21:1211–9.

40. Lamas GA, Mitchell GF, Flaker GC, et al. Clinical significance of mitral regurgitation after acute myocardial infarction. Survival and Ventricular Enlargement Investigators. Circulation 1997;96:827–33.

41. Bursi F, Enriquez-Sarano M, Nkomo VT, et al. Heart failure and death after myocardial infarction in the community: the emerging role of mitral regurgitation. Circulation 2005;111:295–301.

42. Grigioni F, Detaint D, Avierinos JF, Scott C, Tajik J, Enriquez-Sarano M. Contribution of ischemic mitral regurgitation to congestive heart failure after myocardial infarction. J Am Coll Cardiol 2005;45:260–7.

43. Grigioni F, Enriquez-Sarano M, Zehr KJ, Bailey KR, Tajik AJ. Ischemic mitral regurgitation: long-term outcome and prognostic implications with quantitative Doppler assessment. Circulation 2001;103:1759–64.

44. Brookes CI, Kemp MW, Hooper J, Oldershaw PJ, Moat NE. Plasma brain natriuretic peptide concentrations in patients with chronic mitral regurgitation. J Heart Valve Dis 1997;6:608–12.

45. Haggstrom J, Hansson K, Karlberg BE, Kvart C, Olsson K. Plasma concentration of atrial natriuretic peptide in relation to severity of mitral regurgitation in Cavalier King Charles Spaniels. Am J Vet Res 1994;55:698–703.

46. Rossi A, Enriquez-Sarano M, Abel M, et al. Natriuretic peptide levels in atrial fibrillation: a prospective hormonal and Doppler-echocardiographic study. J Am Coll Cardiol 2000;35:1256–62.

47. Detaint D, Messika-Zeitoun D, Avierinos JF, et al. B-type natriuretic peptide in organic mitral regurgitation: determinants and impact on outcome. Circulation 2005;111:2391–7.

48. Detaint D, Messika-Zeitoun D, Chen HH, et al. Association of B-type natriuretic peptide activation to left ventricular end-systolic remodeling in organic and functional mitral regurgitation. Am J Cardiol 2006;97:1029–34.

49. Pedersen HD, Koch J, Poulsen K, Jensen AL, Flagstad A. Activation of the renin-angiotensin system in dogs with asymptomatic and mildly symptomatic mitral valvular insufficiency. J Vet Intern Med 1995;9:328–31.

50. Dell'Italia LJ, Meng QC, Balcells E, et al. Increased ACE and chymase-like activity in cardiac tissue of dogs with chronic mitral regurgitation. Am J Physiol 1995;269:H2065–73.

51. Dell'Italia LJ, Meng QC, Balcells E, et al. Compartmentalization of angiotensin II generation in the dog heart. Evidence for independent mechanisms in intravascular and interstitial spaces. J Clin Invest 1997;100:253–8.

52. Nkomo VT, Gardin JM, Skelton TN, Gottdiener JS, Scott CG, Enriquez-Sarano M. Burden of valvular heart diseases: a population-based study. Lancet 2006;368:1005–11.

53. Singh JP, Evans JC, Levy D, et al. Prevalence and clinical determinants of mitral, tricuspid, and aortic regurgitation (the Framingham Heart Study). Am J Cardiol 1999;83:897–902.

54. Ling LH, Enriquez-Sarano M, Seward JB, et al. Clinical outcome of mitral regurgitation due to flail leaflet. N Engl J Med 1996;335:1417–23.

55. Marijon E, Ou P, Celermajer DS, et al. Prevalence of rheumatic heart disease detected by echocardiographic screening. N Engl J Med 2007;357:470–6.

56. Kligfield P, Hochreiter C, Niles N, Devereux RB, Borer JS. Relation of sudden death in pure mitral regurgitation, with and without mitral valve prolapse, to repetitive ventricular arrhythmias and right and left ventricular ejection fractions. Am J Cardiol 1987;60:397–9.

57. Forrester JS, Diamond G, Freedman S, et al. Silent mitral insufficiency in acute myocardial infarction. Circulation 1971;44:877–83.

58. Antman EM, Angoff GH, Sloss LJ. Demonstration of the mechanism by which mitral regurgitation mimics aortic stenosis. Am J Cardiol 1978;42:1044–8.

59. Desjardins VA, Enriquez-Sarano M, Tajik AJ, Bailey KR, Seward JB. Intensity of murmurs correlates with severity of valvular regurgitation. Am J Med 1996;100:149–56.

60. Folland ED, Kriegel BJ, Henderson WG, Hammermeister KE, Sethi GK. Implications of third heart sounds in patients with valvular heart disease. The Veterans Affairs Cooperative Study on Valvular Heart Disease. N Engl J Med 1992;327:458–62.

61. Glick BN, Roberts WC. Usefulness of total 12-lead QRS voltage in diagnosing left ventricular hypertrophy in clinically isolated, pure, chronic, severe mitral regurgitation. Am J Cardiol 1992;70:1088–92.

62. Scott-Jupp W, Barnett NL, Gallagher PJ, Monro JL, Ross JK. Ultrastructural changes in spontaneous rupture of mitral chordae tendineae. J Pathol 1981;133:185–201.

63. Enriquez-Sarano M, Freeman WK, Tribouilloy CM, et al. Functional anatomy of mitral regurgitation: accuracy and outcome implications of transesophageal echocardiography. J Am Coll Cardiol 1999;34:1129–36.

64. Mellino M, Salcedo EE, Lever HM, Vasudevan G, Kramer JR. Echographic-quantified severity of mitral anulus calcification: prognostic correlation to related hemodynamic, valvular, rhythm, and conduction abnormalities. Am Heart J 1982;103:222–5.

65. Shively BK, Gurule FT, Roldan CA, Leggett JH, Schiller NB. Diagnostic value of transesophageal compared with transthoracic echocardiography in infective endocarditis. J Am Coll Cardiol 1991;18:391–7.

66. Boltwood CM, Tei C, Wong M, Shah PM. Quantitative echocardiography of the mitral complex in dilated cardiomyopathy: the mechanism of functional mitral regurgitation. Circulation 1983;68:498–508.

67. Mohty D, Orszulak TA, Schaff HV, Avierinos JF, Tajik JA, Enriquez-Sarano M. Very long-term survival and durability of mitral valve repair for mitral valve prolapse. Circulation 2001;104:I1–I7.

68. Hung J, Papakostas L, Tahta SA, et al. Mechanism of recurrent ischemic mitral regurgitation after annuloplasty: continued LV remodeling as a moving target. Circulation 2004;110:II85–90.

69. Monin JL, Dehant P, Roiron C, et al. Functional assessment of mitral regurgitation by transthoracic echocardiography using standardized imaging planes diagnostic accuracy and outcome implications. J Am Coll Cardiol 2005;46:302–9.

70. Zoghbi WA, Enriquez-Sarano M, Foster E, et al. Recommendations for evaluation of the severity of native valvular regurgitation with two-dimensional and Doppler echocardiography. J Am Soc Echocardiogr 2003;16:777–802.

71. Spain MG, Smith MD, Grayburn PA, Harlamert EA, DeMaria AN. Quantitative assessment of mitral regurgitation by Doppler color flow imaging: angiographic and hemodynamic correlations. J Am Coll Cardiol 1989;13:585–90.

72. Tribouilloy C, Shen WF, Quere JP, et al. Assessment of severity of mitral regurgitation by measuring regurgitant jet width at its origin with transesophageal Doppler color flow imaging. Circulation 1992;85:1248–53.

73. Mele D, Vandervoort P, Palacios I, et al. Proximal jet size by Doppler color flow mapping predicts severity of mitral regurgitation. Clinical studies. Circulation 1995;91:746–54.

74. Klein AL, Obarski TP, Stewart WJ, et al. Transesophageal Doppler echocardiography of pulmonary venous flow: a new marker of mitral regurgitation severity. J Am Coll Cardiol 1991;18:518–26.

75. Enriquez-Sarano M, Dujardin KS, Tribouilloy CM, et al. Determinants of pulmonary venous flow reversal in mitral regurgitation and its usefulness in determining the severity of regurgitation. Am J Cardiol 1999;83:535–41.

76. Vandervoort PM, Rivera JM, Mele D, et al. Application of color Doppler flow mapping to calculate effective regurgitant orifice area. An in vitro study and initial clinical observations. Circulation 1993;88:1150–6.

77. Enriquez-Sarano M, Bailey KR, Seward JB, Tajik AJ, Krohn MJ, Mays JM. Quantitative Doppler assessment of valvular regurgitation. Circulation 1993;87:841–8.

78. Enriquez-Sarano M, Avierinos JF, Messika-Zeitoun D, et al. Quantitative determinants of the outcome of asymptomatic mitral regurgitation. N Engl J Med 2005;352:875–83.

79. Dujardin KS, Enriquez-Sarano M, Bailey KR, Nishimura RA, Seward JB, Tajik AJ. Grading of mitral regurgitation by quantitative Doppler echocardiography: calibration by left ventricular angiography in routine clinical practice. Circulation 1997;96:3409–15.

80. Enriquez-Sarano M, Tajik AJ, Schaff HV, Orszulak TA, Bailey KR, Frye RL. Echocardiographic prediction of survival after surgical correction of organic mitral regurgitation. Circulation 1994;90:830–7.

81. Wisenbaugh T, Skudicky D, Sareli P. Prediction of outcome after valve replacement for rheumatic mitral regurgitation in the era of chordal preservation. Circulation 1994;89:191–7.

82. Zile MR, Gaasch WH, Carroll JD, Levine HJ. Chronic mitral regurgitation: predictive value of preoperative echocardiographic indexes of left ventricular function and wall stress. J Am Coll Cardiol 1984;3:235–42.

83. Schiller NB, Shah PM, Crawford M, et al. Recommendations for quantitation of the left ventricle by two-dimensional echocardiography. American Society of Echocardiography Committee on Standards, Subcommittee on Quantitation of Two-Dimensional Echocardiograms. J Am Soc Echocardiogr 1989;2:358–67.

84. Thomson HL, Basmadjian AJ, Rainbird AJ, et al. Contrast echocardiography improves the accuracy and reproducibility of left ventricular remodeling measurements: a prospective, randomly assigned, blinded study. J Am Coll Cardiol 2001;38:867–75.

85. Quinones MA, Waggoner AD, Reduto LA, et al. A new, simplified and accurate method for determining ejection fraction with two-dimensional echocardiography. Circulation 1981;64:744–53.

86. Amico AF, Lichtenberg GS, Reisner SA, Stone CK, Schwartz RG, Meltzer RS. Superiority of visual versus computerized echocardiographic estimation of radionuclide left ventricular ejection fraction. Am Heart J 1989;118:1259–65.

87. Enriquez-Sarano M, Schaff HV, Orszulak TA, Bailey KR, Tajik AJ, Frye RL. Congestive heart failure after surgical correction of mitral regurgitation. A long-term study. Circulation 1995;92:2496–503.

88. Bonow RO, Carabello BA, Chatterjee K, et al. ACC/AHA 2006 guidelines for the management of patients with valvular heart disease: a report of the American College of Cardiology/American Heart Association Task Force on Practice Guidelines (writing Committee to revise the 1998 guidelines for the management of patients with valvular heart disease) developed in collaboration with the Society of Cardiovascular Anesthesiologists endorsed by the Society for Cardiovascular Angiography and Interventions and the Society of Thoracic Surgeons. J Am Coll Cardiol 2006; 48:e1–148.

89. Messika-Zeitoun D, Bellamy M, Avierinos JF, et al. Left atrial remodelling in mitral regurgitation – methodologic approach, physiological determinants, and outcome implications: a prospective quantitative Doppler-echocardiographic and electron beam-computed tomographic study. Eur Heart J 2007;28:1773–81.

90. Zaret BL, Wackers FJ. Nuclear cardiology (2). N Engl J Med 1993;329:855–63.

91. Boucher CA, Bingham JB, Osbakken MD, et al. Early changes in left ventricular size and function after correction of left ventricular volume overload. Am J Cardiol 1981;47:991–1004.

92. Gelfand EV, Hughes S, Hauser TH, et al. Severity of mitral and aortic regurgitation as assessed by cardiovascular magnetic resonance: optimizing correlation with Doppler echocardiography. J Cardiovasc Magn Reson 2006;8:503–7.

93. Leung D, Griffin B, Snader C, Luthern L, JD T, Marwick T. Determinants of functional capacity in chronic mitral regurgitation unassociated with coronary artery disease or left ventricular dysfunction. Am J Cardiol 1997;79:914–20.

94. Lancellotti P, Troisfontaines P, Toussaint AC, Pierard LA. Prognostic importance of exercise-induced changes in mitral regurgitation in patients with chronic ischemic left ventricular dysfunction. Circulation 2003;108:1713–7.

95. Le Tourneau T, de Groote P, Millaire A, et al. Effect of mitral valve surgery on exercise capacity, ventricular ejection fraction and neurohormonal activation in patients with severe mitral regurgitation. J Am Coll Cardiol 2000;36:2263–9.

96. Sellers RD, Levy MJ, Amplatz K, Lillehei CW. Left retrograde cardioangiography in acquired cardiac disease: technique, indications and interpretations in 700 cases. Am J Cardiol 1964;14:437–47.

97. Croft CH, Lipscomb K, Mathis K, et al. Limitations of qualitative angiographic grading in aortic or mitral regurgitation. Am J Cardiol 1984;53:1593–8.

98. Sandler H, Dodge HT, Hay RE, Rackley CE. Quantitation of valvular insufficiency in man by angiocardiography. Am Heart J 1963;65:501–13.

99. Borow KM, Green LH, Mann T, et al. End-systolic volume as a predictor of postoperative left ventricular performance in volume overload from valvular regurgitation. Am J Med 1980;68:655–63.

100. Enriquez-Sarano M, Klodas E, Garratt KN, Bailey KR, Tajik AJ, Holmes DR, Jr. Secular trends in coronary atherosclerosis – analysis in patients with valvular regurgitation. N Engl J Med 1996;335:316–22.

101. Freeman WK, Schaff HV, Khandheria BK, et al. Intraoperative evaluation of mitral valve regurgitation and repair by transesophageal echocardiography: incidence and significance of systolic anterior motion. J Am Coll Cardiol 1992;20:599–609.

102. Leitch JW, Mitchell AS, Harris PJ, Fletcher PJ, Bailey BP. The effect of cardiac catheterization upon management of advanced aortic and mitral valve disease. Eur Heart J 1991;12:602–7.

103. Rapaport E. Natural history of aortic and mitral valve disease. Am J Cardiol 1975;35:221–7.

104. Munoz S, Gallardo J, Diaz-Gorrin JR, Medina O. Influence of surgery on the natural history of rheumatic mitral and aortic valve disease. Am J Cardiol 1975;35:234–42.

105. Horstkotte D, Loogen F, Kleikamp G, Schulte HD, Trampisch HJ, Bircks W. [Effect of prosthetic heart valve replacement on the natural course of isolated mitral and aortic as well as multivalvular diseases. Clinical results in 783 patients up to 8 years following implantation of the Bjork-Shiley tilting disc prosthesis]. Z Kardiol 1983;72:494–503.

106. Wilson MG, Lim WN. The natural history of rheumatic heart disease in the third, fourth, and fifth decades of life. I. Prognosis with special reference to survivorship. Circulation 1957;16:700–12.

107. Delahaye JP, Gare JP, Viguier E, Delahaye F, De Gevigney G, Milon H. Natural history of severe mitral regurgitation. Eur Heart J 1991;12(Suppl B):5–9.

108. Rosenhek R, Rader F, Klaar U, et al. Outcome of watchful waiting in asymptomatic severe mitral regurgitation. Circulation 2006;113:2238–44.

109. Avierinos JF, Gersh BJ, Melton LJ, III, et al. Natural history of asymptomatic mitral valve prolapse in the community. Circulation 2002;106:1355–61.

110. Grigioni F, Tribouilloy C, Avierinos JF, et al. Outcomes in mitral regurgitation due to flail leaflets. J Am Coll Cardiol Img 2008;1:133–141.

111. Rosen SE, Borer JS, Hochreiter C, et al. Natural history of the asymptomatic/minimally symptomatic patient with severe mitral regurgitation secondary to mitral valve prolapse and normal right and left ventricular performance. Am J Cardiol 1994;74:374–80.

112. Grigioni F, Avierinos JF, Ling LH, et al. Atrial fibrillation complicating the course of degenerative mitral regurgitation: determinants and long-term outcome. J Am Coll Cardiol 2002;40:84–92.
113. Enriquez-Sarano M, Basmadjian AJ, Rossi A, Bailey KR, Seward JB, Tajik AJ. Progression of mitral regurgitation: a prospective Doppler echocardiographic study. J Am Coll Cardiol 1999;34:1137–44.
114. Grigioni F, Enriquez-Sarano M, Ling LH, et al. Sudden death in mitral regurgitation due to flail leaflet. J Am Coll Cardiol 1999;34:2078–85.
115. Hammermeister KE, Fisher L, Kennedy W, Samuels S, Dodge HT. Prediction of late survival in patients with mitral valve disease from clinical, hemodynamic, and quantitative angiographic variables. Circulation 1978;57:341–9.
116. Ling LH, Enriquez-Sarano M, Seward JB, et al. Early surgery in patients with mitral regurgitation due to flail leaflets: a long-term outcome study. Circulation 1997;96:1819–25.
117. Tischler MD, Rowan M, LeWinter MM. Effect of enalapril therapy on left ventricular mass and volumes in asymptomatic chronic, severe mitral regurgitation secondary to mitral valve prolapse. Am J Cardiol 1998;82:242–5.
118. Marcotte F, Honos GN, Walling AD, et al. Effect of angiotensin-converting enzyme inhibitor therapy in mitral regurgitation with normal left ventricular function. Can J Cardiol 1997;13:479–85.
119. Host U, Kelbaek H, Hildebrandt P, Skagen K, Aldershvile J. Effect of ramipril on mitral regurgitation secondary to mitral valve prolapse. Am J Cardiol 1997;80:655–8.
120. Rothlisberger C, Sareli P, Wisenbaugh T. Comparison of single dose nifedipine and captopril for chronic severe mitral regurgitation. Am J Cardiol 1994;73:978–81.
121. Wisenbaugh T, Sinovich V, Dullabh A, Sareli P. Six month pilot study of captopril for mildly symptomatic, severe isolated mitral and isolated aortic regurgitation. J Heart Valve Dis 1994;3:197–204.
122. Chua YL, Schaff HV, Orszulak TA, Morris JJ. Outcome of mitral valve repair in patients with preoperative atrial fibrillation. Should the maze procedure be combined with mitral valvuloplasty? J Thorac Cardiovasc Surg 1994;107:408–15.
123. Dajani A, Taubert K, Ferrieri P, Peter G, Shulman S. Treatment of acute streptococcal pharyngitis and prevention of rheumatic fever: a statement for health professionals. Committee on Rheumatic Fever, Endocarditis, and Kawasaki Disease of the Council on Cardiovascular Disease in the Young, the American Heart Association. Pediatrics 1995;96:758–64.
124. Wilson W, Taubert KA, Gewitz M, et al. Prevention of infective endocarditis: guidelines from the American Heart Association: a guideline from the American Heart Association Rheumatic Fever, Endocarditis, and Kawasaki Disease Committee, Council on Cardiovascular Disease in the Young, and the Council on Clinical Cardiology, Council on Cardiovascular Surgery and Anesthesia, and the Quality of Care and Outcomes Research Interdisciplinary Working Group. Circulation 2007;116:1736–54.
125. Enriquez-Sarano M, Schaff HV, Orszulak TA, Tajik AJ, Bailey KR, Frye RL. Valve repair improves the outcome of surgery for mitral regurgitation. A multivariate analysis. Circulation 1995;91:1022–8.
126. Perier P, Deloche A, Chauvaud S, et al. Comparative evaluation of mitral valve repair and replacement with Starr, Bjork, and porcine valve prostheses. Circulation 1984;70:I187–92.
127. Cohn LH, Allred EN, Cohn LA, et al. Early and late risk of mitral valve replacement. A 12 year concomitant comparison of the porcine bioprosthetic and prosthetic disc mitral valves. J Thorac Cardiovasc Surg 1985;90:872–81.
128. Detaint D, Sundt TM, Nkomo VT, et al. Surgical correction of mitral regurgitation in the elderly: outcomes and recent improvements. Circulation 2006;114:265–72.
129. Carabello BA, Nolan SP, McGuire LB. Assessment of preoperative left ventricular function in patients with mitral regurgitation: value of the end-systolic wall stress-end-systolic volume ratio. Circulation 1981;64:1212–7.
130. Tribouilloy CM, Enriquez-Sarano M, Schaff HV, et al. Impact of preoperative symptoms on survival after surgical correction of organic mitral regurgitation: rationale for optimizing surgical indications. Circulation 1999;99:400–5.
131. Handa N, Schaff HV, Morris JJ, Anderson BJ, Kopecky SL, Enriquez-Sarano M. Outcome of valve repair and the Cox maze procedure for mitral regurgitation and associated atrial fibrillation. J Thorac Cardiovasc Surg 1999;118:628–35.
132. Vahanian A, Baumgartner H, Bax J, et al. Guidelines on the management of valvular heart disease: The task force on the management of valvular heart disease of the European Society of Cardiology. Eur Heart J 2007;28:230–68.
133. Gillinov AM, Wierup PN, Blackstone EH, et al. Is repair preferable to replacement for ischemic mitral regurgitation? J Thorac Cardiovasc Surg 2001;122:1125–41.
134. Bax JJ, Braun J, Somer ST, et al. Restrictive annuloplasty and coronary revascularization in ischemic mitral regurgitation results in reverse left ventricular remodeling. Circulation 2004;110:II103–8.
135. Braun J, Bax JJ, Versteegh MI, et al. Preoperative left ventricular dimensions predict reverse remodeling following restrictive mitral annuloplasty in ische q mic mitral regurgitation. Eur J Cardiothorac Surg 2005;27:847–53.

11 Tricuspid Stenosis and Regurgitation

Charles J. Bruce, Patricia A. Pellikka, and Heidi M. Connolly

CONTENTS

The normal tricuspid valve anatomy is characterized by three leaflets: anterior, posterior, and septal (Fig. 1). The anterior leaflet is the most anatomically constant of the three, the other leaflets varying more often in size and position. The leaflets are attached to the tricuspid valve annulus. Similar to the mitral valve leaflets, the tricuspid valve leaflets are restrained by chordae tendinea attached to papillary muscles, which are in turn inserted into the right ventricular wall.

Tricuspid valve disease presents most commonly as tricuspid regurgitation. Tricuspid valve stenosis is rare and is seen primarily in countries where rheumatic heart disease is common. Even when tricuspid stenosis is present, it is often accompanied by regurgitation and thus in these instances more commonly presents as a "mixed" lesion. This chapter will concentrate primarily on tricuspid regurgitation, describing the clinical presentation, diagnostic evaluation, etiology, pathophysiology, natural history, and treatment.

TRICUSPID REGURGITATION

Etiology

Tricuspid regurgitation is a common incidental echocardiographic finding and is readily detected using color-flow Doppler imaging (1). Some degree of tricuspid regurgitation is appreciated in most patients with and without cardiovascular disease. In fact, its detection permits a noninvasive echocardiographic Doppler estimate of right ventricular systolic pressure by using the peak tricuspid regurgitant velocity in the modified Bernoulli equation to determine the systolic gradient between the right atrium and the right ventricle. The right atrial pressure is estimated and added to this gradient, yielding an estimation of right ventricular systolic pressure. In healthy individuals, the severity of tricuspid regurgitation is usually trivial or mild and considered physiologic, not warranting routine follow-up.

Tricuspid regurgitation has traditionally assumed a lower priority than other valve disease because it is often a secondary phenomenon. However, in recent years, it has become increasingly appreciated that severe tricuspid regurgitation is not a benign lesion accounting for significant adverse morbidity

From: *Contemporary Cardiology: Valvular Heart Disease*
Edited by: Andrew Wang, Thomas M. Bashore, DOI 10.1007/978-1-59745-411-7_11
© Humana Press, a part of Springer Science+Business Media, LLC 2009

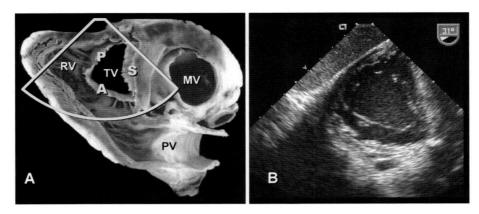

Fig. 1A. (A) Pathology image demonstrating right ventricle (RV) with tricuspid valve (TV) in short axis. The pathologic section is oriented to replicate the classical transesophageal transgastric view obtained at a transducer angle of 31° (Fig. 1B). Note septal, anterior, and posterior leaflets. P, posterior leaflet; S, septal leaflet; A, anterior leaflet; PV, pulmonary valve; MV, mitral valve. (Pathologic image courtesy of Dr William D. Edwards, Department of Laboratory Medicine and Pathology, Mayo Clinic College of Medicine). (B) Transesophageal transgastric echocardiographic image using same imaging plane (defined by the border in Fig. 1A) demonstrating the right ventricle with tricuspid valve septal, anterior, and posterior leaflets.

and mortality regardless of etiology and that early clinical recognition and treatment is warranted *(2)*. Nevertheless, due to the frequent functional nature of the lesion as well as the long latent period of mild or easily controllable symptoms with medications, early intervention of mild to moderate tricuspid valve disease is not recommended.

Tricuspid regurgitation that is at least moderate or greater in severity is most frequently "functional" in nature, and not related to specific tricuspid leaflet pathology but rather secondary to another disease process causing right ventricular dilatation, distortion of the subvalvular apparatus, tricuspid annular dilatation, or all three *(3)*. Less commonly, it may reflect a pathological process involving the tricuspid leaflets themselves. Causes of clinically significant tricuspid regurgitation are outlined in Table1.

Functional tricuspid regurgitation, secondary to annular dilatation, is the most common mechanism of tricuspid regurgitation (Table 1). By definition, when tricuspid regurgitation is functional, the tricuspid valve leaflets are morphologically normal. Tricuspid regurgitation results from leaflet tip malcoaptation secondary to annular dilatation. The tricuspid regurgitation itself results in progressive right ventricular diastolic volume overload, additional right ventricular dilatation, and further annular dilatation that ultimately results in a cycle of progressive worsening tricuspid regurgitation. Initial annular dilatation is a consequence of right ventricular enlargement resulting from any condition that directly affects the right ventricle such as right ventricular myocardial infarction or dilated cardiomyopathy. Right ventricular enlargement may also be secondary to right ventricular pressure overload in patients with pulmonary hypertension or right ventricular volume overload in patients with an increased flow state (e.g., atrial septal defects or anomalous pulmonary venous drainage). Functional tricuspid regurgitation is also commonly seen in patients with rheumatic left-sided valvular heart disease with associated pulmonary hypertension. As a general rule, when systolic pulmonary artery pressures increase beyond 55 mmHg, tricuspid regurgitation can occur despite anatomically normal tricuspid leaflets, whereas more than mild tricuspid regurgitation occurring in the setting of lower systolic pulmonary pressures (less than 40 mmHg) likely reflects a structural abnormality of the valve leaflets or the subvalvular apparatus *(4, 5)*.

Direct injury to the leaflets resulting in tricuspid regurgitation may be either iatrogenic secondary to device leads or endomyocardial biopsy or related to specific disease processes. When caused by

Table 1
Causes of Tricuspid Valve Regurgitation

Congenital
Ebstein's anomaly
Tricuspid valve dysplasia
Tricuspid valve hypoplasia
Tricuspid valve cleft
Double orifice tricuspid valve
Unguarded tricuspid valve orifice

Right ventricular disease
Right ventricular dysplasia
Endomyocardial fibrosis
Increased right heart pressure

Acquired
Annular dilatation
Left-sided valvular heart disease
Endocarditis
Trauma
Carcinoid heart disease
Rheumatic heart disease
Tricuspid valve prolapse
Iatrogenic (radiation, drugs, biopsy, pacemaker, ICD)

Right ventricular dilatation
Pulmonary hypertension
   Primary pulmonary hypertension
   Secondary to left-sided heart disease (valvular heart disease; cardiomyopathy, etc.)

Right ventricular volume overload
   Atrial septal defect
   Anomalous pulmonary venous drainage

permanent pacemaker or internal cardiac defibrillator leads, the mechanism of valve injury is variable, related to lead entrapment in the tricuspid apparatus, direct leaflet perforation at the time of lead insertion, fibrotic adhesion of the lead to the leaflet, or avulsion or laceration of the tricuspid valve leaflets upon lead removal *(6)*. As leaflet injury may be underappreciated in patients having undergone prior lead implants, a high clinical index of suspicion is warranted, particularly when these patients present with worsening right heart failure.

Direct trauma from transvenous endomyocardial biopsy is also a concern, particularly in cardiac transplantation patients who undergo repeated biopsies for rejection surveillance *(7)*. In an effort to reduce the frequency of this complication, echocardiographic guidance during the biopsy procedure may avert accidental damage to the tricuspid valve or subvalvular apparatus.

The tricuspid leaflets and supporting structures may also be damaged indirectly by blunt chest trauma, most often following a motor vehicle accident. Damage may also occur by infective and marantic endocarditis *(7, 8)*. Right-sided infective endocarditis is usually a manifestation of intravenous drug abuse *(4, 9)*. It is also seen in patients with indwelling venous catheters used for dialysis or chemotherapy, or infected pacemaker or defibrillator devices. *Staphylococcus aureus* is responsible for 80% of these tricuspid valve infections *(4)*. Infrequently, marantic or noninfective endocarditis may occur in the setting of connective tissue diseases such as systemic lupus erythematosus, rheumatoid arthritis, or antiphospholipid antibody syndrome *(10)*.

Serotonin-active drugs may also induce tricuspid regurgitation by directly damaging the valve leaflets. This association was first described with the ergot alkaloids, ergotamine and methysergide, used for migraine therapy. The anorectic drugs, fenfluramine and dexfenfluramine, were subsequently implicated and have since been withdrawn from the market. Pergolide and cabergoline are both dopamine agonists used in the treatment of Parkinson's disease and restless leg syndrome. These agents may also induce tricuspid regurgitation by a similar mechanism to fenfluramine and dexfenfluramine and have also been voluntarily withdrawn *(11–13)*. The histopathological changes seen in these valves include a fibroproliferative response that appears to be mediated by the 5-HT$_{2B}$ receptor. These pathologic features are similar to those seen in carcinoid heart disease.

Carcinoid heart disease is a rare but distinctive form of valve disease affecting primarily the right-sided cardiac valves. Carcinoid is a rare tumor arising from argentaffin cells. The primary tumor is usually located in the small bowel and metastasizes to the liver. The primary tumor and metastases produce active substances, including serotonin. Serotonin is recognized to be an agent involved in the development and progression of valve disease in patients with carcinoid syndrome *(14)*. Carcinoid heart disease involves a combination of tricuspid valve regurgitation with rare stenosis as well as pulmonary valve regurgitation and stenosis (Fig. 2). Left-sided valvular abnormalities can also be seen and occur in approximately 10% of patients with carcinoid valve disease *(15)*. Characteristically, left-sided carcinoid valve disease occurs due to shunting of blood from right to left atrium through a patent foramen ovale. Less commonly, left-sided valve disease occurs in patients with bronchial carcinoid or very active carcinoid disease with high levels of circulating serotonin.

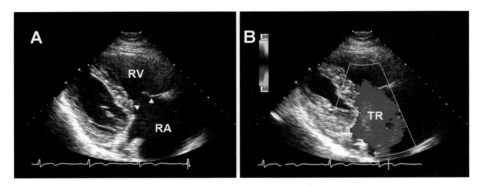

Fig. 2. (A) Two-dimensional echocardiographic systolic image of right ventricular inflow view demonstrates thickened septal and anterior tricuspid valve leaflets (*arrowheads*) and enlargement of the right ventricle (RV) and right atrium (RA) in a patient with carcinoid heart disease. (B) Color-flow Doppler image demonstrates severe tricuspid valve regurgitation (TR) in the same patient. Note laminar color flow (*blue*) filling an enlarged right atrium.

Mediastinal radiation can directly damage the tricuspid leaflets. The associated post-inflammatory fibrosis and calcification, usually manifest five or more years following the radiation insult, result in distortion of the leaflets causing tricuspid regurgitation *(4, 16, 17)*. Assessment and treatment of tricuspid regurgitation in this setting may be complicated by concomitant dysfunction of other cardiac valves as well as pericardial, myocardial, and coronary artery involvement.

Congenital causes of tricuspid regurgitation are rare and include congenital tricuspid valve prolapse, which may occur as an isolated abnormality or be associated with mitral valve prolapse and other connective tissue disorders. The most common congenital cause of tricuspid regurgitation is Ebstein's anomaly *(18)*. In Ebstein's anomaly there is inferior displacement of the septal and posterior tricuspid valve leaflets into the right ventricle and variable tethering of the anterior leaflet. The severity of tricuspid regurgitation depends on whether there is significant adherence of the leaflets to the right ventricular wall, the degree of annular tethering, and valve leaflet fenestrations.

Clinical Manifestations and Assessment

At the time of diagnosis, patients with severe tricuspid regurgitation may either be asymptomatic, remaining so for prolonged periods, or present with symptoms and signs of right heart failure. Characteristic symptoms include fatigue and exertional dyspnea. As symptoms progress, lower extremity edema, early satiety and right upper quadrant pain related to hepatic congestion and capsular distension, as well as increasing abdominal girth as a result of abdominal ascites develop. Rarely, patients may have severe symptoms of fatigue and dyspnea with minimal peripheral findings. Also, since tricuspid regurgitation is often secondary to pulmonary hypertension, symptoms of coexisting valvular heart disease or pulmonary hypertension may predominate. Symptoms of edema are usually relieved with administration of diuretics. However, dyspnea and fatigue often persist since these symptoms are due to reduced cardiac output.

In patients with severe tricuspid regurgitation, the physical examination is notable for distended jugular veins and elevated venous pressure with a prominent "CV" wave. Marked right atrial enlargement may mask the venous pressure elevation and abnormal waveform. If significant pulmonary hypertension is present, a prominent "a" wave will also be seen. On auscultation, a systolic murmur is appreciated at the lower left sternal border that characteristically increases with inspiration (Carvallo's sign). The murmur is pansystolic or less than pansystolic depending on the severity. If tricuspid regurgitation is severe, an associated third sound may be present which may also vary in intensity with inspiration. Often, however, little or no murmur is appreciated despite torrential tricuspid regurgitation due to equalization of pressures between the right atrium and ventricle. A fourth heart sound may be heard when severe right ventricular hypertrophy due to pulmonary hypertension is present.

Chest palpation may reveal a volume overloaded dilated right ventricle with a prominent parasternal impulse or lift. Examination of the lungs may reveal a pleural effusion, and that of the abdomen may reveal pulsatile hepatomegaly with or without ascites. In untreated patients, bilateral lower extremity edema is often present. In severe cases, anasarca may be present with edema extending to the thigh, lumbar sacral level, and abdominal wall. Rarely, severe tricuspid regurgitation may cause systolic propulsion of the eyeballs, pulsatile varicose veins, or a venous systolic thrill and murmur in the neck *(4, 19–21)*.

The chest radiographic findings in severe tricuspid regurgitation include cardiomegaly due to right ventricular enlargement. This is manifest by loss of the retrosternal airspace appreciated on the lateral projection. Right atrial enlargement is also noted and identified as prominence of the right heart border on the anteroposterior view. The azygos vein may be prominent if the right-sided pressures are increased. Furthermore, prominent pulmonary hilar segments may be seen if significant pulmonary hypertension is present. Unilateral or bilateral pleural effusions as well as elevated hemi diaphragms secondary to ascites may also be seen.

Transthoracic echocardiography is the test of choice to confirm and document the presence of tricuspid regurgitation and define its severity and etiology. Tricuspid regurgitation can be readily assessed by comprehensive echo-Doppler techniques using color-flow Doppler as well as continuous wave Doppler, providing a semi-quantitative assessment of severity (Fig. 3). A characteristic dense systolic continuous wave Doppler signal is appreciated when tricuspid regurgitation is severe. Severe tricuspid regurgitation also results in a triangular or "dagger-shaped" early peaking tricuspid regurgitant jet profile due to early equilibration of pressures between the right atrium and right ventricle (Fig. 4). The vena contracta can be measured using color-flow Doppler; this indirectly reflects the effective regur-

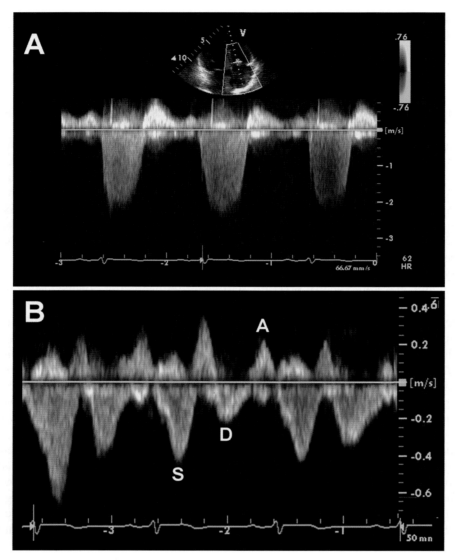

Fig. 3. (A) Continuous wave Doppler signal across the tricuspid valve demonstrates a low-velocity systolic jet (2 m/s) with a symmetrical rounded appearance consistent with mild tricuspid valve regurgitation. Measurement of the systolic velocity provides an indirect assessment of right ventricular systolic pressure using the modified Bernoulli equation. (B) Hepatic vein pulsed wave Doppler signal with accompanying ECG tracing demonstrating normal hepatic vein flow in the patient with mild tricuspid regurgitation in Fig. 3A. Systolic flow (S) and diastolic flow (D) is seen emanating from the hepatic veins into the inferior vena cava (flow seen displayed below the baseline) and atrial reversal flow (A) representing normal flow refluxing into the hepatic veins resulting from atrial contraction.

gitant orifice area. When this measures greater than 0.7 cm, severe tricuspid regurgitation is present *(4, 22)*. Quantitative assessment is also feasible and can be performed with the proximal isovelocity surface area (PISA) method. If severe tricuspid regurgitation is present, interrogation of the inferior vena cava and hepatic vein provides ancillary information. With severe tricuspid regurgitation, the inferior vena cava is usually dilated greater than 2 cm and systolic flow reversals are seen in the hepatic veins *(22–24)* (Fig. 4). These systolic reversals reflect retrograde flow in the hepatic veins that

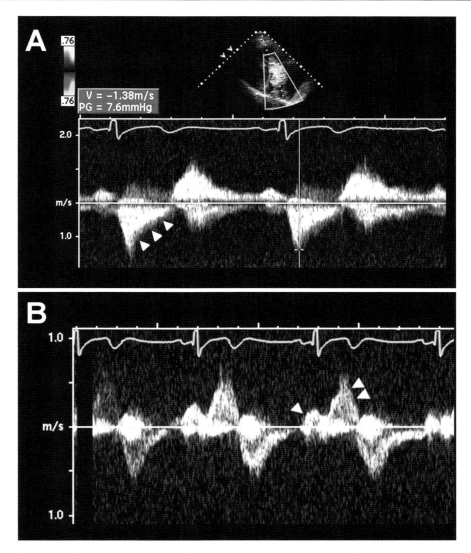

Fig. 4. (A) A dense systolic continuous wave Doppler signal is demonstrated in a patient with severe tricuspid valve regurgitation. Severe tricuspid regurgitation results in a triangular or "dagger-shaped" (*arrowheads*) early peaking tricuspid regurgitant jet profile due to early equilibration of pressures between the right atrium and right ventricle. (B) Hepatic vein pulsed wave Doppler signal demonstrating both atrial (*single arrowhead*) and systolic reversed flow (*double arrowhead*), indicating elevation in right atrial pressure and severe tricuspid valve regurgitation in a patient in sinus rhythm. These systolic reversals reflect retrograde flow in the hepatic veins that can be appreciated clinically as a pulsatile liver. Hepatic vein systolic reversals may not be specific for severe tricuspid regurgitation when atrial fibrillation is present.

can be appreciated clinically as a pulsatile liver. Hepatic vein systolic reversals may not be specific for severe tricuspid regurgitation when atrial fibrillation is present *(22)*.

The assessment of the consequences of tricuspid regurgitation on right ventricular size and function is important. Although two-dimensional echocardiography can provide a morphologic assessment of right ventricular dimensions and function *(25)*, accurate measurement of right ventricular dimensions, volumes, and function are difficult due to the complex three-dimensional anatomy of the right ventricular chamber. Three-dimensional echocardiographic imaging offers promise of feasible clinical measures of right ventricular size and systolic function in the future *(26)*. Echocardiography can also provide Doppler-derived surrogate measures of right ventricular function that have been shown to have prognostic value in patients with pulmonary hypertension. These measures include the right-sided index of myocardial performance (Tei index) *(27)* and measurements of the peak systolic velocity and displacement of the tricuspid annulus using tissue Doppler imaging *(28–30)*. Measures of change in pressure over time (dP/dt) have also been reported in the assessment of right heart function *(31)*. In addition, myocardial acceleration during isovolumic contraction, also known as isovolumic acceleration (IVA), a tissue Doppler index of systolic contractile function, has been validated using conductance catheters *(32)* and demonstrates reduced right ventricular contractile function *(33)*.

Transthoracic echocardiography confirms not only presence and severity of tricuspid regurgitation but also provides important information regarding the etiology. Determination of the etiology requires a careful assessment of tricuspid leaflet morphology, tricuspid annular dimension, the subvalvular apparatus, and right ventricular size and function. The presence of an intracardiac device, e.g., pacer or defibrillation lead, should prompt careful assessment of leaflet mobility. Also, presence of pulmonary hypertension can be determined and coexisting left-sided valvular heart disease can be identified.

Transesophageal echocardiography compliments transthoracic echocardiography in the assessment of tricuspid valve regurgitation. Although the tricuspid valve is often difficult to visualize by transesophageal imaging due to the location of the valve relative to the esophagus, complimentary data regarding the cause of tricuspid valve regurgitation may be obtained. Intra-operative transesophageal echocardiography can be used to assess tricuspid valve morphology prior to operation and should be used to evaluate the results of tricuspid repair immediately after cardiopulmonary bypass to detect residual tricuspid regurgitation or the development of tricuspid stenosis. Following tricuspid valve replacement, assessment of prosthetic valve function and prosthetic or periprosthetic regurgitation can be performed permitting prompt surgical revision if necessary. It should be remembered that prevailing hemodynamic conditions related to general anesthesia in the operating room may result in underestimation of tricuspid regurgitation severity.

Cardiac catheterization is rarely required for the assessment of tricuspid valve regurgitation alone, but may be required to assess the contribution of pulmonary hypertension to the causation of regurgitation and the likelihood of successful repair. Hemodynamically, severe tricuspid regurgitation is characterized by elevated right atrial pressure with the presence of a "C-V" wave or nearly identical right atrial and right ventricular waveforms; elevated right ventricular diastolic pressure when right ventricular dysfunction is present; and reduced cardiac output. Cardiac MRI can be used to quantify right ventricular size and function *(34, 35)*. It may provide complimentary data to facilitate decision regarding timing of tricuspid valve operative intervention.

Pathophysiology

Tricuspid regurgitation is characterized by the backflow of blood from the right ventricle into the right atrium during systole reducing cardiac output. Since the right atrium is relatively compliant there are often no major hemodynamic consequences with acute or chronic mild, moderate, or even moderately severe tricuspid regurgitation. However, when the regurgitation is severe mean right atrial pressure rises. Regurgitant flow produces a "C-V" wave that is reflected through the venous system. Chronically, the volume overload causes progressive dilatation of the right ventricle and movement of the intraventricular septum toward the left ventricle during diastole. Right ventricular failure ensues secondary to right ventricular dysfunction further increasing the mean right atrial pressure resulting in systemic venous congestion manifest as hepatic congestion, ascites, lower extremity edema, and reduced cardiac output.

Natural History

The natural history of tricuspid regurgitation varies based on the underlying etiology and pathophysiology. For example, patients with severe tricuspid regurgitation secondary to pulmonary hypertension will have a variable clinical course depending on whether the pulmonary hypertension is primary or secondary. As a general rule, when tricuspid regurgitation accompanies other diseases, the prognosis is usually less favorable than when it is not present. Due to the adverse hemodynamic consequence of right ventricular volume overload, tricuspid regurgitation of at least moderate degree usually begets tricuspid regurgitation resulting in a slow and steadily inexorable clinical and hemodynamic deterioration.

The natural history of severe tricuspid regurgitation is one of a prolonged latent period with eventual progressive right ventricular and later right atrial volume overload. Atrial arrhythmias are common secondary to right atrial enlargement and may be difficult to treat in the presence of persistent tricuspid regurgitation. Symptoms of right heart failure can be palliated with diuretic use. As the disease progresses, increasing doses of diuretics are needed. This may result in decreased forward flow, reducing cardiac output resulting in increasing fatigue and worsening renal function. Due to hepatic congestion and resultant anorexia, patients may become nutritionally depleted.

Severe tricuspid valve regurgitation has an important impact on clinical outcome and survival in patients with cardiovascular disease. Groves et al. *(36)* reported that patients with severe tricuspid valve regurgitation had a significant reduction in exercise capacity caused by impaired cardiac output response to exercise and therefore experienced a poor functional outcome (Fig. 5). Sagie et al. *(37)* demonstrated that tricuspid regurgitation was an independent predictor of long-term survival after percutaneous balloon mitral valvuloplasty (Fig. 6) and Koelling et al. *(38)* showed that the degree of tricuspid valve regurgitation was an independent predictor of survival in patients with left ventricular systolic dysfunction. Patients with severe mitral or tricuspid valve regurgitation represent a high-risk subset of patients with left ventricular systolic dysfunction.

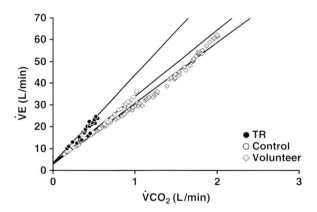

Fig. 5. Relation between minute ventilation (VE) and CO_2 production (VCO_2) during exercise in patients following percutaneous mitral balloon valvuloplasty (PMBV) with and without severe tricuspid regurgitation compared with healthy volunteers. The linear relation between VE and VCO_2 is significantly steeper in the patients with clinically significant tricuspid regurgitation reflecting an exaggerated hyperpneic response. Exercise duration, maximal oxygen consumption, and anaerobic threshold were also significantly lower in this group *(36)*.

The independent effect of tricuspid valve regurgitation on prognosis was evaluated by Messika-Zeitoun et al. They reported the outcome of flail tricuspid valve leaflets in 60 patients who were seen at Mayo Clinic over a 20-year period *(7)*. The 60 patients with tricuspid valve flail were divided into

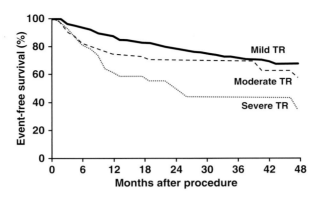

Fig. 6. Kaplan–Meyer surgical curve demonstrates survival probability after percutaneous balloon mitral valvuloplasty among 318 patients with mild, moderate, or severe tricuspid valve regurgitation. These patients should be referred for operative intervention *(37)*.

three groups depending on symptoms and associated cardiovascular disease. Half of the patients underwent operative intervention (27 repair, 6 tricuspid valve replacement). The natural history of tricuspid regurgitation from flail leaflets without associated cardiovascular disease demonstrated an increased risk of atrial fibrillation, symptoms, heart failure, surgery, or death (Fig. 7). Symptomatic improvement was noted in 88% of operated patients. Long-term survival of patients with unoperated tricuspid regurgitation caused by flail leaflets compared with expected survival in a US matched population demonstrated excess mortality (4.5% yearly, $p < 0.01$).

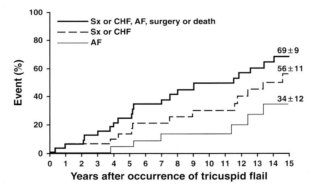

Fig. 7. Kaplan–Meyer curves depict the incidence of new atrial fibrillation (AF), Class III or IV symptoms(Sx), or congestive heart failure (CHF), and the composite endpoint of first occurrence of symptoms, CHF, new AF, tricuspid surgery, or death.

The effect of right-sided chamber enlargement in patients with severe tricuspid valve regurgitation, even in asymptomatic patients, was noteworthy in this series. The clinical outcome stratified according to the degree of right-sided cardiac chamber enlargement demonstrated a marked difference in events when severe enlargement of the right heart chambers was present (Fig. 8).

In summary, tricuspid valve regurgitation due to a flail leaflet causes an increase in cardiovascular morbidity and mortality. An increase in morbidity was noted even in asymptomatic patients who had right heart enlargement. The operative risk for tricuspid valve repair or replacement is low for these patients and symptomatic improvement can be expected. Unfortunately, arrhythmia risks persist even after successful repair since surgery is mostly performed at an advanced stage.

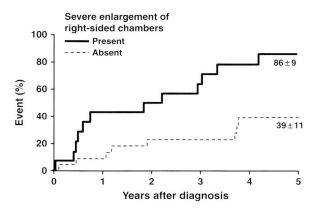

Fig. 8. Kaplan–Meyer curves depict the incidence of combined endpoints of symptoms or heart failure, new atrial fibrillation, cardiac surgery, or death in patients initially conservatively managed. Note that patients with severe right-sided cardiac chamber enlargement had a higher incidence of events *(7)*.

Management

GENERAL

The patient's clinical status and the cause of the tricuspid valve abnormality usually determine the appropriate therapeutic strategy (Table 2) *(4)*. Initial treatment is geared at identifying the etiology and treating this if possible. Symptomatic treatment involves the use of diuretics. Oral diuretics are effective if combined with fluid and sodium restriction. On occasion, if significant fluid accumulation has occurred, intravenous diuresis is needed since there may be concomitant bowel edema rendering oral diuretics ineffective.

Table 2
Key Points to Clinical Management of Tricuspid Regurgitation

---

(1) Symptoms and signs of severe tricuspid valve regurgitation may be subtle and increase gradually over years
(2) Echocardiography is the diagnostic test of choice to assess tricuspid valve regurgitation
(3) Severe tricuspid valve regurgitation causes right heart enlargement, right ventricular dysfunction, and increase in the risk of atrial fibrillation
(4) Severe tricuspid regurgitation is associated with excess mortality, especially when associated with right heart enlargement
(5) With improved surgical expertise and survival, classical indications for operative intervention for tricuspid regurgitation should be reconsidered
(6) Tricuspid valve repair or replacement should be performed for symptomatic patients with severe tricuspid valve regurgitation

---

Although diuretics improve edema, this therapy may decrease cardiac output and thus worsen fatigue and dyspnea. There are no data on the efficacy of various medical treatment modalities in patients with severe tricuspid valve regurgitation.

Endocarditis prophylaxis recommendations have changed and impact management of patients with tricuspid valve disease *(39)*. Endocarditis prophylaxis is no longer recommended for all patients with valvular heart disease undergoing routine dental, gastrointestinal, or genitourinary procedures.

High-risk patients, i.e., those with prosthetic tricuspid valves, prior endocarditis, or complex or palliated congenital tricuspid valve disease undergoing high-risk procedures, should use endocarditis prophylaxis.

SURGERY

Tricuspid valve surgery is the only demonstrated effective treatment for symptomatic tricuspid valve regurgitation. At our institution, where operative outcomes for tricuspid valve disease are excellent, tricuspid valve repair or replacement is recommended for patients with severe tricuspid valve regurgitation and (1) symptoms of reduced cardiac output which include fatigue and exertional dyspnea or persistent right heart failure despite medical therapy, (2) mitral valve disease or other cardiac disease that requires operative intervention, (3) progressive right ventricular enlargement or dysfunction, and (4) select asymptomatic patients, such as patients with traumatic tricuspid valve flail with severe tricuspid valve regurgitation. Tricuspid valve operation is also recommended in patients with moderate tricuspid valve regurgitation undergoing other cardiac surgery.

Surgical options include tricuspid valve repair with a purse-string annuloplasty. This is most commonly performed for functional tricuspid regurgitation in patients with a dilated annulus related to other valvular heart disease. It is often combined with valve replacement on the left side of the heart and, importantly, should not be performed in patients with severe pulmonary hypertension due to the risk of recurrent severe tricuspid valve regurgitation.

Ringed annuloplasty is another surgical option for patients with tricuspid valve regurgitation. This is most commonly performed when tricuspid regurgitation is the main operative indication and only mild to moderate pulmonary hypertension is present. In patients with functional tricuspid regurgitation, the degree of tricuspid valve tethering has been shown to predict residual tricuspid regurgitation following tricuspid annuloplasty (40).

Tricuspid valve repair options are possible for patients with Ebstein's anomaly; the most commonly described procedure involves a specialized monocusp repair (18). This procedure requires appropriate patient selection and congenital cardiac surgical expertise and should be performed at an experienced center.

Tricuspid valve replacement is indicated for patients with symptomatic tricuspid regurgitation and pulmonary hypertension or for patients who have abnormal tricuspid valves that are not amenable to repair. These include patients with carcinoid heart disease, rheumatic heart disease, Ebstein's anomaly with valves not amenable to repair or recurrent tricuspid valve regurgitation after repair. When there is marked annular dilatation, tricuspid valve replacement should also be considered. Most commonly, a bioprosthesis is placed in the tricuspid position as this obviates the need for long-term anticoagulation. In addition, the durability of bioprostheses placed in the right heart is generally better than bioprostheses placed in the left heart, likely related to the lower transvalvular pressure gradients (41). It is also noteworthy that pericardial bioprostheses are not usually used in the tricuspid position due to the increased stiffness of the prosthesis and concern regarding increased risk of obstruction. Indications for mechanical tricuspid valve replacement include an established need for long-term anticoagulation (mechanical left-sided prostheses or atrial fibrillation).

Patients with severe tricuspid valve regurgitation being referred for operative intervention should be considered for concomitant partial or full Maze procedure. Although this may not alleviate atrial fibrillation, it may decrease the clinical impact (42).

Ratnatunga et al. (43) reported from the UK registry on prosthetic valves, the outcome of 425 tricuspid valve prostheses and 63,000 valve replacements. They noted no significant difference in survival among 200 patients with mechanical prostheses versus 225 with bioprosthetic valves. In a study by Rizzoli, data from 11 studies with 646 mechanical and 514 bioprosthetic tricuspid valves were pooled. The hospital mortality for tricuspid valve replacement was 19%. There was no difference in late survival, thrombosis or structural valve deterioration between the two types of prostheses *(44)*. In the current era, the operative risk for tricuspid valve replacement or repair is considerably lower.

The AHA/ACC guidelines for the timing of tricuspid valve repair and replacement have been recently revised and published. These are summarized in Table 3.

Table 3
Management of Patients with Severe Tricuspid Regurgitation (AHA/ACC 2006 Guidelines)

Class I
   Tricuspid valve repair is beneficial for severe TR in patients with MV disease requiring MV surgery.
   (Level of Evidence: B)

Class IIa
1. Tricuspid valve replacement or annuloplasty is reasonable for severe primary TR when symptomatic.
   (Level of Evidence: C)
2. Tricuspid valve replacement is reasonable for severe TR secondary to diseased/abnormal tricuspid valve
   leaflets not amenable to annuloplasty or repair. *(Level of Evidence: C)*

Class IIb
Tricuspid annuloplasty may be considered for less than severe TR in patients undergoing MV surgery when
   there is pulmonary hypertension or tricuspid annular dilatation. *(Level of Evidence: C)*

Class III
1. Tricuspid valve replacement of annuloplasty is not indicated in asymptomatic patients with TR whose
   pulmonary artery systolic pressure is less than 60 mmHg in the presence of a normal MV. *(Level of
   Evidence: C)*
2. Tricuspid valve replacement or annuloplasty is not indicated in patients with mild primary TR. *(Level of
   Evidence: C)*

Classification of recommendations and level of evidence are expressed in the ACC/AHA format as follows:

- **Class I**: Conditions for which there is evidence for and/or general agreement that the procedure or treatment is beneficial, useful, and effective.
- **Class II**: Conditions for which there is conflicting evidence and/or a divergence of opinion about the usefulness/efficacy of a procedure or treatment.
  - **Class IIa**: Weight of evidence/opinion is in favor of usefulness/efficacy.
  - **Class IIb**: Usefulness/efficacy is less well established by evidence/opinion.
- **Class III**: Conditions for which there is evidence and/or general agreement that the procedure/treatment is not useful/effective and in some cases may be harmful.
- **Level of Evidence B**: Data derived from a single randomized trial or nonrandomized studies.
- **Level of Evidence C**: Only consensus opinion of experts, case studies, or standard-of-care.

SPECIFIC SURGICAL CONSIDERATIONS BASED ON ETIOLOGY

Early surgery should be considered for patients with severe tricuspid regurgitation from blunt chest trauma since the long-term prognosis of flail tricuspid leaflets is poor *(7)*.

When severe symptomatic tricuspid regurgitation is secondary to leaflet perforation or lead impingement from a pacemaker lead, removal or repositioning of the lead may decrease the degree of tricuspid regurgitation *(6)*. If this is not possible, tricuspid valve repair or replacement should be performed. Repair in this setting involves excluding the lead from the affected leaflets, suture repair of a defect in the leaflet; or by positioning the pacemaker lead by suture fixation in the recess of either the posteroseptal or anteroposterior commissure. With tricuspid valve replacement, the pacemaker lead is placed outside the sewing ring. These patients can be expected to have symptomatic improvement following tricuspid valve repair or replacement.

Carcinoid heart disease is best treated surgically with valve replacement and operative intervention has a beneficial impact on patient survival (45). Indications for operative intervention include progressive symptoms of fatigue, dyspnea or right heart failure, and progressive enlargement or dysfunction of the right heart. Asymptomatic patients with severe carcinoid heart disease may be candidates for valve replacement to allow partial hepatic resection or liver transplantation.

For patients with pulmonary hypertension secondary to pulmonary thromboembolic disease pulmonary thromboendarterectomy has been shown to reduce pulmonary hypertension and severe tricuspid regurgitation without tricuspid annuloplasty despite a dilated tricuspid valve annulus. Twenty-seven patients with moderate to severe pulmonary hypertension and severe tricuspid regurgitation underwent pulmonary thromboendarterectomy. In 19 patients (70%) the tricuspid regurgitation resolved completely following the procedure (46). Compared to the eight patients with persistent severe tricuspid regurgitation, those with diminished tricuspid regurgitation were more likely to have had a reduction in pulmonary artery pressure below 40 mmHg. Tricuspid regurgitation secondary to severe primary pulmonary hypertension not amenable to surgical therapy is usually treated with diuretic therapy and pulmonary vasodilators.

In the setting of left-sided valvular heart disease, according to 2006 ACC/AHA Valvular Heart Disease Guidelines, tricuspid valve annuloplasty should be considered at the time of left-sided valve surgery even when only mild tricuspid regurgitation is present if there is associated annular dilatation. Interestingly, a number of observational studies have documented improvement in tricuspid regurgitation severity when percutaneous balloon mitral valvuloplasty is performed in patients with mitral stenosis, severe pulmonary hypertension, and significant functional tricuspid regurgitation (47, 48). Unfortunately, the outlook for patients who have undergone prior left-sided valvular heart disease surgery who subsequently present with symptomatic severe tricuspid regurgitation is dismal. Repeat surgery to address the tricuspid valve regurgitation alone in these patients can be performed with acceptable early mortality (8.8%). However, late mortality remains high (event-free survival 41.6 + 9.2%) predicted by age and the number of previous cardiac operations. In the survivors, however, significant symptomatic improvement can be expected (49).

DILEMMAS IN MANAGEMENT

Coexisting disease makes treatment of tricuspid regurgitation difficult and is often influenced by the severity of the underlying disease. Simply fixing the tricuspid regurgitation may not result in an overall satisfactory outcome. Patients who have already undergone prior cardiac surgery may be poor candidates for isolated repeat cardiac surgery to abolish tricuspid valve regurgitation. Thus, it is important to scrutinize the tricuspid valve at the time of the index surgery and undertake tricuspid valve repair or replacement at that time to avoid the problem of worsening tricuspid valve regurgitation postoperatively.

Timing of tricuspid valve surgery for tricuspid regurgitation remains controversial (4). This controversy has diminished somewhat with the advent of preoperative and intra-operative two-dimensional and Doppler echocardiographic assessment. Intra-operative transesophageal echocardiography Doppler allows refinement of annuloplasty techniques to optimize outcome (50–52). However, the assessment of the tricuspid valve with transesophageal echocardiography may be difficult due to suboptimal angles of interrogation and hemodynamic alterations which occur under anesthesia. A comprehensive assessment of the severity of tricuspid regurgitation is usually better undertaken by careful preoperative transthoracic echocardiography (4). Patients undergoing surgery for mitral stenosis who have coexisting tricuspid regurgitation usually have pulmonary hypertension. In this situation it is difficult to predict whether the tricuspid regurgitation will improve following relief of mitral stenosis and subsequent drop in pulmonary artery pressure *(53)*. If the pulmonary hypertension is severe, the tricuspid valve anatomy is not grossly distorted and annular dilatation is absent, improvement in tricuspid regurgitation can be expected following relief of mitral stenosis alone. However, if there is severe tricuspid regurgitation, the valve is deformed or there is dilatation of the tricuspid annulus, tricuspid valve surgery is necessary *(4)*. When patients with multivalvular disease have severe tricuspid regurgitation, tricuspid annuloplasty or replacement is often performed. Also, it is reasonable to consider tricuspid annuloplasty in patients with mild tricuspid regurgitation who are undergoing mitral valve surgery for mitral regurgitation when there is pulmonary hypertension or tricuspid annular dilatation *(4)*.

Adult patients with an atrial septal defect or other shunt lesion causing tricuspid annular dilatation and more than moderate tricuspid regurgitation should be considered for operative intervention rather than device closure. Patients with an atrial septal defect referred to surgery should have tricuspid valve repair in conjunction with atrial septal defect closure if there is moderate or more tricuspid regurgitation, given the unpredictable reduction in regurgitation following surgical atrial septal defect closure alone. Operation should include abolition of the cardiac shunt, tricuspid valve repair to decrease the degree of right heart enlargement, and when appropriate and feasible Maze procedure. This may have an impact on late atrial arrhythmias *(42)*.

TRICUSPID STENOSIS

Tricuspid stenosis is rare and is usually post-inflammatory in nature resulting from rheumatic heart disease. It is commonly associated with tricuspid regurgitation and also accompanied by mitral stenosis. Additional causes of tricuspid stenosis include right-sided endocarditis with large bulky vegetations and right atrial tumors which may cause functional tricuspid stenosis by obstructing the tricuspid orifice. Causes of TR outlined in Table 4 etiologies of tricuspid stenosis are included in Table 4. These acquired conditions often result in mixed stenosis and regurgitation.

Table 4
Etiology of Tricuspid Stenosis

Rheumatic heart disease
Congenital tricuspid stenosis
Right atrial tumors
Carcinoid heart disease
Endomyocardial fibrosis
Valvular vegetations
Extracardiac tumors

In tricuspid stenosis, flow into the right ventricle from the systemic veins and the right atrium is impaired resulting in a diastolic pressure gradient between the right atrium and right ventricle. The normal tricuspid valve area is 7 cm^2. Significant impairment of right ventricular filling occurs when the valve area is less than 1.5 cm^2 and severe tricuspid stenosis is defined as a tricuspid valve area of less than 1 cm^2 *(4)*. When the right atrial pressure exceeds 10 mmHg peripheral edema develops *(54, 55)*.

Symptoms of isolated tricuspid stenosis are nonspecific but may include fatigue, dyspnea, edema, and ascites. Right atrial pressure elevation causes hepatic congestion, and patients often present with early satiety, right upper quadrant pain, and peripheral edema. The physical examination is notable for a giant "a" wave and diminished rate of "y" descent in the jugular venous pulse. On auscultation an opening snap may be appreciated in valvular tricuspid stenosis and mid-diastolic rumble that increases with inspiration. Treatment of tricuspid stenosis is directed at the underlying etiology and most commonly requires tricuspid valve replacement.

COMBINED/MIXED TRICUSPID STENOSIS AND REGURGITATION

Tricuspid regurgitation and tricuspid stenosis may coexist, particularly in patients with rheumatic heart disease, carcinoid heart disease, and tricuspid valve endocarditis. These conditions present with symptoms and signs of both tricuspid stenosis and regurgitation, and treatment is aimed at the specific etiology.

CONCLUSION

Tricuspid valve disease, particularly tricuspid regurgitation, is an important clinical problem associated with significant morbidity and mortality. Unfortunately, minimal evidence-based data are currently available to guide choice of optimal intervention and its timing. An increased awareness of its presence and predisposing factors as well as earlier intervention may be associated with improved outcomes in the future.

REFERENCES

1. Singh, J.P., et al., *Prevalence and clinical determinants of mitral, tricuspid, and aortic regurgitation (the Framingham Heart Study)*. Am J Cardiol, 1999. 83(6): 897–902.
2. Nath, J., E. Foster, and P.A. Heidenreich, *Impact of tricuspid regurgitation on long-term survival*. J Am Coll Cardiol, 2004. 43(3): 405–9.
3. Behm, C.Z., J. Nath, and E. Foster, *Clinical correlates and mortality of hemodynamically significant tricuspid regurgitation*. J Heart Valve Dis, 2004. 13(5): 784–9.
4. Bonow, R., et al., *American College of Cardiology/American Heart Association Task Force on Practice Guidelines; Society of Cardiovascular Anesthesiologists; Society for Cardiovascular Angiography and Interventions; Society of Thoracic Surgeons ACC/AHA 2006 guidelines for the management of patients with valvular heart disease: A report of the American College of Cardiology American Heart Association Task Force on Practice Guidelines (writing committee to revise the 1998 Guidelines for the Management of Patients With Valvular Heart Disease): Developed in collaboration with the Society of Cardiovascular Anesthesiologists: Endorsed by the Society for Cardiovascular Angiography and Interventions and the Society of Thoracic Surgeons*. Circulation, 2006. 114(5): e84–231.
5. Waller, B.F., et al., *Etiology of pure tricuspid regurgitation based on annular circumference and leaflet area: analysis of 45 necropsy patients with clinical and morphologic evidence of pure tricuspid regurgitation*. J Am Coll Cardiol, 1986. 7(5): 1063–74.
6. Lin, G., et al., *Severe symptomatic tricuspid valve regurgitation due to permanent pacemaker or implantable cardioverter-defibrillator leads*. J Am Coll Cardiol, 2005. 45(10): 1672–5.
7. Messika-Zeitoun, D., et al., *Medical and surgical outcome of tricuspid regurgitation caused by flail leaflets*. J Thorac Cardiovasc Surg, 2004. 128: 296–302.
8. van Son, J.A., et al., *Traumatic tricuspid valve insufficiency. Experience in thirteen patients*. J Thorac Cardiovasc Surg, 1994. 108(5): 893–8.
9. Chan, P., J.D. Ogilby, and B. Segal, *Tricuspid valve endocarditis*. Am Heart J, 1989. 117(5): 1140–6.
10. Waller, B.F., W.S. Knapp, and J.E. Edwards, *Marantic valvular vegetations*. Circulation, 1973. 48(3): 644–50.
11. Zanettini, R., et al., *Valvular heart disease and the use of dopamine agonists for Parkinson's disease*. N Engl J Med, 2007. 356(1): 39–46.
12. Schade, R., et al., *Dopamine agonists and the risk of cardiac-valve regurgitation*. N Engl J Med, 2007. 356(1): 29–38.
13. Pritchett, A.M., et al., *Valvular heart disease in patients taking pergolide*. Mayo Clin Proc, 2002. 77(12): 1280–6.
14. Moller, J.E., et al., *Factors associated with progression of carcinoid heart disease*. N Engl J Med, 2003. 348(11): 1005–15.
15. Connolly, H.M., et al., *Surgical management of left-sided carcinoid heart disease*. Circulation, 2001. 104(12 Suppl 1): I36–40.
16. Adams, M.J., et al., *Radiation-associated cardiovascular disease*. Crit Rev Oncol Hematol, 2003. 45(1): 55–75.
17. Crestanello, J.A., et al., *Mitral and tricuspid valve repair in patients with previous mediastinal radiation therapy*. Ann Thorac Surg, 2004. 78(3): 826–31; discussion 831.
18. Attenhofer Jost, C.H., et al., *Ebstein's anomaly*. Circulation, 2007. 115(2): 277–85.
19. Naylor, C.D., *Systolic propulsion of the eyeballs in tricuspid regurgitation*. Lancet, 1995. 346(8991–8992): 1706.
20. Hollins, G.W. and J. Engeset, *Pulsatile varicose veins associated with tricuspid regurgitation*. Br J Surg, 1989. 76(2): 207.

21. Amidi, M., et al., *Venous systolic thrill and murmur in the neck: a consequence of severe tricuspid insufficiency.* J Am Coll Cardiol, 1986. 7(4): 942–5.

22. Zoghbi, W.A., et al., *Recommendations for evaluation of the severity of native valvular regurgitation with two-dimensional and Doppler echocardiography.* J Am Soc Echocardiogr, 2003. 16(7): 777–802.

23. Sakai, K., et al., *Evaluation of tricuspid regurgitation by blood flow pattern in the hepatic vein using pulsed Doppler technique.* Am Heart J, 1984. 108(3 Pt 1): 516–23.

24. Pennestri, F., et al., *Assessment of tricuspid regurgitation by pulsed Doppler ultrasonography of the hepatic veins.* Am J Cardiol, 1984. 54(3): 363–8.

25. Lang, R.M., et al., *Recommendations for chamber quantification: a report from the American Society of Echocardiography's Guidelines and Standards Committee and the Chamber Quantification Writing Group, developed in conjunction with the European Association of Echocardiography, a branch of the European Society of Cardiology.* J Am Soc Echocardiogr, 2005. 18(12): 1440–63.

26. Lang, R.M., et al., *Three-dimensional echocardiography: the benefits of the additional dimension.* J Am Coll Cardiol, 2006. 48(10): 2053–69.

27. Tei, C., et al., *Doppler echocardiographic index for assessment of global right ventricular function.* J Am Soc Echocardiogr, 1996. 9(6): 838–47.

28. LaCorte, J.C., et al., *Correlation of the Tei index with invasive measurements of ventricular function in a porcine model.* J Am Soc Echocardiogr, 2003. 16(5): 442–7.

29. Meluzin, J., et al., *Pulsed Doppler tissue imaging of the velocity of tricuspid annular systolic motion; a new, rapid, and non-invasive method of evaluating right ventricular systolic function.* Eur Heart J, 2001. 22(4): 340–8.

30. Miller, D., et al., *The relation between quantitative right ventricular ejection fraction and indices of tricuspid annular motion and myocardial performance.* J Am Soc Echocardiogr, 2004. 17(5): 443–7.

31. Imanishi, T., et al., *Validation of continuous wave Doppler-determined right ventricular peak positive and negative dP/dt: effect of right atrial pressure on measurement.* J Am Coll Cardiol, 1994. 23(7): 1638–43.

32. Vogel, M., et al., *Validation of myocardial acceleration during isovolumic contraction as a novel noninvasive index of right ventricular contractility: comparison with ventricular pressure-volume relations in an animal model.* Circulation, 2002. 105(14): 1693–9.

33. Frigiola, A., et al., *Pulmonary regurgitation is an important determinant of right ventricular contractile dysfunction in patients with surgically repaired tetralogy of Fallot.* Circulation, 2004. 110(11 Suppl 1): II153–7.

34. Beygui, F., et al., *Routine breath-hold gradient echo MRI-derived right ventricular mass, volumes and function: accuracy, reproducibility and coherence study.* Int J Cardiovasc Imaging, 2004. 20(6): 509–16.

35. Davlouros, P.A., et al., *The right ventricle in congenital heart disease.* Heart, 2006. 92(Suppl 1): i27–38.

36. Groves, P., et al., *Reduced exercise capacity in patients with tricuspid regurgitation after successful mitral valve replacement for rheumatic mitral valve disease.* Br Heart J, 1991. 66: 295–301.

37. Sagie, A., et al., *Significant tricuspid regurgitation is a marker for adverse outcome in patients undergoing percutaneous balloon mitral valvuloplasty.* J Am Coll Cardiol, 1994. 24: 696–702.

38. Koelling, T., et al., *Prognostic significance of mitral regurgitation and tricuspid regurgitation in patients with left ventricular systolic dysfunction.* Am Heart J, 2002. 144: 524–9.

39. Wilson, W., et al., American Heart Association Rheumatic Fever, Endocarditis, and Kawasaki Disease Committee; American Heart Association Council on Cardiovascular Disease in the Young; American Heart Association Council on Clinical Cardiology; American Heart Association Council on Cardiovascular Surgery and Anesthesia; Quality of Care and Outcomes Research Interdisciplinary Working Group. *Prevention of infective endocarditis. Guidelines from the American Heart Association. A Guideline From the American Heart Association Rheumatic Fever, Endocarditis, and Kawasaki Disease Committee, Council on Cardiovascular Disease in the Young, and the Council on Clinical Cardiology, Council on Cardiovascular Surgery and Anesthesia, and the Quality of Care and Outcomes Research Interdisciplinary Working Group.* Circulation, 2007. 116(15): 1736–54.

40. Fukuda, S., et al., *Tricuspid valve tethering predicts residual tricuspid regurgitation after tricuspid annuloplasty.* Circulation, 2005. 111(8): 975–9.

41. Ohata, T., et al., *Comparison of durability of bioprostheses in tricuspid and mitral positions.* Ann Thorac Surg, 2001. 71(5 Suppl): S240–3.

42. Stulak, J.M., et al., *Right-sided Maze procedure for atrial tachyarrhythmias in congenital heart disease.* Ann Thorac Surg, 2006. 81(5): 1780–4; discussion 1784–5.

43. Ratnatunga, C., et al., *Tricuspid valve replacement: UK Heart Valve Registry mid-term results comparing mechanical and biological prostheses.* Ann Thorac Surg, 1998. 66: 1940–7.

44. Rizzoli, G., et al., *Biological or mechanical prostheses in tricuspid position? A meta-analysis of intra-institutional results.* Ann Thorac Surg, 2004. 77(5): 1607–14.

45. Moller, J.E., et al., *Prognosis of carcinoid heart disease: analysis of 200 cases over two decades.* Circulation, 2005. 112(21): 3320–7.

46. Sadeghi, H.M., et al., *Does lowering pulmonary arterial pressure eliminate severe functional tricuspid regurgitation? Insights from pulmonary thromboendarterectomy.* J Am Coll Cardiol, 2004. 44(1): 126–32.

47. Song, J.M., et al., *Outcome of significant functional tricuspid regurgitation after percutaneous mitral valvuloplasty.* Am Heart J, 2003. 145(2): 371–6.

48. Hannoush, H., et al., *Regression of significant tricuspid regurgitation after mitral balloon valvotomy for severe mitral stenosis.* Am Heart J, 2004. 148(5): 865–70.

49. Staab, M.E., R.A. Nishimura, and J.A. Dearani, *Isolated tricuspid valve surgery for severe tricuspid regurgitation following prior left heart valve surgery: analysis of outcome in 34 patients.* J Heart Valve Dis, 1999. 8(5): 567–74.

50. Yada, I., et al., *Preoperative evaluation and surgical treatment for tricuspid regurgitation associated with acquired valvular heart disease. The Kay-Boyd method vs the Carpentier-Edwards ring method.* J Cardiovasc Surg (Torino), 1990. 31(6): 771–7.

51. Pellegrini, A., et al., *Evaluation and treatment of secondary tricuspid insufficiency.* Eur J Cardiothorac Surg, 1992. 6(6): 288–96.

52. De Simone, R., et al., *Adjustable tricuspid valve annuloplasty assisted by intraoperative transesophageal color Doppler echocardiography.* Am J Cardiol, 1993. 71(11): 926–31.

53. Fawzy, M.E., et al., *Immediate and long-term effect of mitral balloon valvotomy on severe pulmonary hypertension in patients with mitral stenosis.* Am Heart J, 1996. 131(1): 89–93.

54. el-Sherif, N., *Rheumatic tricuspid stenosis. A haemodynamic correlation.* Br Heart J, 1971. 33(1): 16–31.

55. Killip, T., III and D.S. Lukas, *Tricuspid stenosis; physiologic criteria for diagnosis and hemodynamic abnormalities.* Circulation, 1957. 16(1): 3–13.

12 Pulmonary Valve Stenosis and Regurgitation

Carlos E. Ruiz and Laurence M. Schneider

CONTENTS

INTRODUCTION

Congenital pulmonary valve stenosis with intact ventricular septum is by far the most common cause of obstruction to the right ventricular outflow and is a relatively common lesion with an estimated prevalence of about 10% of children born with congenital heart disease, approximately 1 in 1,500 births *(1–4)*. There are other congenital and acquired causes of right ventricular outflow obstruction, such as double-chamber right ventricle, asymmetric septal hypertrophy with infundibular obstruction, supravalvular pulmonary stenosis, or pulmonary branch stenosis, all of which do have in common an intact interventricular septum. The extreme of pulmonary valve stenosis is pulmonary atresia with or without ventricular septal defect. Congenital pulmonary valve regurgitation is a rare anomaly, usually accompanying other anomalies such as tetralogy of Fallot with absent pulmonary valve or idiopathic dilatation of the pulmonary arteries *(5)*, but by far the most common cause of pulmonary regurgitation is secondary to pulmonary hypertension.

From: *Contemporary Cardiology: Valvular Heart Disease*
Edited by: Andrew Wang, Thomas M. Bashore, DOI 10.1007/978-1-59745-411-7_12
© Humana Press, a part of Springer Science+Business Media, LLC 2009

ETIOLOGY OF PULMONARY VALVE STENOSIS

Congenital

The pulmonary valve derives from the two endocardial cushions within the truncus arteriosus, the intercalated valve cushions and the major truncus cushions, once they fuse to form the truncus septum *(6)*. The cause of congenital pulmonary stenosis is not known, although genetic factors may play an important role. However, there are many documented associations of right ventricular outflow obstruction with multiple somatic abnormalities *(7–12)*. Perhaps the most commonly recognized is the Noonan syndrome, an autosomal dominant trait with a pleiomorphic phenotype for which a high percentage of affected individuals have cardiac involvement, pulmonary valve stenosis by far being the most common form, although hypertrophic cardiomyopathy is the second most common cardiac abnormality. This syndrome is thought to be closely tight to the PTPN11 gene which encodes a non-membranous protein tyrosine phosphate (SHP-2) with diverse roles in signal transduction via the RAS-mitogen-activated protein kinase (MAPK) pathway, relevant in the epidermal growth factor signaling in semilunar valve morphogenesis *(13)*. A closely related (allelic disorder) syndrome is the LEOPARD syndrome which is an autosomal dominant syndrome characterized by multiple lentigines and "café au lait" spots with electrocardiographic conduction abnormalities, hypertelorism, hypertrophic obstructive cardiomyopathy, pulmonary stenosis, abnormal male genitalia, growth retardation, and deafness *(14)*. Alagille syndrome results from a JAG1 gene mutation, consists of a paucity of intrahepatic bile ducts and vertebral anomalies such as hemivertebrae, dysmorphia, and is commonly associated with pulmonary branch stenosis, but pulmonary valvar stenosis and tetralogy of Fallot, as well as ASD and VSD, are also seen.

Acquired

Ninety-five percent of all cases of pulmonary valve stenosis are congenital or associated with congenital heart disease *(15)*. The acquired causes may be divided into conditions with valvular involvement causing stenosis and intrinsic obstruction to the right ventricular outflow tract or conditions causing external compression with right ventricular outlet obstruction or main pulmonary artery narrowing. Table 1 summarizes the etiological classification.

Table 1
Etiological Classification of Acquired Pulmonary Valve Stenosis

Valvular	Carcinoid heart disease
	Radiation-induced valvular disease
	Rheumatic heart disease
Intrinsic	Primary cardiac tumors
	Twin–twin transfusion syndrome
	Pericardial band/ring—chronic pericarditis
External	Unruptured aneurysms of the sinus of Valsalva
	Pericardial/myocardial abscess
	Mediastinal mass

Carcinoid is the most common cause of acquired valvular pulmonary stenosis *(15)* with the remainder of the valvular causes limited to reports. Carcinoid heart disease may occur in up to 50% of cases of carcinoid *(16)* with pulmonary valve involvement causing stenosis ranging from 32 to 49% of those cases *(17)*. Radiation-induced valvular disease has been well described many years after mediastinal radiation for Hodgkin and non-Hodgkin's lymphoma. The majority of cases remain asymptomatic with up to 6% developing significant valvular dysfunction *(18, 19)*. Rheumatic disease has the least affinity for the pulmonary valve, being the rarest of all the rheumatic valve diseases with only very few reported cases.

Intrinsic and progressive obstruction to the right ventricular outflow tract may rarely be caused by primary cardiac tumors such as leiomyosarcoma *(20, 21)*, rhabdomyoma *(22)*, and myxoma *(23)*. Pregnancies complicated by twin–twin transfusion syndrome may have up to a 9% incidence of the recipient twin developing right ventricular outflow tract obstruction in utero. The cause is unclear but may be related to altered fetal circulation causing right ventricular hypertrophy which may directly obstruct pulmonary blood flow *(24, 25)*.

Extrinsic compression of the right ventricular outflow tract or pulmonary valve has a number of reported causes. A fibrocalcified pericardial band/ring, usually as a result of chronic pericarditis, may result in pulmonary stenosis *(26–29)*. Unruptured aneurysms of the sinus of valsalva, congenital and acquired, usually remain asymptomatic and undetected; however, in rare instances those originating from the right coronary sinus have been reported as producing right ventricular outflow obstruction *(30–33)*. Both pericardial and myocardial abscesses, from sources such as tuberculosis, are able to obstruct the right ventricular outflow tract *(34, 35)*. Mediastinal masses such as Hodgkin and non-Hodgkin lymphoma, teratoma, thymic carcinoid tumor, and metastatic pleomorphic adenocarcinoma can all rarely cause infravalvular, valvular, or supravalvular pulmonary valve compression *(36–40)*.

PATHOPHYSIOLOGY OF PULMONARY STENOSIS

All patterns and causes of pulmonary stenosis result in an increase in the afterload of the right ventricle with progressive, compensatory right ventricular hypertrophy, the degree of which depends on the severity *(41)* and the duration of the pulmonary stenosis. If the stenosis is not severe, or the cause of the obstruction gradual, as in the majority of acquired cases, right ventricular hypertrophy will usually will be minimal or not occur. Severe pulmonary stenosis always results in right ventricular hypertrophy. The greater the severity of the pulmonary stenosis the greater the right ventricular hypertrophy and the smaller the right ventricular cavity size. This tends to cause progressive right ventricular diastolic dysfunction with increased filling pressures in the right atrium. This phenomena may ultimately result in shunting of desaturated blood across the patent foramen ovale into the left atrium *(42)*. In neonates with critical pulmonary valve stenosis and the right-to-left shunt at the atrial level, a patent ductus arteriosus is essential to provide pulmonary blood flow, and therefore these patients behave as ductal dependent. The ultimate degree of pulmonary valve stenosis is pulmonary valvar atresia and there are two types of pulmonary atresia with intact ventricular septum. Type I: pulmonary atresia leads to massive right ventricular hypertrophy and obliteration of the chamber. Suprasystemic right ventricular pressure results in retrograde flow of blood through feeding sinusoids into the coronary artery circulation. Type II: tricuspid insufficiency allows retrograde flow of blood into the right atrium and through an atrial septal defect that is almost invariably present. Right ventricular chamber diameter is normal or enlarged. More moderate degrees of pulmonary stenosis lead to right ventricular hypertrophy with a normal sized right ventricular cavity. The left ventricle and aortic diameters are usually enlarged secondary to increased flow. The tricuspid valve is almost always anomalous. Frequent presentations include hypoplastic valve leaflets, fibrotic valve leaflets, fused commissures, reduced number of chordae tendinae, abnormal attachments to papillary muscles, and frank Ebstein's anomaly *(43)*. Hypertrophy of the right ventricle leads to hypokinesis of the ventricular free wall which further deteriorates the ventricular function *(44)*.

Outside of the neonatal critical pulmonary stenosis-atresia severe right ventricular dysfunction is relatively rare and usually occurs in patients who have had severe pressure overload for a long period of time *(42)*. However, myocardial fibrosis, due to a number of potential mechanisms *(45)*, may ultimately develop, and in these patients they will continue to have significantly impaired systolic and diastolic functions even after intervention. Furthermore, right ventricular hypertrophy may cause right ventricular outflow obstruction that may be inadvertent prior to release of the valvar obstruction.

With exertion, excessive right ventricular afterload can limit right ventricular systolic performance reducing the left ventricular preload and hence limit cardiac output.

NATURAL HISTORY OF PULMONARY STENOSIS

The natural history of pulmonary valve stenosis is dependant, primarily, on the severity of the gradient. The majority of studies (46) and reported cases seem to confirm that newborns and children with mild pulmonary stenosis and systolic pressure gradients less than 50 mmHg were asymptomatic and remained so into their seventh and eighth decades (47). They usually present with asymptomatic cardiac murmurs that are detected on routine examination. However, infants with initial systolic pressure gradients greater than 50 mmHg have an annual increase in the gradient of 8.6 mmHg (48). Nevertheless, there are studies showing that even mild pulmonary stenosis may not be static and between 10 and 28% (49–51) of infants may progress to moderate or severe pulmonary stenosis. Predicting which of these mildly affected newborns or infants will progress is difficult, but progression tends to occur more often and more rapidly in younger infants than in older infants and children (51). Progression may be related to thickened and dysmorphic valvar leaflets, as seen in patients with Noonan syndrome (49). Infants with even moderate pulmonary stenosis as defined by systolic pressure gradients between 30 and 50 mmHg may actually improve as was demonstrated in a follow-up study (52). Other studies seem to have found similar improvements in their subjects (49). Patients with moderate or severe pulmonary stenosis may have mild exertional dyspnea. Adults may be asymptomatic irrespective of the severity of their obstruction.

Adult patients with severe or critical obstruction may present with signs of systemic venous congestion, which are usually interpreted as signs of CHF. The signs are due to severe right ventricular dysfunction or to cyanosis secondary to a right-to-left shunt across a patent foramen ovale or an atrial septal defect. Lightheadedness, syncope, and chest pain that resemble angina pectoris are rare, even in patients with severe obstruction.

SYMPTOMS AND SIGNS IN PULMONARY STENOSIS

The occurrence of symptoms in valvar pulmonary valve stenosis is usually related to the severity of the gradient across the pulmonary valve (46). Patients with gradients <30 mmHg are most often asymptomatic and have no significant progression of the disease.

Neonates

In critical valvar pulmonary stenosis or pulmonary atresia, right-to-left shunting across a patent foramen ovale (PFO) or atrial septal defect (ASD) results in cyanosis. This is usually associated with a hypertrophied right ventricle. If prompt intervention does not occur, gradual closure of the patent ductus arteriosus (PDA) over 12–48 h leads to progressive hypoxemia as pulmonary blood flow is diminished. After successful balloon intervention, right ventricular afterload is normalized and, over a course of weeks to months, returns to normal function. During that period right ventricular compliance remains impaired with ongoing right-to-left shunting via a PFO or ASD resulting in lesser degrees of cyanosis and hypoxemia. Rarely, persistent desaturations may occur with ongoing right ventricular non-compliance and this can be alleviated by closure of the PFO or ASD.

Children

Most children present with an asymptomatic heart murmur. Surprisingly, high gradients do not always equate to considerable symptoms. Young children often maintain patency of the PFO which, during peak exercise, allows for a right-to-left shunt and hence produces exercise-induced cyanosis. Few children may have cyanosis at rest. Severe right ventricular hypertrophy and dysfunction is uncommon *(48)*.

Adolescents/Adults

If symptoms are present they may include exercise intolerance, breathlessness, and fatigue. Exercise testing may reveal subnormal exercise tolerance but rarely causes electrocardiographic ST changes *(53)*. Right heart failure with peripheral edema, jugular venous distention, and ascites is an uncommon occurrence, usually indicating a near premorbid state.

EXAMINATION FINDINGS OF PULMONARY STENOSIS

Visible and palpable signs reflect the effects of right ventricular hypertrophy and include a prominent jugular venous a-wave (due to forceful atrial contraction against a hypertrophied RV), an RV precordial lift or heave, and a left parasternal systolic thrill at the second intercostal space. On auscultation, the first heart sound (S1) is normal and the second heart sound (S2) splitting is widened because of prolonged pulmonic ejection (pulmonic component of S2 [P2] is delayed). The P2 component is soft and in severe pulmonic stenosis may be absent—single second sound. In RV failure and hypertrophy, the third and fourth heart sounds (S3 and S4) are rarely audible at the left parasternal fourth intercostal space. A click in congenital PS is thought to result from abnormal ventricular wall tension. The click occurs early in systole (very near S1) and is not affected by hemodynamic changes. The degree of prematurity of this ejection click during held expiration also correlates well with the severity of the transvalvular gradient. Ejection clicks are not present in subvalvar stenosis.

A harsh crescendo–decrescendo ejection murmur is audible and is heard best at the left parasternal second (valvular stenosis) or fourth (infundibular stenosis) intercostal space with the diaphragm of the stethoscope when the patient leans forward. Unlike the aortic stenosis murmur, a PS murmur does not radiate, and the crescendo component lengthens as stenosis progresses. The murmur grows louder immediately with Valsalva release and with inspiration; the patient may need to be standing for this effect to be heard.

Subvalvular infundibular pulmonary stenosis, on the other hand, causes a splitting interval of 100 ms or more with little or no respiratory variation. The respiratory variation of the wide split S2, normally seen in valval stenosis, may be significantly diminished or absent in patients with a severe poststenotic dilatation of the main pulmonary artery *(54)*.

DIAGNOSTIC FINDINGS OF PULMONARY STENOSIS

Electrocardiogram

With pulmonary stenosis the ECG reflects the degree of right ventricular hypertrophy. The rhythm is sinus with normal ECG intervals. The P-wave frontal plane axis is normal. The QRS frontal plane axis tends to be in the lower left quadrant, or up to +120° in cases of small right ventricle, while it is usually very rightward, greater than +120° in cases of large right ventricles. Mild degrees of obstruction have a normal ECG pattern, but with moderate to severe obstruction right-axis deviation and right ventricular hypertrophy (qR-wave in lead V1). An rSr morphology may also occur in lead V1. Of note is that older children and adults appear to have a left preponderance which may mask slight right ventricular hypertrophy *(55)*. Right atrial abnormalities are reflected as peaked P-waves (P-pulmonale) in leads II and III.

Chest X-Ray

The most consistent radiologic feature is a prominent main pulmonary artery secondary to post-stenotic dilatation of the main pulmonary artery and frequently the left pulmonary artery may be seen on CXR with severe pulmonary obstruction. This may be related to the direction of the high-velocity jet through the stenotic pulmonary valve. With mild to moderate stenosis, heart size remains normal; however, with severe stenosis right ventricular hypertrophy causes the apex to lift off the left hemidiaphragm and in the lateral chest X-ray there is filling-in of the retrosternal space. In severe stenosis it is not rare to observe decreased pulmonary vascular markings. With infundibular stenosis, the pulmonary artery is normal sized. Right atrial enlargement is relatively uncommon unless significant right ventricular dysfunction and/or tricuspid regurgitation are present. Calcified pericardial rings/bands and intrinsic and extrinsic masses may be seen on CXR.

Echocardiography and Doppler

The sine qua non of diagnosis is two-dimensional and Doppler echocardiography (55). During systole, the leaflets do not lie parallel to the margins of the pulmonary artery wall, but rather curve inward toward the midpoint of the main pulmonary artery—the so-called doming of the valve. The visualization of thickened leaflets, normal diameter of the pulmonary valve annulus, dilated pulmonary trunk, and hypertrophied right ventricle are hallmarks of this anomaly. Generally, calcification of the leaflets is not prominent. In contrast, dysplastic pulmonary valves have thickened, nodular, immobile leaflets with minimal or no commissure fusion (no doming); small annulus; and minimal or absent pulmonary artery dilation.

The pressure gradient across the right ventricular outflow tract is estimated by continuous wave Doppler using the modified Bernoulli equation which, unlike left-sided stenoses, correlates well with catheter-based peak-to-peak gradients (41). Right ventricular pressure overload causes shifting of the interventricular septum toward the left ventricle during systole causing the characteristic D-shape with flattened septum (44). Assessment of right ventricular size and contractility can be made. Obstruction at the valvular, subvalvular, or supravalvular level may be seen as well as localization of masses intrinsic to the myocardium or extrinsic to the heart.

Cardiac Catheterization

Cardiac catheterization is nowadays seldom used for the diagnosis of pulmonary stenosis and reserved for the few patients in whom hemodynamic status was unable to be assessed accurately with non-invasive techniques. However, since the standard of care treatment for the majority of patients with severe valvar pulmonary stenosis is balloon valvuloplasty, this diagnostic tool remains important. The oximetry data obtained depends on the severity of the obstruction and the associated intracardiac or extracardiac shunts present, such as atrial septal defect and patent ductus arteriosus. The most important parameters obtained are the measurements of right ventricular pressure, simultaneously with the main pulmonary artery pressure (transvalvular gradient) and the RV/LV ratio. The right ventricular end-diastolic pressure may be normal or increased in patients with severe stenosis. The right atrial pressure curve usually shows tall A-waves in severe stenosis. A prominent V-wave may be present if there is concomitant tricuspid regurgitation. When the pressure gradient is adjusted for heart rate, the inclusion of cardiac output does not improve the accuracy of prediction of severity (56). The calculation of the valve area using the Gorlin formula has several problems, making it unacceptable as an index of severity. Thus, severity is routinely assessed by the transvalvular gradient. Mild stenosis is considered to be present if the systolic gradient is less than 40 mmHg and/or the right ventricular pressure is less than one-half of the left ventricular pressure. Moderate stenosis is defined as a gradient grater than 40 mmHg and/or right ventricular pressure greater than one-half of the systemic pressure. Severe stenosis is classified as a transvalvular gradient greater than 80 mmHg and/or a right ventricular pressure equal or greater than the systemic pressure. These definitions assume a normal cardiac output under resting conditions and, therefore is important to measure cardiac output, even though valve area will not be taken into account.

Right ventricular angiography, preferably in a biplane mode, can facilitate imaging of the anatomical structures and the level of the obstruction. The best orthogonal views are in the anteroposterior position with a 40−50° cephalad angulation and in the lateral view (Fig. 1). These views will allow assessment of the annular size, the presence of infundibular narrowing as well as the characterization and degree of dysplastic leaflets, all of them important to determine the feasibility of an intervention.

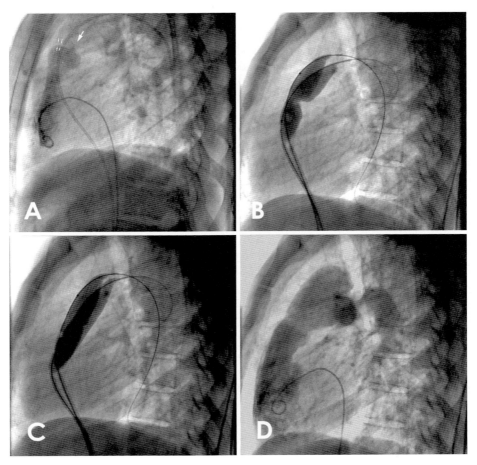

Fig. 1. (A) Right ventricular angiography in a lateral projection, showing the thickness of the pulmonary valve cusps (*small arrows*), the jet through the stenotic and domed pulmonary valve (*large arrow*), and the unobstructed right ventricular outflow tract. **(B)** Waist on the balloon catheters from the stenotic valve. **(C)** Balloon fully inflated with disappearance of the waist. **(D)** Right ventricular angiography postdouble balloon pulmonary valvuloplasty, showing the wider jet from the right ventricle to the dilated main pulmonary artery.

TREATMENT OF PULMONARY STENOSIS

Balloon valvuloplasty is the preferred method for the treatment of pulmonary stenosis in children *(57)* and adults *(58, 59)*. The valve should be pliable and adequately mobile for balloon valvuloplasty to be adequately successful. In Noonan syndrome, due to the degree of immobility of the dysplastic pulmonary valve, a surgical approach may be preferred *(60)*. Various techniques of balloon valvuloplasty are used such as single, double, and the Inoue two-component balloon.

Many investigators over the last two decades have described excellent acute *(60–63)* and long-term results *(64–66)* from balloon valvuloplasty. The valvuloplasty and angioplasty of Congenital Anomalies registry is the largest published clinical series of percutaneous pulmonary valvuloplasties available *(67)*, reporting the acute results of dilations performed in 784 patients. The overall results of these procedures showed a reduction of the peak systolic pulmonary valve gradient from 71 to 28 mmHg with few serious complications. A residual gradient of 30 mmHg or more was associated with more severe initial obstruction and a dysplastic pulmonary valve. Over 860 infants, children, and adolescents have been followed up for between 1 and 14 years in multiple trials *(68)*. Approximately 80% of these patients were free from clinically significant stenosis at final follow-up and only 15−18% required additional procedures because of clinically significant stenosis at final follow-up. Recently, the long-term results of balloon valvuloplasty in adults with concomitant severe infundibular stenosis and tricuspid regurgitation have shown to be excellent with regression of the severe infundibular stenosis and tricuspid regurgitation *(69)*. Results of balloon valvuloplasty appear to be similar to surgical valvotomy over 10 years *(66)*. Survival after 25 years of follow-up for 90 patients after surgery for pulmonary stenosis showed 93% survival with moderate to severe pulmonary regurgitation in 37% and re-operation for pulmonary regurgitation necessary in 9%. Sixty-seven percent of the patients were in NYHA Class I *(70)*.

Factors determining immediate and long-term results of balloon valvuloplasty are lower prevalvuloplasty pulmonary gradients, lower right ventricular systolic pressures, and lower right ventricular voltage electrocardiogram (R-wave amplitude in V1) *(71)*. The Second Natural History Study of Congenital Heart Defects showed that in medically managed children followed over 5–21 years, a transpulmonary valve gradient of <50 mmHg showed no increase in gradient whereas pressure gradients >50 mmHg showed a significant increase *(46)*. Due to the excellent safety of balloon valvuloplasty there are recommendations to perform percutaneous balloon valvuloplasty with resting peak systolic gradients greater than 40 mmHg *(68)*. Factors that may lead to poor long-term outcome include higher initial pulmonary valvar gradient, higher early residual gradient, smaller ratio of balloon to valve, smaller valvar diameter, younger age at initial presentation, and dysplastic pulmonary valve *(68)*.

ETIOLOGY OF PULMONARY VALVE REGURGITATION

The etiology of pulmonary regurgitation can be divided into conditions associated with anatomically normal valve cusps, anatomically abnormal cusps *(15)*, and iatrogenic after valvular intervention, surgical or otherwise, such as postballoon valvuloplasty (Table 2). Iatrogenic etiology is the most common and among those the leading cause is the residual regurgitation encountered in patients with post-tetralogy of Fallot repair, especially patients that had a transannular patch repair *(72)*.

PATHOPHYSIOLOGY OF PULMONARY REGURGITATION

The pathophysiologic consequences of pulmonary regurgitation are perhaps less well understood. In severe pulmonary regurgitation, forward pulmonary blood flow can be maintained indirectly by the work of the left heart via the systemic venous return and by right atrial contraction. In these right ventricles a late diastolic forward flow in the pulmonary trunk coincident with atrial systole is seen and the right ventricle temporarily acts as a conduit. Furthermore, the pulmonary microvasculature is of low resistance. The importance of this is that with each right ventricular systole blood moves readily forward through the pulmonary microvessels whose slight resistance acts as a "watershed" into the pulmonary veins, which in turn are maintained at low pressure by action of the left heart. Flow that passes forward through alveolar capillaries in systole is unlikely to pass back again

Table 2
Etiological Classification of Acquired Pulmonary Valve Regurgitation

Normal pulmonary valve cusps	Elevated pulmonary artery systolic pressures
	Idiopathic-dilated pulmonary trunk
	Marfan's syndrome
	Infective endocarditis
Abnormal pulmonary valve cusps	Congenital—absent pulmonary valve syndrome
	Rheumatic
	Carcinoid
	Trauma
	Infective endocarditis
Iatrogenic	Surgical repair of tetralogy of Fallot
	Percutaneous balloon angioplasty—stenting

in diastole, there being no significant reversal of gradient. The pulmonary microvascular bed, therefore, has a valve-like effect in the setting of severe PR. This is evidenced by the fact that severe or free regurgitation is usually associated with a measured regurgitant fraction of only about 40% *(73, 74)* which is generally well tolerated for a long period of time. However, pulmonary regurgitation can worsen by conditions that lead to elevated pulmonary artery pressure such as pulmonary artery branch stenosis, bronchopulmonary disease (COPD), left ventricular dysfunction, or pulmonary vascular disease *(75)*.

Right ventricular adaptation and response to pulmonary regurgitation depends on the degree and duration of the regurgitant flow *(76)*, as well as the properties of the right ventricle and pulmonary arteries. Worsening degrees of pulmonary regurgitation cause right ventricular volume overload which increases end-diastolic volumes followed by a gradual rise in end-systolic volumes and eventual deterioration of myocardial function. Historically it has been said that the right ventricle tolerates volume loading well for a long time *(77)*; however, this concept is in reality poorly understood and is being challenged. Acute volume overload can occur postoperative repair of a pulmonary valve. Infants and children tend to have more compliant right ventricles and hence tolerate acute pulmonary regurgitation better than adults, who may progress to right ventricular decompensation due to a hypertrophied and relatively non-compliant right ventricle *(72)*.

NATURAL HISTORY OF PULMONARY REGURGITATION

Pulmonary regurgitation is usually well tolerated for many years with patients remaining free of symptoms until marked right ventricular dilatation and systolic dysfunction occur. Symptoms are usually associated with established right ventricular dysfunction which may be irreversible *(72)*. Pulmonary regurgitation is common after surgical or percutaneous relief of pulmonary stenosis and following repair of tetralogy of Fallot. Pulmonary regurgitation in these patients is shown to relate to the use of a transannular patch—more extensively performed in an earlier surgical era to reconstruct the right ventricular outflow tract (RVOT). Furthermore, transannular patching and/or aggressive infundibulectomy predispose to RVOT aneurysms or akinetic regions. The latter, combined with chronic regurgitation, has an adverse effect on right ventricular function and overall prognosis *(73)*. As a result, routine and generous transannular patch type of repair has now been abandoned and limited RVOT patching with preservation of pulmonary valve function have become key therapeutic goals during primary repair of tetralogy in infancy. It is usually well tolerated in childhood. However, recent long-term studies have demonstrated that this condition leads to progressive right ventricular dilatation and, with time, to right ventricular dysfunction, exercise intolerance, ventricular tachycardia, and sudden cardiac death *(78–82)*. Furthermore, recent advances in non-invasive imaging, and in particular wider availability of cardiovascular magnetic resonance, have improved the assessment of pulmonary regurgitation and right ventricular function in these patients.

SYMPTOMS AND SIGNS IN PULMONARY REGURGITATION

The great majority of patients remain symptom free for many years, until right ventricular dilatation with significant systolic dysfunction appears. In the early stages of right ventricular dysfunction, most patients remain as NYHA-FC I; however, when tested by different exercise test protocols, certain exercise intolerance is evident *(78, 79)*. The serious problem with these patients is that when they become overly symptomatic, there is always a high degree of right ventricular dysfunction, and usually at this stage it is irreversible.

Patients under the age of 30 with isolated congenital pulmonary regurgitation and otherwise normal cardiac structures, also remain symptom free. However, after this, they tend to manifest symptoms of failure and can also present as a sudden cardiac death *(77, 83)*.

The symptoms manifestations of these patients mostly are exercise intolerance, congestive heart failure, atrial and ventricular arrhythmias, and also sudden cardiac death.

When the right ventricular function is adversely affected to a significant degree, the physical examination may reveal elevated jugular venous pressure, distended liver with sometimes a pulsatile sensation (depending on the amount of tricuspid regurgitation), and positive hepato-jugular reflux. They also present with peripheral edema of variant degrees.

Palpable signs are attributable to pulmonary hypertension and RV hypertrophy. They include a palpable pulmonic component (P2) of the second heart sound (S2) at the left upper sternal border and a sustained RV impulse that is increased in amplitude at the left middle and lower sternal border.

On auscultation, the first heart sound (S1) is normal. The S2 may be split or single. When split, P2 may be loud and audible shortly after the aortic component of S2 (A2) because of pulmonary hypertension, or P2 may be delayed because of increased RV stroke volume. S2 may be single because of prompt pulmonic valve closing with a merged A2–P2 or, rarely, because of congenital absence of the pulmonic valve. An RV third heart sound (S3), fourth heart sound (S4), or both may be audible with RV dysfunction; these sounds can be distinguished from left ventricular heart sounds because they are located at the left parasternal fourth intercostal space and because they grow louder with inspiration (Carvallo sign).

The murmur of PR due to pulmonary hypertension is a high-pitched, early diastolic decrescendo murmur that begins with P2 and ends before S1 and that radiates toward the mid-right sternal edge (Graham Steell's murmur); it is heard best at left upper sternal border with the diaphragm of the stethoscope while the patient holds the breath at end-expiration and sits upright. The murmur of PR without pulmonary hypertension is shorter, lower-pitched, and rougher in quality and begins after P2. Both murmurs may resemble the murmur of aortic regurgitation but can be distinguished by inspiration (which makes the pulmonary regurgitation murmur louder) and by Valsalva release. After Valsalva release, the pulmonary regurgitation murmur immediately becomes loud (because of immediate venous return to the right side of the heart), but the aortic regurgitation murmur requires 4 or 5 beats to do so (delay time in feeling the pulmonary bed). Also, a soft pulmonary regurgitation murmur may sometimes become even softer during inspiration because this murmur is usually best heard at the second left intercostal space, where inspiration pushes the stethoscope away from the heart. A pansystolic murmur of tricuspid regurgitation can commonly be heard, and typically this murmur increases during inspiration (Rivero-Carvallo sign) in distinction of the mitral regurgitation murmur.

DIAGNOSTIC FINDINGS OF PULMONARY REGURGITATION

Electrocardiogram

With pulmonary regurgitation most patients are in sinus rhythm. A volume overloaded right ventricle may cause QRS prolongation with rSr morphology in the precordial leads. Patients who previously underwent tetralogy of Fallot repair via a right ventriculotomy often have a right bundle branch block *(72)*. As the right ventricle enlarges, so the QRS lengthens. This may also reflect right ventricular dysfunction and have prognostic implications for malignant arrhythmias and sudden cardiac death.

Chest X-Ray

Severe pulmonary regurgitation causes dilatation of the pulmonary trunk and central pulmonary arteries as well as right ventricular dilatation, as evidenced by filling of the retrosternal space in a lateral view.

Echocardiography and Doppler

Echocardiography remains the most widely used imaging method for pulmonary regurgitation; however, cardiac magnetic resonance (CMR) imaging is now considered the gold standard for both pulmonary regurgitant quantification and right ventricular volumetric analysis *(41)*. Using echocardiography, right ventricular size and function can be evaluated, and volume overload produces characteristic paradoxical motion of the interventricular septum *(72)*. Using continuous wave Doppler a ratio of pulmonary regurgitant flow to total diastolic duration can be measured which yields a sensitivity of 100% and specificity of 85% for identifying patients who have significant pulmonary regurgitation *(84)*. A pulmonary regurgitant pressure half-time of <100 ms also correlates with hemodynamically significant regurgitation *(85)*. Right ventricular restrictive physiology is commonly present after repair of tetralogy of Fallot. Restrictive ventricular physiology can be detected by pulsed wave as well as tissue Doppler. In these patients, a non-compliant RV acts as a conduit between the right atrium and the pulmonary artery at the end of diastole, counteracting the effect of the regurgitation and contributing to forward pulmonary flow, and therefore to effective cardiac output. Echocardiography is also able to visualize traumatized or infected pulmonary valves which have been damaged leading to regurgitation.

Cardiac Catheterization

Nowadays both hemodynamic assessment and angiography play no role in the diagnosis and management of patients with pulmonary regurgitation.

Cardiac Magnetic Resonance

This is a non-invasive modality which is now considered the gold standard for evaluation and follow-up of patients with pulmonary regurgitation *(41, 86)*. There are distinctive advantages of this technology over echocardiography in that magnetic resonance is independent of geometrical assumptions for evaluation of right ventricular volume, mass, and function, and its wide field of views allows an unrestricted evaluation of the right ventricular outflow aneurismal or akinetic regions. Velocity mapping allows for accurate quantification of systolic and diastolic flows through the pulmonary valve allowing for calculation of the regurgitant fraction *(87)*. Due to the highly accurate measurements of right ventricular volumes that are able to be measured by CMR, optimal timing of pulmonary valve replacement can be better decided *(88)*. CMR can also better assess extracardiac lesions *(89)*.

TREATMENT OF PULMONARY REGURGITATION

Definitive treatment of pulmonary regurgitation, especially that caused by repair of tetralogy of Fallot, is replacement of the pulmonary valve (PVR). Xenografts, homografts, or stented prostheses are all options; however, the longevity of these treatments remains similar with finite life spans (77). Operating too early results in multiple redo procedures whereas the danger of delaying PVR is late right ventricular dysfunction, arrhythmia, and sudden cardiac death. Perioperative risk is higher in patients with established right ventricular dysfunction (90). Those patients with established mild to moderate right ventricular dysfunction should still be considered for PVR but usually require longer postoperative intensive care (72). PVR has a perioperative mortality of 1–4% and 10-year actuarial survival of 86–95% (91). In a mixed group of adults and children, freedom from further valve replacement was 81, 58, and 41% at 5, 10, and 15 years, respectively (92). In adults, the life span of the pulmonary valve prosthesis ranges between 15 and 30 years. Patients should be considered for PVR when both moderate to severe or severe pulmonary regurgitation and progressive right ventricular dilatation are present.

Following timely PVR right ventricular end-diastolic volume rapidly decreases over 6 months (88) with possible improvement in systolic function. Normalization of right ventricular function and mass by PVR appears to be largely dependant on the preexisting right ventricular end-diastolic volume with an end-diastolic volume below 150 ml/m^2 and above 200 ml/m^2 as the cut-offs for prompt remodeling of the right ventricle (93). With reduction in right ventricular volumes a reduction in QRS duration has been observed (91). If PVR is performed late, right ventricular recovery is incomplete (94). It remains of utmost importance to know the proper time span that the right ventricle can endure pulmonary regurgitation before irreversible dysfunction occurs.

Newer techniques for replacing pulmonary valves include a percutaneous valve delivery approach (limited to a right ventricular outflow tract of <22 mm) and a transventricular-stented bioprosthesis without cardiopulmonary bypass that allows for implantation of prosthesis with diameters greater than 22 mm. Results of 58 patients with a percutaneous approach have been encouraging early results showing lower morbidity than surgery and significant early symptomatic improvement (95–97). The transventricular approach has been successfully used in a limited number of patients (98).

If pulmonary regurgitation has a primary condition such as endocarditis or pulmonary hypertension from left-sided cardiac conditions as a cause, treatment of these conditions is indicated.

REFERENCES

1. Abrahams DG, Wood P. Pulmonary stenosis with normal aortic root. Br Heart J 1951; 13: 519.
2. Campbell M. Simple pulmonary stenosis: Pulmonary stenosis with closed ventricular septum Br Heart J 1954; 16: 273.
3. Keith JD. Prevalence, incidence and epidemiology. In Keith JD, Rowe RD, Vlad P (eds.): Heart Disease in Infancy and Childhood. 3rd ed. New York, Macmillan, p. 5, 1978.
4. Mitchell SC, Korones SB, Berendes HW. Congenital heart disease in 56,109 births: Incidence and natural history. Circulation 1971; 43: 323–332.
5. Collins NP, Braunwald E, Morrow AG. Isolated congenital pulmonic valvular regurgitation. Am J Med 1960; 28: 159.
6. Van Mierop LHS. Anatomy and embryology of the right ventricle. International Academy of Pathology Monograph 15, Baltimore, Williams & Wilkins, 1974.
7. Klinge T, Laursen HB. Familial pulmonary stenosis with underdeveloped or normal right ventricle. Br Heart J 1975; 37: 60
8. Nora JJ, Torres FG, Sinha AK, McNamara DG. Characteristic cardiovascular anomalies of XO Turner syndrome, XX and XY phenotype and XO/XX Turner mosaic. Am J Cardiol 1970; 25: 639.
9. Patterson DF, Haskins ME, Schnarr WR. Hereditary dysplasia of the pulmonary valve in beagle dogs: Pathologic and genetic studies. Am J Cardiol 1981; 47: 631.
10. Nora JJ, Nora AH. Recurrence risk in children having one parent with a congenital heart disease. Circulation 1976; 53: 701.
11. Noonan JA. Hypertelorism with Turner phenotype: A new syndrome with associated congenital heart disease. Am J Dis Child 1968; 116(4): 373–380.

12. Linde LM, Turner SW, Sparkes RS. Pulmonary valvular dysplasia: A cardiofacial syndrome. Br Heart J 1973; 35: 301.

13. Ogata T, Yoshida R. PTPN11 mutations and genotype-phenotype correlations in Noonan and LEOPARD syndromes. Ped Endocrinol Rev 2005; 2: 669–674.

14. Diglio MC, Sarkozy A, de Zorzi A et al. LEOPARD syndrome: clinical diagnosis in the first year of life. Am J Med Genet. Part A. 2006; 140: 740–746.

15. Waller BF, Howard J, Fess S. Pathology of pulmonic valve stenosis and pure regurgitation. Clin Cardiol Jan 1995; 18: 45–50.

16. Quaedvlieg PF, Lamers CB, Taal BG. Carcinoid heart disease: An update. Scand J Gastroenterol Suppl. 2002; 236: 66–71.

17. Pellikka PA, Tajik AJ, Khandheria BK et al. Carcinoid heart disease. Clinical and echocardiographic spectrum in 74 patients. Circulation 1993; 87: 1188–1196.

18. Tetsuo I, Yuji N, Hiroshi M, Toro K et al. Severe infundibular pulmonary stenosis and coronary artery stenosis with ventricular tachycardia 24 years after mediastinal irradiation. Int Medicine Sep 2005; 44: 963–966.

19. Rummeny E, Hausen W, Lorbacher P, Willems D. Acquired infundibular pulmonary stenosis. Possible late complication following radiotherapy of Hodgkin disease. Z Kardiol Oct 1984; 73: 641–645.

20. Masayasu E, Kensaku K, Toshiyuki N, Kazuhiko N et al. Primary cardiac leiomyosarcoma growing rapidly and causing right ventricular outflow obstruction. Int Medicine Apr 1998; 37: 370–375.

21. Rastan AJ, Walther T, Mohr FW, Kostelka M. Leiomyosarcoma – an unusual cause of right ventricular outflow tract obstruction. Thorac Cardiovasc Surg. Dec 2004; 52: 376–377.

22. De Almeida EC, Leite MS, de Silva MA, Rassi L Jr. Right ventricular rhabdomyoma causing pulmonary stenosis. Arq Bras Cardiol Jun 1993; 60: 417–419.

23. Riera JM, Vila IC, Serrano JM, Aleixandre LM, Baliarda XR, de Auta GM, Ruiz FE, Domenech JP, Garriga JR. Right ventricular myxoma. A rare case of pulmonary stenosis. Rev Esp Cardiol Feb 1996; 49: 153–154.

24. Lougheed J, Sinclair BG, Fung K, Bigras JL, Ryan G, Smallhorn JF, Hornberger LK. Acquired right ventricular outflow tract obstruction in the recipient twin in twin-twin transfusion syndrome. J Am Coll Cardiol Nov 2001; 38: 1533–1538.

25. Nizard J, Bonnet D, Fermont L, Ville Y. Acquired right heart outflow tract anomaly without systemic hypertension in recipient twins in twin-twin transfusion syndrome. Ultrasound Obstet Gynecol Dec 2001; 18: 669–672.

26. Kang WC, Park CH, Chung WJ, Han SH, Ahn TH, Shin EK. Images in cardiovascular medicine. Severe pulmonary artery stenosis caused by extrinsic compression of a calcified circular ring. Circulation Aug 2005; 112: e76–e78.

27. Kawata M, Kataoka T, Kuramoto E, Adachi K, Matsuura A, Sakamoto S, Tobe S, Yamaji S. Pulmonary artery stenosis due to external compression by a calcified pericardial band. Jpn Heart J May 2004; 45: 527–533.

28. Hwang YJ, Park CH, Jeon YB, Park KY. Severe pulmonary artery stenosis by a calcified pericardial ring. Eur J Cardio-thorac Surg Apr 2006; 29: 619–621.

29. Tartarini G, Balbarini A, Gherarducci G, Mengozzi G, Barsotti A, Mariani M. Right ventricular outflow obstruction due to a fibrocalcified pericardial band. J Nuc Med Allied Sci Jan 1984; 28: 47–52.

30. Feldman DN, Roman MJ. Aneurysms of the sinuses of valsalva. Cardiology 2006; 106: 73–81.

31. Liau CS, Chu IT, Ho FM. Unruptured congenital aneurysm of the sinus of valsalva presenting with pulmonary stenosis. Catheter Cardiovasc Interv Feb 1999; 36: 210–213.

32. Haraphongse M, Ayudhya RK, Jugdutt B, Rossall RE. Isolated unruptured sinus of valsalva aneurysm producing right ventricular outflow obstruction. Cathet Cardiovasc Diagn Feb 1990; 19: 98–102.

33. Kerber RE, Ridges JD, Kriss JP, Silverman JF, Anderson ET, Harrison DC. Unruptured aneurysm of the sinus of valsalva producing right ventricular outflow obstruction. Am J Med Dec 1972; 53: 775–783.

34. Rawls WJ, Shuford WH, Logan WD, Hurst JW, Schlant RC. Right ventricular outflow tract obstruction produced by a myocardial abscess in a patient with tuberculosis. Am J Cardiol May 1968; 21: 738–745.

35. Upward JW, Daly K, Jackson G. Pericardial abscess causing right ventricular outflow tract obstruction. Successful surgical correction. Br Heart J May 1983; 49: 507–509.

36. Flint EJ, Wright C, Singh A. Acquired pulmonary stenosis due to pleomorphic adenocarcinoma. Br Heart J Apr 1984; 51: 457–461.

37. Lynch M, Blevins LS, Martin RP. Acquired supravalvular pulmonary stenosis due to extrinsic compression by a metastatic thymic carcinoid tumour. Int J Card Imaging Mar 1996; 12: 61–63.

38. Baduini G, Paolillo V, Di Summa M. Echocardiographic findings in a case of acquired pulmonic stenosis from extrinsic compression by a mediastinal cyst. Chest Oct 1981; 80: 507–509.

39. Viseur P, Unger P. Doppler echocardiographic diagnosis and follow-up of acquired pulmonary stenosis due to external cardiac compression. Cardiology 1995; 86: 80–82.

40. Mandysova E, Neuzil P, Niederle P, Belohlavek O, Kozak T, Mandys V. Pulmonary stenosis caused by external compression of non-Hodgkin lymphoma. Echocardiography. Aug 2004; 21: 565–567.

41. Davlouros PA, Niwa K, Webb G, Gatzoulis MA. The right ventricle in congenital heart disease. BMJ Apr 2006; 92(supp 1): i27–i38.

42. Graham TP. Ventricular performance in congenital heart disease. Circulation Dec 1991; 84(6): 2259–2274.
43. Marvin W, Mahoney LT. Pulmonary atresia with intact ventricular septum. Heart Disease in Infants, Children, and Adolescents, 4th ed. Baltimore, Williams and Wilkins, 1989, p. 338.
44. Bleeker GB, Holman ER, Yu CM, Breithardt OA, Kaandorp TA, Schalij MJ, van der Wall EE, Bax JJ, Nihoyannopoulos. Acquired right ventricular dysfunction. BMJ Apr 2006; 92(supp 1): i14–i18.
45. Babu-Narayan SV, Goktekin O, Moon J, Broberg C, Pantely G, Pennell D, Gatzoulis M, Kilner PJ. Late gadolinium enhancement cardiovascular magnetic resonance of the systemic right ventricle in adults with previous atrial redirection surgery for transposition of the great arteries. Circ Apr 2005; 111(16): 2091–2098.
46. Weidman W H. Report from the second joint study on the natural history of congenital heart defects (NHS-2): Second natural history study of congenital heart defects. Circ Feb 1993; 87(2S): 1–13.
47. Perloff J. Postpediatric congenital heart disease: Natural survival patterns. Cardiovasc Clin 1979; 10: 27–51.
48. Lange PE, Onnasch DG, Heintzen PH. Valvular pulmonary stenosis. Natural history and right ventricular function in infants and children. Eur Heart J Aug 1985; 6(8): 706–709.
49. Gielen H, Daniels O, van Lier H. Natural history of congenital pulmonary valvar stenosis: an echo and Doppler cardiographic study. Cardiol Young Mar 1999; 9(2): 129–135.
50. Anand R, Mehta AV. Natural history of asymptomatic pulmonary stenosis diagnosed in infancy. Clin Cardiol Apr 1997; 20(4): 377–380.
51. Rowland DG, Hamill WW, Allen HD, Gutgesell HP. Natural course of isolated pulmonary valve stenosis in infants and children utilizing Doppler Echocardiography. Am J Cardiol Feb 1997; 79(3): 344–349.
52. Hideshi T, Kazuo I, Kazuki I, Shunzo C. Mild to moderate pulmonary valvular stenosis in infants sometimes improves to the condition unnecessary to do PTPV: Doppler echocardiographic observation. Tohoku J Exp Med 1995; 176: 155–162.
53. Driscoll DJ, Wolfe RR, Gersony WM, Hayes CJ, Keane JF, Kidd L, O'Fallon WM, Pieroni DR, Weidman WH. Cardiorespiratory responses to exercise of patients with aortic stenosis, pulmonary stenosis, and ventricular septal defect. Circulation Feb 1993; 87: I102–I113.
54. Singh SP et al. Unusual splitting of the second heart sound in pulmonary stenosis. Am J Cardiol 1970; 25: 28.
55. Dore A, Gatzoulis M, Webb G, Daubeney P. Diagnosis and management of adult congenital heart disease. Philadelphia, Churchill Livingstone, 2003: 299–303.
56. Ellison R.C et al. Indirect assessment of severity in pulmonary stenosis. Circulation 1977, 56(Suppl. I): 114.
57. Stanger P, Cassidy SC, Girod DA, Kan JS, Lababidi Z, Shapiro SR. Balloon pulmonary valvuloplasty: results of the valvuloplasty and angioplasty of congenital anomalies registry. Am J Cardiol 1990; 65: 775–783.
58. Kaul UA, Singh B, Tyagi S, Bhargava M, Arora R, Khalilullah M. Long term results after balloon pulmonary valvuloplasty in adults. Am Heart J 1993; 126: 1152–1155.
59. Chen CR, Cheng TO, Huang T. Percutaneous balloon valvuloplasty for pulmonic stenosis in adolescents and adults. N Engl J Med 1996; 335: 21–25.
60. Almeda FQ, Kavinsky CJ, Pophal G, Klein LW. Pulmonic valvular stenosis in adults: Diagnosis and treatment. Cath Cardiovasc Interv 2003; 60: 546–557.
61. Sullivan ID, Robinson PJ, Macartney FJ. Percutaneous balloon valvuloplasty for pulmonary valve stenosis in infants and children. Br Heart J 1985; 54: 435–441.
62. Rocchini AP, Kveselis DA, Crowley D, Dick M, Rosenthal A. Percutaneous balloon valvuloplasty for treatment of congenital pulmonary valvular stenosis in children. J Am Coll Cardiol 1984; 3: 1005–1012.
63. Beekman RH, Rocchini AP, Rosenthal A. Therapeutic cardiac catheterization for pulmonary valve and pulmonary artery stenosis. Cardiol Clin 1989; 7: 331–340.
64. Rao PS, Galal O, Patnana M, Buck SH, Wilson AD. Results of 3 to 10 year follow-up of balloon dilatation of the pulmonary valve. Heart 1998; 80: 591–595.
65. McCrindle BW, Kan JS. Long term results after balloon pulmonary valvuloplasty. Circulation 1991; 83: 1915–1922.
66. McCridle BW. Independent predictors of long-term results after balloon pulmonary valvuloplasty. Valvuloplasty and angioplasty of congenital anomalies registry investigators. Circulation 1994; 89: 1751–1759.
67. Stanger P, Cassidy SC, Girod DA, Kan JS, Lababidi Z, Shapiro SR. Balloon pulmonary valvuloplasty: Results of the valvuloplasty and angioplasty of congenital anomalies registry. Am J Cardiol 1990; 65: 775–783.
68. Gudausky TM, Beekman RH. Current options, and long-term results for interventional treatment of pulmonary valvar stenosis. Cardiol Young. 2006; 16: 418–427.
69. Fawzy ME, Hassan W, Fadel BM, Sergani H, El Shaer F, El Widaa, Al Sanei A. Long-term results (up to 17 years) of pulmonary balloon valvuloplasty in adults and its effects on concomitant severe infundibular stenosis and tricuspid regurgitation. Am Heart J Mar 2007; 153(3): 422–8.
70. Roos-Hesselink JW, Meijboom FJ, Spitaels SEC, vanDomburg RT, vanRijen EHM, Utens EMWJ, Bogers AJJC, Simoons ML. Long-term outcome after surgery for pulmonary stenosis (a longitudinal study of 22–33 years). Eur Heart J 2006; 27: 482–488.
71. Silvilairat S, Pongprot Y, Sittiwangkul R, Phornphutkul C. Factors determining immediate and medium-term results after pulmonary balloon valvuloplasty. J Med Assoc Thai Sep 2006; 89(9): 1404–1411.

72. Beatriz B, Philip J.K, Michael A.G. Pulmonary regurgitation: not a benign lesion. European Heart J 2005; 26: 433–439.
73. Davlouros PA, Kilner PJ, Hornung TS et al. Right ventricular function in adults with repaired tetralogy of Fallot assessed with cardiovascular magnetic resonance imaging: detrimental role of right ventricular outflow aneurysms or akinesia and adverse right-to-left ventricular interaction. J Am Coll Cardiol 2002; 40: 2044–2052.
74. Rebergen SA, Chin JG, Ottenkamp J et al. Pulmonary regurgitation in the late postoperative follow-up of tetralogy of Fallot. Volumetric quantitation by nuclear magnetic resonance velocity mapping. Circulation 1993; 88: 2257–2266
75. Ilbawi MN, Idriss FS, DeLeon SY et al. Factors that exaggerate the deleterious effects of pulmonary insufficiency on the right ventricle after tetralogy repair. Surgical implications. J Thorac Cardiovasc Surg 1987; 93: 36–44.
76. Laneve S, Uesu CT, Taguchi JT. Isolated pulmonary valvular regurgitation. Am J Med Sci 1962; 244 : 446.
77. Shinebourne E, Babu-Narayan S, Carvalho JS. Tetralogy of Fallot: From fetus to adult. Heart 2006; 92: 1353–1359.
78. Wessel HU, Cunningham WJ, Paul MH et al. Exercise performance in Tetralogy of Fallot after intracardiac repair. J Thorac Cardiovasc Surg 1980; 80: 582–593.
79. Carvalho JS, Shinebourne EA, Busst C et al. Exercise capacity after complete repair of Tetralogy of Fallot: deleterious effects of residual pulmonary regurgitation. Br Heart J 1992; 67: 470–473.
80. Redington AN, Oldershaw PJ, Shinebourne EA et al. A new technique for the assessment of pulmonary regurgitation and its application to the assessment of right ventricular function before and after repair of Tetralogy of Fallot. Br Heart J 1988; 60: 57–65.
81. Marie PY, Marcon F, Brunotte F et al. Right ventricular overload and induced sustained ventricular tachycardia in operatively "repaired" Tetralogy of Fallot. Am J Cardiol 1992; 69: 785–789.
82. Gatzoulis MA, Balaji S, Webber SA et al. Risk factors for arrhythmia and sudden cardiac death late after repair of Tetralogy of Fallot: A multicentre study. Lancet 2000; 356: 975–981.
83. Shimazaki Y, Blackstone EH, Kirklin JW. The natural history of isolated congenital pulmonary valve incompetence: Surgical implications. Thorac Cardiovasc Surg 1984; 32: 257–259.
84. Li W, Davlouros PA, Kilner PJ. Doppler-echocardiographic assessment of pulmonary regurgitation in adults with repaired Tetralogy of Fallot: comparison with cardiovascular magnetic resonance imaging. Am Heart J 2004; 147: 165–172.
85. Silversides CK, Veldtman GR, Crossin J. Pressure half-time predicts hemodynamically significant pulmonary regurgitation in adults with repaired Tetralogy of Fallot. J Am Soc Echocardiogr 2003; 16: 1057–1062.
86. Geva T, Sandweiss BM, Gauvreau K. Factors associated with impaired clinical status in long-term survivors of Tetralogy of Fallot repair evaluated by magnetic resonance imaging. J AM Coll Cardiol 2004; 43: 1068–1074.
87. Helbring WA, de Roos A. Optimal imaging in assessment of right ventricular function in Tetralogy of Fallot with pulmonary regurgitation. Am J Cardiol 1998; 82: 1561–1562.
88. Vliegen HW, van Straten A, de Roos A. Magnetic resonance imaging to assess the hemodynamic effects of pulmonary valve replacement in adults late after repair of Tetralogy of Fallot. Circualtion 2002; 106: 1703–1707.
89. Helbring WA, Niezen RA, Le Cessie S. Right ventricular diastolic function in children with pulmonary regurgitation after repair of Tetralogy of Fallot: Volumetric evaluation by magnetic resonance velocity mapping. J Am Coll Cardiol 1996; 28: 1827–1835.
90. Therrien J, Siu SC, Harris L. Impact of pulmonary valve replacement on arrhythmia propensity late after repair of Tetralogy of Fallot. Circulation 2001; 103: 2489–2494.
91. van der Wall E, Mulder B. Pulmonary valve replacement in patients with Tetralogy of Fallot and pulmonary regurgitation: Early surgery similar to optimal timing of surgery. Eur Heart J 2005; 26: 2614–2615.
92. Caldarone CA, McCrindle BW, Van Arsdell GS. Independent factors associated with longevity of prosthetic valves and valved conduits. J Thrac cardiovasc Surg 2000; 120: 1022–1030.
93. Valsangiacomo B, Dave HH, Kellenberger CJ, Dodge-Khatami A, Pretre R, Berger F, Bauersfeld U. Remodeling of the right ventricle after early pulmonary valve replacement in children with repaired Tetralogy of Fallot: Assessment by cardiovascular magnetic resonance. Eur Heart J 2005; 26: 2721–2727.
94. Therrien J, Siu SC, McLaughlin PR. Pulmonary valve replacement in adults late after repair of Tetralogy of Fallot: Are we operating too late? J AM Coll Cardiol 2002; 39: 1664–1669.
95. Khambadkone S, Coats L, Taylor A, Boudjemline Y, Derrick G, Tsang V. Percutaneous pulmonary valve implantation in humans: Results in 59 consecutive patients. Circulation 2005; 112: 1189–1197.
96. Nordmeyer J, Coats L, Bonhoeffer P. Current experience with percutaneous pulmonary valve implantation. Semin Thorac Cardiovasc Surg 2006; 18(2): 122–125.
97. Khambadkone S. Bonhoeffer P. Percutaneous pulmonary valve implantation. Semin Thorac Cardiovasc Surg Pediatr Card Surg Annu 2006;9: 23–8.
98. Schreiber C, Horer J, Vogt M, Fratz S, Kunze M, Galm C, Eicken A, Lange R. A new treatment option for pulmonary valvar insufficiency: first experience with implantation of a self-expanding stented valve without use of cardiopulmonary bypass. Eur J cardiothorac Surg 2007; 31(1): 26–30.

13 Contemporary Considerations in Aortic Valve Surgery

B. Zane Atkins, Neal D. Kon, and G. Chad Hughes

CONTENTS

PREOPERATIVE EVALUATION

The aortic valve must be viewed as a complex of the aorto-ventricular junction, aortic annulus, valve leaflets, aortic root (sinus of Valsalva segment), and the sinotubular junction (Fig. 1). In so doing, surgery for the aortic valve can be approached in a manner similar to that for the mitral valve complex *(1)*, such that the corrective operation may be individually tailored to the patient's underlying disease and anatomy.

Aortic stenosis (AS) is the most common valvular heart lesion affecting adults in the United States and contributes significantly to the more than 40,000 aortic valve replacements (AVR) performed annually in the United States alone *(2, 3)*. Rheumatic heart disease is the main cause of valvular heart disease worldwide, but fewer than 10% of AS cases in the United States and Western Europe are rheumatic *(4)*. In contrast, senile, calcific disease of the aortic valve is responsible for the vast majority of AS cases *(4)*. Since the incidence of AS increases with age and the US population as a whole is aging, increased numbers of patients presenting with AS are expected in the near future *(5)*. Currently, the incidence of AS is estimated to be 1−2% among those over 65 years of age and 4% among octagenarians *(6)*.

The remainder of the non-rheumatic cases of AS are found in the context of congenital bicuspid aortic valve (BAV) disease. BAV is the most common congenital cardiac defect, present in approximately 1−2% of the population *(7)*. BAV may be associated with AS (75%), aortic regurgitation (AR) (15%), or mixed AS/AR (10%) *(8, 9)*. BAV should be considered the likely diagnosis in patients younger than 65 years of age presenting with aortic valve disease *(10)*. Importantly, with a sensitivity of approximately 80%, transthoracic echocardiography may not accurately identify BAV *(11)*. Nevertheless, it is important to recognize BAV since it is an autosomal dominant trait with variable penetrance. Consequently, first-order relatives of affected patients should undergo screening echocardiography *(10)*.

Further, preoperative identification of BAV should prompt consideration of CT or MRI scanning of the chest to rule out ascending aortic dilation, which is frequently seen in association with BAV. In fact,

From: *Contemporary Cardiology: Valvular Heart Disease*
Edited by: Andrew Wang, Thomas M. Bashore, DOI 10.1007/978-1-59745-411-7_13
© Humana Press, a part of Springer Science+Business Media, LLC 2009

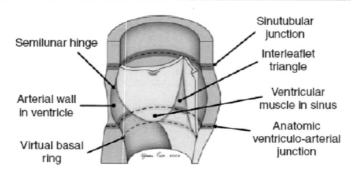

Fig. 1. Anatomy of the aortic valve and root. Note that the aortic root (sinus of Valsalva segment) extends from the anatomic ventriculo-aortic junction to the sinotubular junction (STJ). The tubular ascending aorta then begins at the level of the STJ. The sinus of Valsalva segment is important anatomically as this section of aorta includes the area of attachment of the valve cusps to the aortic wall, the ostia of the left and right coronary arteries, and is the region where eddy currents are formed which promote normal systolic opening as well as diastolic closure of the aortic valve as well as normal coronary blood flow patterns. Reproduced with permission from Asante-Korang A and Anderson RH *(175)*.

more than half of patients with BAV will develop some degree of ascending aortic dilation, even with a normally functioning bicuspid valve *(12)*. Specific pathophysiologic mechanisms leading to ascending aortic dilation in BAV are similar to associated connective tissue disorders of the ascending aorta with histologic abnormalities of the aortic media such as decreased extracellular matrix *(fibrillin 1)*, increased matrix degradation enzymes *(matrix metalloproteinase 2)*, thinner elastic lamellae, increased severity of cystic medial necrosis, elastic fragmentation, and smooth muscle cell reorientation *(13)*. These distinctive pathologic alterations have recently been linked to identifiable genetic mutations including *NOTCH1* missense variants *(14)*. In sum, these abnormalities confer increased fragility of the aortic media predisposing to aneurysm formation and aortic dissection *(15)*. Therefore, as addressed below, one should have a low threshold for concomitant ascending aortic replacement at the time of AVR in patients with BAV.

As noted, BAV can also be an important cause of AR. Other etiologies of AR include endocarditis with perforated or flail aortic valve leaflets, congenital abnormalities such as ventricular septal defect with associated aortic cusp prolapse, aortic root anomalies, most frequently aortic root aneurysm in patients with either congenital (e.g. the Marfan syndrome) or acquired aneurysms of the aortic root, rheumatic disease, and idiopathic causes *(8)*. In addition, patients with aortic aneurysms limited to the tubular ascending aorta above the sinotubular junction frequently have some degree of central AR due to outward displacement of the commissural posts from the dilated ascending aorta and sinotubular junction (STJ) (Fig. 2).

Prior to undertaking operation for aortic valve disease, whether for AR or AS, preoperative left and right heart catheterization is suggested for men over the age of 35, premenopausal women over the age of 35 with risk factors for coronary disease, postmenopausal women *(16)*, and those with evidence of reduced ventricular function *(17)*. Specifically, left heart catheterization is useful to directly measure transvalvular pressure gradients, estimate aortic valve area using the Gorlin formula, as well as to rule out concomitant coronary disease requiring adjunctive bypass surgery and identify any associated coronary anomalies. For example, patients with BAV frequently have a non-dominant right coronary artery, which may have important surgical implications with regard to perioperative right ventricular protection or coronary button reimplantation if aortic root replacement is required. An ascending thoracic aortogram performed at the time of left heart catheterization is useful in patients with aortic valve disease in association with an ascending aneurysm to give additional information with regard to aortic root (sinus of Valsalva segment) diameter and sinotubular junction definition, both of which

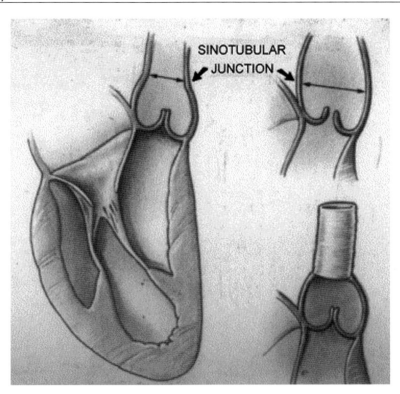

Fig. 2. Aneurysm of the tubular ascending aorta with secondary development of aortic insufficiency (AR). The normal anatomic situation is demonstrated on the *left* and that of a dilated STJ secondary to ascending aortic aneurysm is seen on the *top right*. In the latter case, the typically central AR jet is due to outward distraction of the valve commissures (dilated STJ). If the sinus of Valsalva segment (aortic root) and aortic valve leaflets below the STJ are otherwise relatively normal, the AR can frequently be corrected by replacing the aneurysmal ascending aorta with a properly sized Dacron graft to downsize the STJ to a normal diameter approximately equal to that of the aortic annulus *(bottom right)*. This STJ downsizing properly repositions the commissural posts to improve aortic cusp coaptation. Reproduced with permission from Feindel CM and David TE *(176)*.

are critical in deciding whether or not formal aortic root replacement (button Bentall procedure) is required (Fig. 3). Coronary CT angiography (CTA) may provide an alternative to left heart catheterization, especially in patients felt to be at low risk of having associated CAD *(18)*. CTA, especially with 3-D reconstruction, may also provide useful data with regard to aortic root and ascending aortic dimensions and anatomy.

Right heart catheterization provides important information with regard to left- and right-sided filling pressures as well as cardiac index, all of which help the surgeon and cardiac anesthesiologist anticipate possible issues with perioperative myocardial function, including potential difficulty weaning from cardiopulmonary bypass (CPB) and the need for post-CPB support such as inotropic agents, intra-aortic balloon pump, or inhaled pulmonary vasodilators such as nitric oxide.

Aortic Stenosis

The normal aortic valve area (AVA) in the adult is 3–4 cm^2; this value must be reduced to approximately one-fourth of normal before symptoms occur *(19)*. Patients with AS are frequently asymptomatic at the time of initial clinical presentation, with the diagnosis being suspected secondary to a murmur detected on physical examination. The disease is typically gradually progressive with a long

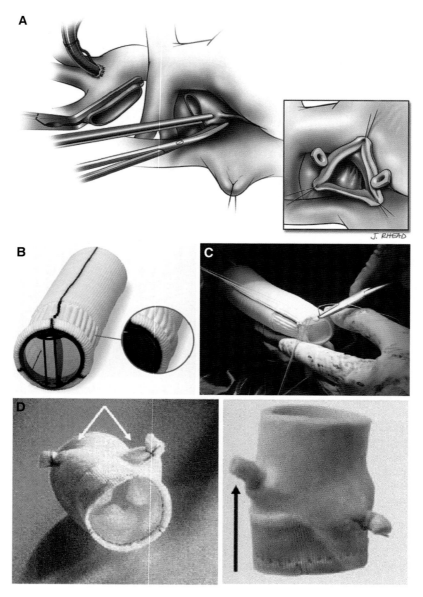

Fig. 3. Aortic root replacement (button Bentall procedure). In this procedure, the aortic valve leaflets as well as the entire aortic root are removed down to the level of the ventriculo-aortic junction (**panel A**). Buttons containing the left and right main coronary arteries are then fashioned for reimplantion (**panel A** *inset*) into a valved conduit, which may contain either a mechanical (**panel B**) or bioprosthetic valve (**panel C**). The bioprosthetic valved conduit shown has been "hand-made" by sewing a bovine pericardial valve into a Dacron graft incorporating premade sinuses of Valsalva (Gelweave Valsalva conduit, Sulzer Vascutek, Refrewshire, Scotland), as this type of bioprosthetic valved conduit is not commercially available. Other options include a stentless full porcine aortic root (**panel D**) or a homograft (not shown). Our preference is to avoid the use of homografts, except in the setting of severe endocarditis with root abscess, due to their limited durability as compared to any of the preceding options. Regardless of the valved conduit chosen, the technique for implantation is similar and the final result is demonstrated in **panel E**. **Panel A** reproduced with permission from Doty JR *(177)*. **Panels B**, **D**, and **E** in public domain.

E

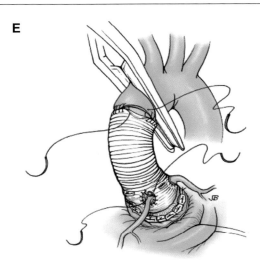

Fig. 3. *(Continued).*

asymptomatic latent period. Obstruction to left ventricular outflow results in left ventricular pressure overload. The physiologic response to this pressure overload includes the development of left ventricular hypertrophy (LVH) in an attempt to normalize wall stress and left ventricular work according to the law of Laplace (wall stress = pressure × radius/2 × wall thickness). The result is a thick-walled, non-compliant chamber with initial diastolic dysfunction and, eventually, systolic dysfunction when the chronic pressure load overcomes left ventricular contractile reserve *(20)*.

LVH is frequently detectable by electrocardiography (ECG); ECG may also reveal signs of left ventricular strain such as inverted T-waves. Development of LVH has been strongly linked with complications of AS including sudden death, neurologic events such as syncope, and congestive heart failure *(21)*. Angina results from an imbalance between the oxygen demands of the hypertrophied left ventricle and reduced coronary blood supply secondary to the transvalvular gradient. As mentioned, excessive afterload (afterload mismatch) often leads to reduced ventricular function and forward cardiac output, in which case the transvalvular gradient may appear low despite the presence of severe AS. This phenomenon has been termed "low-gradient AS," and low-gradient AS has been associated with worse outcomes after AVR compared with typical, high-gradient AS *(22)*.

Echocardiography is the most convenient method to confirm the diagnosis of aortic valvular disorders, including AS. Transvalvular gradients are determined from peak systolic velocity across the aortic valve using the modified Bernoulli equation (pressure gradient = 4 × aortic jet velocity^2). The mean gradient may also be determined echocardiographically from the integral of instantaneous pressure gradients over the systolic ejection period. However, estimation of transvalvular gradients is based on several assumptions, not direct measurements. Therefore, if uncertainty remains as to gradient severity based on echocardiographic findings, direct measurement of gradients at cardiac catheterization should be considered if the findings will affect clinical decision making *(16)*. Finally, estimation of AVA by echocardiography may be performed using the continuity principle. Data such as these derived by echocardiographic means correlate reasonably well with those obtained at cardiac catheterization *(23)*. Cardiovascular MRI has also emerged as an accurate method for evaluating aortic valve area as determined by planimetry, and this technique appears comparable to cardiac catheterization as well *(24, 25)*.

In assessing patients with asymptomatic AS, quantitative exercise Doppler echocardiography may be more useful than exercise ECG or resting echocardiography for predicting those at higher risk for cardiac events (including need for AVR) in the short-term (26). Therefore, this technique may help to determine which asymptomatic AS patients may benefit from earlier AVR. Using exercise Doppler echocardiography, Lancellotti et al. found that independent predictors of cardiac events were an increase in the mean transaortic pressure gradient by more than 18 mmHg during exercise, abnormal exercise testing, and an AVA <0.75 cm^2. In contrast, absolute values for peak or mean transaortic pressure gradients may not always be predictive of adverse events (26).

In those with low gradient/low output AS, some have proposed the use of echocardiography during dobutamine infusion (22, 27) or therapeutic sodium nitroprusside infusion (28) to determine which low-gradient AS patients might benefit from AVR. Monin et al. demonstrated that when LV contractile reserve was present (defined by increased SV of >20% during dobutamine infusion), AVR could be performed safely. However, without LV contractile reserve, AVR was associated with an operative mortality of nearly one-third (22). Similar results have been seen by Quere et al. more recently, who found that patients with contractile reserve on preoperative DSE had an operative mortality of 6% versus 33% if contractile reserve was absent (29). In addition, patients in whom the transvalvular gradient increased during dobutamine infusion were felt more likely to benefit following aortic valve replacement (27). Finally, serum concentrations of B-type natriuretic peptide (BNP) appear to be elevated in cases of low gradient/low output AS with preserved contractility when compared to low gradient/low output AS without preserved contractility (30). In addition, BNP concentrations strongly correlated with survival after AVR in this patient population.

The onset of symptoms marks a turning point in the disease, and once symptoms occur, clinical outcome is very poor without surgical treatment in the BAV population (31) (Fig. 4). Consequently, indications for surgical intervention for severe AS include symptoms such as angina, syncope, or congestive heart failure (16). However, the triad of syncope, dyspnea on exertion, and angina is seen in only about one-third of patients and it appears that any of the symptoms is significant in the more common calcific AS patients. In addition, surgical intervention should be considered in *asymptomatic* patients with moderate-to-severe aortic valve calcification and either an aortic jet velocity greater than 4.0 m/s (32, 33) or a rapid increase in aortic jet velocity (>0.3 m/s/year), as prior work has suggested this may represent a subset of asymptomatic patients at high risk for death or complication due to their disease (32). Furthermore, a small (≤1%) incidence of sudden death in previously asymptomatic AS patients may justify AVR prior to the development of symptoms, especially in good surgical candidates. This latter issue, though, remains contentious (16, 34). Other indications for AVR in asymp-

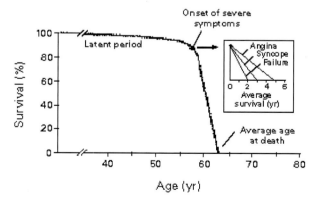

Fig. 4. Natural history curve for unoperated aortic stenosis. A relatively long latent phase with minimal symptoms precedes the development of severe symptoms, which may arise in the form of heart failure, syncope, or angina. With development of these symptoms, survival decreases rapidly if aortic valve replacement is not performed. Reproduced with permission from Carabello BA and Crawford FA (178).

tomatic AS include an abnormal response to exercise testing, extremely severe AS (AV area <0.6 cm^2, mean transvalvular gradient >60 mmHg, and jet velocity >5.0 m/s), extensive aortic valve calcification such that rapid progression of AS and symptoms are expected, and when the expected mortality from AVR is <1% *(16)* (Table 1).

Table 1

Indications for Aortic Valve Replacement for Aortic Stenosis and Aortic Insufficiency, Based on 2006 Guidelines of the ACC/AHA for Management of Patients with Valvular Heart Disease *(17)*. EDD = End-Diastolic Dimension; ESD = End-Systolic Dimension

	Aortic stenosis (AS)	Aortic regurgitation (AR)
Class I (AVR *should* be performed)	– Symptomatic, severe AS (Level B) – Severe AS undergoing CABG, aortic surgery, or other cardiac valvular procedure (Level C) – Severe AS with LV systolic dysfunction (EF <50%, Level C)	– Symptomatic, severe AR (Level B) – Asymptomatic, severe AR with LV systolic dysfunction (EF <50%) at rest (Level B) – Severe AR undergoing CABG, aortic surgery, or other cardiac valvular procedure (Level C)
Class IIa (AVR *is reasonable* to consider)	– Moderate AS undergoing CABG, aortic surgery, or other cardiac valvular procedure (Level B)	– Asymptomatic, severe AR with normal LV function but severe LV dilation (EDD >75 mm or ESD >55 mm, Level B)
Class IIb (AVR *may be* considered)	– Asymptomatic, severe AS, abnormal exercise testing (Level C) – Asymptomatic, severe AS with high likelihood of rapid progression or if AVR may be delayed at symptom onset (Level C) – Mild AS undergoing CABG if high likelihood of progression (Level C) – Asymptomatic, extremely severe AS if predicted operative mortality is ≤1% (Level C)	– Moderate AR undergoing CABG or ascending aortic surgery (Level C) – Asymptomatic, severe AR with normal resting LV function when LV dilation exceeds EDD 70 mm or ESD 50, if progressive LV dilation, worsening exercise tolerance, or abnormal hemodynamic response to exercise (Level C)
Class III (AVR is *not* recommended)	– Asymptomatic AS for the prevention of sudden death (Level B)	– Asymptomatic, mild, moderate, or severe AR with normal LV systolic resting function without moderate or severe LV dilation (Level B)

Aortic Regurgitation

Relative to AS, patients with AR are even more likely to be asymptomatic at diagnosis, reflecting the long latency period between the development of AR and the demonstration of symptoms. When symptoms of AR finally develop, life expectancy is dramatically reduced. The chief symptoms of AR at the time of initial clinical presentation are those of congestive heart failure.

With the prolonged left ventricular volume overload characteristic of AR, eccentric cardiac hypertrophy develops as a compensatory mechanism *(35)*. In addition, reduced coronary blood flow secondary to decreased pulse pressure/diastolic blood pressure contributes to the pathophysiolgy of AR, and global myocardial fibrosis may develop.

As with AS, the examination and echocardiography establish the diagnosis of AR. The severity of AR can be assessed using the vena contracta (VC) of the regurgitant jet. Willett et al. reported that VC obtained with TEE intraoperatively correlated well with aortic flow probe measurements *(36)*. Chin et al. demonstrated that an "aortic regurgitation index," comprised of five echocardiographically derived parameters, provides a more comprehensive assessment of AR severity *(37)*. Finally, an eccentric AR jet should always raise concern about associated aortic cusp pathology *(1)*, which may have important surgical implications.

Indications for surgical intervention for AR include severe regurgitation with symptoms of heart failure, evidence of left ventricular systolic dysfunction, or increasing left ventricular dimensions (Table 1). Since symptoms may be a late finding, any evidence for LV dysfunction should prompt surgical intervention. Recent ACC/AHA guidelines suggest that anytime the echocardiographic LV end-systolic dimension is >5.0 cm or the LV ejection fraction is <55%, then that is case enough to warrant surgical AVR. In cases of aortic valve endocarditis, additional indicators for surgery include heart block, recurrent septic emboli, and failure of medical therapy *(16)*.

Since aortic root pathology often accompanies AR, it is critical to obtain echocardiographic measurements at the level of the aortic annulus, aortic root (sinus of Valsalva segment), sinotubular junction, and tubular ascending aorta (Fig. 5) to assist with surgical planning. This preoperative evaluation will help to ensure that the most appropriate procedure to correct the underlying pathology is planned and performed. For example, echocardiography can help define the severity and mechanisms of AR and lend information regarding the likelihood for valve repair and aortic leaflet preservation in disorders such as Type A aortic dissection *(38)* and annuloaortic ectasia.

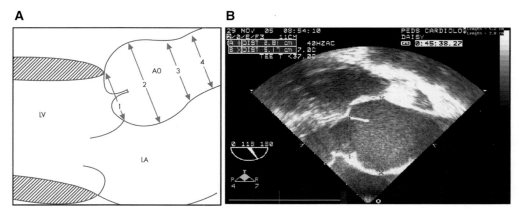

Fig. 5. Aortic root dimensions. Drawing (**A**) demonstrating important aortic root dimensions determined echocardiographically at the level of the annulus (1), sinus of Valsalva segment (2), sinotubular junction (STJ) (3), and tubular ascending aorta (4). Reproduced with permission from Erbel R et al. *(179)*. (**B**) Representative transesophageal echocardiographic image from a patient with the Marfan syndrome and an aortic root aneurysm. Markers indicate measurements taken at level of the aortic annulus and sinus of Valsalva segment.

SURGICAL DECISION MAKING

Aortic Valve Replacement

When planning AVR, the chief issues related to surgical decision making involve the type of valve prosthesis to be inserted, the timing of surgery (see above), and issues related to concomitant procedures. The ideal prosthesis for AVR is characterized by excellent hemodynamics, minimal residual transvalvular pressure gradient, and laminar flow through the prosthesis. In addition, the valvular prosthesis should be durable, easy to implant, quiet, biocompatible, and resistant to thromboembolism *(39)*. Unfortunately, the ideal aortic valvular prosthesis does not presently exist. Thus, patients and physicians must choose among a variety of options, each with their own inherent advantages and disadvantages, which will be outlined in the following section.

The two major categories of valvular prostheses, which account for the vast majority of implanted aortic valves, include mechanical and bioprosthetic valves. Regarding the decision between bioprosthetic and mechanical valves, the primary advantage of mechanical valves is their durability and reliable performance *(40, 41)*. Conversely, the primary disadvantage of mechanical valves relates to the need for lifelong warfarin anticoagulation and attendant lifestyle limitations and thromboembolic (TE) and bleeding risks *(41, 42)*. When anticoagulation is managed appropriately, the risk of TE with mechanical valves is similar to that for bioprosthetic valves *(43)*. Bileaflet mechanical valves are the standard in current practice, with the St. Jude Medical (St. Jude Medical, Inc., St. Paul, MN) prosthesis the modern prototype, having been first implanted in 1977. Most of these valves are constructed using carbon strengthened with silicon carbide additives. Other examples of bileaflet mechanical valves include those manufactured by CarboMedics (Austin, TX); Advancing the Standard Medical (ATS, Minneapolis, MN); Medtronic, Inc. (Minneapolis, MN); and Medical Carbon Research Institute, LLC (MCRI, Austin, TX). Modifications to the standard mechanical valves have been made, primarily involving sewing cuff alteration, as with the SJM high performance (HP) valve, or to the valve housing, as with the SJM Regent valve, such that a larger effective orifice area can be achieved *(40)*. This allows implantation of larger valves with improved hemodynamics and more effective LV mass regression after AVR *(44)*. The On-X® mechanical valve (MCRI) was introduced in Europe in 1996 and differs from other bileaflet mechanical valves in that it is made from pure pyrolytic carbon. The PROACT (Prospective Randomized On-X® Valve Anticoagulation Trial) study is an FDA-approved multicenter trial, sponsored by MCRI, currently enrolling patients to determine whether or not defined patient groups receiving AVR (low versus high risk for TE events) with the On-X® valve may be safely maintained on lower doses of warfarin or, for patients in the low-risk aortic valve arm, on antiplatelet drugs (aspirin plus clopidogrel) alone compared with standard anticoagulation regimens. No single mechanical valve has shown superior patient outcomes, and all demonstrate extremely low rates of structural valve deterioration, the major advantage of mechanical valves.

Conversely, the primary advantage of bioprosthetic valves is that systemic anticoagulation with warfarin is not required. As a result, patients receiving tissue valves have a lower rate of anticoagulation-related bleeding complications *(45)*. However, their limited durability (freedom from structural valve deterioration and need for reoperation) and suboptimal hemodynamics, due to a generally smaller effective orifice area size-for-size as compared to mechanical valves, have historically been the Achilles' heel of bioprosthetic valves. As a result, use of bioprosthetic valves has generally been recommended for patients older than 65 years of age or with reduced life expectancy *(46)*. These tendencies may be changing in light of improved tissue engineering and the increased lifespan of newer generation tissue valves *(45, 47, 48)*. Recently, it has been recognized that metabolic syndromes with hypercholesterolemia are associated with more rapid progression of aortic stenosis *(49)* as well as more rapid deterioration of bioprosthetic valves *(50, 51)*. Consequently, aggressive lipid-lowering strategies, including statin therapy, may deter structural deterioration of bioprosthetic valves and prolong their lifespan *(52)*. Other independent risk factors for bioprosthetic valvular degeneration are female sex, smoking, and diabetes mellitus *(51, 53)*.

Stented bioprosthetic valves, which incorporate a semi-rigid external support structure for the valve leaflets, represent the majority of tissue valves implanted in clinical practice. The external support provides accurate valve mounting, improving ease of implantation. Two types of stented bioprosthetic valves are currently available in the United States: porcine aortic valves, which incorporate chemically stabilized porcine valve leaflets mounted on a stented structure or frame, and bovine pericardial valves. The leaflets of the latter valve type are constructed from bovine pericardium and subsequently mounted on a stented frame. Available porcine valves include the Medtronic Mosaic valve

(Medtronic Inc., Minneapolis, MN), the St. Jude Medical Biocor and Biocor Supra valves (St. Jude Medical, Inc., St. Paul, MN), and the Carbomedics Mitroflow valve (Carbomedics, Inc., Austin, TX). Bovine pericardial valves include the Carpentier–Edwards (C–E) Perimount (Edward Lifesciences, Irvine, CA) and the CE Perimount Magna valves as well as the Sorin Soprano (Sorin Group, Saluggia, Italy) valves. At present, based on the best available data, no one bioprosthetic valve appears superior with regard to patient outcomes and none requires systemic anticoagulation with warfarin, which is their major advantage. Their major disadvantage is the incidence of structural valve deterioration and subsequent need for reoperation, although the lifespan of the latest generation of tissue valves is unknown.

Physicians involved in educating patients regarding the choice of bioprosthetic versus mechanical aortic valve prostheses should be familiar with several important studies. Peterseim et al. compared 841 patients who underwent first-time AVR. The C–E bovine pericardial valve was used in 429 patients and the SJM bileaflet tilting disc valve in 412 patients (46). Importantly, 10-year survival was not affected by the choice of prosthesis. Further, there was no difference in TE event rates or endocarditis at 10 years, although the risk of major bleeding events was higher with mechanical AVR. The need for reoperation was significantly higher with bioprosthetic valves in patients ≤65 years of age at the time of AVR, although there was no difference in reoperation rates at 10 years in patients >65 years of age. Further, patients of any age with renal disease, coronary artery disease, or an ejection fraction <40%, as well as patients with lung disease over the age of 60 years, rarely required reoperation due to poor 10-year survival and thus bioprosthetic valves were recommended in these patients as well (45) (Fig. 6). Results similar to those reported by Peterseim et al. have been noted by others (54–56). For instance, the Department of Veterans Affairs randomized study of bioprosthetic versus mechanical heart valves made their final report with 15-year follow-up in 2000. All-cause mortality and reoperative rates were lower following mechanical AVR. Primary valve failure rate did not differ between prostheses in patients ≥ 65 years of age. Bleeding risk was lower with bioprostheses, although other valve-related complications were similar (55).

	Ten-year survival (%)	Actual 10-year freedom from reoperation on CE aortic valve (%)
Renal disease, any age	27 ± 8	100 ± 0
Lung disease (patient older than 60 y)	30 ± 6	96 ± 2
Ejection fraction < 40%, any age	35 ± 6	95 ± 2
Coronary artery disease, any age	35 ± 5	98 ± 0.8
Age > 65 y	41 ± 4	98 ± 0.7

Fig. 6. Ten-year survival and actual freedom from reoperation following bioprosthetic aortic valve replacement in certain high-risk subsets. The data suggest implantation of bioprosthetic aortic valves should be strongly considered for all patients >65 years of age, patients >60 years of age with pulmonary disease, as well as for patients of any age with renal disease, coronary artery disease, or an ejection fraction <40% due to poor 10-year survival and infrequent need for reoperation in these subgroups due to their comorbid conditions. Reproduced with permission from Peterseim DS et al. (46).

The decision between tissue and mechanical valve should be made by the patient with educated input regarding the pros and cons of each option from the patient's physicians. We do not hesitate to implant tissue valves in younger patients who wish to avoid anticoagulation due to lifestyle concerns (e.g. young, active individual, desire to become pregnant, etc.), although we generally will guide patients toward a mechanical option at the time of redo-AVR if their life expectancy exceeds 10–15 years at that time. The latter is especially true if the patient will require aortic root replacement (button Bentall procedure) as their second operation, given the difficulty of redo-root replacement. This is supported by data from Lau et al., who recently reported a survival advantage for those patients receiving a mechanical prosthesis at the time of redo-AVR as compared to those receiving another biologic valve *(57)*. An algorithm to assist physicians and patients with the choice of valve is presented in Fig. 7.

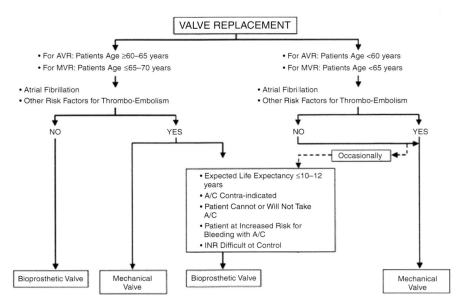

Fig. 7. Algorithm to assist with the decision between bioprosthetic and mechanical AVR. These recommendations are not absolute, and the ultimate decision rests with the patient with educated physician input. Reproduced with permission from Rahimtoola SH *(180)*.

The hemodynamic results with all aortic valve prostheses, mechanical or bioprosthetic, are affected by the effective orifice area (EOA) of the implanted valve. The EOA represents the area available for blood flow through the valve and generally increases with increasing valve size. When the EOA of the implanted valve is too small relative to the body surface area (BSA) of the patient, patient–prosthesis mismatch (PPM), a concept originally introduced by Rahimtoola *(58)*, is considered to exist. When PPM is present, the postoperative transvalvular gradient remains high and may even approach levels seen with severe AS. Persistent transvalvular gradients are associated with increased LV work requirements, failure of LV mass regression, and persistent symptoms of AS. PPM is considered severe if the prosthetic valvular effective orifice area indexed to the patient's body surface area (EOAI) is ≤ 0.65 cm^2/m^2; moderate if EOAI is ≤ 0.85 cm^2/m^2 but ≥ 0.65 cm^2/m^2; and absent if the EOAI is ≥ 0.85 cm^2/m^2 *(59)*. Although some have disputed the importance of PPM *(60)*, most now agree that PPM adversely affects patient outcomes after AVR *(59, 61, 62)*.

Due to concerns over PPM, stentless bioprosthetic valves, which generally have a larger EOA size-for-size compared with mechanical or stented bioprosthetic valves, have been increasingly utilized for AVR. In initial evaluation, stentless valves had better hemodynamics and improved survival rates relative to stented biological or mechanical valves and were more durable than stented biological valves *(63)*. Stentless valves may be preferred in patients with a small aortic root, and arguments have been made that wider utilization of stentless valves may minimize PPM *(64)*. Stentless valves also appear to have better hemodynamic profiles than stented valves during exercise testing *(65)*. Technical reasons for not implanting stentless valves include extensive aortic root calcification, coronary ostia opposed by 180, presence of the two coronary ostia in close proximity, or unusual disproportion between the sinotubular junction and the aortic annulus *(21)*. Whereas stented valves allow perfect valve mounting within the aortic annulus, thus reducing the risk of implanting an incompetent valve, postoperative AR and limited durability remain a concern with the free-hand stentless valve insertion technique. This issue may be circumvented with full aortic root replacement using a stentless porcine root *(39)* (Fig. 3C).

Recent evidence also suggests that stentless biological valves may have better coronary flow reserve compared to stented valves *(66)*. Additionally, compared with stented bovine pericardial valves, stentless valves have been associated with increased transvalvular EOA and decreased pressure gradients during extended follow-up *(67)*. However, as seen in other studies, LV mass regression after stentless valve implantation was not different from stented aortic bioprostheses *(67)*. The ASSERT (Aortic Stentless versus Stented valve assessed by Echocardiography Randomized Trial) randomized patients with severe AS with an aortic annular diameter ≤25 mm and no other contraindications to stentless valve implantation to receive either a stentless valve or a stented bioprosthetic valve *(21)*. In this study, LV mass index fell significantly in both groups at 6 and 12 months relative to baseline, but no differences in LV mass were found between the groups at either time point. Further, there were no differences in clinical outcomes *(21)*. Similar findings have been reported by others *(68–70)*.

At the present time, there is no clear evidence that stentless valves are superior to stented bioprosthetic valves, and thus the decision regarding the type of bioprosthetic valve should mainly depend on surgeon preference and experience. This is especially true now that supra-annular expanded EOA stented bioprostheses are available that offer acceptable gradients even in small sizes. However, the duration of long-term follow-up with stentless bioprostheses is not as extensive as for stented valves, and there is no guarantee that long-term durability will be similar to stented bioprostheses.

Concomitant Procedures with AVR

Concomitant AVR may be advisable among patients presenting for coronary artery bypass grafting who are also determined to have aortic valve disease. In asymptomatic patients with mild-to-moderate AS or AR, AVR at the time of coronary surgery avoids future aortic valve surgery *(71)*. Using the Society of Thoracic Surgeons database, Smith et al. further defined those patients undergoing CABG who might benefit from concomitant AVR for mild-to-moderate AS based on patient-specific factors including age, peak transvalvular gradient, and the rate of progression of the transvalvular gradient *(72)* (Fig. 8). Other studies have suggested that mild aortic valve disease can be safely observed based on information that reoperative AVR can be performed fairly safely in this context *(73)*. Given the choice of mechanical versus bioprosthetic AVR and concomitant CABG, mechanical AVR may be associated with worse long-term survival and more valve-related complications, likely due to anticoagulation-related difficulties *(74)*. In addition, as mentioned previously, data from our own institution suggest that a minority of patients with significant CAD will actually outlive a tissue valve *(46)*. To summarize, it is recommended that patients with moderate-to-severe AS or severe AR, regardless of symptoms, who are undergoing CABG should also undergo AVR *(16)*. In addition, patients with mild-to-moderate AS should undergo AVR if they meet the criteria outlined by Smith et al. *(72)* (Fig. 8). Finally, patients with moderate AR should be considered for AVR if undergoing concomitant CABG *(16)* (Table 1).

When mitral valve regurgitation (MR) accompanies aortic valve disease, the decision must be made as to whether or not the mitral valve requires surgical intervention as well. Vanden Eynden et al. recently evaluated the effect of AVR for AS on moderate-to-severe MR and found that the primary predictor of persistent MR postoperatively was the underlying pathology of the mitral valve *(75)*.

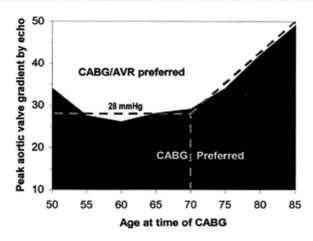

Fig. 8. Decision analysis approach to concomitant AVR in patients with mild-to-moderate aortic stenosis undergoing CABG. Using this model, concomitant AVR is preferred in patients of all ages undergoing CABG with peak gradient >50 mmHg and in patients <70 years of age with peak gradient of 25−30 mmHg. However, for older patients, competing mortalities increase the gradient threshold by 1−2 mmHg/year. Reproduced with permission from Smith WT IV *(72)*.

Specifically, significant MR due to rheumatic or myxomatous valve disorders were unlikely to improve after AVR, while those with degenerative (e.g., dilated mitral annulus) or ischemic mitral disorders might improve after AVR. Ruel et al. also examined which patients with double valve disease were at increased risk for postoperative morbidity due to persistent MR after AVR *(76)*. Patients with AS and peak aortic gradient <60 mmHg, MR >2+, and a left atrial diameter >5 cm had increased rates of CHF and persistent MR after AVR. Patients with AR and LV end-systolic diameter <45 mm predicted an increased risk of CHF and persistent MR after AVR. Similarly, Barreiro et al. found that moderate MR was an independent risk factor impacting long-term survival when the mitral disorder was not addressed at the time of AVR *(77)*.

Patients with preoperative atrial fibrillation undergoing AVR should be considered for concomitant atrial ablation procedure to include, at a minimum, pulmonary vein isolation and left atrial appendage resection. The Mayo Clinic group has shown that preoperative atrial fibrillation is associated with worse outcomes after AVR compared to a well-matched cohort in normal sinus rhythm *(78)*. This strategy has been shown to be effective in reducing the thromboembolic complications of atrial fibrillation after AVR *(79)*.

Aortic Valve Repair

Aortic valve-sparing techniques were introduced by Wolfe in 1980 for ascending aortic dissection *(80)* and by David et al. in 1992 for ascending aortic aneurysm with associated deformation of the aortic annulus, aortic leaflet malalignment, and AR *(81)*. These valve-sparing approaches rivaled the gold-standard Bentall procedure, which historically involved AVR with a mechanical valved conduit and required lifelong anticoagulation *(82)*. Since these early descriptions, aortic valve-sparing procedures have gained in popularity, allowing patients to avoid mechanical or biologic prostheses and associated issues of anticoagulation therapy, TE phenomena, or structural valve deterioration *(1)*. Consequently, the indications for aortic valve-sparing operations on the aortic root, as well as operations aimed at repair of the aortic valve leaflets themselves, have expanded to include selected patients with bicuspid aortic valves, aortic cusp prolapse, and the Marfan syndrome, among others. These operations have also been applied to a broader age range of patients (83).

In terms of the techniques for aortic valve-sparing root replacement, available options include either the remodeling (Fig. 9) or reimplantation technique (84) (Fig. 10). The reimplantation technique is now preferred by most surgeons performing these procedures due to lower rates of postoperative bleeding and better stabilization of the aortic annulus, since the graft is telescoped outside the annulus (Fig. 10). This maneuver reinforces the annulus and prevents late annular dilation. Consequently, the risk of late AR development appears less with the reimplantation technique. This is especially important in patients with the Marfan syndrome, who are prone to continued annular dilation if the remodeling technique is used (85).

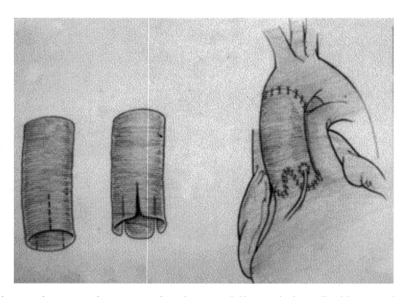

Fig. 9. Valve-sparing aortic root replacement using the remodeling technique. In this procedure, the entire aorta of the sinus of Valsalva segment (aortic root) is removed leaving a rim of aorta of approximately 4—5 mm in width around the valve and commissures. Coronary buttons are fashioned as in a traditional button Bentall procedure. A Dacron graft is then anastomosed to the residual aorta and the coronary buttons re-implanted, thus removing the entire aneurysmal aorta, yet preserving the native aortic valve. Perioperative bleeding complications are increased with this procedure as compared to the reimplantation technique and late annular dilation and recurrent AR have been problematic, making this procedure less favored by the majority of surgeons now performing valve-sparing root replacement. Reproduced with permission from Feindel CM and David TE (176).

In cases of isolated aortic valve cusp prolapse, techniques for correction include free edge plication or reinforcement, triangular resection, or resuspension with PTFE (86). These procedures are often associated with aortic valve annuloplasty for the normal aortic root or with a valve-sparing root operation if the root is dilated (86). In fact, external aortic prosthetic annuloplasty has been shown to improve the reproducibility of aortic root remodeling procedures (87). Techniques for correcting AR associated with BAV include resection of the median raphe or leaflet plication, subcommissural annuloplasty, reinforcement of the leaflet free edge, and sinotubular junction plication (88). Due to the strong association of BAV with proximal aortic dilation, aortic root procedures are also commonly required (88). In the context of BAV, there is increased movement for concomitant ascending aortic or aortic root replacement when the ascending aortic diameter is ≥4.5 cm (Fig. 11) (89, 90).

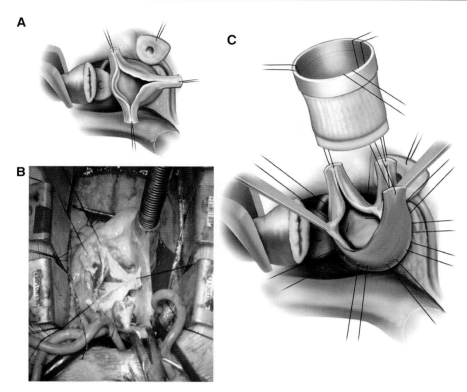

Fig. 10. Valve-sparing aortic root replacement. Valve-sparing aortic root replacement using the modified T. David-V reimplantation technique with the Gelweave Valsalva conduit (Sulzer Vascutek, Refrewshire, Scotland), which incorporates premade sinuses of Valsalva into the Dacron graft. (Drawing **panel A** and intraoperative photo **panel B**) As with the remodeling technique, the entire aorta of the sinus of Valsalva segment (aortic root) is removed leaving a rim of aorta approximately 4–5 mm in width around the valve and commissures. Coronary buttons are fashioned as in a traditional button Bentall procedure. (**Panel C**) Next, sutures are placed from inside to out in the LVOT below the level of the spared aortic valve. These sutures then are used to anchor an appropriately sized Dacron graft, which will function as the new aortic root. Because this graft is telescoped down outside the residual aorta and annulus, it serves to reinforce the annulus, thus preventing the late annular dilation which has proven problematic with the remodeling technique. As mentioned, in the example demonstrated, the graft has prefashioned sinuses of Valsalva, although one can also create neo-sinuses utilizing a standard straight Dacron graft. (**Panel D**) A second suture line is then run along the rim of retained aorta, suturing it to the Dacron graft after the commissural posts have been re-suspended to the appropriate height. This second suture line represents the hemostatic suture line of the repair. The preserved aortic valve (intraoperative photo **panel E**) is competent, holding a column of water (intraoperative photo **panel F**). Finally, the coronary buttons are re-implanted into the graft as in a standard button Bentall procedure (intraoperative photo panel G), followed by the distal anastomosis of the graft to the tubular ascending aorta to complete the repair (**panel H**). Reproduced with permission from Hughes GC et al. *(181)*.

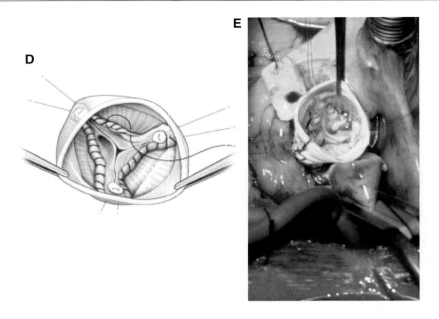

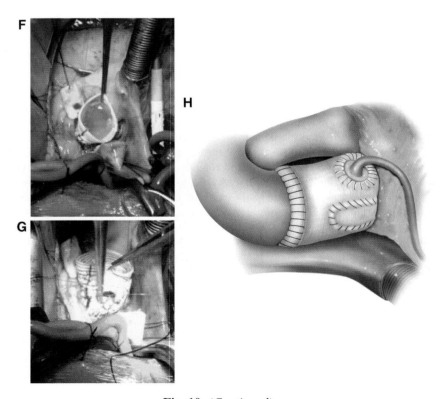

Fig. 10. *(Continued).*

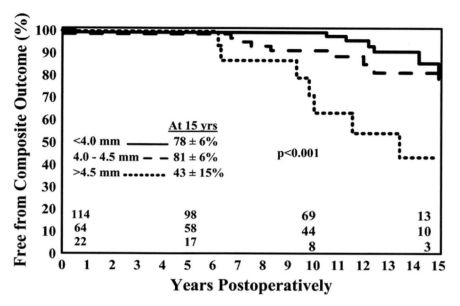

Fig. 11. Prophylactic aortic root replacement. Data supporting prophylactic ascending aortic replacement at the time of AVR for patients with bicuspid aortic valve (BAV) and ascending aortic diameter ≥ 4.5 cm. This study retrospectively examined $n = 201$ patients with BAV undergoing isolated AVR and found that freedom from complications relating to the ascending aorta or need for reoperation for ascending aortic replacement was only 43% at 15 years in those with an ascending aortic diameter ≥ 4.5 cm at the time of surgery. Consequently, concomitant ascending aortic replacement in patients with BAV undergoing AVR is recommended at this diameter. Reproduced with permission from Borger MA et al. *(182)*.

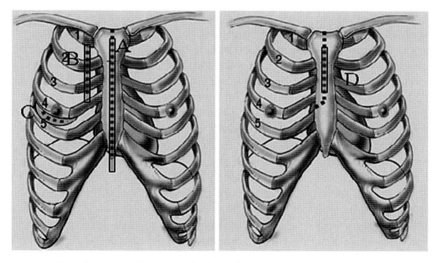

Fig. 12. Surgical approaches. These include standard median sternotomy (**A**), right parasternal incision (**B**), right anterior mini-thoracotomy (**C**), and partial upper sternotomy (**D**). Reproduced with permission from Kim BS et al. *(183)*.

TECHNICAL ASPECTS AND CONSIDERATIONS DURING SURGERY
Incision

Similar outcomes have been noted for full median sternotomy compared with partial upper sternotomy *(91)*, with some demonstrated advantages for lesser incisions *(92, 93)* (Fig. 12). Intraoperative TEE is critical when minimized incisions are planned, as this modality helps to ensure accurate placement of cannulae and other support devices *(94)*. Routine use of carbon dioxide insufflation of the operative field is considered important when smaller incisions are used to reduce problems with de-airing the heart upon completion of the operation *(95)*.

Regardless of the incision utilized, the aorta and right atrium are cannulated for cardiopulmonary bypass after access to the heart is obtained. If concomitant mitral valve surgery is planned, dual venous cannulation is preferred. A cardioplegia needle is inserted in the aortic root for delivery of antegrade cardioplegia, and a retrograde cardioplegia catheter is usually introduced through the right atrium into the coronary sinus. Cold blood cardioplegia has been associated with less ischemic stress and myocardial injury than warm blood cardioplegia in patients undergoing AVR *(96)*. Similar degrees of myocardial injury/protection have been noted whether antegrade or retrograde cardioplegia is given during AVR *(97)*, but retrograde cardioplegia may aid in reducing aortic cross-clamp time by allowing a more efficient flow of the operation, particularly when concomitant procedures are performed *(98, 99)*. Additionally, combined antegrade and retrograde cold blood cardioplegia provides better myocardial protection during AVR than cold crystalloid cardioplegia or continuous, retrograde warm blood cardioplegia *(100)*. Finally, among patients with ischemic heart disease, postoperative morbidity is reduced when a strategy of combined antegrade and retrograde cold blood cardioplegia is used instead of antegrade crystalloid cardioplegia *(101)*.

Prior to systemic cooling, a left ventricular vent is placed via the right superior pulmonary vein in order to prevent distension of the LV during delivery of cardioplegia or with the development of ventricular fibrillation, particularly if AR is prominent. Moderate systemic hypothermia is recommended, generally cooling to 28–30 C *(102)*. The aorta is then cross-clamped and antegrade cardioplegia given down the aortic root, provided the degree of AR is not excessive. In cases of severe AR, arrest may not be achievable with antegrade cardioplegia, and retrograde delivery of cardioplegia may be required. However, if retrograde cardioplegia is unable to induce cardiac arrest, aortotomy should be performed expeditiously, especially with LV distension, and additional cold blood cardioplegia then given down the individual coronary ostia. We prefer to monitor myocardial temperature via a temperature probe in the septum and administer cardioplegia until a septal temperature $<10°C$ has been achieved. Continuous cold blood can be administered via the coronary sinus to help maintain myocardial cooling between doses of cardioplegia during the procedure.

Once adequate arrest has been achieved, the aortic valve is inspected. When replacement is being performed, the aortic valve leaflets are excised, taking care to preserve the structural integrity of the aortic annulus. Calcium deposits must be carefully and thoroughly debrided, but overly aggressive manipulation in the area of the right non-coronary commisure is cautioned to avoid injury to the His bundle and risk of postoperative heart block *(103)*.

Recent evidence suggests that insertion of the aortic valve prosthesis in the supra-annular position may have advantages with regard to postoperative transvalvular gradients and other indices of hemodynamic performance relative to an intra-annular prosthesis *(104)*. However, these results may reflect inherent advantages of the bovine pericardial valve construct, since the CE Perimount valve showed better hemodynamics when inserted in the intra-annular position compared with the intra-annular porcine Mosaic valve. In vitro studies have also corroborated the better hemodynamics of pericardial valves *(105)*. In addition, supra-annular positioning of the valve generally allows placement of a larger prosthesis than is possible in the intra-annular position. However, with supra-annular valve placement, one must be cognizant of occlusion of either coronary ostium by the valve prosthesis, especially if the ostia have a particularly low takeoff within the sinus of Valsalva segment. Regardless, we find this technique quite useful in the patient with a small aortic annulus.

When concomitant coronary artery surgery is planned, the distal coronary artery anastomoses are performed prior to addressing the aortic valve. Once the distal coronary anastomoses are completed, attention is turned to the aortic valve. After AVR completion and closure of the aortotomy, the proximal vein graft anastomoses are performed where applicable. These are often done under a single cross-clamp, as this has been associated with improved neurologic outcomes (106).

Stentless valve insertion as a complete aortic root has been described (107) (Fig. 3C). Insertion of a stentless full root should be performed using an oversizing technique, whereby a valve one size larger than the diameter of the aortic annulus is chosen (107, 108). Problems with insertion of a stentless full root can arise with regard to coronary reimplantation and subsequent coronary insufficiency. These difficulties occasionally arise due to differences in the angle of orientation of the pig coronary arteries on the porcine root and the human coronary arteries. This may be especially problematic in patients with "true" bicuspid aortic valves and 180° opposite coronary ostia. When performing full stentless porcine root replacement, it is crucial to line up the left coronary artery with that of the porcine root, and if the RCA does not line up well, a RSVG bypass to the RCA should be performed (39). Alternatively, the porcine root may be rotated such that the human left coronary artery is anastomosed to the porcine right coronary and the human right coronary attached to the non-coronary sinus of the pig root.

If the aortic valve is being spared during supracoronary ascending aortic replacement, it is important to downsize the STJ to a diameter similar to the native aortic annulus so as to bring the commissural posts back into their normal position; this will generally restore aortic valve competence by increasing leaflet coaptation if the valve and root are otherwise normal (109). However, if the root (sinus of Valsalva segment) is significantly dilated, a formal valve-sparing root replacement (Fig. 11) will better correct the underlying pathology if the valve is otherwise suitable for preservation.

SURGICAL OUTCOMES

Following AVR for AS, one can expect resolution of symptoms, LVH regression, and improved LV systolic function secondary to reduced afterload (110). Importantly, postoperative survival is similar to age-matched controls after AVR for AS when performed prior to the development of LV dysfunction or CHF (111). Similarly, incomplete regression of LVH after AVR has been associated with adverse outcomes such as reduced long-term survival (112, 113). Contrary to the immediate improvement in systolic performance, diastolic dysfunction may persist for several more years after AVR (114). In fact, Gjertsson et al. recently evaluated diastolic dysfunction in AS and found that the proportion of patients with moderate-to-severe diastolic dysfunction actually increased with time after AVR despite normalization of LV mass and appropriate adjustments for senile diastolic dysfunction (115). Finally, AVR is associated with improved quality of life scores, particularly among the elderly, and has been found to be similar to age-matched individuals without heart disease (116, 117).

Following AVR for severe AR, results are chiefly dependent upon preoperative LV function, although severity of symptoms is also important (118). Patients with AR and LV dysfunction can expect reversal of dysfunction after AVR provided the dysfunction is not chronic, i.e., longer than 15 months (119). Conversely, when LV dysfunction has been present for an extended period of time, when the EF is <40%, and when end-systolic LV diameter is greater than 50 mm, the risk of postoperative heart failure is increased substantially, especially in patients older than 50 years of age (16, 120, 121). Those with evidence for LV dilation and heart failure preoperatively, even if severe, can still successfully undergo AVR as the management of CHF will be facilitated by removing the chronic volume overload (16). Finally, despite increased operative risk, patients with AR and severe left ventricular dysfunction can expect significant long-term survival (122, 123).

Reported 30-day mortality rates for isolated AVR in low-risk patients are as low as 1% *(124)*, whereas overall mortality rates for isolated AVR range from 2 to 6% *(125–133)*. Female patients generally have higher unadjusted mortality and cardiac morbidity than males following isolated AVR *(127, 129, 134, 135)*. Given the aging of the population as a whole, attention has been paid recently to the effects of AVR on more elderly patients, especially those older than 80 years of age. Several studies have documented significantly higher 30-day mortality rates (8–10%) among patients of more advanced age undergoing elective, isolated AVR *(116, 127, 136, 137)*. Identified risks for increased mortality among the elderly are small body surface area, longer duration of cardiopulmonary bypass, postoperative renal failure, postoperative stroke, and need for IABP *(137, 138)*.

Several studies have evaluated independent risk factors for operative mortality after AVR (Table 2) *(127–132)*. Five variables predictive of increased mortality risk after AVR are common to each of these analyses: preoperative renal failure, urgency of AVR, preoperative heart failure, presence of CAD or recent MI, and redo cardiac operation. Other factors independently associated with operative mortality from the individual studies include preoperative atrial fibrillation, active endocarditis, preoperative stroke, advanced age, lower body surface area, multiple valve procedures, and hypertension *(127–132)*. Lastly, data from two of these analyses have been used to formulate risk stratification models for AVR based on simple scoring systems *(130, 132)*. These models have been subsequently and independently validated to accurately predict operative mortality for individuals undergoing AVR *(139)*.

Table 2
Synopsis of Individual Studies Assessing Operative Mortality Risk Associated with Aortic Valve Replacement

Study	Years	No. of patients	Identified risk factors	Comments
Maganti et al. *(127)*	1990–2003	2,255	Renal failure Urgent AVR Stroke Heart failure Previous cardiac surgery Hypertension Small aortic valve	Single center (Toronto)
Kuduvalli et al. *(125)*	1997–2004	4,550	Age >70 years Renal failure NYHA class IV Hypertension Atrial fibrillation EF <30% Previous cardiac surgery Non-elective AVR Cardiogenic shock Concomitant CABG	NWQIP in Cardiac Intervention database (UK)
Edwards et al. *(128)*	1994–1997	49,073	Emergency/salvage AVR Recent MI Previous cardiac surgery Renal failure Endocarditis Preoperative IABP	STS database

Table 2
(Continued)

Study	Years	No. of patients	Identified risk factors	Comments
Nowicki et al. *(129)*	1991–2001	5,793	Advanced age Lower BSA Previous cardiac surgery Increased creatinine Previous stroke NYHA class IV Heart failure Atrial fibrillation Urgent AVR Coronary artery disease	Northern New England Cardiovascular Disease Study Group
Rankin et al. *(124)*	1993–2004	409,904	Urgent AVR Age >70 years Previous cardiac surgery Coronary artery disease Endocarditis	STS database
Astor et al. *(126)*	1994	46,397	Advanced age Female sex Renal failure Stroke Heart failure Previous cardiac surgery Coronary artery disease	National Inpatient Sample (AHRQ)

Complications

Complications occurring after AVR are similar in scope and frequency to those seen after other cardiac surgery procedures. Recently reported rates of common complications after AVR include atrial fibrillation 25–35%; cardiac failure 1–4%; respiratory failure 5–8%; neurologic events 2.5–5.5%; renal dysfunction 1.2–7%; infection 2.5–4.6%; and overall morbidity 7.9% *(127, 134, 140)*.

One complication more specific to valvular heart surgery, including AVR, is that of heart block requiring permanent pacemaker. This has been reported to occur in 3–5% of cases *(141–143)*. Risk factors for this complication have been assessed and include heavy annular calcification, bicuspid aortic valve, female sex, and longer perfusion times *(141, 142)*. By multivariate analysis, Limongelli et al. found that AR, preoperative MI, baseline pulmonary hypertension, and postoperative electrolyte imbalance were all independently associated with heart block and the need for pacemaker *(143)*. Other identified risks for need for permanent pacing include preexisting bundle branch block, prior valve surgery, and multiple valve surgery, particularly when the tricuspid valve is involved *(144)*. The size and type of aortic valve prosthesis does not appear to influence need for PPM after AVR with a stented prosthesis *(142)*, but stentless valves may be associated with reduced need for PPM compared with stented valves *(145)*.

The low cardiac output syndrome (LCOS) is another complication after AVR that bears special mention. Maganti et al. recently reported a series of over 2,200 patients who underwent isolated AVR between 1990 and 2003. LCOS was defined as hemodynamic instability requiring inotropic support for ≥30 min postoperatively or intra-aortic balloon pump therapy. This was seen in 3.9% of study patients *(130)*. Independent predictors for LCOS included preoperative renal insufficiency, earlier year of AVR, EF less than 40%, preoperative cardiogenic shock, female gender, and increasing age *(130)*. Not surprisingly, LCOS was associated with significantly higher rates of other complications (MI, stroke, postoperative renal failure, bleeding) and postoperative mortality compared with patients from the same cohort who did not experience LCOS *(130)*. Using similar definitions and study design, Vanky et al. evaluated LCOS after AVR for AS *(146)*. By multivariate analysis, independent risks for LCOS included preoperative hemodynamic instability, hypertension, CHF, LV dysfunction, pulmonary hypertension, prolonged aortic cross-clamp times, and intraoperative MI (146).

Patients undergoing AVR for low-gradient aortic stenosis (LGAS) require careful consideration prior to any decision to proceed with surgical intervention, as mentioned previously. These patients have reduced ejection fraction and, thus, transvalvular gradient is felt to underestimate the severity of AS. Operative mortality in this subset is higher than reported for patients with higher transvalvular gradients despite reduced left ventricular systolic function. For example, the Mayo Clinic reported a 21% 30-day mortality rate in a group of 52 low gradient/low output AS patients undergoing AVR *(147)*. Mortality rates were higher in patients receiving smaller prostheses, suggesting PPM may be particularly important in this high-risk subset, as has been corroborated more recently *(148)*. However, for patients surviving the procedure, the vast majority experienced significant improvements in their NYHA class as well as ejection fraction, suggesting these patients should not be denied AVR given the potential clinical benefit.

Results of AVR with Mechanical Prostheses

Several long-term reports are available to document the results of AVR with mechanical prostheses *(40, 41, 149–151)*. Emery et al. reported 25-year follow-up with the St. Jude Medical bileaflet prosthesis for 2,982 isolated AVR cases *(40)*. Follow-up was complete in 95%, with a mean of 7 ± 5 years (range 1 month to 24.8 years). At 10 years, freedom from valve-related mortality was 93%; freedom from reoperation was 98%; freedom from TE events was 86%; freedom from bleeding events was 81%; freedom from endocarditis was 99%; and freedom from valve thrombosis was 99% *(40)*. No cases of structural failure occurred with the SJM valve in the aortic position. Causes of valve-related mortality included neurologic events from bleeding or TE phenomena, other bleeding complications, and endocarditis. Although valve-related deaths are most frequent in the first 3 months after mechanical AVR *(133)*, sudden, unexplained death was the most frequent cause of death attributed to valve-related causes in the Emery study, as per the published guidelines regarding heart valve reporting *(152)*. Hence, an overestimation of valve-related mortality in this study is possible. Very similar data were reported by Ikonomidis et al., who also reported a 20-year experience with the SJM valve *(41)*, as well as by other groups reporting on different mechanical aortic valve prostheses *(149–151)*.

In light of observations that much of the morbidity and mortality of AVR is related to anticoagulation, suggestions for safer institution of anticoagulation have been put forth. For instance, home INR monitoring appears to reduce the complications of warfarin anticoagulation *(43)*. Furthermore, by slowly bringing INR levels into the therapeutic range, early hemorrhagic complications are reduced *(41)*. Finally, several have noted that TE risk increases steadily after mechanical AVR, and this is often associated with "patient-related factors," including various comorbidities *(40, 54, 153)*.

Results of AVR with Bioprostheses

Glower et al. reported results with the C–E porcine valve at 15 years, including 531 AVR *(154)*. Mean age at AVR was 63 ± 13 years. Actuarial freedom from reoperation at 15 years was 48% ± 6%, whereas *actual* freedom from reoperation at 15 years was 86% ± 2%. This is the preferred analysis since some patients inevitably died without valve degeneration necessitating reoperation *(155)*. Freedom from TE at 15 years was 77% ± 4%; from hemorrhage 95% ± 2%; and from endocarditis 94% ± 1% *(154)*. More recently, Jamieson et al. reported 20-year data for the C–E supra-annular porcine aortic bioprosthesis, which included an 86.4% ± 1.2% freedom from structural valve deterioration at 18 years and an 85.0% ± 1.2% freedom from reoperation at 18 years *(156)*. Similar data are available for other types of pericardial and porcine bioprostheses, although, for these newer prostheses, follow-up has not reached that of the aforementioned studies *(46, 47, 157–159)*.

Results of AVR with Concomitant Cardiac Surgery Procedures

Kobayashi et al. recently reviewed the results for AVR/CABG and found that emergency procedures, EF <30%, age >65 years, obstructive pulmonary disease, and NYHA class III/IV were predictive of mortality. Interestingly, severity of coronary disease and the number of bypass grafts performed did not affect survival *(160)*. Similar observations have been previously made *(161, 162)*. In contrast, grafting the left anterior descending (LAD) coronary artery with the internal mammary artery (IMA) confers a survival benefit compared to those undergoing CABG/AVR not involving IMA to LAD *(162)*.

Regarding double valve surgery, Gillinov et al. have demonstrated that, where feasible, AVR with mitral valve repair is associated with improved long-term survival compared with AVR with mitral valve replacement *(163)*. In addition, MV repair was associated with 86% freedom from MV replacement at 15 years for non-rheumatic pathologies and 75% 15-year freedom from MV replacement for rheumatic disease. However, others have advocated MV replacement for double valve disease, particularly for rheumatic pathology, citing an increased risk for reoperation with mitral repairs and similar rates of TE complications between mitral repair and replacement in concert with AVR *(164, 165)*. When double valve replacement is performed, it appears that long-term results, including all valve-related complications, are better with mitral bioprostheses as compared to mechanical prostheses *(164, 166)*.

Results of AVR with Stentless Valves

Ten-year data have been reported for the Medtronic Freestyle stentless valve, which was evaluated in eight different North American centers *(167)*. Actuarial freedom from structural valve deterioration was 96.0% ± 4.5% for the full root method of implantation and freedom from reoperation was 92.3% ± 6.0% using this technique. In addition, 10-year freedom from moderate AR was 97.7% ± 1.6%. Comparable outcomes were seen with the subcoronary technique of stentless bioprosthetic AVR implantation as well *(167)*. In addition, similar results have been achieved in Europe using the Sorin Pericarbon Freedom stentless valve, although the data are limited to 7 years of follow-up *(168)*.

Results of Aortic Root Replacement

David et al. recently reported long-term results for 220 patients undergoing aortic valve-sparing root procedures for aortic root aneurysm *(169)*. Survival at 10 years was 88% ± 3%, and freedom from moderate or severe AR was 85% ± 5% at 10 years. However, for patients who underwent root reimplantation as opposed to the remodeling root procedure, freedom from moderate-to-severe AR was 94% ± 4% at 10 years. Freedom from redo valve replacement was 95% ± 3% at 10 years *(169)*. Therefore, these data form the basis of this group's preference for the reimplantation technique over the remodeling technique for valve-sparing root replacement. A similar position has been advocated by other groups as well *(83, 170)*.

Karck et al. reported their experience with composite mechanical valved conduit root replacement (Bentall procedure) as compared with the valve-sparing root reimplantation procedure in 119 Marfan syndrome patients with aortic dissection or aneurysm *(171)*. Despite longer operative times for valve-sparing operations, mid- and long-term results were comparable between the two techniques, including 5-year freedom from reoperation and death. As expected, TE and bleeding complications were significantly greater in the mechanical composite group, leading the authors to recommend the valve-sparing root reimplantation technique as the procedure of choice in these cases *(171)*.

Mid-term results for valve-sparing root replacement in patients with the Marfan syndrome using the Gelweave Valsalva conduit (Sulzer Vascutek, Refrewshire, Scotland), which incorporates premade sinuses of Valsalva into the Dacron graft (Fig. 10), have recently been reported *(172)*. In this study, the 5-year freedom from structural deterioration was 88.9% ± 8%. Similar results were reported by Jeanmart et al., who performed either root reimplantation or root remodeling procedures for a variety of aortic root pathologies and also used the Gelweave Valsalva graft in 40% of the reimplantation procedures *(1)*. Only one case of recurrent AR requiring reoperation was encountered after 5 years of follow-up *(1)*. The St. Jude Medical mechanical valved conduit has also been shown to be comparable to aortic homografts for aortic root replacement *(173)*.

Finally, Etz et al. evaluated their results with bioprosthetic valved conduits in 275 patients treated over 12 years *(174)*. The conduits were "hand-made," constructed at the time of surgery, since these devices are not yet available commercially. Freedom from aortic valve reoperation was 86% at 10 years; freedom from TE was 96% at 10 years; and freedom from endocarditis was 99% at 15 years. There was a 3% rate of bleeding complications over 15 years of follow-up.

REFERENCES

1. Jeanmart H, de Kerchove L, Glineur D, et al. Aortic valve repair: the functional approach to leaflet prolapse and valve-sparing surgery. Ann Thorac Surg 2007;83:S746–51.
2. Schelbert EB, Rosenthal GE, Welke KF, Vaughan-Sarrazin MS. Treatment variation in older black and white patients undergoing aortic valve replacement. Circulation 2005;112:2347–53.
3. Konsari S, Sintek CF. Surgery of the Aortic Valve. In: Cardiac Surgery: Safeguards and pitfalls in operative technique (3rd ed.). Lippincott Williams and Wilkins, Philadelphia, pp 45–74.
4. Davies MJ, Treasure T, Parker DJ. Demographic characteristics of patients undergoing aortic valve replacement for stenosis: relation to valve morphology. Heart 1996;75:174–8.
5. Population Projections Program PD. Projections of the total resident population by 5-year age groups, and sex with special age categories: 1999 to 2050. Washington, DC: US Census Bureau; January 13, 2000.
6. Stewart BF, Siscovick D, Lind BK, et al. Clinical factors associated with calcific aortic valve disease: cardiovascular health study. J Am Coll Cardiol 1997;29:630–4.
7. Sievers H-H, Schmidtke C. A classification system for the bicuspid aortic valve from 304 surgical specimens. J Thorac Cardiovasc Surg 2007;133:1226–33.
8. Roberts WC, Ko JM, Moore TR, Jones WH Jr. Causes of pure aortic regurgitation in patients having isolated aortic valve replacement at a single US tertiary hospital (1993 to 2005). Circulation 2006;114:422–9.
9. Roberts WC, Ko JM. Frequency of decades of unicuspid, bicuspid, and tricuspid aortic valves in adults having isolated aortic valve replacement for aortic stenosis, with or without associated aortic regurgitation. Circulation 2005;111:920–5.
10. Lewin MB, Otto CM. The bicuspid aortic valve: adverse outcomes from infancy to old age. Circulation 2005;111:832–4.
11. Brandenburg RO Jr, Tajik AJ, Edwards WD, et al. Accuracy of 2-dimensional echocardiography diagnosis of congenitally bicuspid valve: echocardiographic-anatomic correlation in 115 patients. Am J Cardiol 1973;83:1469–73.
12. Nistri S, Sorbo MD, Marin M, Palisi M, Scognamiglio R, Thiene G. Aortic root dilatation in young men with normally functioning bicuspid aortic valves. Heart 1999;82:19–22.
13. Fedak PW, Verma S, David TE, Leask RL, Weisel RD, Butany J. Clinical and pathophysiological implications of a bicuspid aortic valve. Circulation 2000;102(Suppl III):III-35–9.
14. McKellar SH, Tester DJ, Yagubyan M, Majumdar R, Ackerman MJ, Sundt TM III. Novel *NOTCH1* mutations in patients with bicuspid aortic valve disease and thoracic aortic aneurysms. J Thorac Cardiovasc Surg 2007; 134:290–6.
15. Roberts CS, Roberts WC. Dissection of the aorta associated with congenital malformation of the aortic valve. J Am Coll Cardiol 1991; 17:712–6.
16. Bonow RO, Carabello BA, Chatterjee K, et al. ACC/AHA 2006 guidelines for the management of patients with valvular heart disease: a report of the American College of Cardiology/American Heart Association Task Force on Practice

Guidelines (Writing Committee to develop guidelines for the management of patients with valvular heart disease). Circulation 2006;114:e84–e231.

17. Bermudez GA, Abdelnur R, Midell A, DeMeester T. Coronary artery disease in aortic stenosis: importance of coronary arteriography and surgical implications. Angiology 1983;34:591–6.

18. Ferencik M, Ropers D, Abbara S, et al. Diagnostic accuracy of image postprocessing methods for the detection of coronary artery stenoses by using multidetector CT. Radiology 2007;243:696–702.

19. Fullerton DA. Aortic valve replacement. In Mastery of Cardiothoracic Surgery (2nd ed.) Kaiser LR, Kron IL, Spray TL. (Eds.). Lippincott Williams and Wilkins, Philadelphia, pp 410–23.

20. Gjertsson P, Caidahl K, Farasati M, Oden A, Bech-Hanssen O. Preoperative moderate to severe diastolic dysfunction: a novel Doppler echocardiographic long-term prognostic factor in patients with severe aortic stenosis. J Thorac Cardiovasc Surg 2005;129:890–6.

21. Perez de Arenaza D, Lees B, Flather M, et al. Randomized comparison of stentless versus stented valves for aortic stenosis: effects on left ventricular mass. Circulation 2005;112:2696–702.

22. Monin JL, Quere JP, Monchi M, et al. Low-gradient aortic stenosis: operative risk stratification and predictors for long-term outcome: a multicenter study using dobutamine stress hemodynamics. Circulation 2003; 108:319–24.

23. Stoddard MF, Arce J, Liddell NE, Peters G, Dillon S, Kupersmith J. Two-dimensional transesophageal echocardiographic determination of aortic valve area in adults with aortic stenosis. Am Heart J 1991;122:1415–22.

24. Kupfahl C, Honold M, Meinhardt G, et al. Evaluation of aortic stenosis by cardiovascular magnetic resonance imaging: comparison with established routine clinical techniques. Heart 2004;90:893–901.

25. John AS, Dill T, Brandt RR, et al. Magnetic resonance to assess the aortic valve area in aortic stenosis: how does it compare to current diagnostic standards? J Am Coll Cardiol 2003;42:519–26.

26. Lancellotti P, Lebois F, Simon M, Tombeux C, Chauvel C, Pierard LA. Prognostic importance of quantitative exercise Doppler echocardiography in asymptomatic valvular aortic stenosis. Circulation 2005;112(Suppl I):I-377–82.

27. Nishimura RA, Grantham JA, Connolly HM, Schaff HV, Higano ST, Holmes DR Jr. Low-output, low-gradient aortic stenosis in patients with depressed left ventricular systolic function: the clinical utility of the dobutamine challenge in the catheterization laboratory. Circulation 2002; 106:809–13.

28. Khot UN, Novaro GM, Popovic ZB, et al. Nitroprusside in critically ill patients with left ventricular dysfunction and aortic stenosis. N Engl J Med 2003;348:1756–63.

29. Quere J-P, Monin J-L, Petit H, et al. Influence of preoperative left ventricular contractile reserve on postoperative ejection fraction in low-gradient aortic stenosis. Circulation 2006;113:1738–44.

30. Bergler-Klein J, Mundigler G, Pibarot P, et al. B-type natriuretic peptide in low-flow, low-gradient aortic stenosis: relationship to hemodynamics and clinical outcome: results from the Multicenter Truly or Pseudo-severe Aortic Stenosis (TOPAS) study. Circulation 2007;115:2848–55.

31. Ross J, Braunwald E. Aortic stenosis. Circulation 1968;38(Suppl 5):61–7.

32. Rosenhek R, Binder T, Porenta G, et al. Predictors of outcome in severe, asymptomatic aortic stenosis. NEJM 2000;343:611–7.

33. Otto CM, Burwash IG, Leggett ME, et al. Prospective study of asymptomatic valvular aortic stenosis: clinical, echocardiographic, and exercise predictors of outcome. Circulation 1997;95:2262–70.

34. Otto CM. Aortic stenosis-listen to the patient, look at the valve. NEJM 2000;343:652–4.

35. McCarthy PM. Aortic valve surgery in patients with left ventricular dysfunction. Semin Thorac Cardiovasc Surg 2002;14:137–43.

36. Willett DA, Hall SA, Jessen ME, Wait MA, Grayburn PA. Assessment of aortic regurgitation by transesophageal color Doppler imaging of the vena contracta: validation against an intraoperative aortic flow probe. J Am Coll Cardiol 2001;37:1450–5.

37. Chin CH, Chen CH, Chen CC, Chen TH, Chang ML, Chiou HC. Prediction of severity of isolated aortic regurgitation by echocardiography: an aortic regurgitation index study. J Am Soc Echocardiogr 2005;18:1007–13.

38. Movsowitz HD, Levine RA, Hilgenberg AD, Isselbacher EM. Transesophageal echocardiographic description of the mechanisms of aortic regurgitation in acute type A aortic dissection: implications for aortic valve repair. J Am Coll Cardiol 2000;36:884–90.

39. Kon ND. Invited commentary. Ann Thorac Surg 1999;68:2344.

40. Emery RW, Krogh CC, Arom KV, et al. The St. Jude Medical cardiac valve prosthesis: a 25-year experience with single valve replacement. Ann Thorac Surg 2005;79:776–83.

41. Ikonomides JS, Krantz JM, Crumbley AJ, et al. Twenty-year experience with the St. Jude Medical valve prosthesis. J Thorac Cardiovasc Surg 2003;126:2022–31.

42. Butchart EG, Ionescu A, Payne N, Giddings J, Grunkemeier GL, Fraser AG. A new scoring system to determine thromboembolic risk after heart valve replacement. Circulation 2003;108(Suppl 1):II-68–74.

43. Koertke H, Zittermann A, Minami K, et al. Low-dose international normalized ratio self-management: a promising tool to achieve low complication rates after mechanical heart valve replacement. Ann Thorac Surg 2005;79:1909–14.

44. Bach DS, Sakwa MP, Goldbach M, Patracek MR, Emery RW, Mohr FW. Hemodynamics and early clinical performance of the St. Jude Medical Regent mechanical aortic valve. Ann Thorac Surg 2002;74:2003–9.

45. Riess F-C, Bader R, Cramer E, et al. Hemodynamic performance of the Medtronic Mosaic porcine bioprosthesis up to ten years. Ann Thorac Surg 2007;83:1310–8.

46. Peterseim DS, Cen YY, Cheruvu S, et al. Long-term outcome for biologic versus mechanical aortic valve replacement in 841 patients. J Thorac Cardiovasc Surg 1999;117:890–7.

47. Fradet G, Bleese N, Busse E, et al. The Mosaic valve clinical performance at seven years: results from a multicenter prospective clinical trial. J Heart Valve Dis 2004;13:239–47.

48. Rieder K, Kasimir MT, Silberhumer G, et al. Decellularization protocols of porcine heart valves differ importantly in efficiency of cell removal and susceptibility of the matrix to recellularization with human vascular cells. J Thorac Cardiovasc Surg 2004;127:399–405.

49. Briand M, Lemieux I, Dumesnil JG, et al. Metabolic syndrome negatively influences disease progression and prognosis in aortic stenosis. J Am Coll Cardiol 2006;47:2229–36.

50. Briand M, Pibarot P, Despres J-P, et al. Metabolic syndrome is associated with faster degeneration of bioprosthetic valves. Circulation 2006;114(suppl 1):I-512–7.

51. Nollert G, Miksch J, Kreuzer E, Reichart B. Risk factors for atherosclerosis and the degeneration of pericardial valves after aortic valve replacement. J Thorac Cardiovasc Surg 2003;126:965–8.

52. Moura LM, Ramos SF, Zamorano JL, et al. Rosuvastatin affecting aortic valve endothelium to slow the progression of aortic stenosis. J Am Coll Cardiol 2007;49:562–4.

53. Ruel M, Kulik A, Rubens FD, et al. Late incidence and determinants of reoperation in patients with prosthetic heart valves. Eur J Cardiothorac Surg 2004;25:364–70.

54. Khan SS, Trento A, DeRobertis M, et al. Twenty-year comparison of tissue and mechanical valve replacement. J Thorac Cardiovasc Surg 2001;122:257–69.

55. Hammermeister K, Sethi GK, Henderson WG, Grover FL, Oprian C, Rahimtoola SH. Outcomes 15 years after valve replacement with a mechanical versus a bioprosthetic valve: final report of the Veterans Affairs randomized trial. J Am Coll Cardiol 2000;36:1152–8.

56. Carrier M, Pellerin M, Perrault LP, et al. Aortic valve replacement with mechanical and biologic prostheses in middle-aged patients. Ann Thorac Surg 2001;71:S253–6.

57. Lau L, Jamieson WR, Hughes C, Germann E, Chan F. What prosthesis should be used at valve re-replacement after structural valve deterioration of a bioprosthesis? Ann Thorac Surg 2006;82:2123–32.

58. Rahimtoola SH. The problem of valve prothesis-patient mismatch. Circulation 1978;58:20–4.

59. Blais C, Dumesnil JG, Baillot R, Simard S, Doyle D, Pibarot P. Impact of valve prosthesis-patient mismatch on short-term mortality after aortic valve replacement. Circulation 2003;108:983–8.

60. Medalion B, Blackstone EH, Lytle BW, White J, Arnold JH, Cosgrove DM. Aortic valve replacement: is valve size important? J Thorac Cardiovas Surg 2000;119:963–74.

61. Blackstone EH, Cosgrove DM, Jamieson WRE, et al. Prosthesis size and long-term survival after aortic valve replacement. J Thorac Cardiovas Surg 2003;126:783–96.

62. Walther T, Rastan A, Falk V, et al. Patient prosthesis mismatch affects short- and long-term outcomes after aortic valve replacement. Eur J Thorac Cardiovasc Surg 2006;30:15–9.

63. Thomson HL, O'Brien MF, Almeida AA, Tesar PJ, Davison MB, Burstow DJ. Hemodynamics and left ventricular mass regression: a comparison of the stentless, stented and mechanical aortic valve replacement. Eur J Cardiothorac Surg 1998;13:572–5.

64. Bach DS, Cartier PA, Kon ND, Johnson KG, Dumesnil JG, Doty DB. Impact of high transvalvular to subvalvular velocity ratio early after aortic valve replacement with Freestyle stentless aortic bioprosthesis. Semin Thorac Cardiovasc Surg 2001;13(Suppl 1):75–81.

65. Pibarot P, Demesnil JG, Jobin J, Cartier P, Honos G, Durant L-G. Hemodynamic and physical performance during maximal exercise in patients with an aortic bioprosthetic valve. J Am Coll Cardiol 1999;34:1609–17.

66. Bakhtiary F, Schiemann M, Dzemali O, et al. Impact of patient-prosthesis mismatch and aortic valve design on coronary flow reserve after aortic valve replacement. J Am Coll Cardiol 2007;49:790–6.

67. Tsialtas D, Bolognesi R, Beghi C, et al. Stented versus stentless bioprostheses in aortic valve stenosis: effect on left ventricular remodeling. Heart Surg Forum 2007;10:E205–10.

68. Milano AD, Blanzola C, Mecozzi G, et al. Hemodynamic performance of stented and stentless aortic bioprostheses. Ann Thorac Surg 2001;72:33–8.

69. Doss M, Martens S, Wood JP, et al. Performance of stentless versus stented aortic valve bioprostheses in the elderly patient: a prospective randomized trial. Eur J Cardiothorac Surg 2003;23:299–304.

70. Ali A, Halstead JC, Cafferty F, et al. Are stentless valves superior to modern stented valves? Circulation 2006;114(Suppl 1):I-535–40.

71. Hochrein J, Lucke JC, Harrison JK, et al. Mortality and need for reoperation in patients with mild-to-moderate asymptomatic aortic valve disease undergoing coronary artery bypass graft alone. Am Heart J 1999;138:791–7.

72. Smith WT IV, Ferguson TB Jr, Ryan T, Landolfo CK, Peterson ED. Should coronary artery bypass graft surgery patients with mild or moderate aortic stenosis undergo concomitant aortic valve replacement? A decision analysis approach to the surgical dilemma. J Am Coll Cardiol 2004;44:1241–7.

73. Sundt TM III, Murphy SF, Barzilai B, et al. Previous coronary artery bypass grafting is not a risk factor for aortic valve replacement. Ann Thorac Surg 1997;64:651–7.

74. Akins CW, Hilgenberg AD, Vlahakes GJ, MacGillivray TE, Torchiana DF, Madsen JC. Results of bioprosthetic versus mechanical aortic valve replacement performed with concomitant coronary artery bypass grafting. Ann Thorac Surg 2002;74:1098–106.

75. Vanden Eynden F, Bouchard D, El-Hamamsy I, et al. Effect of aortic valve replacement for aortic stenosis on severity of mitral regurgitation. Ann Thorac Surg 2007;83:1279–84.

76. Ruel M, Kapila V, Price J, Kulik A, Burwash IG, Mesana TG. Natural history and predictors of outcome in patients with concomitant functional mitral regurgitation at the time of aortic valve replacement. Circulation 2006;114(Suppl 1):I-541–6.

77. Barreiro CJ, Patel ND, Fitton TP, et al. Aortic valve replacement and concomitant mitral valve regurgitation in the elderly. Circulation 2005;112(Suppl I):I-443–7.

78. Ngaage DL, Schaff HV, Barnes SA, et al. Prognostic implications of preoperative atrial fibrillation in patients undergoing aortic valve replacement: is there an argument for concomitant arrhythmia surgery? Ann Thorac Surg 2006;82:1392–9.

79. Bando K, Kobayashi J, Sasako Y, Tagusari O, Niwaya K, Kitamura S. Effect of maze procedure in patients with atrial fibrillation undergoing valve replacement. J Heart Valve Dis 2002;11:719–24.

80. Wolfe WG. Acute ascending aortic dissection. Ann Surg 1980;192:658–66.

81. David TE, Feindel CM. An aortic valve-sparing operation for patients with aortic incompetence and aneurysm of the ascending aorta. J Thorac Cardiovasc Surg 1992;103:617–22.

82. Bentall H, DeBono A. A technique for complete replacement of the ascending aorta. Thorax 1968;23:338–9.

83. Kallenbach K, Karck M, Pak D, et al. Decade of aortic valve sparing reimplantation: are we pushing the limits too far? Circulation 2005;112(Suppl I):I-253–9.

84. David TE, Feindel DM, Webb GD, Colman JM, Armstrong S, Maganti M. Aortic valve preservation in patients with aortic root aneurysm: results of the reimplantation technique. Ann Thorac Surg 2007;83:S732–5.

85. de Oliveira NC, David TE, Ivanov J, et al. Results of surgery for aortic root aneurysm in patients with Marfan syndrome. J Thorac Cardiovasc Surg 2003;125:789–96.

86. El Khoury G, Vanoverschelde JL, Glineur D, et al. Repair of aortic valve prolapse: experience with 44 patients. Eur J Cardiothorac Surg 2004;26:628–33.

87. Lansac E, Di Centa I, Bonnet N, et al. Aortic prosthetic ring annuloplasty: a useful adjunct to standardized aortic valve-sparing procedure? Eur J Cardiothorac Surg 2006;29:537–44.

88. El Khoury G, Vanoverschelde JL, Glineur D, et al. Repair of bicuspid aortic valves in patients with aortic regurgitation. Circulation 2006;114(Suppl I):I610–16.

89. Russo CF, Mazzetti S, Garatti A, et al. Aortic complications after bicuspid aortic valve replacement: long-term results. Ann Thorac Surg 2002;74:S1773–6.

90. Gleason TG. Current perspective on aortic valve repair and valve-sparing aortic root replacement. Semin Thorac Cardiovasc Surg 2006;18:154–64.

91. Mihaljevic T, Cohn LH, Unic D, Aranki SF, Couper GS, Byrne JG. One-thousand minimally invasive valve operations: early and late results. Ann Surg 2004;240:529–34.

92. Bakir I, Casselman FP, Wellens F, et al. Minimally invasive versus standard approach aortic valve replacement: a study in 506 patients. Ann Thorac Surg 2006;81:1599–604.

93. Bonacchi M, Prifti E, Giunit G, Frati G, Sani G. Does ministernotomy improve postoperative outcome in aortic valve operation? A prospective randomized study. Ann Thorac Surg 2002;73:460–5.

94. Applebaum RM, Cutler WM, Bhardwaj N, et al. Utility of transesophageal echocardiography during port-access minimally invasive cardiac surgery. Am J Cardiol 1998;15:183–8.

95. Svenarud P, Persson M, van der Linden J. Effect of CO_2 insufflation on the number and behavior of air microemboli in open-heart surgery: a randomized clinical trial. Circulation 2004;109:1127–32.

96. Ascione R, Caputo M, Gomes WJ, et al. Myocardial injury in hypertrophic hearts of patients undergoing aortic valve surgery using cold or warm blood cardioplegia. Eur J Cardiothorac Surg 2002;21:440–6.

97. Lotto AA, Ascione R, Caputo M, Bryan AJ, Angelini GD, Suleiman MS. Myocardial protection with intermittent cold blood during aortic valve operation: antegrade versus retrograde delivery. Ann Thorac Surg 2003;76:1227–33.

98. Dagenais F, Pelletier LC, Carrier M. Antegrade/retrograde cardioplegia for valve replacement: a prospective study. Ann Thorac Surg 1999;68:1681–5.

99. Menasche P, Subayi JB, Piwnica A. Retrograde coronary sinus caridoplegia for aortic valve operations: a clinical report on 500 patients. Ann Thorac Surg 1990;49:556–63.

100. Jin XY, Gibson DG, Pepper JR. Early changes in regional and global left ventricular function after aortic valve replacement. Comparison of crystalloid, cold blood, and warm blood cardioplegias. Circulation 1995;92(Suppl 9):II155–62.
101. Flack JE III, Cook JR, May SJ, et al. Does cardioplegia type affect outcome and survival in patients with advanced left ventricular dysfunction? Results from the CABG Patch Trial. Circulation 2000;102(Suppl III):III-84–9.
102. Vazquez-Jimenez JF, Qing M, Hermanns B, et al. Moderate hypothermia during cardiopulmonary bypass reduces myocardial cell damage and myocardial cell death related to cardiac surgery. J Am Coll Cardiol 2001; 38:1216–23.
103. El-Khally Z, Thibault B, Staniloae C, et al. Prognostic significance of newly acquired bundle branch block after aortic valve replacement. Am J Cardiol 2004;94:1008–11.
104. Wagner IM, Eichinger WB, Bleiziffer S, et al. Influence of completely supra-annular placement of bioprostheses on exercise hemodynamics in patients with a small aortic annulus. J Thorac Cardiovasc Surg 2007;133:1234–41.
105. Gerosa G, Tarzia V, Rizzoli G, Bottio T. Small aortic annulus: the hydrodynamic performances of 5 commercially available tissue valves. J Thorac Cardiovasc Surg 2006;131:1058–64.
106. Hammon JW, Stump DA, Butterworth JF, et al. Single crossclamp improves 6-month cognitive outcome in high-risk coronary bypass patients: the effect of reduced aortic manipulation. J Thorac Cardiovasc Surg 2006;131:114–21.
107. Kon ND, Cordell R, Adair SM, Dobbins JE, Kitzman DW. Aortic root replacement with the Freestyle stentless porcine aortic root bioprosthesis. Ann Thorac Surg 1999;67:1609–16.
108. David TE, Feindel CM, Bos J, Sun Z, Scully HE, Rakowski H. Aortic valve replacement with a stentless porcine aortic valve. A six-year experience. J Thorac Cardiovasc Surg 1994;108:030–6.
109. David TE, Feindel CM, Armstrong S, Maganti M. Replacement of the ascending aorta with reduction of the diameter of the sinotubular junction to treat aortic insufficiency in patients with ascending aortic aneurysm. J Thorac Cardiovasc Surg 2007;133:414–18.
110. Connolly HM, Oh JK, Orszulak TA, et al. Aortic valve replacement for aortic stenosis with severe left ventricular dysfunction: prognostic indicators. Circulation 1997;95:2395–400.
111. Lund O. Preoperative risk evaluation and stratification of long-term survival after valve replacement for aortic stenosis: reasons for earlier operative intervention. Circulation 1990;82:124–39.
112. Lund O, Kristensen LH, Baandrup U, et al. Myocardial structure as a determinant of pre- and postoperative ventricular function and long-term prognosis after valve replacement for aortic stenosis. Eur Heart J 1998;19:1099–108.
113. Levy D. Clinical significance of left ventricular hypertrophy: insights from the Framingham Study. J Cardiovasc Pharmacol 1991;17(Suppl 2):S1–6.
114. Villari B, Vassalli G, Monrad ES, Chiariello M, Turina M, Hess OM. Normalization of diastolic dysfunction in aortic stenosis late after valve replacement. Circulation 1995;91:2353–8.
115. Gjertsson P, Caidahl K, Bech-Hanssen O. Left ventricular diastolic dysfunction late after aortic valve replacement in patients with aortic stenosis. Am J Cardiol 2005;96:722–7.
116. Tseng EE, Lee CA, Cameron DE, et al. Aortic valve replacement in the elderly: risk factors and long-term results. Ann Surg 1997;225:793–804.
117. Huber CH, Goeber V, Berdat P, Carrel T, Eckstein F. Benefits of cardiac surgery in octogenarians-a postoperative quality of life assessment. Eur J Cardiothorac Surg 2007;31:1099–105.
118. Bonow RO, Borer JS, Rosing DR, et al. Preoperative exercise capacity in symptomatic patients with aortic regurgitation as a predictor of postoperative left ventricular function and long-term prognosis. Circulation 1980;62:1280–90.
119. Bonow RO, Rosing DR, Maron BJ, et al. Reversal of left ventricular dysfunction after aortic valve replacement for chronic aortic regurgitation: influence of duration of preoperative left ventricular dysfunction. Circulation 1984;70:570–9.
120. Tornos MP, Olona M, Permanyer-Miralda G, et al. Heart failure after aortic valve replacement for aortic regurgitation; prospective 20-year study. Am Heart J 1998;136:681–7.
121. Turina J, Milincic J, Seifert B, Turina M. Valve replacement in chronic aortic regurgitation. True predictors of survival after extended follow-up. Circulation 1998;98(Suppl 19):II100–6.
122. Rothenburger M, Drebber K, Tjan TDT, et al. Aortic valve replacement for aortic regurgitation and stenosis in patients with severe left ventricular dysfunction. Eur J Cardiothorac Surg 2003;23:703–9.
123. Chaliki HP, Mohty D, Avierinos J-F, et al. Outcomes after aortic valve replacement in patients with severe aortic regurgitation and markedly reduced left ventricular function. Circulation 2002;106:2687–93.
124. Bridgewater B, Adult Cardiac Surgeons of North West England. Mortality data in adult cardiac surgery for named surgeons: retrospective examination of prospectively collected date on coronary artery surgery and aortic valve replacement. BMJ 2005;330:506–10.
125. Hannan EL, Racz MJ, Jones RH, et al. Predictors of mortality for patients undergoing cardiac valve replacements in New York State. Ann Thorac Surg 2000;70:1212–18.
126. Jamieson WRE, Edwards FH, Schwartz M, Bero JW, Clark RE, Grover FL, Database Committee of the Society of Thoracic Surgeons. Risk stratification for cardiac valve replacement. National cardiac surgery database. Ann Thorac Surg 1999;67:943–51.

127. Rankin JS, Hammill BG, Ferguson TB Jr, et al. Determinants of operative mortality in valvular heart surgery. J Thorac Cardiovasc Surg 2006;131:547–57.

128. Kuduvalli M, Grayson AD, Au J, et al. A multi-centre additive and logistic risk model for in-hospital mortality following aortic valve replacement. Eur J Cardiothorac Surg 2007;31:607–13.

129. Astor BC, Kaczmarek RG, Hefflin B, Daley WR. Mortality after aortic valve replacement: results from a nationally representative database. Ann Thorac Surg 2000;70:1939–45.

130. Maganti MD, Rao V, Borger MA, Ivanov J, David TE. Predictors of low cardiac output syndrome after isolated aortic valve surgery. Circulation 2005;112(Suppl I):I-448–52.

131. Edwards FH, Peterson ED, Coombs LP, et al. Prediction of operative mortality after valve replacement surgery. J Am Coll Cardiol 2001;37:885–92.

132. Nowicki ER, Birkmeyer NJO, Weintraub RW, et al. Multivariable prediction of in-hospital mortality associated with aortic and mitral valve surgery in Northern New England. Ann Thorac Surg 2004;77: 1966–77.

133. Verheul HA, van den Brink RBA, Bouma BJ, et al. Analysis of risk factors for excess mortality after aortic valve replacement. J Am Coll Cardiol 1995;26:1280–6.

134. Duncan AR, Lin J, Koch CG, Gillinov AM, Xu M, Starr NJ. The impact of gender on in-hospital mortality and morbidity after isolated aortic valve replacement. Anesth Analg 2006;103:800–8.

135. Lytle BW, Cosgrove DM, Taylor PC, et al. Primary isolated aortic valve replacement: early and late results. J Thorac Cardiovasc Surg 1989;97:675–94.

136. Chiappini B, Camurri N, Loforte A, Di Marco L, Di Bartolomeo R, Marinelli G. Outcome after aortic valve replacement in octogenarians. Ann Thorac Surg 2004;78:85–9.

137. Melby SJ, Zierer A, Kaiser SP, et al. Aortic valve replacement in octogenarians: risk factors for early and late mortality. Ann Thorac Surg 2007;83:1651–6.

138. Bloomstein LZ, Gielchinsky I, Bernstein AD, et al. Aortic valve replacement in geriatric patients: determinants of in-hospital mortality. Ann Thorac Surg 2001;71:597–600.

139. Jin R, Grunkemeier GL, Starr A. Validation and refinement of mortality risk models for heart valve surgery. Ann Thorac Surg 2005;80:471–9.

140. Mehta RH, Bruckman D, Das S, et al. Implications of increased left ventricular mass index on in-hospital outcomes in patients undergoing aortic valve surgery. J Thorac Cardiovasc Surg 2001;122:919–28.

141. Erdogan HB, Kayalar N, Ardal H, et al. Risk factors for requirement of permanent pacemaker implantation after aortic valve replacement. J Card Surg 2006;21:211–15.

142. Elahi MM, Osman KA, Bhandari M, Dhanapuneni RR. Does the type of prosthesis influence the incidence of permanent pacemaker implantation following isolated aortic valve replacement? Heart Surg Forum 2005;8:E396–400.

143. Limongelli G, Ducceschi V, D'Andrea A, et al. Risk factors for pacemaker implantation following aortic valve replacement: a single centre experience. Heart 2003;89:901–4.

144. Koplan BA, Stevenson WG, Epstein LM, Aranki SF, Maisel WH. Development and validation of a simple risk score to predict the need for permanent pacing after cardiac valve surgery. J Am Coll Cardiol 2003; 41:795–801.

145. Elahi M, Usmann K. The bioprosthesis type and size influence the postoperative incidence of permanent pacemaker implantation in patients undergoing aortic valve surgery. J Interv Card Electrophysiol 2006;15:113–18.

146. Vanky FB, Hakanson E, Tamas E, Svedjeholm R. Risk factors for postoperative heart failure in patients operated on for aortic stenosis. Ann Thorac Surg 2006;81:1297–304.

147. Connolly HM, Oh JK, Schaff HV, et al. Severe aortic stenosis with low transvalvular gradient and severe left ventricular dysfunction: result of aortic valve replacement in 52 patients. Circulation 2000;101:1940–6.

148. Kulik A, Burwash IG, Kapila V, Mesana TG, Reul M. Long-term outcomes after valve replacement for low-gradient aortic stenosis: impact of prosthesis-patient mismatch. Circulation 2006;114(Suppl 1):I553–8.

149. Baykut D, Grize L, Schindler C, Keil AS, Bernet F, Zerkowski H-R. Eleven-year single-center experience with the ATS Open Pivot bileaflet heart valve. Ann Thorac Surg 2006;82:847–52.

150. Palatianos GM, Laczkovics AM, Simon P, et al. Multicentered European study on safety and effectiveness of the On-X prosthetic heart valve: intermediate follow-up. Ann Thorac Surg 2007;83:40–6.

151. Gillinov AM, Blackstone EH, Alster JM, et al. The Carbomedics Top Hat supra-annular aortic valve: a multicenter study. Ann Thorac Surg 2003;75:1175–80.

152. Edmunds LH, Clark RE, Cohn LH, Grunkemeier GL, Miller DL, Weisel RD. Guidelines for reporting morbidity and mortality after cardiac valvular operations. J Thorac Cardiovasc Surg 1988;96:351–3.

153. Jamieson WRE, Moffatt-Bruce SD, Skarsgard P, et al. Early antithrombotic therapy for aortic valve bioprostheses: is there an indication for routine use? Ann Thorac Surg 2007;83:549–57.

154. Glower DD, Landolfo KP, Cheruvu, et al. Determinants of 15-year outcome with 1,119 standard Carpentier-Edwards porcine valves. Ann Thorac Surg 1998;66:S44–8.

155. Grunkemeier GL, Jamieson WRE, Miller DC, Starr A. Actuarial versus actual risk of porcine structural valve deterioration. J Thorac Cardiovasc Surg 1994;108:709–18.

156. Jamieson WRE, Burr LH, Miyagishima RT, et al. Carpentier-Edwards supra-annular aortic porcine bioprosthesis: clinical performance over 20 years. J Thorac Cardiovasc Surg 2005;130:994–1000.

157. Minami K, Zitterman A, Schulte-Eistrup S, Koertze H, Korfer R. Mitroflow Synergy prostheses for aortic valve replacement: 19 years experience with 1,516 patients. Ann Thorac Surg 2005;80:1699–705.

158. Dellgren G, David TE, Raanani E, Armstrong S, Ivanov J, Rakowski H. Late hemodynamic and clinical outcomes of aortic valve replacement with the Carpentier-Edwards Perimount pericardial bioprosthesis. J Thorac Cardiovasc Surg 2002;124:146–54.

159. Bottio T, Rizzoli G, Thiene T, Nesseris G, Casarotto D, Gerosa G. Hemodynamic and clinical outcomes with the Biocor valve in the aortic position: an 8-year experience. J Thorac Cardiovasc Surg 2004;127:1616–23.

160. Kobayashi KJ, Williams JA, Nwakanma L, Gott VL, Baumgartner WA, Conte JV. Aortic valve replacement and concomitant coronary artery bypass: assessing the impact of multiple grafts. Ann Thorac Surg 2007;83:969–78.

161. Stassano P, Di Tommaso L, Vitale DF, et al. Aortic valve replacement and coronary artery surgery: determinants affecting early and long-term results. Thorac Cardiovasc Surg 2006;54:521–7.

162. Gall S Jr, Lowe JE, Wolfe WW, Oldham HN Jr, Van Trigt P III, Glower DD. Efficacy of the internal mammary artery in combined aortic valve replacement-coronary artery bypass grafting. Ann Thorac Surg 2000;69:524–30.

163. Gillinov AM, Blackstone EH, Cosgrove DM III, et al. Mitral valve repair with aortic valve replacement is superior to double valve replacement. J Thorac Cardiovasc Surg 2003;125:1372–87.

164. Hamamoto M, Bando K, Kobayashi J, et al. Durability and outcome of aortic valve replacement with mitral valve repair versus double valve replacement. Ann Thorac Surg 2003;75:28–33.

165. Kuwaki K, Kawaharada N, Morishita K, et al. Mitral valve repair versus replacement in simultaneous mitral and aortic valve surgery for rheumatic disease. Ann Thorac Surg 2007;83:558–63.

166. Kuwaki K, Tsukamoto M, Komatsu K, Morishita K, Sakata J, Abe T. Simultaneous aortic and mitral valve replacement: predictors of adverse outcomes. J Heart Valve Dis 2003;12:169–76.

167. Bach DS, Kon ND, Demesnil JG, Sintek CF, Doty DB. Ten-year outcome after aortic valve replacement with the Freestyle stentless bioprosthesis. Ann Thorac Surg 2005;80:480–7.

168. D'Onofrio A, Auriemma S, Magagna P, et al. Aortic valve replacement with the Sorin Pericarbon Freedom stentless prosthesis: 7 years' experience in 130 patients. J Thorac Cardiovasc Surg 2007; 134:491–5.

169. David TE, Feindel CM, Webb GD, Colman JM, Armstrong S, Maganti M. Long-term results of aortic valve-sparing operation for aortic root aneurysm. J Thorac Cardiovasc Surg 2006;132:347–54.

170. Erasmi AW, Sievers H-H, Bechtel M, Hanke T, Stierle U, Misfeld M. Remodeling or reimplantation for valve-sparing aortic root surgery. Ann Thorac Surg 2007;83:S752–6.

171. Karck M, Kallenbach K, Hagl C, Rhein C, Leyh R, Haverich A. Aortic root surgery in Marfan syndrome: comparison of aortic valve-sparing reimplantation versus composite grafting. J Thorac Cardiovasc Surg 2004;127:391–8.

172. Settepani F, Szeto WY, Pacini D, et al. Reimplantation valve-sparing aortic root replacement in Marfan syndrome using the Valsalva conduit: an intercontinental multicenter study. Ann Thorac Surg 2007;83:S769–73.

173. Lima B, Hughes GC, Lemair A, Jaggers J, Glower DD, Wolfe WG. Short-term and intermediate-term outcomes of aortic root replacement with St. Jude mechanical conduits and aortic allografts. Ann Thorac Surg 2006;82:579–85.

174. Etz CD, Homann TM, Rane N, et al. Aortic root reconstruction with a bioprosthetic valved conduit: a consecutive series of 275 procedures. J Thorac Cardiovasc Surg 2007;133:1455–63.

175. Asante-Korang A, Anderson RH. Echocardiographic assessment of the aortic valve and left ventricular outflow track. Cardiol Young 2005;15(Suppl 1):27–36.

176. Feindel CM, David TE. Aortic valve sparing operations: basic concepts. Int J Cardiol 2004;97(Suppl 1):61–6.

177. Doty JR, Doty DB. Stentless aortic bioprosthesis for disease of the aortic valve, root, and ascending aorta. Oper Tech Thorac Cardiovasc Surg 2006;11:185–99.

178. Carabello BA, Crawford FA. Valvular heart disease. N Engl J Med 1997;337:32–41.

179. Erbel R, Eggebrecht H. Aortic dimensions and risk of dissection. Heart 2006;92:137–42.

180. Rahimtoola SH. Choice of prosthetic heart valve for adult patients. J Am Coll Cardiol 2003;41:893–904.

181. Hughes GC, Swaminathan M, Wolfe WG. Reimplantation technique (David operation) for multiple sinus of Valsalva aneurysms. Ann Thorac Surg 2006;82:e14–16.

182. Borger MA, Preston M, Ivanov S, et al. Should the ascending aorta be more frequently in patients with bicuspid aortic valve disease? J Thorac Cardiovasc Surg 2004;128:677–83.

183. Kim BS, Soltesz EG, Cohn LH. Minimally invasive approaches to aortic valve surgery: Brigham experience. Semin Thorac Cardiovasc Surg 2006;18:148–53.

14 Contemporary Considerations in Mitral Valve Surgery

Donald D. Glower

CONTENTS

PATIENT EVALUATION AND PATIENT SELECTION

Perhaps the most powerful determinant of outcome in mitral valve surgery is patient selection. Because outcomes are different, patient selection differs slightly for mitral replacement versus mitral repair and for mitral stenosis versus mitral regurgitation. The ACC/AHA guidelines continue to evolve but do reflect conventional wisdom and current evidence in selecting patients for operation (1).

Mitral Stenosis

The ACC/AHA guidelines for intervention for mitral stenosis are shown in Fig. 1. Patients must have at least moderate mitral stenosis to warrant mitral replacement or balloon valvuloplasty. Patients also should be reasonably symptomatic with NYHA class III or IV symptoms. Other indications include significant pulmonary hypertension (peak pulmonary pressure >50 mm Hg) and/or recent onset atrial fibrillation. Patients with mitral valve morphology suitable for balloon valvuloplasty ideally should be referred for balloon valvuloplasty, given the good results and lower morbidity and mortality than mitral commissurotomy (2). An established echocardiographic scoring system is generally used to decide favorable valve morphology for balloon valvuloplasty, and it includes an evaluation of mitral valve leaflet thickness, calcification, and mobility as well as an assessment of submitral chordal fusion (3). Contraindications for balloon valvuloplasty include left atrial thrombus and more than moderate degree of mitral regurgitation. In the current era in the United States, mitral stenosis implies a high probability of mitral replacement, given that percutaneous balloon valvuloplasty is usually preferable treatment for mitral stenosis patients with valve morphology suitable for repair.

From: Contemporary Cardiology: Valvular Heart Disease
Edited by: Andrew Wang, Thomas M. Bashore, DOI 10.1007/978-1-59745-411-7_14
© Humana Press, a part of Springer Science+Business Media, LLC 2009

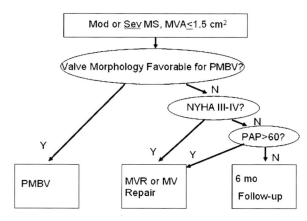

Fig. 1. Algorithm for intervention in mitral stenosis from ACC/AHA guidelines for management of mitral stenosis *(1)*. PMBV = percutaneous mitral balloon valvotomy, PAP = pulmonary arterial pressure.

Mitral Regurgitation

The indications for intervention in mitral regurgitation are more difficult than in mitral stenosis. Patients should have at least moderate mitral regurgitation (generally at least moderate to severe regurgitation). Patients anticipating mitral replacement generally have either NYHA class III–IV symptoms or an EF <60% or left ventricular end-systolic dimension (LVESD) >40 mm by echocardiography. Significant pulmonary hypertension and recent onset atrial fibrillation are relative indications for operation anticipating replacement (Fig. 2) *(1)*.

Most patients in the United States with mitral regurgitation have valves that are amenable to surgical repair. This presumes that the patient has access to a center with experience performing durable

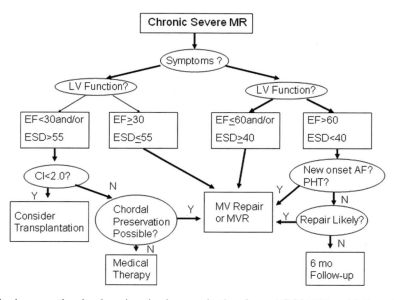

Fig. 2. Algorithm for intervention in chronic mitral regurgitation from ACC/AHA guidelines for management of mitral regurgitation *(1)*. EF = ejection fraction, PHT = pulmonary hypertension, ESD = end-systolic dimension by echocardiography.

mitral repair; otherwise referral would be appropriate given the added mortality and morbidity of either replacement or delayed operation.Because the outcomes from mitral repair are better than those of replacement, the threshold for operating is lower for repair than replacement *(4, 5)*. Many are now advocating that patients with severe mitral regurgitation and a repairable valve should proceed with elective repair regardless of symptoms or hemodynamics *(6)*. Stress testing may be helpful in patients with borderline indications (for instance, to evaluate peak systolic pulmonary artery pressure during exercise), but the exact role of stress testing remains controversial. The use of BNP as a surrogate for exercise testing to reveal underlying LV dysfunction is promising, but remains under evaluation *(7, 8)*.

Concurrent Operation

An additional controversial area is how to manage the mitral valve in patients with mitral valve disease not meeting criteria for operation, but in whom cardiac surgery is indicated for another procedure such as coronary bypass grafting *(9)* or aortic valve replacement *(10, 11)*. The consensus is that any mitral valve with moderate or more stenosis or regurgitation should at least be considered for concurrent operation, whether it be replacement or repair. Most would agree that severe mitral regurgitation or at least moderate mitral stenosis should be dealt with intraoperatively. More controversy surrounds those patients with only moderate mitral regurgitation *(12)*. Here the surgeon must balance the additional morbidity and mortality of concurrent mitral repair versus the additional morbidity and mortality of continued moderate mitral regurgitation. Unfortunately, isolated coronary bypass or aortic valve replacement alone in these patients on average does little to improve the severity of moderate mitral regurgitation. While the relationship between surgical volume and outcomes remains controversial *(13)*, low-risk patients in experienced centers with low morbidity in mitral repair are appropriate for more aggressive use of concurrent mitral repair. High-risk patients or patients in centers less experienced in mitral repair should not have the mitral valve repaired.

Contraindications

Relative contraindications for any mitral surgery include relative contraindications to any cardiac operation in general. A patient's operative risk can be calculated using either of 2 online tools: www.euroscore.org or www.sts.org/sections/stsnationaldatabase/riskcalculator. These sites provide validated estimates to assess risk for an individual patient when a number of comorbid variables are introduced. Major areas for the latter include extreme older age, reoperation, pulmonary hypertension, and concurrent life-threatening lung, renal, or cerebrovascular disease. A somewhat unique relative contraindication to surgery for mitral regurgitation might be those patients with low ejection fraction <30% and cardiac index <2.0 L/min/m^2. These patients have very high surgical risk, tend to have relative little symptomatic or survival benefit, and might be considered for alternative therapy such as cardiac transplantation *(14)*.

Mechanism of Mitral Valve Disease

When evaluating a mitral regurgitation patient for mitral repair, the mechanism of regurgitation has implications. Valves with active infection, extensive calcification, prior repair, or extensive anterior leaflet fibrosis (difficult to assess on echo) are inherently more likely to need replacement. Carpentier *(15)* has classified the mechanisms of mitral leaflet dysfunction as Class I (annular dilation), Class II (leaflet prolapse), Class IIIa (diastolic restriction or stenosis), or Class IIIb (systolic restriction) (Fig. 3). These mechanisms are not mutually exclusive in any one patient, and they also affect the probability and facility of obtaining a repair. Class I patients may often need only an annuloplasty which

Carpentier Classification of Mitral Pathology

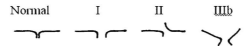

Fig. 3. Carpentier classification of mitral valve pathology. The linear schematic on the *left* represents the anterior leaflet and on the *right* the posterior leaflet. Shown are normal leaflets, Type I annular dilation, Type II leaflet prolapse, Type IIIb systolic restriction *(15)*.

is relatively safe, fast, and can even be done with ventricular fibrillation instead of cardioplegic arrest. Class II patients require more complex leaflet or chordal repair which in turn require more operative time and better exposure generally with cardioplegic arrest. Anterior leaflet prolapse is more difficult to repair that posterior prolapse and has lower success rates depending on the surgeon's experience, along with a higher rate of recurrent regurgitation relative to posterior prolapse. In experienced hands, however, anterior prolapse can receive a durable repair in 85−90% of patients. Class IIIa patients referred for surgery usually need mitral replacement. Finally, Class IIIb patients are generally sicker with either ischemic or dilated cardiomyopathy as etiologies. The repair in type IIIb is often a simple and quick annuloplasty that can be done with ventricular fibrillation or cardioplegic arrest, but more recurrence of late mitral regurgitation is well documented in this group due to continued underlying ventricular pathology (*see* Surgical Outcomes below).

ALTERNATIVE APPROACHES TO THE MITRAL VALVE

Once operation is chosen as the appropriate therapy, the next decision in mitral valve operation may be choice of incisional approach. Choices include full median sternotomy, partial superior sternotomy, partial inferior sternotomy, right full anterolateral thoracotomy, right mini-thoracotomy, left thoracotomy, and totally endoscopic approach. Differences between approaches do exist but should be of secondary importance to obtaining an appropriate and lasting result for the mitral valve. The full median sternotomy has advantages of reproducibility and ability to perform any additional cardiac procedure. All alternative incisions have a learning curve and limit the operating field to exclude most concurrent procedures *(16)*. Like any new technology, most of these alternative incisions can, in large centers, have the mentioned advantages over standard sternotomy. Early in the learning curve in lower volume centers there can actually have higher morbidity and mortality than standard sternotomy.

Percutaneous

A number of approaches to the mitral valve may be taken in patients undergoing mitral surgery. First, percutaneous balloon valvuloplasty may be appropriate in patients with isolated mitral stenosis and suitable valve morphology as defined by the echocardiographic scoring system. Percutaneous mitral repair with devices such as the Evalve mitral clip *(17)* or other percutaneous mitral repair devices *(18)* are currently investigational but might have a future role. Until long-term data are available, the newer percutaneous techniques will at first be considerations in those patients with higher surgical risk and lesser life expectancy.

Median Sternotomy

Median sternotomy is the standard approach for any cardiac operation because of its flexibility to handle most any cardiac pathology with excellent cardiac exposure. All surgical teams are experienced in this approach, and little special equipment or cost is associated. Disadvantages are the relatively large incision, additional blood loss due to the vascularity of the bone marrow, and additional risk of sternal nonunion or sternal infection associated with operating on any bone.

Partial Sternotomy

Partial sternotomy (either superior, inferior, or transverse) may provide excellent exposure to the mitral valve *(19–21)*. These approaches offer access to the mitral valve through the right atrium and the interatrial septum (so-called transeptal approach). Advantages are smaller and more cosmetic incisions, less blood loss, similar speed, and lack of additional equipment over standard sternotomy. The major disadvantage is less access to the rest of the heart, although the aortic valve and tricuspid valve are easily accessible here.

Standard Thoracotomy

Standard right thoracotomy can provide excellent mitral valve exposure, as well as exposure of the tricuspid valve and both atria. Advantages are primarily avoidance of the sternum in patients with prior sternotomy or risk factors for sternal wound complications. Disadvantages include potential compromise of the right lung and limited access to the remaining heart. Little special equipment is needed, and most surgeons are familiar with this approach. Left thoracotomy offers access only to the mitral valve with exposure only adequate enough for annuloplasty or mitral replacement in most cases.

Right Mini-Thoracotomy

Right mini-thoracotomy can provide excellent mitral exposure with all the advantages of standard right thoracotomy *(22)*. Further advantages include an even smaller cosmetic incision, even less blood loss, and even less dissection of previously operated fields in previously operated patients. Disadvantages include limited access to the rest of the heart (only concurrent tricuspid or atrial surgery is routinely facile), need for additional equipment, often need for peripheral arterial access, and increased operating times over sternotomy. These approaches lend themselves to the use of robotic methods as well *(23, 24)*.

Endoscopic

Finally, totally endoscopic (defined as no incision larger than 1 cm) mitral repair has been reported, but to date is not routinely available. Potential advantages include better cosmesis and faster patient rehabilitation. Disadvantages include extended operative times, need for peripheral arterial access, and limited technical facility with all cases reported to date requiring robotic assistance and modified repair techniques *(25)*.

INTRAOPERATIVE DECISION MAKING

Mitral Repair Versus Replacement

An important issue in surgical decision making is the decision to repair versus replace the mitral valve *(4, 5, 26)*. The primary concern is the likelihood of a durable and properly functioning mitral valve. A leaking but repaired mitral valve is worse than a functional prosthetic valve replacement. The potential advantages of a repaired mitral valve over a replaced mitral valve are avoidance of anticoagulation, avoidance of perivalvular leaks and valvular thrombosis, better durability than current bioprostheses, better preservation of ventricular function, lower operative mortality, possibly better late survival, and elimination of posterior ventricular-annular rupture (which carries a 40% mortality). Disadvantages of mitral repair include a longer operating time and the lower possibility of an adequate depending on the patient selected and the institutional experience. In short, mitral repair is generally to be preferred in mitral regurgitation, as long as a durable result can be obtained.

Many risk factors for a mitral valve repair to fail must be considered (Table 1). In mitral stenosis, as mentioned above, surgical repair is only an issue if percutaneous valvuloplasty is not available. If percutaneous balloon valvuloplasty is not available in an otherwise suitable mitral stenosis patient, then surgical mitral repair (open mitral commissurotomy) has the same advantages as mitral repair in mitral regurgitation, but mitral commissurotomy has the additional disadvantage of potential restenosis and thus, reoperation in the future (similar to bioprosthetic mitral replacement) *(27, 28)*.

Table 1
Risk Factors for Failed Mitral Repair

Ejection fraction <40%
Any anterior leaflet pathology
Active endocarditis
Rheumatic disease
Prior mediastinal irradiation
Low volume institution

Several technical issues are relevant to mitral replacement. First is obtaining a leak-free suture line between the valve prosthesis and the mitral annulus. Most surgeons use interrupted, pledgetted sutures to achieve this goal. Other techniques such as running suturelines have been associated with problematic incidences of perivalvular regurgitation. Second is the issue of mitral valve sizing. Although controversy exists, data suggest that most mitral prostheses of 25 mm or greater size will be adequate and provide an orifice area well over 2 cm^2.

Mitral Valve Repair Technique

Mitral repair can be very simple (annuloplasty alone) or can be quite complex. The wide variety of mitral pathology and the relatively low volume of mitral patients coming to surgery in the United States (40,000/year) can make mitral repair a bit more challenging for the 4,600 practicing thoracic surgeons in the United States. Mitral valve repair involves many continuously evolving techniques being applied by many operators for the many differing mitral pathologies. The Carpentier classification of mitral pathology is helpful in matching repair technique to the mitral pathology.

In any mitral repair, leaflet clefts often need to be closed. To assess this, the valve is tested using saline with the heart arrested, and again using transesophageal echocardiography off cardiopulmonary bypass. The vasodilatory effects of general anesthesia reduce mitral regurgitation by about one grade. Thus, one should leave the operating room with no more that 1+ mitral regurgitation by intraoperative echo. Mitral repair without intraoperative transesophageal echo (TEE) has had less optimal results than when TEE guidance is available.

REPAIR OF ANNULAR DILATION

Annular dilation (Carpentier type I pathology) is treated by mitral annuloplasty (Fig. 4). Although it is difficult to make absolute generalizations, several retrospective series have shown a significantly greater rate of recurrent mitral regurgitation if an annuloplasty ring is not used in surgical mitral repair. Thus, the so-called Kay annuloplasty (a suture placed in the commissures only) or the placement of a pericardial band instead of an annular ring has been associated with excessive early recurrent or residual mitral regurgitation. Many types of rings are available, but they fall in to several general categories: flexible versus rigid/semiflexible, complete rings versus partial rings, and finally ventricular remodeling rings.

Mitral Valve Repair

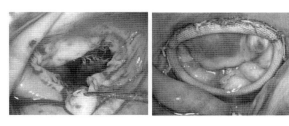

Before Repair   **After Repair**

Fig. 4. A typical mitral valve with P2 mid-posterior leaflet prolapse and ruptured chords before repair *(left panel)* and after repair by triangular resection of P2 and ring annuloplasty *(right panel)*.

Flexible rings have the advantage of reducing suture tension by matching the ring to annular geometry, with the disadvantage that flexible rings have less impact on matching annular shape to anterior leaflet geometry. While controversial, some data suggest that flexible rings may have higher rates of recurrent regurgitation in patients with severe ventricular dysfunction (e.g., EF < 40) *(29)*. *Partial rings* have the advantage of rapid implantation requiring fewer sutures, with the primary disadvantages of more tension on the trigonal/commissural sutures, being more sensitive to mis-sizing due to commissural suture misplacement, and more recurrent regurgitation in patients with significant ventricular dysfunction. A number of ventricular *remodeling rings* are now available that are usually rigid or semirigid rings designed to address mitral regurgitation due to ventricular dysfunction or posterior prolapse. Data directly comparing these various types of rings is currently lacking.

REPAIR OF PROLAPSE

Type II leaflet dysfunction or prolapse can be considered as either posterior leaflet prolapse or anterior leaflet prolapse. Posterior prolapse usually occurs in the P2 (mid) region, next most commonly in the P3 (inferior) region, and rarely in the P1 (superior) region. Treatment options include leaflet resection, leaflet plication, chordal transfer, chordal replacement, and edge-to-edge repairs (Fig. 5). Leaflet resection (either quadrangular or triangular) is commonly used in addition and can include up to about 50% of the posterior leaflet circumference. Leaflet reconstruction can be done either by primary annular plication or by sliding leaflet valvuloplasty. Height of the posterior leaflet can be reduced to ≤1.5 cm by either sliding leaflet plasty or by folding plasty. Leaflet resection has the advantage of being reasonably reproducible though the disadvantage of causing distortion of the remaining leaflet tissues, particularly in larger resections.Secondary posterior leaflet chords can be transferred to the

Mitral Repair Techniques

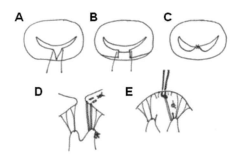

Fig. 5. Techniques of mitral valve repair: triangular resection of P2 (**panel A**), quadrangular resection of P2 and sliding leaflet plasty (**panel B**), Alfieri edge-to-edge repair A2 to P2 (**panel C**), replacement of ruptured chords with artificial Gortex chords (**panel D**), and transfer of secondary anterior leaflet chords to the edge of the anterior leaflet (**panel E**).

posterior leaflet segment, or 4-0 or 5-0 Gortex chords can be placed to the prolapsed segment. Finally, an edge-to-edge repair can be done (Alfieri stitch) as long as the ring used is at least 30 mm.

Anterior prolapse can be repaired by chordal transfer, artificial chords, triangular resection, plication, or edge-to-edge repair. Here the size of the resection is limited to less that 10 mm of leaflet length in most cases. Chordal transfer can use chords either from the corresponding segment of the posterior leaflet (then handled as a quadrangular resection) or from secondary chords under the anterior leaflet. The primary difficulty in Gortex chord placement is careful selection of chordal length, for which several techniques have been developed and continue to be under investigation.

REPAIR OF SYSTOLIC RESTRICTION

Systolic restriction (Carpentier type IIIb) implies LV dilation and/or dysfunction. Here rigid, complete rings are favored, and rings tend to be undersized by at least 2−4 mm (usually 24−26 mm sizes) to compensate for the fact that the leaflets and subvalvular apparatus are pulled into the ventricle. Specialty rings that compress the septal-free wall diameter or attempt to treat restriction in the P2–P3 area can be used. Newer techniques addressing the ventricular remodeling include the Myocor Myosplint® *(30)* placing a bar through the left ventricle at the time of mitral repair to reduce the antero-posterior annular dimension and the ACORN Dacron mesh *(31)* surrounding the heart to reduced overall chamber size. Both are being evaluated in trials as additional means to favorably alter ventricular dimensions by systolic restriction.

REPAIR OF DIASTOLIC RESTRICTION (STENOSIS)

Diastolic restriction (Carpentier type IIIa or mitral stenosis) is often relatively unsuited for mitral repair, given that most patients referred for operation for mitral stenosis are also unsuitable for balloon valvuloplasty. In those patients undergoing repair for mitral stenosis, repair techniques include mitral commissurotomy, debulking and refenestration of fused mitral leaflets, and replacement of diseased mitral chords with artificial 4-0 or 5-0 Gortex sutures. Annuloplasty rings less than 30 mm in size should not be used in these patients because of the likelihood of accelerating recurrent stenosis.

Unfortunately, the underlying rheumatic disease process continues, and most of these patients will have recurrent stenosis and/or regurgitation within 10–15 years.

Mechanical Versus Biological Prostheses

GENERAL CONSIDERATIONS

All patients undergoing mitral operation need to have a discussion about the appropriate choice of mitral prosthesis should the mitral valve need to be replaced, because every patient has some likelihood of needing mitral replacement *(26)*. The basic choice is one of mechanical versus biological prostheses. The ACC/AHA guidelines *(1)* recommend a bioprostheses for those patients who cannot or will not take anticoagulation. This might, for example, include the young female desiring several more years of childbearing potential. Mechanical prostheses are recommended for patients under age 65 or with chronic atrial fibrillation. Otherwise, patients over age 65 without other need for anticoagulation could have biological prostheses. Patients with other indications for anticoagulation will do better with mechanical prostheses to avoid unnecessary reoperation.In the average patient, there will be an initial advantage of biological prostheses up to about 9 years, whereupon mechanical prostheses have better freedom from valve-related morbidity/mortality *(32, 33)* (Fig. 6).

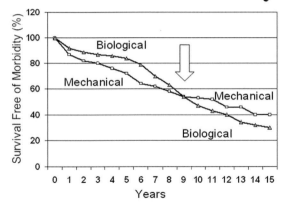

Fig. 6. Survival free of valve-related morbidity following mechanical versus biological mitral valve replacement *(33)*. Note less morbidity from biological valve replacement until about 9 years when degeneration of the biological valve material begins to be manifest.

Retrospective and randomized studies have shown that the survival after mechanical versus biological replacement is similar *(33)* (Fig. 7). The difference is that mechanical patients have a higher incidence of hemorrhagic complications *(33)* (Fig. 8), while the biological patients have more reoperations *(32)* (Fig. 9). Biological prostheses clearly have decreased durability in younger patients, those with hypercalcemia, and those with renal insufficiency on dialysis *(26)*.

HYPERTROPHIC CARDIOMYOPATHY

Besides age and ability to safely take anticoagulation, several specific issues in prosthesis choice merit consideration in patients with hypertrophic cardiomyopathy. Those patients with classic hypertrophic cardiomyopathy (not just hypertrophy due to hypertension or aortic stenosis) have a narrow

Survival

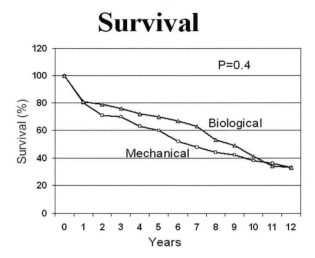

Fig. 7. Patient survival after randomization to mechanical versus biological mitral valve replacement *(33)*. Note at 12 years survival is quite similar.

Hemorrhage

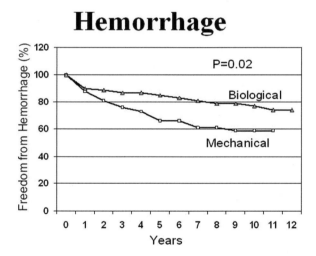

Fig. 8. Freedom hemorrhage after randomization to mechanical versus biological mitral valve replacement *(33)*. Obviously the warfarin requirement for mechanical prostheses increases hemorrhagic risk.

LV outflow tract during systole to where even the lowest profile and correctly oriented biological prosthesis in the mitral position may produce a fixed left ventricular outflow tract obstruction. Stented biological mitral prostheses are therefore relatively contraindicated in patients with hypertrophic cardiomyopathy *(34)*.

HYPERPARATHYROIDISM AND RENAL FAILURE

Second, patients with dialysis-dependent renal failure and patients with known hyperparathyroidism are at increased risk of premature calcification of implanted biological valve prostheses, even in periods as short as 6 months *(35, 36)*. However, mechanical prostheses are associated with a high incidence

Reoperation

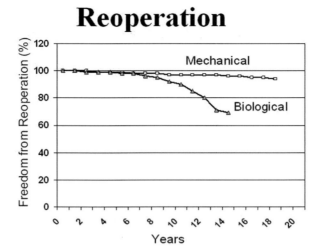

Fig. 9. Freedom from mitral valve reoperation after mechanical versus biological mitral valve replacement *(32)*. Again after about 9 years degenerative changes in the biological valve tissue begins to result in hemodynamic changes requiring reoperation.

of hemorrhage and death in dialysis patients (Fig. 10). In fact, the average life expectancy of a dialysis valve replacement patient is only 2–4 years, while the actual incidence of premature biological valve degeneration in dialysis patients is no more than 10%, as long as the parathyroid hormone level is well under 1,000 ng/L. Therefore, most groups are tending to use biological prostheses in dialysis-dependent patients despite recommendations that mechanical valves be the first line option *(36)*. Alternatives might be surgical or chemical parathyroidectomy to allow biological valve replacement in hyperparathyroidism patients.

Survival on Dialysis

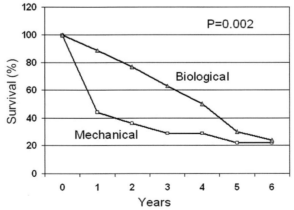

Fig. 10. Patient survival after mechanical versus biological mitral valve replacement in patients on renal dialysis at Duke University 1985–2002. Note that survival is similar at 6 years, with worse outcomes initially for patients in whom a mechanical valve is selected.

CALCIFICATION AND LEAFLET DEGENERATION

Several factors are becoming clear to delay calcification of native valve tissue, and these factors may be associated with improved durability of biological prostheses also (though as yet unproven). These factors are avoidance of oral and intravenous calcium supplementation in patients with biological valve prostheses *(37)* and use of statins in patients with biological prostheses *(38, 39)*. Oral calcium supplementation, though, may be critically important to help prevent osteoporosis in women, so its recommendation must be quite tempered. Evidence may be growing that current pericardial valves tend to fail by calcification and stenosis, while porcine prostheses (particularly in larger sizes) tend to fail by degeneration and valvular regurgitation. Thus patients with significant disorders of calcium metabolism might do somewhat better with porcine bioprostheses (other factors being equal), while patients requiring large bioprostheses might do better with pericardial valves.

CURRENT TRENDS IN VALVE REPLACEMENT CHOICE

While there have been many changes in the cyclical fashions of decision making, the current trend is to make increasing use of bioprostheses in the mitral position, although mechanical mitral prostheses still dominate in the United States (Fig. 11). This trend is related to the growing dissatisfaction among patients regarding the use of anticoagulation, the aging of the general population, the improved durability of current bioprostheses, and the growing possibility that percutaneous bioprostheses may be available in 5–10 years to replace a failed bioprosthetic valve.

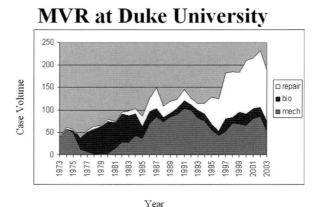

Fig. 11. Volume of mitral valve surgery at Duke University by mitral repair, biological mitral replacement, or mechanical mitral replacement. These data are similar to most large centers where mitral valve repair has progressively become more commonplace.

Concurrent Surgical Procedures

Several concomitant cardiac surgical procedures merit consideration at the time of mitral valve operation. These might include coronary bypass grafting, maze procedures, aortic valve operation, and tricuspid operation.

CORONARY ARTERY BYPASS GRAFTING

The indications for concurrent coronary bypass grafting are essentially the same as for isolated coronary bypass grafting. Any major coronary vessel with a 70% or greater diameter stenosis of a graftable coronary should generally receive coronary bypass grafting at the time of mitral valve operation. Ignoring significant coronary disease has NOT decreased the risk of operation, due to increased risk of perioperative myocardial infarction when the vessel is ignored *(40)*. The role for angioplasty of selected coronary arteries followed by less invasive approaches to the mitral valve (so-called "hybrid" procedures) has yet to be established but might exist in selected, older, higher risk patients *(41)*. These kinds of hybrid procedures may become more of the norm in the future.

MAZE PROCEDURES

While no standardized guidelines exist, possible indications for a concomitant maze procedure might be desired to avoid anticoagulation or failure of medical therapy to control symptoms in patients who either have a history of atrial fibrillation or to prevent atrial fibrillation in those at high risk for developing the arrhythmia. Risk factors for developing new postoperative atrial fibrillation include a history of prior atrial fibrillation, right or left atrial diameter over 5 cm by echocardiography, and age over 75 years. The maze procedure may have some theoretical benefit in restoring some degree of atrial transport function with further improvement of symptoms, but this is probably a more minor factor that has yet to be conclusively demonstrated. The downsides to a concomitant maze procedure are longer procedure times and higher likelihood of bradyarrhythmias that might require permanent pacemaker placement.

Many forms of maze procedure exist with different degrees of success and different morbidities. In general, the full Cox cut and sew maze III procedure will have the highest success rates, but also the highest morbidity and mortality *(42)*. The so-called "modified maze" procedures using cryotherapy, electrodiathermy/RF, laser, or microwave generally have lower success than the cut and sew maze *(43)*. Basic elements of any maze procedure include isolation of the four pulmonary veins with connecting lines between all 4 veins, exclusion of the left atrial appendage, connection of the pulmonary veins to the mitral annulus, connection of the superior vena cava to the inferior vena cava, and connection of the inferior vena cava to the tricuspid annulus near the coronary sinus. More extensive procedures involving multiple lines in left and right atria tend to have more success than simple pulmonary vein isolation. Factors favoring a more extensive maze procedure are persistent atrial fibrillation, severe atrial dilation, and a long prior history of atrial fibrillation. There are some data that restoring sinus rhythm by use of the maze procedure improves functional tricuspid regurgitation *(44)*.

ASSOCIATED AORTIC VALVE DISEASE

Concurrent aortic valve disease, either moderate aortic regurgitation or stenosis should be addressed at the time of mitral valve surgery to avoid the likelihood of early reoperation for residual aortic valve disease. Concurrent aortic and mitral valve replacement can compromise the ability to place an adequate sized aortic prosthesis (due to compression by the mitral prosthesis). This can be avoided by not oversizing the mitral prosthesis and by careful use of low profile, supra-annular aortic prostheses using simple, unpledgeted sutures.

ASSOCIATED TRICUSPID VALVE DISEASE

Indications. The operative indications for tricuspid valve disease remain poorly defined. In many, the TR is associated with RV dysfunction and pulmonary hypertension. With repair/replacement of the mitral valve, the volume load on the LV and the elevated PCWP should both be improved with a resultant improvement in functional TR. Though most TR is functional in nature, even mitral valve surgery may not restore the condition to normal. Severe tricuspid regurgitation should be addressed at the time of mitral operation to avoid early reoperation, to avoid persistent perioperative right heart failure, and to improve perioperative and postoperative hemodynamics *(45)*. Many patients in need of tricuspid valve operation today have already undergone prior mitral valve surgery, thus raising the issue of whether these patients should have had tricuspid operation at the time of their original mitral operation. Several factors predict a higher likelihood of at least moderate tricuspid regurgitation progressing after surgery *(45)*. These factors include intrinsic tricuspid leaflet pathology, placement of a transvenous pacing wire across the tricuspid valve, pulmonary hypertension, chronic atrial fibrillation, and prior sternotomy (Table 2).

Table 2
Risk Factors for Recurrent Tricuspid Regurgitation After
Mitral Valve Surgery

Tricuspid leaflet pathology
Transvenous pacing wires across tricuspid
Pulmonary hypertension
Chronic atrial fibrillation
Poor right ventricular function
Prior sternotomy

Tricuspid Repair Versus Replacement.   The factors predicting need for a tricuspid operation may also predict a higher likelihood of the tricuspid repair failing *(46)* (Table 2). In general, tricuspid repair will have advantages over tricuspid replacement as there is a lower incidence of heart block due to surgical injury, the avoidance of prosthesis durability issues in young patients, and the avoidance of anticoagulation. On the other hand, recurrent tricuspid regurgitation after failed tricuspid repair results in far more morbidity than tricuspid replacement. Tricuspid repair is generally the best approach in those with functional tricuspid regurgitation, in those with few if any of the above risk factors, and when the tricuspid valve that appears competent upon opening the right atrium during the surgical intervention.

Mechanical Versus Biological Tricuspid Replacement.   Bioprostheses are indicated for almost all adult tricuspid replacements *(47)*. Mechanical tricuspid prostheses should be reserved for the very young and healthy patient who can tolerate a high degree of anticoagulation *(48)*. Concern exists that mechanical tricuspid prostheses may have a higher but yet unquantified risk of sudden death due to thrombosis, low pressure gradients across the hinge wash jet, and relatively low flow velocities *(49)*. Mechanical tricuspid prostheses also exclude future use of transvenous pacing leads, unless placed in the coronary sinus, and make any invasive assessment of right heart and pulmonary function difficult to obtain.

Left Atrial Incisions

As with the chest wall incision, several approaches to the mitral valve have been used. The most common is to go directly into the left atrium in the right lateral wall anterior to the right pulmonary veins but posterior to the interatrial groove. This approach is most common in either anterior or right lateral chest wall incisions and has advantages of being very flexible, allowing wide opening of the left atrium, and being readily incorporated into pulmonary vein isolation for the maze procedure. The left atrium may also be opened through the interatrial septum exposed via the right atrium. This approach is limited to sternotomy incisions, provides a more limited opening in the left atrium, but needs less dissection and retraction of the heart. The left atrium can also be exposed through the so-called superior approach through the superior dome of the left atrium between the aorta and the superior vena cava.

This approach provides even more limited exposure, a short distance to the mitral, and a reasonable alternative for the superior partial sternotomy, for example. The left atrium may also be opened through the left atrial appendage via left thoracotomy, but the view of the subvalvular apparatus is poor enough to only allow mitral replacement or annuloplasty in most cases.

Chordal Preservation

There is now abundant animal and human literature to suggest that, in general, as many anterior and posterior mitral chords should be preserved as possible. Preservation of the posterior mitral chords has essentially eliminated the otherwise 2−3% incidence of intraoperative ventricular-annular disruption which carries up to a 40% mortality. Preservation of the posterior chords alone also improves postoperative ejection fraction, contractility and decreases left ventricular size *(50)* (Fig. 12). Preservation of anterior chords in addition to posterior chords further preserves overall left ventricular contractility. Disadvantages and caveats about chordal preservation include the avoidance of perivalvular leak around the preserved chordal tissue, avoidance of left ventricular outflow tract obstruction by bulky chords, and avoidance of prosthesis dysfunction by leaflet distortion from preserved tissue. A controversial but probably reasonable alternative to chordal preservation is to place artificial Gortex chords between the papillary muscles and the mitral annulus in the place of missing chords. This technique is under investigation at a number of centers and early results are quite promising *(51, 52)*.

Chordal Preservation in MVR

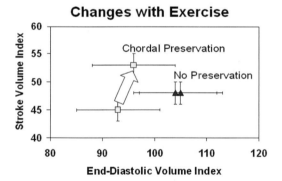

Fig. 12. Left ventricular performance after mitral valve replacement either with or without chordal preservation *(50)*. MVR after chordal preservation results in a normal exercise response with an increase in both LV end-diastolic volume index and stroke volume index with stress. Without chordal preservation the LV end-diastolic volume index is elevated at rest and neither the diastolic volume index nor stroke volume index increase with stress.

POSTOPERATIVE MANAGEMENT

General Considerations

In the current era, patients generally emerge from the operating room fully anesthetized and having just been weaned form cardiopulmonary bypass. Both general anesthesia and cardiopulmonary bypass have many physiological effects. First, the heart itself often has some degree of altered systolic and/or diastolic dysfunction due to hemodilution and the effects of incomplete myocardial preservation. These factors are in addition to the altered hemodynamics emerging from cardiopulmonary bypass of lowered systemic vascular resistance, hemodilution with lowered oxygen delivery to tissues, and elevated systemic catecholamines. Patients with any degree of preoperative contractility impairment therefore often benefit from 4–12 h of moderate inotropic stimulation in combination with light systemic vasoconstriction using agents like epinephrine or dopamine. By 12–24 h postoperatively, these agents are less often needed, and the effects of general anesthesia and cardiopulmonary bypass are largely reversed. Hemodilution leads to volume overload and hypoalbuminemia. Thus, most patients require more oral diuretic therapy postoperatively than preoperatively for 2–4 weeks after discharge. The most common cause of patient readmission after mitral surgery is fluid retention.

Atrial Arrhythmias

The second most common cause of readmission after mitral operation is atrial arrhythmias. Postoperative pericarditis develops in all patients to some degree over the first 3–6 weeks, with possible resultant clinical effects of atrial fibrillation, fever, leukocytosis, and pain. Anti-inflammatory medication like acetaminophen, ibuprofen, and steroids can ameliorate most of these effects with the exception of atrial fibrillation. Atrial fibrillation unfortunately seems to respond little to anti-inflammatory agents and is often exacerbated by the fact that most mitral valve patients come to surgery with some degree of preoperative atrial enlargement and/or atrial pathology. About 15–20% have had pre-op atrial fibrillation (53, 54). Beta blockade alone decreases the incidence of new postoperative atrial fibrillation from 70 to 50%, but it remains still at unacceptable levels on beta blockers alone. Transient use of an antiarrhythmic agent over the first 3–6 weeks can decrease the incidence of new postoperative atrial fibrillation to about 25% (55). There are some data that statin agents may also be effective (56). Inotropic agents clearly aggravate postop atrial arrhythmias (57). Antiarrhythmic agents all have side effects and must be individualized to the patient. Antiarrhythmic agents may be loaded preoperatively (58) (preferable but often impractical) or perioperatively. Common postop regimens include intravenous loading with either amiodarone or procainamide in the operating room, then conversion to oral amiodarone or other oral agents like sotalol for 3–6 weeks. Thereby, patients with little postoperative atrial fibrillation may be discharged safely with aspirin alone and no other anticoagulation (with no attendant risks of bleeding). Those patients felt at risk for atrial fibrillation after discharge may be placed on 1–3 months of warfarin depending on the duration of the postoperative atrial fibrillation.

Vasoactive Agents

Cardiopulmonary bypass and general anesthesia affect the entire body and circulatory system. Preoperative calcium channel blockers and angiotensin converting enzyme (ACE) inhibitors should to be stopped 24–48 h preoperatively to minimize postoperative vasodilation which can otherwise require potent vasoconstrictors as to cause visceral/renal injury. To minimize acute renal dysfunction, calcium channel blockers and ACE inhibitors are best initiated only after 2–4 days postoperatively.

SURGICAL OUTCOMES

Survival

Remarkably few randomized trials have compared mitral valve surgery to medical therapy. However, available retrospective data do suggest several conclusions. First, severe mitral valve disease by itself is associated with lower survival than the general age-matched population. Second, patient survival after mitral surgery is usually (but not always) less than that of the general age-matched population, but appears to exceed that of age-matched medical patients in the similar patient groups. Third, postoperative patient survival is heavily dependent on patient characteristics, including the nature and stage of the mitral valve disease. Evidence therefore suggests that mitral operation can offer survival value over continued medical therapy once mitral disease is significant enough to warrant operation but not severe enough that survival remains poor after operation.

Quality of Life

In addition to survival, patient symptoms and quality of life are factors of next importance that have been incorporated into the ACCAHA guidelines. Given the lack of randomized data, most surgical series show significant improvement in patient symptoms and quality of life by 3–6 months postoperatively relative to their preoperative condition after mitral valve surgery (59, 60). The greater the preoperative symptoms, the more the postoperative benefit, up to the point where the patients are so high risk that little benefit is obtained (usually due to irreversible organ dysfunction or irreversible deconditioning).

Ventricular Function

The effects of mitral surgery on left ventricular function have long been controversial but are better understood today than 30 years ago (60). Mitral surgery always carries some risk of cardiac injury and worsening of left and/or right ventricular contractility by a variety of mechanisms including perioperative myocardial infarction, air embolism, or inadequate myocardial protection. Fortunately, the likelihood of this occurring is low today, especially in higher volume centers. Another rare mechanism of postoperative ventricular dysfunction after mitral replacement is excessive resection of mitral chords (61). Finally, we now know that left ventricular ejection fraction is a load-dependent measure of contractility. Thus, postoperatively those with severe mitral regurgitation might be expected to have a fall in the ejection fraction simply as a result of altered loading postoperatively (60).

Reoperation

The likelihood of the need for reoperation depends very much on whether the mitral valve is repair or replaced, the age of the patient, the degree of underlying mitral pathology, and other comorbidity. The need for mitral reoperation after mechanical mitral replacement is <1%/pt-year (generally due to endocarditis, perivalvular leak, and thrombosis), as it is for mitral repair for posterior leaflet prolapse in most centers (1). The reoperation rate for biological mitral replacement increases over time, depending on the age of the patient, with most biological mitral prostheses having a 50% failure rate in the mitral position in 65-year-old patients at about 12–17 years (33) (Fig. 9). Mitral repair for anterior prolapse, ischemic disease, and rheumatic disease all have successively higher reoperation rates. Freedom from recurrent mitral regurgitation after mitral repair is less well quantified than reoperation. Several prospective series place the incidence at 80–90% freedom from 3 to 4+ mitral regurgitation at 10 years after mitral repair, depending on the preoperative pathology (1) (Fig. 13).

Perioperative Morbidity

Other perioperative risks of morbidity after mitral valve surgery are shown in Table 3. These risks have diminished with time and are very dependent on the procedure performed, patient characteristics, and the experience of the center performing the operation.

Recurrent 3-4+ MR

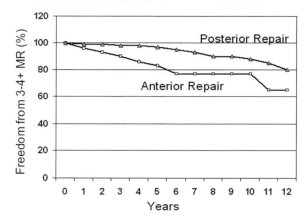

Fig. 13. Freedom from 3+ to 4+ mitral valve regurgitation after mitral valve repair *(70).* Recurrent significant mitral regurgitation is more common over time with anterior mitral valve repair than posterior.

Table 3
Perioperative Morbidity of Mitral Valve Operation. Modified from the STS Database 2002 (www.sts.org/sections/stsnationaldatabase/riskcalculator)

Complication	MV replacement ($n = 4,046$) (%)	MV repair ($n = 3,558$) (%)
Perioperative MI	0.4	0.3
Tamponade	1.0	0.8
Septicemia	2.4	1.0
Stroke – permanent	2.1	1.2
Reoperation – bleeding	5.1	3.2
Reoperation – valve	0.5	0.6
Reoperation – other cardiac	3.7	2.1
Renal failure	5.1	2.5
Deep wound infection	0.3	0.2
Ventilation > 24 h	12.9	5.0
GI Bleed or infarction	4.2	1.8
Any major complication or operative mortality	24.7	12.1

Atrial Fibrillation

Long-term, atrial fibrillation remains a risk for mitral valve surgery patients despite mitral operation *(53, 54).* This risk can be as high as 50% at 5 years in patients with sinus rhythm preoperatively (Fig. 14). The risk again varies tremendously upon the degree of atrial pathology and patient characteristics such as age. Atrial fibrillation can be less of an issue for the patient already on anticoagulation for mechanical mitral replacement, but anticoagulation (and probably even atrial fibrillation itself) is associated with a small but real morbidity and mortality in those patients who otherwise would not need anticoagulation. These are the arguments that have been made for concurrent maze procedures

Atrial Fibrillation

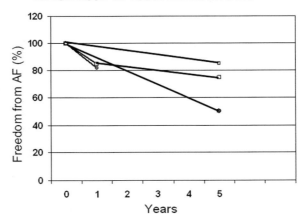

Fig. 14. Freedom new atrial fibrillation after mitral valve operation in patients with preoperative sinus rhythm. Data represent 4 contemporary studies with variable follow-up duration.

Maze in Mitral Operation

Randomized Trial, 35 patients with AF

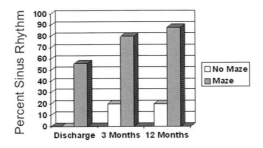

Fig. 15. Advantage of concurrent maze procedure on maintenance of sinus rhythm in patients with preoperative atrial fibrillation *(71)*. These data suggest an advantage for a maze procedure in these individuals.

in mitral patients, even in those without preoperative atrial fibrillation *(62, 63)*. The extent to which the maze procedure can decrease the likelihood of late atrial fibrillation is confounded by the lack of randomized trials, by the diversity of patient characteristics, but the varying definitions of recurrent atrial fibrillation, and by the diversity of maze procedures performed, each with varying success rates. Some series have documented 1-year freedom from atrial fibrillation rates as high as 98% for a full cut and sew Cox maze III to 60–80% for modified maze procedures (Fig. 15).

Permanent Pacing

Valve patients also carry an inherent risk of requiring permanent pacemaker placement both pre-operatively and late postoperatively. The late need for a new pacemaker again may vary, being more with mitral replacement than repair. After mitral replacement, the need is about 1%/pt-year, and about

0.5%/pt-year for mitral repair. Preoperative atrial fibrillation and concurrent maze procedure increase this risk due to increased likelihood of unmasking sinus node dysfunction *(62)*.

Endocarditis

Endocarditis is a long-term risk after mitral valve operation *(64)*. The risk is increased in the first 90 days after any valve operation to about 2−5%/pt-year versus 0.1−0.3%/pt-year thereafter. Thus elective dental work should be discouraged in this time period, and bacterial infections should be treated aggressively the first 90 days, with consideration of a 48-h period of intravenous antibiotics to achieve rapid control of bacteremia during any significant infection. Best evidence suggests that the long-term endocarditis risks of mechanical replacement versus biological replacement versus mitral repair versus native mitral valve disease all are about 0.1−0.3%/pt-year.

Thromboembolism and Hemorrhage

The risk of thromboembolism is greatest in those with a mechanical mitral replacement at about 0.5%/pt-year when on standard anticoagulation with an INR 2.5–3.5. The thromboembolic risk of a mechanical mitral prosthesis on aspirin alone is poorly documented but most certainly is more than the 5%/pt-year for a mechanical aortic valve on aspirin alone (Fig. 16). No data have convincingly shown that any of the modern bileaflet mitral mechanical prostheses have significantly different thromboembolic risk than any other. The thromboembolic risk is less at about 0.5%/pt-year for biological mitral replacement, and less for mitral repair *(65)*. The risk of hemorrhage depends heavily on the degree of anticoagulation used. Most series quote hemorrhage rates of 1–2%/pt-year after mechanical replacement *(66)* or atrial fibrillation. Several methods of bridging patients with transient removal of warfarin are available once the mechanical prosthesis is in place *(67)*. In general low molecular weight heparin is a satisfactory option to fractionated heparin *(68)* except in the instance where the patient is pregnant *(69)*. This generally allows for more easily administered therapy at home rather than requiring hospitalization and the need for serial aPTTs.

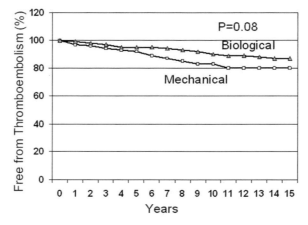

Fig. 16. Freedom thromboembolism after mechanical valve replacement and warfarin versus biological mitral valve replacement without warfarin *(72)*. Note relatively similar risks of thromboembolism.

REFERENCES

1. Bonow RO, Carabello BA, Chatterjee K, et al. ACC/AHA 2006 guidelines for the management of patients with valvular heart disease: a report of the American College of Cardiology/American Heart Association Task Force on Practice Guidelines (Writing Committee to revise the 1998 guidelines for the management of patients with valvular heart disease) developed in collaboration with the Society of Cardiovascular Anesthesiologists endorsed by the Society for Cardiovascular Angiography and Interventions and the Society of Thoracic Surgeons. *J Am Coll Cardiol* 2006 August 1;48(3):e1–148.

2. Reyes VP, Raju BS, Wynne J, et al. Percutaneous balloon valvuloplasty compared with open surgical commissurotomy for mitral stenosis. *N Engl J Med* 1994 October 13;331(15):961–7.

3. Abascal VM, Wilkins GT, O'Shea JP, et al. Prediction of successful outcome in 130 patients undergoing percutaneous balloon mitral valvotomy. *Circulation* 1990 August;82(2):448–56.

4. Ailawadi G, Swenson BR, Girotti ME, et al. Is mitral valve repair superior to replacement in elderly patients? *Ann Thorac Surg* 2008 July;86(1):77–85.

5. Jokinen JJ, Hippelainen MJ, Pitkanen OA, Hartikainen JE. Mitral valve replacement versus repair: propensity-adjusted survival and quality-of-life analysis. *Ann Thorac Surg* 2007 August;84(2):451–8.

6. Schaff HV, Suri RM, Enriquez-Sarano M. Indications for surgery in degenerative mitral valve disease. *Semin Thorac Cardiovasc Surg* 2007;19(2):97–102.

7. Sayar N, Lutfullah OA, Cakmak N, et al. Correlation of the myocardial performance index with plasma B-type natriuretic peptide levels in patients with mitral regurgitation. *Int J Cardiovasc Imaging* 2008 February;24(2):151–7.

8. Shimamoto K, Kusumoto M, Sakai R, et al. Usefulness of the brain natriuretic peptide to atrial natriuretic peptide ratio in determining the severity of mitral regurgitation. *Can J Cardiol* 2007 March 15;23(4):295–300.

9. Fundaro P, Tartara P, Vitali E. Moderate mitral regurgitation repair at the time of coronary bypass: when is it required? *J Thorac Cardiovasc Surg* 2004 November;128(5):796–7.

10. Waisbren EC, Stevens LM, Avery EG, Picard MH, Vlahakes GJ, Agnihotri AK. Changes in mitral regurgitation after replacement of the stenotic aortic valve. *Ann Thorac Surg* 2008 July;86(1):56–62.

11. Torracca L, Verzini A, De BM, Alfieri O. Influence of concomitant mitral valve dysfunction on survival after aortic valve replacement. *J Cardiovasc Surg (Torino)* 2007 December;48(6):797–800.

12. Srivastava AR, Banerjee A, Jacob S, Dunning J. Should patients undergoing coronary artery bypass grafting with mild to moderate ischaemic mitral regurgitation also undergo mitral valve repair or replacement? *Interact Cardiovasc Thorac Surg* 2007 August;6(4):538–46.

13. Kazui T, Osada H, Fujita H. An attempt to analyze the relation between hospital surgical volume and clinical outcome. *Gen Thorac Cardiovasc Surg* 2007 December;55(12):483–92.

14. Wu AH, Aaronson KD, Bolling SF, Pagani FD, Welch K, Koelling TM. Impact of mitral valve annuloplasty on mortality risk in patients with mitral regurgitation and left ventricular systolic dysfunction. *J Am Coll Cardiol* 2005 February 1;45(3):381–7.

15. Carpentier A. Cardiac valve surgery – the "French correction". *J Thorac Cardiovasc Surg* 1983 September;86(3):323–37.

16. Glower DD, Siegel LC, Galloway AC, et al. Predictors of operative time in multicenter port-access valve registry: institutional differences in learning. *Heart Surg Forum* 2001;4(1):40–6.

17. Feldman T, Wasserman HS, Herrmann HC, et al. Percutaneous mitral valve repair using the edge-to-edge technique: six-month results of the EVEREST Phase I Clinical Trial. *J Am Coll Cardiol* 2005 December 6;46(11):2134–40.

18. Block PC. Percutaneous transcatheter repair for mitral regurgitation. *J Interv Cardiol* 2006 December;19(6):547–51.

19. Svensson LG. Minimally invasive surgery with a partial sternotomy "J" approach. *Semin Thorac Cardiovasc Surg* 2007;19(4):299–303.

20. Rodriguez JE, Cortina J, Perez de la SE, Maroto L, Ginestal F, Rufilanchas JJ. A new approach to cardiac valve replacement through a small midline incision and inverted L shape partial sternotomy. *Eur J Cardiothorac Surg* 1998 October;14(Suppl 1):S115–S116.

21. Doty DB, Flores JH, Doty JR. Cardiac valve operations using a partial sternotomy (lower half) technique. *J Card Surg* 2000 January;15(1):35–42.

22. Chiu KM, Lin TY, Li SJ, Chen JS, Chu SH. Less invasive mitral valve surgery via right minithoracotomy. *J Formos Med Assoc* 2006 September;105(9):715–21.

23. Woo YJ, Rodriguez E, Atluri P, Chitwood WR, Jr. Minimally invasive, robotic, and off-pump mitral valve surgery. *Semin Thorac Cardiovasc Surg* 2006;18(2):139–47.

24. Folliguet T, Vanhuyse F, Constantino X, Realli M, Laborde F. Mitral valve repair robotic versus sternotomy. *Eur J Cardiothorac Surg* 2006 March;29(3):362–6.

25. Greco E, Zaballos JM, Alvarez L, et al. Video-assisted mitral surgery through a micro-access: a safe and reliable reality in the current era. *J Heart Valve Dis* 2008 January;17(1):48–53.

26. Rahimtoola SH. Choice of prosthetic heart valve for adult patients. *J Am Coll Cardiol* 2003 March 19;41(6):893–904.

27. Doenst T, Borger MA, David TE. Long-term results of bioprosthetic mitral valve replacement: the pericardial perspective. *J Cardiovasc Surg (Torino)* 2004 October;45(5):449–54.

28. Kulik A, Bedard P, Lam BK, et al. Mechanical versus bioprosthetic valve replacement in middle-aged patients. *Eur J Cardiothorac Surg* 2006 September;30(3):485–91.

29. Spoor MT, Geltz A, Bolling SF. Flexible versus nonflexible mitral valve rings for congestive heart failure: differential durability of repair. *Circulation* 2006 July 4;114(Suppl 1):I67–I71.

30. Mishra YK, Mittal S, Jaguri P, Trehan N. Coapsys mitral annuloplasty for chronic functional ischemic mitral regurgitation: 1-year results. *Ann Thorac Surg* 2006 January;81(1):42–6.

31. Acker MA, Bolling S, Shemin R, et al. Mitral valve surgery in heart failure: insights from the Acorn Clinical Trial. *J Thorac Cardiovasc Surg* 2006 September;132(3):568–77.

32. Hammermeister K, Sethi GK, Henderson WG, Grover FL, Oprian C, Rahimtoola SH. Outcomes 15 years after valve replacement with a mechanical versus a bioprosthetic valve: final report of the Veterans Affairs randomized trial. *J Am Coll Cardiol* 2000 October;36(4):1152–8.

33. Hammermeister KE, Sethi GK, Henderson WG, Oprian C, Kim T, Rahimtoola S. A comparison of outcomes in men 11 years after heart-valve replacement with a mechanical valve or bioprosthesis. Veterans Affairs Cooperative Study on Valvular Heart Disease. *N Engl J Med* 1993 May 6;328(18):1289–96.

34. McIntosh CL, Greenberg GJ, Maron BJ, Leon MB, Cannon RO, III, Clark RE. Clinical and hemodynamic results after mitral valve replacement in patients with obstructive hypertrophic cardiomyopathy. *Ann Thorac Surg* 1989 February;47(2):236–46.

35. Gultekin B, Ozkan S, Uguz E, et al. Valve replacement surgery in patients with end-stage renal disease: long-term results. *Artif Organs* 2005 December;29(12):972–5.

36. Herzog CA, Ma JZ, Collins AJ. Long-term survival of dialysis patients in the United States with prosthetic heart valves: should ACC/AHA practice guidelines on valve selection be modified? *Circulation* 2002 March 19;105(11):1336–41.

37. Izutani H, Shibukawa T, Kawamoto J, Mochiduki S, Nishikawa D. Early aortic bioprosthetic valve deterioration in an octogenarian. *Ann Thorac Surg* 2008 October;86(4):1369–71.

38. Brockbank KG, Song YC. Mechanisms of bioprosthetic heart valve calcification. *Transplantation* 2003 April 27;75(8):1133–5.

39. Moura LM, Maganti K, Puthumana JJ, Rocha-Goncalves F, Rajamannan NM. New understanding about calcific aortic stenosis and opportunities for pharmacologic intervention. *Curr Opin Cardiol* 2007 November;22(6):572–7.

40. Kasimir MT, Bialy J, Moidl R, et al. EuroSCORE predicts mid-term outcome after combined valve and coronary bypass surgery. *J Heart Valve Dis* 2004 May;13(3):439–43.

41. Byrne JG, Leacche M, Unic D, et al. Staged initial percutaneous coronary intervention followed by valve surgery ("hybrid approach") for patients with complex coronary and valve disease. *J Am Coll Cardiol* 2005 January 4;45(1):14–8.

42. Kosakai Y, Kawaguchi AT, Isobe F, et al. Cox maze procedure for chronic atrial fibrillation associated with mitral valve disease. *J Thorac Cardiovasc Surg* 1994 December;108(6):1049–54.

43. McCarthy PM, Gillinov AM, Castle L, Chung M, Cosgrove D, III. The Cox-Maze procedure: the Cleveland Clinic experience. *Semin Thorac Cardiovasc Surg* 2000 January;12(1):25–9.

44. Stulak JM, Schaff HV, Dearani JA, Orszulak TA, Daly RC, Sundt TM, III. Restoration of sinus rhythm by the Maze procedure halts progression of tricuspid regurgitation after mitral surgery. *Ann Thorac Surg* 2008 July;86(1):40–4.

45. Wang G, Sun Z, Xia J, et al. Predictors of secondary tricuspid regurgitation after left-sided valve replacement. *Surg Today* 2008;38(9):778–83.

46. Matsuyama K, Matsumoto M, Sugita T, Nishizawa J, Tokuda Y, Matsuo T. Predictors of residual tricuspid regurgitation after mitral valve surgery. *Ann Thorac Surg* 2003 June;75(6):1826–8.

47. Kuwaki K, Morishita K, Tsukamoto M, Abe T. Tricuspid valve surgery for functional tricuspid valve regurgitation associated with left-sided valvular disease. *Eur J Cardiothorac Surg* 2001 September;20(3):577–82.

48. Scully HE, Armstrong CS. Tricuspid valve replacement. Fifteen years of experience with mechanical prostheses and bioprostheses. *J Thorac Cardiovasc Surg* 1995 June;109(6):1035–41.

49. Shapira Y, Sagie A, Jortner R, Adler Y, Hirsch R. Thrombosis of bileaflet tricuspid valve prosthesis: clinical spectrum and the role of nonsurgical treatment. *Am Heart J* 1999 April;137(4 Pt 1):721–5.

50. David TE, Burns RJ, Bacchus CM, Druck MN. Mitral valve replacement for mitral regurgitation with and without preservation of chordae tendineae. *J Thorac Cardiovasc Surg* 1984 November;88(5 Pt 1):718–25.

51. Boon R, Hazekamp M, Hoohenkerk G, et al. Artificial chordae for pediatric mitral and tricuspid valve repair. *Eur J Cardiothorac Surg* 2007 July;32(1):143–8.

52. Gillinov AM. Artificial chordae for chordal replacement: commentary. *J Card Surg* 2008 May;23(3):207–8.

53. Jongnarangsin K, Oral H. Postoperative atrial fibrillation. *Med Clin North Am* 2008 January;92(1):87–99, x–xi.

54. Patel D, Gillinov MA, Natale A. Atrial fibrillation after cardiac surgery: where are we now? *Indian Pacing Electrophysiol J* 2008;8(4):281–91.

55. Echahidi N, Pibarot P, O'Hara G, Mathieu P. Mechanisms, prevention, and treatment of atrial fibrillation after cardiac surgery. *J Am Coll Cardiol* 2008 February 26;51(8):793–801.

56. Kourliouros A, De SA, Roberts N, et al. Dose-related effect of statins on atrial fibrillation after cardiac surgery. *Ann Thorac Surg* 2008 May;85(5):1515–20.

57. Fleming GA, Murray KT, Yu C, et al. Milrinone use is associated with postoperative atrial fibrillation after cardiac surgery. *Circulation* 2008 October 14;118(16):1619–25.

58. Khanderia U, Wagner D, Walker PC, Woodcock B, Prager R. Amiodarone for atrial fibrillation following cardiac surgery: development of clinical practice guidelines at a university hospital. *Clin Cardiol* 2008 January;31(1):6–10.

59. Sedrakyan A, Vaccarino V, Elefteriades JA, et al. Health related quality of life after mitral valve repairs and replacements. *Qual Life Res* 2006 September;15(7):1153–60.

60. Carabello BA. Indications for mitral valve surgery. *J Cardiovasc Surg (Torino)* 2004 October;45(5):407–18.

61. Rozich JD, Carabello BA, Usher BW, Kratz JM, Bell AE, Zile MR. Mitral valve replacement with and without chordal preservation in patients with chronic mitral regurgitation. Mechanisms for differences in postoperative ejection performance. *Circulation* 1992 December;86(6):1718–26.

62. Bando K, Kobayashi J, Kosakai Y, et al. Impact of Cox maze procedure on outcome in patients with atrial fibrillation and mitral valve disease. *J Thorac Cardiovasc Surg* 2002 September;124(3):575–83.

63. Ad N. The Cox-Maze procedure: history, results, and predictors for failure. *J Interv Card Electrophysiol* 2007 December;20(3):65–71.

64. Bashore TM, Cabell C, Fowler V, Jr. Update on infective endocarditis. *Curr Probl Cardiol* 2006 April;31(4):274–352.

65. Kulik A, Rubens FD, Baird D, et al. Early postoperative anticoagulation after mechanical valve replacement: a Canadian survey. *J Heart Valve Dis* 2006 July;15(4):581–7.

66. Hering D, Piper C, Bergemann R, et al. Thromboembolic and bleeding complications following St. Jude Medical valve replacement: results of the German experience with low-intensity anticoagulation study. *Chest* 2005 January;127(1):53–9.

67. Steger V, Bail DH, Graf D, Walker T, Rittig K, Ziemer G. A practical approach for bridging anticoagulation after mechanical heart valve replacement. *J Heart Valve Dis* 2008 May;17(3):335–42.

68. Meurin P, Tabet JY, Weber H, Renaud N, Ben DA. Low-molecular-weight heparin as a bridging anticoagulant early after mechanical heart valve replacement. *Circulation* 2006 January 31;113(4):564–9.

69. Mahesh B, Evans S, Bryan AJ. Failure of low molecular-weight heparin in the prevention of prosthetic mitral valve thrombosis during pregnancy: case report and a review of options for anticoagulation. *J Heart Valve Dis* 2002 September;11(5):745–50.

70. David TE, Ivanov J, Armstrong S, Christie D, Rakowski H. A comparison of outcomes of mitral valve repair for degenerative disease with posterior, anterior, and bileaflet prolapse. *J Thorac Cardiovasc Surg* 2005 November;130(5):1242–9.

71. Jessurun ER, van Hemel NM, Defauw JJ, et al. A randomized study of combining maze surgery for atrial fibrillation with mitral valve surgery. *J Cardiovasc Surg (Torino)* 2003 February;44(1):9–18.

72. Cen YY, Glower DD, Landolfo K, et al. Comparison of survival after mitral valve replacement with biologic and mechanical valves in 1139 patients. *J Thorac Cardiovasc Surg* 2001 September;122(3):569–77.

15 Surgery of the Tricuspid and Pulmonary Valves

Sapan S. Desai and Andrew J. Lodge

CONTENTS

Compared to aortic and mitral valve surgery, procedures on the tricuspid and pulmonary valves are relatively uncommon (Fig. 1). Consequently there is comparatively sparse literature on tricuspid and pulmonary valve surgery. The lack of large trials therefore requires greater clinician experience and decision making. This chapter will focus on the current issues in surgical decision making for the patient with tricuspid or pulmonary valve diseases.

TRICUSPID VALVE

Indications for Intervention

The decision to intervene on tricuspid valve disease is complex *(1)*. Isolated TR is typically well tolerated for many years until complications such as progressive right atrial and/or ventricular dilation, right ventricular dysfunction, congestive heart failure symptoms, or the development of arrhythmias arise *(2–5)*. TR may occur in the setting of other surgical valvular disease, such as mitral or pulmonary valve disorders; this secondary TR is the most common indication for tricuspid valve surgery *(2)*. Other indications include rheumatic in 11%, congenital in 9%, and other etiologies such as endocarditis, trauma, and papillary muscle rupture in 6% *(6)*.

In cases of severe TR with symptoms, intervention on the tricuspid valve is generally required. Assessment of right ventricular function is an important but not standardized variable for considering surgical treatment. The ACC/AHA indications for tricuspid valve surgery consider the presence of symptoms, pulmonary artery systolic pressure, and concomitant mitral valve disease (Table 1). If TR is mild, the general practice is to follow the tricuspid valve disease with the expectation that it will improve with relief of the volume or pressure load on the right ventricle that results from pulmonary or mitral valve intervention *(2, 4, 5)*. In cases where the TR is moderate or moderate to severe, there is

From: *Contemporary Cardiology: Valvular Heart Disease*
Edited by: Andrew Wang, Thomas M. Bashore, DOI 10.1007/978-1-59745-411-7_15
© Humana Press, a part of Springer Science+Business Media, LLC 2009

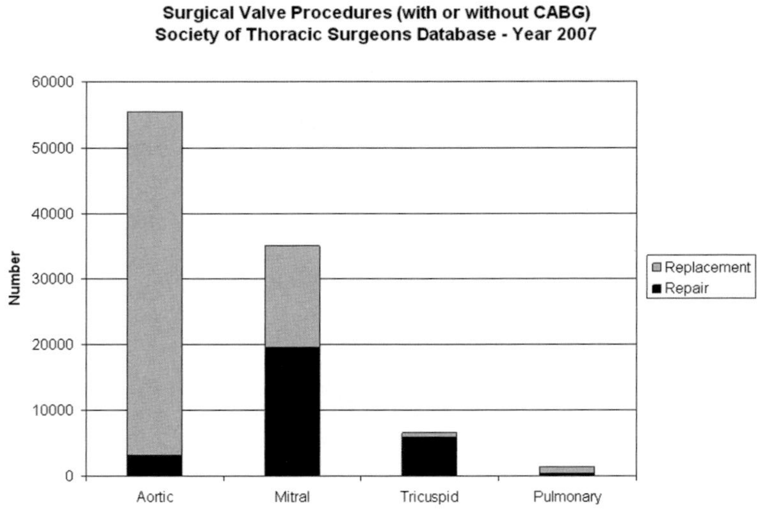

Surgical Valve Procedures (with or without CABG)
Society of Thoracic Surgeons Database - Year 2007

Fig. 1. This graph shows the number and type of valve procedures, either repair or replacement, performed (with or without coronary artery bypass) in the United States in 2007 according to the Society of Thoracic Surgeons database. There are many fewer tricuspid and pulmonary valve surgeries performed compared to aortic and mitral valve procedures.

more controversy *(2)*. If there is an identifiable lesion of the tricuspid valve besides annular dilation, then surgical intervention may be beneficial. Otherwise, the decision to operate on the tricuspid valve depends on the overall condition of the patient, their ability to tolerate additional cardiopulmonary bypass time, and the surgeon's expectation that a successful repair can be performed. These decisions require considerable surgical judgment and experience as there are no good outcome studies to guide

Table 1
ACC/AHA Guidelines for Surgical Intervention in Tricuspid Valve Regurgitation. Adapted from Bonow RO et al. *(7)*

Class 1A
- Annuloplasty for severe TR and pulmonary hypertension in patients with mitral valve disease requiring mitral valve surgery.

Class 2A
- Valve replacement for severe TR secondary to diseased/abnormal tricuspid valve leaflets not amenable to annuloplasty or repair.
- Valve replacement or annuloplasty for severe TR with mean pulmonary artery pressure <60 mmHg when symptomatic.

Class 2B
- Annuloplasty for mild TR in patients with pulmonary hypertension secondary to mitral valve disease requiring mitral valve surgery.

Class 3
- Valve replacement or annuloplasty with pulmonary artery systolic pressure < 60 mmHg in the presence of a normal mitral valve, in asymptomatic patients or in symptomatic patients who have not had a trial of diuretic.

therapy. It is important to realize that the intraoperative TEE may be deceiving as the degree of TR with the patient under anesthesia may be significantly reduced *(8–10)*. Greater reliance should be placed on the degree of TR on the preoperative TTE, although anatomic details may be more clearly delineated on the intraoperative study *(11, 12)*.

It has been suggested that one reason why primary tricuspid valve repair and replacement has a failure rate out of proportion to its perceived technical difficulty and anatomic accessibility is due to the preexisting comorbidities and level of decompensation that exists in such a heart *(13–15)*. The end result is that by the time patients are found to be a surgical candidate for tricuspid valve interventions, they tend to have advanced cardiac dysfunction, emphasizing the importance of diagnosis of tricuspid valve disease earlier in the course *(16)*.

Tricuspid valve degeneration necessitating surgery typically occurs in the setting of severe valve regurgitation that is easily detected on echocardiogram *(17)*. Precisely quantifying the tricuspid valve defect is important in order to opt for the appropriate surgical intervention, if one is even necessary *(17)* Minimizing the morbidity and mortality following tricuspid valve surgery may involve identifying patients who are eligible for this procedure while they are still in early stages of heart failure and prior to deterioration of the LVEF *(18–22)*.

The decision to repair or replace the tricuspid valve is based on many factors *(23–27)*. These include the etiology of the tricuspid valve disease, the degree of tricuspid valve pathology, the patient's age, the urgency of the operation, and other procedures that are required at the same setting. In general, repair is favored over replacement as all prostheses have their limitations *(28, 29)*. Since tricuspid regurgitation is most commonly functional in origin due to RV volume or pressure overload, repair is often possible.

Tricuspid Valve Repair

The tricuspid valve is relatively close to a number of important intracardiac structures. It is in fibrous continuity with the aortic and mitral valves and sutures placed too deeply can compromise the function of these structures. The right coronary artery runs along the anterior portion of the tricuspid annulus and is at risk of injury during tricuspid repair or replacement. Careful attention to placing sutures accurately and utilizing as much of the native tricuspid valve as possible will help to avoid injury to the mitral and aortic valves. The atrioventricular node is also in close proximity to the septal portion of the tricuspid annulus and is the most frequently injured structure in tricuspid valve surgery. The septal leaflet should generally be preserved and used to anchor sutures for valve replacement.

The tricuspid valve is in a favorable position for primary repair due to the lower pressures associated with the right heart in the absence of significant pulmonary hypertension. Replacement operations are typically reserved only for those patients who have demonstrated severe cardiac pathologies or have disease refractory to primary reconstruction. The large size and accessibility of the tricuspid valve also makes it particularly amenable to primary repair. Tricuspid valve repair is performed if the leaflets and chordal apparatus are normal or well preserved. This is the case in virtually all instances of functional or secondary tricuspid regurgitation. In this situation the main problem is annular dilation, and reduction annuloplasty is usually sufficient *(30)*.

There are a number of different options for tricuspid valve annuloplasty. The simplest is some form of suture annuloplasty where sutures only are used to reduce the annular diameter. This can take the form of a plication-type procedure such as the Kay annuloplasty, which is typically performed in the portion of the annulus corresponding to the posterior leaflet *(31)*. One or more pledgeted sutures are used to plicate the annulus such that the diameter is reduced and the anterior and septal leaflets become the primary functional leaflets (Fig. 2a). This type of repair may be particularly useful if regurgitation is limited to a particular commissure.

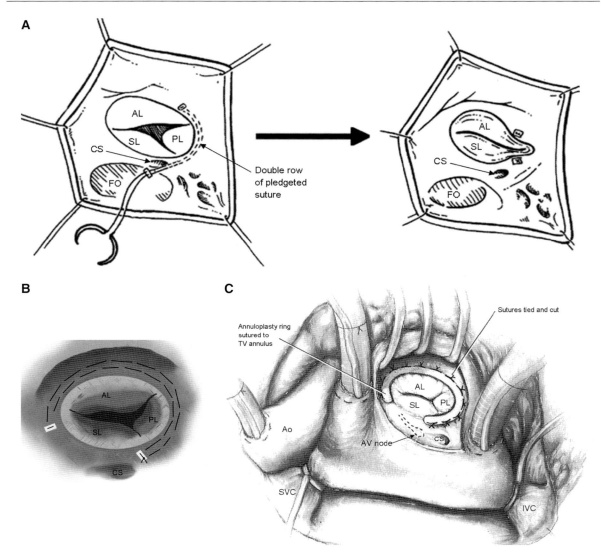

Fig. 2. (a) A suture annuloplasty resulting in "bicuspidization" of the tricuspid valve is illustrated. A double of row of suture has been used to plicate the annulus such that the anterior and septal leaflets become the functional portion of the valve. AL, anterior leaflet; SL, septal leaflet; PL, posterior leaflet; CS, coronary sinus; FO, fossa ovalis. Modified and reproduced by permission from Ghanta RK et al. *(50)* in p. 120. (b) A DeVega-type suture annuloplasty is illustrated. A double row of horizontal mattress suture, usually a nonabsorbable monofilament, is used to reduce the annular diameter to the desired size. AL, anterior leaflet; SL, septal leaflet; PL, posterior leaflet; CS, coronary sinus. (c) A ring annuloplasty is shown, in this case using a partial annuloplasty ring. Note that in this case as in Fig. 2b it is important that the annuloplasty extend to beyond the antero-septal and postero-septal commissures to prevent recurrent dilation of the annulus. Avoiding the remainder of the septal portion of the annulus avoids injury to the conduction system. AL, anterior leaflet; SL, septal leaflet; PL, posterior leaflet; CS, coronary sinus; Ao, aorta; SVC, superior vena cava; IVC, inferior vena cava; AV, atrioventricular. Modified and reproduced by permission from Douglas JM *(166)* in p. 388.

Another approach that is more commonly employed is the De Vega annuloplasty in which a double row of running suture is placed around approximately two-thirds of the circumference of the tricuspid annulus *(32, 33)*. The suture is usually buttressed on both ends with a pledget (Fig. 2b). The portion of the annulus corresponding to the septal leaflet is left bare to avoid the conduction system. It is important when performing this type of repair to ensure that the encircling suture extends just beyond the antero-septal and postero-septal commissures with the theory being that the non-septal portion of the annulus is more prone to re-dilation and that anchoring the suture in the fibrous septal portion will help prevent this. The degree of annular reduction can be individualized and calibrated by tying the suture over a dilator of known diameter. In general, it is difficult to downsize the annulus excessively and produce tricuspid stenosis. A diameter of 25 mm in small adults and 27 mm in larger adults is usually well tolerated *(34)*.

Suture annuloplasty procedures are not durable in the long term *(6, 22, 35–40)*. This may be due to re-dilation of the unbuttressed annulus or to sutures pulling through the tissue or breaking over time *(41, 42)*. For this reason, the utility of these procedures is limited. They may be useful in children who are still growing, with the thought being that the absence of prosthetic material will not excessively restrict annular growth and lead to later tricuspid stenosis *(35, 38, 43)*. They may also be useful in cases of secondary TR associated with lesions such as atrial septal defect or PI where there is moderate or severe TR *(39, 40)*. In this instance, correction of the primary lesion is expected to lead to sufficient unloading and possible remodeling of the right ventricle, thereby marginalizing the role of long-term annuloplasty.

The other alternative for reduction annuloplasty is to use an annuloplasty ring (Fig. 2c). In general these are commercially available products, some of which are designed specifically for the tricuspid valve and some of which can be used for either the mitral or tricuspid valves. In these procedures, the ring is affixed to the tricuspid annulus using a series of horizontally placed sutures. Most surgeons will select the size of the ring based on the distance between the antero-septal and postero-septal commissures or on the area of the anterior leaflet *(44, 45)*. The former measurement is preferred because this portion of the annulus is less prone to dilate and thereby represents a more normal dimension in the patient. The sutures are spaced more widely on the annulus than on the ring such that when they are tied, a reduction of the annular circumference is affected. Many surgeons will use a partial (non-circumferential) ring for tricuspid annuloplasty cases to cover the same portion of the annulus as the De Vega repair *(46–48)*. This avoids the placement of sutures in the area of the conduction system and thus greatly reduces the risk of heart block. It has generally been accepted that ring annuloplasty is more durable than suture annuloplasty, although some recent studies have again questioned this *(6, 49–51)*.

In rheumatic heart disease, the nature of the tricuspid valve disease may be stenosis rather than insufficiency. If the stenosis results primarily from fusion of the commissures and the leaflets remain relatively pliable and uninvolved, the valve can be repaired by commissurotomy. In these cases the chordae must be addressed properly to avoid subsequent significant TR *(52)*. Commissurotomy is typically reserved only for clinically significant rheumatic disease *(53–55)*. Indications for surgery for tricuspid stenosis include NYHA class III or IV congestive heart failure, risk of perpetuating infective endocarditis, significant functional or organic disease, outflow obstruction, or clinically significant congenital disease *(56–59)*.

Because the anatomy of the tricuspid valve is more variable than that of the mitral valve and because organic disease of this valve is less common, there are no standard techniques for complex tricuspid valve repair analogous to those used for repair of the mitral valve. The exception to this is for Ebstein's anomaly for which a number of somewhat standardized techniques have developed *(60–62)*. These techniques generally involve reduction of the annular diameter, plication of the atrialized portion of the right ventricle, and construction of a somewhat monocuspid valve with the anterior leaflet being the primary functional leaflet (Fig. 3). This technique is based on that pioneered by Danielson and Fuster, which includes plication of the free wall of the atrialized portion of the right ventricle, annuloplasty of the posterior tricuspid valve, and reduction of the right atrium *(63)*. Indications for surgery included advanced NYHA congestive heart failure, worsening cyanosis, systemic embolization, and accessory conduction pathways leading to tachyarrhythmias. Long-term results with 42 patients had a 7.1% early death rate typically from ventricular fibrillation; the majority of patients had a long-term improvement to NYHA class I or II.

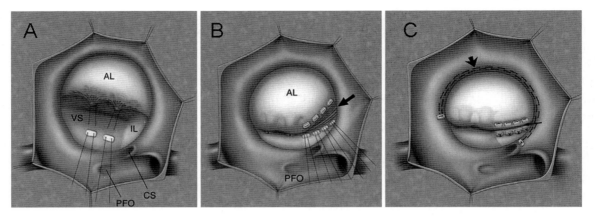

Fig. 3. Tricuspid valve repair for Ebstein's anomaly. **A**. Pledgeted horizontal mattress sutures are used to move the major papillary muscle(s) toward the ventricular septum. **B**. The posterior (inferior) angle of the tricuspid orifice is closed, placating the inferior leaflet. **C**. An anterior annuloplasty, in this case a DeVega-type suture annuloplasty is used to narrow the annulus. All of these maneuvers are designed to create a more functional, essentially monocuspid valve based on the anterior leaflet. AL, anterior leaflet; VS, ventricular septum; IL, inferior (posterior) leaflet; CS, coronary sinus; PFO, patent foramen ovale. Modified and reproduced by permission from Dearani JA et al. *(167)*.

Other forms of complex tricuspid valve repair depend on the individual patient anatomy and valve pathology, and so are left to the discretion of the surgeon. Similar to mitral valve surgery, tricuspid valve surgery should be approached with the intention of repairing rather than replacing the valve whenever feasible. In general, complex repairs such as leaflet resections or the insertion of artificial chordae tendineae are accompanied by a ring annuloplasty, a practice probably reinforced by the mitral repair experience *(64, 65)*.

In cases of traumatic regurgitation or endocarditis, primary repair is also occasionally feasible. There are several reports of successful tricuspid valve repair after traumatic injury, but most of these have been late presentations and the results of repair in the acute setting may not be as favorable *(66, 67)*. Ruptured chordae are often found in the chronic setting, and scarring may facilitate re-implantation or artificial chord placement *(68–71)*. In the acute setting of papillary muscle or chordae tendineae rupture in a patient with multiple injuries, it may be more prudent to perform expeditious valve replacement as the recently injured myocardium may not hold sutures well *(72–75)*. Tricuspid valve endocarditis that requires surgery may be reparable if the vegetations are sufficiently peripheral and the valve leaflets have not been excessively damaged. Debridement, small resections, and even reconstruction with pericardium can be performed. If extensive involvement is encountered, valve replacement may be a better option *(76–78)*.

The results of repair must be carefully assessed at the completion of the procedure to ensure adequate tricuspid valve competence and the absence of stenosis. This is more challenging in tricuspid valve surgery due to both the anterior position of the right ventricle and the tricuspid valve annulus, and the subsequent distortion of the annulus that occurs to sufficiently expose the valve. These features make the standard technique of instilling saline into the ventricle to pressurize it and close the valve somewhat less effective. Regardless, this remains the most useful technique of assessment with the heart still open. The practice of assessing for residual TR by finger palpation through a right atrial appendage purse string suture after weaning from cardiopulmonary bypass has rightfully been replaced by intraoperative TEE. Anything more than mild residual TR by TEE should be addressed as it will likely worsen in the postoperative period when the patient is awake *(79, 80)*.

Tricuspid Valve Replacement

Tricuspid valve replacement is undertaken when the valve is damaged beyond reasonable possibility of durable repair or when primary repair has failed. Specific tricuspid valve prostheses are not manufactured due to the relatively low frequency of use and because mitral prostheses can be used for this purpose. Unlike the case with the mitral valve where there is a relatively well-defined fibrous annulus, the tricuspid valve annulus can be relatively flimsy and difficult to discern. For this reason, as well as to preserve papillary muscle to ventricle continuity, the tricuspid valve leaflets are frequently not excised but instead used to secure the prosthetic valve sewing ring *(81)*.

Valves that are severely stenotic or involved with endocarditis may require excision of leaflets and chordae *(82–84)*. If the septal leaflet is excised, attempts are made to preserve a portion of it adjacent to the annulus to hold the sutures for the valve prosthesis. The valve is usually sized to fit the native annulus and can be quite large. It is not unusual for the annulus to be larger than the largest prosthesis available, in which case the valve sutures are used to downsize it. Braided polyester pledget-supported sutures are used, with the pledgets placed in the supra-annular position. After the valve is secured with the sutures, it should be inspected to ensure the sub-valvular apparatus does not interfere with leaflet opening. The valve implantation can usually be performed with the heart beating. However, in some cases, cardioplegic arrest may be useful initially to inspect the native valve, assess it for possible repair, and size it for the appropriate prosthetic valve or annuloplasty ring. The heart can be reperfused once this is done, and the sutures placed appropriately. The atrium is closed after air is vented from the right heart. The replacement valve is assessed in a similar manner as the repaired valve prior to leaving the operating room. In the case of valve repair, we recommend complete avoidance of suture placement in the septal portion of the annulus, which can virtually always be accomplished.

Finally, there are now early attempts to replace the tricuspid valve using percutaneous techniques *(85)*. At this time, all reports have been in the pre-clinical stage with no human interventions, so it is unclear whether this may be feasible in the future. There is certainly a growing interest in hybrid cath/OR laboratories, and the possibility of percutaneous approaches is of great interest.

The vast majority of tricuspid valve replacements are done with bioprosthetic valves *(3, 13, 15, 86–88)*. There are a variety of reasons for this, but foremost among them is the general feeling that mechanical valve prostheses are more prone to thrombosis in the right side of the heart than the left. This is thought to be due the lower pressure system with lower blood flow velocities and possibly more potential for stagnant flow. Avoiding the use of a mechanical valve also minimizes the limitations to right heart catheterization or transvenous pacemaker placement in the future. The use of mechanical compared to bioprosthetic valves remains controversial, and there are those that advocate the use of mechanical valves in the tricuspid position *(23, 24, 26, 89–92)*. There are a variety of stented bioprosthetic mitral valve prostheses that can be used in the tricuspid position. It has been traditionally felt that these valves are much less durable than their mechanical counterparts when used in the mitral position. However, reliable durability data for these valves when used for tricuspid replacement are not available. The presumption is that longevity will be better than for mitral replacement given the lower hemodynamic stress on the valve *(93, 94)*.

After implantation of a bioprosthetic valve in the tricuspid position, anticoagulation is usually recommended for 3 months, consistent with American Heart Association guidelines for aortic and mitral bioprostheses *(95)*. Patients in sinus rhythm after 3 months may fare well thereafter with only aspirin, but there are no published guidelines for this and the decision should be based on individual patient risk factors.

If a mechanical valve is chosen, postoperative anticoagulation with warfarin is required *(96)*. A postoperative heparin to warfarin bridge is typically reserved for patients who undergo a mechanical tricuspid valve replacement. While there have not been any major studies examining the target INR for patients with mechanical right heart valves, extrapolating from literature on mitral and aortic valves indicates that the target INR for these patients should be 2–3 *(97, 98)*. Limited studies indicate that the risk of thromboembolic events is higher with mechanical valves in the right heart *(99)*.

PULMONARY VALVE

Indications for Intervention

Most patients with clinically significant pulmonary valve disease have congenital heart disease. Pulmonary valvular stenosis is usually readily approached using percutaneous balloon valvotomy. Many dysplastic pulmonary valves require surgical intervention, as do those with a hypoplastic pulmonary annulus, severe PR, severe TR, or those in need of a surgical Maze procedure. Most of these will have had prior surgery such as repair of tetralogy of Fallot or an intervention for congenital pulmonary stenosis. Recent guidelines have been published and are outlined in Table 2.

Table 2
ACC/AHA Guidelines for Intervention in Pulmonary Valve Stenosis and the Surgical Training Required Are Outlined. Adapted from Warnes et al. *(100)*

Indications for intervention
Class 1B
- Balloon valvotomy is indicated in ASYMPTOMATIC patients with domed PS and peak instantaneous gradient by Doppler >60 mmHg or mean gradient >40 mmHg (with < moderate pulmonary regurgitation)

Class 1C
- Balloon valvotomy is indicated in SYMPTOMATIC patients with domed PS and peak instantaneous gradient by Doppoer >50 mmHg or mean >30 mmHg (with < moderate PR)

Class 1C
- Surgical intervention is indicated in severe PS with hypoplastic pulmonary annulus, severe PR or sub-valvular PS. Surgery is preferred for those with a dysplastic pulmonary valve, when there is severe TR or need for surgical Maze procedure

Class 3C
- Balloon valvotomy is not recommended in ASYMPTOMATIC patients with domed PS and peak instantaneous gradient <50 mmHg in the presence of a normal cardiac output.
- Balloon valvotomy is not recommended in patients with PS associated with severe PR.
- Balloon valvotomy is not recommended in SYMPTOMATIC patients with a Doppler peak instantaneous gradient <30 mmHg.

Surgical training
Class 1B
- Surgeons with training and expertise in congenital heart disease should perform operations for the RV outflow tract and pulmonary valve

There is also a growing body of evidence that percutaneous valve replacement, particularly for degenerated bioprosthetic pulmonary valves within conduits, will become a viable option in the near future *(85, 101)*. This section will describe many important aspects of pulmonary valve surgery.

Surgical Approach

Since the pulmonary valve is an anterior structure, exposure of the valve is relatively easy through a sternotomy but difficult through a transverse incision in the artery since the pulmonary artery is oriented in a more anterior to posterior direction. There are some aspects of the exposure that can be challenging. For example, the right ventricular outflow tract, and therefore the pulmonary valve, can be displaced quite leftward under the left hemi-sternum making exposure more challenging. The trajectory of the main pulmonary artery away from the surgeon also compromises visualization of the pulmonary valve. The left anterior descending coronary artery runs just to the left of the right ventricular outflow tract and care must be taken to avoid it, especially in reoperations where it may be obscured by adhesions. Occasionally a large conal branch of the right coronary artery crosses just below the pulmonary annulus and should be avoided during pulmonary valve replacement. More rarely, the left anterior descending may arise from the right coronary artery and follow a similar course.

Pulmonary Valve Repair

Of all the cardiac valves, the pulmonary valve is perhaps the least amenable to surgical repair. The major exception to this is congenital pulmonary stenosis. Here, surgical pulmonary valvotomy can effectively relieve the valvular obstruction. This procedure has increasingly been supplanted with percutaneous transcatheter balloon valvotomy, as noted above. When deemed possible by preoperative imaging, the pulmonary valve can be visualized via a transverse or longitudinal pulmonary arteriotomy. Commissurotomies are performed by incising along the fused commissures back to the pulmonary artery wall. Care should be taken to eliminate the obstruction as completely as possible. This sometimes involves resecting muscle from the infundibulum of the right ventricle to avoid obstruction from right ventricular hypertrophy due to long-standing pulmonary stenosis. Even if pulmonary insufficiency results, this is usually well tolerated over many years, although the patient may need later pulmonary valve replacement if the PR progresses.

In older children with a late presentation, a transannular patch may be necessary to completely relieve right ventricular outflow tract obstruction. This patch, typically constructed from glutaraldehyde fixed autologous pericardium or PTFE, serves to further enlarge the outflow tract by eliminating sub-valvular obstruction thereby reducing the risk of residual stenosis. This results in PR, but is typically well tolerated in the short term. It would rarely be necessary to replace the pulmonary valve during the same setting, as even substantial PR is likely to be tolerated for longer than a prosthetic pulmonary valve would last (102–106). The exception to this would be in a small child who has significant TR where replacement of the tricuspid valve is undesirable since the combination of PR and TR may be poorly tolerated. The decision to perform a transannular patch repair is tailored to the individual situation and dependent on surgeon experience. It is most applicable to growing children.

Pulmonary Valve Replacement

The pulmonary valve is the least frequently replaced cardiac valve (Fig. 1). As such, there are no manufactured valve prostheses designed specifically for the pulmonary position. Instead, valves designed for the aortic position are used. Valved conduits such as pulmonary homografts, bovine jugular vein conduits, and xenograft (porcine) aortic root grafts can be used for more complex right ventricular outflow tract reconstruction (107–109).

Most cardiac valve replacements are performed with interrupted mattress sutures of braided polyester that are initially all placed in the valve annulus, then passed through the valve sewing ring after which the valve is seated and the sutures are tied. Given the exposure to the pulmonary valve as described above, we have chosen to use a running monofilament suture to secure the pulmonary valve prosthesis to the annulus. Using a parachuting technique, multiple bites are taken between the valve

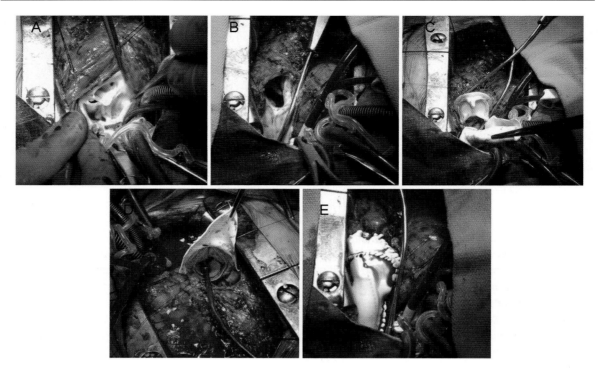

Fig. 4. The technique of pulmonary valve replacement is illustrated here in a series of intraoperative photos of a patient with previous surgery and severe PI. **A**. The pulmonary artery has been opened and the valve is shown with dysplastic and prolapsing leaflets. **B**. The valve has been excised and the RVOT is exposed with the back wall of the main pulmonary artery intact. **C**. A polytetrafluoroethylene (PTFE) patch has been sewn to the cephalad aspect of the pulmonary arteriotomy and a bioprosthetic valve has been seated in the RVOT with the posterior portion of the suture line along the sewing ring completed. **D**. The PTFE patch has been used to augment the main pulmonary artery and is secured to the prosthetic valve sewing ring anteriorly. **E**. The completed repair with the remainder of the patch having been used to augment the distal infundibulum.

and the posterior annulus after which the valve is lowered into the pulmonary artery and the anterior portions of the suture line are completed (Fig. 4). When using this technique, one must be sure that the posterior suture line is tight. This can be checked with a right angle clamp and is best done prior to completion of the most anterior portion. If the annulus is very flimsy or friable, the interrupted mattress suture technique may be preferred. Another potential pitfall when performing pulmonary valve replacement relates to the posteriorly directed main pulmonary artery. Care must be taken to ensure that the valve is oriented properly along the axis of the right ventricular outflow tract – the tendency is to tilt the valve anteriorly which could result in undesirable turbulence and valve wear as well as an increased gradient after implantation.

At the completion of the pulmonary valve replacement procedure, assessment of the result is more difficult than for the other cardiac valves. Due to the anterior and more distal position of the valve, visualization by TEE may be suboptimal. One should be able to determine if there is significant residual insufficiency by this method. If a gradient across the valve cannot be accurately determined and there is concern that residual obstruction is present, pressures can be measured directly in the right ventricle and pulmonary artery by needle puncture. Bioprosthetic valves can have peak gradients as high as 30 mmHg associated with them *(110, 111)*. A gradient higher than this should raise questions about a technical problem.

Pulmonary Valve Prostheses

The choice of prosthesis for pulmonary valve replacement is complex because pulmonary valve disease frequently involves the entire right ventricular outflow tract, and in many cases the patients have had prior surgery. It is not uncommon to address either narrowing or aneurysmal dilation of the infundibulum at the time of valve replacement. Similar arguments about the choice between bioprosthetic and mechanical valve replacement that were made for the tricuspid valve apply to the pulmonary valve as well *(112–115)*. As with the tricuspid valve, most surgeons will replace the pulmonary valve with a biologic prosthesis *(116, 117)*. Data on the longevity of stented bioprostheses in the pulmonary position are lacking as well *(118)*.

In cases where it is not desirable to implant a pulmonary valve prosthesis but that the resultant pulmonary valve insufficiency from a transannular patch-type repair will not be tolerated (i.e., elevated pulmonary vascular resistance), a temporary valve mechanism can be constructed. A variety of means for creating a monocuspid pulmonary valve have been described *(119–122)*. The most common employs an extra piece of PTFE that is sutured to a transannular patch and acts as a flap. It is generally felt that the functionality of these monocuspid valves is short lived, and it is not a viable alternative as a long-term pulmonary valve substitute *(123)*. It is mostly applicable in small children undergoing tetralogy of Fallot repair, but may be useful in other circumstances *(119, 121)*.

Stented bioprostheses are one of the most common substitute valves utilized. When combining this type of valve substitute with augmentation of the right ventricular outflow tract, even small patients can be implanted with a relatively large valve. In smaller children this is an advantage because implantation of an oversized valve is possible. The use of homografts for pulmonary valve replacement has not been as successful in the long term, except when used to reconstruct the RVOT during the Ross procedure *(124)*. This is likely due to the fact than when not used in the Ross procedure, the homograft occupies a somewhat non-orthotopic position. There is relatively little experience with the use of mechanical valve prostheses in the pulmonary position. In those series that have reported on this procedure, the results have been suboptimal *(115, 116)*. At this time we continue to recommend stented bioprostheses as the pulmonary valve substitute of choice.

Homografts and other types of valved conduits such as bioprosthetic valves inside a Dacron conduit, the valved bovine jugular vein, and porcine aortic roots can also be used for more complex right ventricular outflow tract reconstruction. For the smallest patients, homografts tend to be the conduit of choice as they are available in small sizes and have favorable hemodynamic profiles for small prostheses. Aortic as well as pulmonary homografts can be used, but pulmonary homografts are preferred, as their aortic counterparts tend to calcify and become stenotic earlier. The bovine jugular vein conduits can be used for older children and adults, and some studies have compared their performance with the homograft with favorable results *(125–127)*. The Dacron-valved conduits have fallen out of favor as they are less versatile and easy to handle than their tissue counterparts. The experience with the xenograft conduits is relatively young, and long-term studies are still pending. Preliminary results in children and young adults have been favorable *(128, 129)*. These conduits have the advantage, like the bovine jugular vein conduit, that they are readily available in a variety of sizes, which can be an issue with homografts, particularly in smaller sizes.

ADDITIONAL TECHNICAL ASPECTS AND SURGICAL CONSIDERATIONS

Reoperation Issues

Surgery on the tricuspid and pulmonary valves frequently occurs in the setting of reoperation, especially in patients with congenital heart disease. The resultant pulmonary valve pathology may include stenosis, but some degree of pulmonary insufficiency is almost always present. This pulmonary insufficiency is the most common indication for reoperation on the pulmonary valve. Surgical disease of the tricuspid and pulmonary valves frequently results in enlargement of the right atrium, right ventricle, and sometimes the pulmonary arteries. In patients that have had prior surgery involving the RVOT, such as tetralogy of Fallot repair, an outflow tract patch is frequently present across the pulmonary annulus. The enlarged right ventricle is closely opposed and frequently adherent to the anterior chest wall. The presence of prosthetic material may exacerbate the adhesions. This combination of factors can create the potential for significant problems with sternal re-entry. Careful evaluation of the anatomy and attention to the preoperative imaging studies helps to evaluate the risks. Angiography, computed tomography, and magnetic resonance imaging can be helpful in planning the operation. A finding of particular concern on the angiogram or MRI is a portion of the right heart that is immobile against the anterior chest wall, implying the presence of significant adhesions.

With careful planning, catastrophic cardiac injury is uncommon in the current era. A variety of techniques for sternal re-entry have been described. The option we prefer is summarized here. External defibrillator pads are placed on the patient outside of the surgical field. We selectively expose the groin vessels for cannulation depending on the particular anatomy. In practice this is fairly uncommon. Factors that might influence us to do so include multiple prior sternotomies, massive enlargement of the right atrium or ventricle, features on the preoperative images that suggest fixation of the heart to the sternum, prior groin cutdown, or a patient body habitus that would prevent rapid exposure of the femoral vessels should that be required. In smaller children, the iliac vessels may be used to place adequately sized cannulae. We make the sternotomy incision several centimeters below the xiphoid. In most reoperative cases this does not involve extending the original scar. The plane of dissection behind the sternum is established in this space. The oscillating saw is used to divide most of the sternal bone, but not the posterior table. Beginning from the most caudal aspect and working cephalad, the anterior table is elevated bilaterally with bone or skin hooks and the posterior table is divided with the scissors or saw. This is done under direct vision, which is facilitated by using a small sump sucker inserted between the heart and the sternum. Care should be taken to avoid blunt or blind dissection. Using this technique, if the heart is entered the injury should be relatively small. In this case the skin can then be rapidly reapproximated with penetrating towel clips, which usually results in a low level of blood loss that can be managed by the anesthesia team while preparations are made for peripheral cannulation for CPB.

In the absence of cardiac injury, once the sternum is completely divided the right hemi-sternum is elevated and dissection is performed on the right side. This usually facilitates exposure of the aorta and right atrium for cannulation for CPB. Sufficient dissection is performed on the left side to place a chest retractor. Once the cannulation sites have been exposed, as much dissection as feasible is performed before heparinization to minimize bleeding and cardiopulmonary bypass time. In most pulmonary valve procedures, minimal lateral and posterior dissection is required. Limiting this may decrease the potential for bleeding and postoperative tamponade. In tricuspid valve procedures, as in mitral operations, mobilizing the anterior and diaphragmatic surfaces of the heart will improve exposure to the tricuspid valve. At the completion of the operation, if it is anticipated that subsequent surgery is likely, one might choose to use some type of adhesion barrier to facilitate later sternotomy. We have used a PTFE pericardial substitute for this – a technique that does not reduce adhesions but creates a plane between the sternum and the epicardial surface. Other absorbable products to reduce adhesion formation are being developed and studied (130), and there is interest in using an extracellular matrix scaffold in the same manner which may actually help regenerate the pericardium.

Cannulation and Exposure

The tricuspid valve is always exposed by opening the right atrium. This is facilitated by placing venous cannulae in the superior and inferior vena cava, around which snares are placed externally to prevent blood from bypassing the cannula and entering the atrium. Bi-caval cannulation can be achieved by a variety of means. The superior vena cava can be directly cannulated through its anterior wall above the cavo-atrial junction or via the right atrial appendage. Placing the cannula in the appendage may help with retraction of the opened right atrium and facilitate exposure of the valve. In minimally invasive cases, a cannula can be introduced percutaneously via the right internal jugular vein. The inferior vena cava cannula can be placed through the low right atrium or the inferior vena cava itself. The former approach should employ a lateral placement of the cannula so as not to interfere with exposure of the annulus, whereas the latter approach involves dissection of the infra-diaphragmatic inferior vena cava (IVC) and runs the risk of troublesome bleeding after decannulation. The IVC cannula can also be advanced via a percutaneous femoral approach using long venous cannulae. If exposure of the valve is difficult using a transthoracic cannulation approach, the cannulae can be inserted directly into the respective caval vessel after the right atrium is opened, which may result in less tethering of the annulus than external cannulation. Prior to closure of the atrium, the cannulae can be replaced through the original purse string sutures.

When making the right atriotomy to expose the tricuspid valve, different options are available. All should avoid the sinus node area just caudal and slightly lateral to the SVC-RA junction. An oblique or transverse atriotomy can be made from the base of the right atrial appendage toward the space between the right lower pulmonary vein and the IVC. Alternatively, a semicircular incision can be used about 2 cm above the IVC cannula. In any case, a portion of intact right atrium should be left around the atrioventricular junction to provide purchase for a retractor. As stated above, if there are no atrial or ventricular septal defects, this can be done with the heart beating. This introduces the issue of coronary sinus return in the operative field, but this can usually be managed with cardiotomy suction.

Pulmonary Valve Exposure

Cardiopulmonary bypass for pulmonary valve surgery can be established with either aortic and right atrial or bi-caval cannulation. Exposure of the pulmonary valve should proceed by completely dividing the tissue between the aorta and the pulmonary artery. It is usually not necessary to circumferentially mobilize the entire main pulmonary artery. Stay sutures placed in the pulmonary valve annulus can help to elevate it into field and bring it to the midline. A vertical incision is then made in the pulmonary artery as described above. If there is a previous outflow tract or pulmonary artery patch present, the incision is usually begun through this. Occasionally a portion of the patch will have to be excised because of calcification. This type of incision provides good exposure to the pulmonary bifurcation, the annulus and to the sub-valvular area. If the main pulmonary artery is very dilated, a transverse incision can be used. It is occasionally desirable to completely transect the pulmonary artery to improve exposure. When a vertical incision is used, it is closed with a patch. We prefer PTFE for this purpose.

Myocardial Protection

Myocardial protection for operations on the tricuspid and pulmonary valves is rarely a major issue since at least a portion of these procedures can be performed with the heart perfused. If part of a larger operation, the other portion is usually performed using standard cardioplegia techniques. In most cases, if ventricular function is relatively preserved, a combination of antegrade cardioplegia and topical cooling of the heart provides sufficient myocardial protection. If tricuspid valve intervention is planned and retrograde cardioplegia is desired, the right atrium can be opened early on and the coronary sinus can be directly cannulated. If this approach is chosen a purse string suture in the mouth of the coronary sinus helps to stabilize the cannula. Once the procedure involving the left side of the heart is completed the cross-clamp can be released to finish the pulmonary and/or tricuspid valve portions, thereby limiting ischemic time and allowing a period of myocardial reperfusion prior to weaning from bypass. Some surgeons have found it useful to use induced ventricular fibrillation with the heart perfused to limit cardiac motion. If this technique is chosen, mild systemic hypothermia should be used to limit myocardial oxygen consumption. In cases where the heart is left empty and beating, normothermia or mild hypothermia can be employed.

Pacemaker Implantation

An important additional consideration for patients who undergo tricuspid valve surgery involves the need or potential future need for a permanent pacemaker. In patients who develop heart block during tricuspid valve surgery, consideration should be given to the implantation of permanent epicardial leads for dual chamber (or biventricular) pacing. These leads can be left in a subcostal subcutaneous pocket in case they are needed later. Patients that already have a pacemaker should have permanent leads placed and tunneled to their old generator pocket. Alternatively, a new subcostal pocket can be created. It is undesirable to have transvenous pacemaker leads crossing a prosthetic tricuspid valve, although it is possible in the case of a bioprosthetic valve. In certain tricuspid valve replacement cases where there is an existing transvenous ventricular lead and the patient is not expected to need future lead replacement, the lead can be placed between the prosthetic valve and the native annulus with sutures around it to preserve its function. An example of such a case is tricuspid valve replacement during left ventricular assist device implantation.

Alternative Approaches and Minimally Invasive Surgery

It is possible to expose the tricuspid and pulmonary valves through different incisions than a median sternotomy (Fig. 5). These alternative approaches can be so-called minimally invasive approaches and are applicable usually when the procedure is isolated the tricuspid or pulmonary valve only, although there are some exceptions to this. Pulmonary valve replacement can be performed through a partial upper median sternotomy. Tricuspid valve repair or replacement can potentially be performed through a partial lower sternotomy or through a right anterior thoracotomy using an inframammary incision. In these cases, peripheral cannulation for cardiopulmonary bypass may be required. The lack of requirement for aortic cross-clamping and cardioplegia in simple procedures may facilitate these approaches.

Hybrid Approaches

There is a growing interest and investigation into performing percutaneous transcatheter valvuloplasty and valve replacements. Much of the work is focusing on the aortic and mitral valves as these represent larger markets. The pulmonary valve may lend itself to such an approach (101, 131). Challenges to be overcome include the negotiation of a relatively large delivery system into proper position in the right ventricular outflow tract. A hybrid per-ventricular approach, similar to that described for muscular VSD closure, may provide a novel and less invasive strategy to implant such valves when they become available (132). Appropriate communication between the cardiologist and the surgeon will be important to ensure proper patient selection for these procedures, and, as noted earlier, the development of hybrid OR/cath laboratory rooms should facilitate this.

Intracardiac Repairs

As stated above, it is occasionally necessary to address an atrial or ventricular septal defect at the time of tricuspid or pulmonary valve surgery. In the case of an atrial septal defect, which is often a patent foramen ovale, it is a relatively simple matter to close the defect, although it does alter the conduct of the operation. During tricuspid valve surgery, the defect can be closed after the right atrium

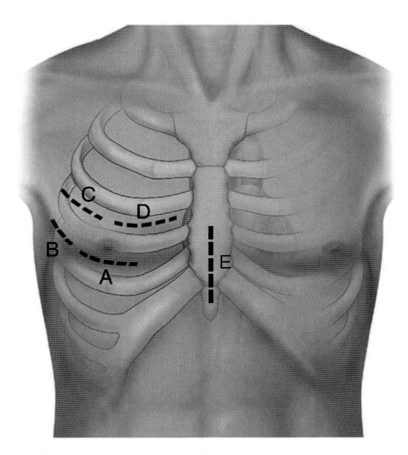

Fig. 5. A variety of incisions can be used for minimally invasive procedures on the tricuspid valve. A–D are thoracotomy incisions. Of these, C and D are used for port access procedures. E is a partial lower median sternotomy incision. F is a partial upper median sternotomy incision. Choice of incision is based on surgeon preference, the planned procedure, and patient anatomy.

is opened but before the valve is addressed using a brief period of cardioplegic or fibrillatory arrest. The heart can then be reperfused or defibrillated and the valve can be repaired or replaced. In these cases cannulation is not altered. In pulmonary valve surgery, however, additional dissection and a cannulation strategy that allows for opening of the right atrium must be added in addition to the period of arrest. Repair of the intracardiac defect can be performed prior to pulmonary valve replacement, which allows the heart a period of time to recover in beating state before the patient is weaned from CPB.

Electrophysiologic Issues

Perhaps some of the most common additional procedures necessary during tricuspid and pulmonary valve surgery are related to electrophysiologic issues. These patients not infrequently have arrhythmias. Given the advances in surgical technology available to treat such problems, as well as the greater recognition of their incidence and significance, such adjunctive procedures may become more common in the future.

Decision making related to such procedures is relatively straightforward. In the case of atrial tachyarrhythmias other than atrial fibrillation such as atrial flutter, a right atrial maze should be considered. In the case of tricuspid valve surgery, the right atrium will be well exposed and the maze lesions can be applied with the traditional cut and sew method or with a number of energy sources used to create the transmural lesions. This would typically be done after the tricuspid valve is implanted. In the case of pulmonary valve surgery, more additional dissection will need to be performed. If atrial fibrillation is present and a decision is made to perform a more standard Cox-maze procedure including the left atrial lesion set, a period of cardioplegia while the left atrium is opened is used. If this procedure is performed with tricuspid valve replacement, serious consideration should be given to the placement of permanent epicardial pacemaker leads given the relatively high incidence of pacemaker requirement in these patients.

SURGICAL OUTCOMES

Morbidity and Mortality

While the paucity of literature specifically examining tricuspid or pulmonary valve repair or replacement limits the conclusions that can be drawn regarding overall morbidity and mortality, certain parallels can be drawn from the extensive literature regarding mitral and aortic valve interventions. Primary repair of the tricuspid valve, while it may appear suitable for reconstruction, has had somewhat poor long-term results. It has been indicated that this may be a reflection of the increased severity of the underlying etiology, rather than limitations in technique or valve amenability to repair *(133)*.

The morbidity and mortality associated with valve repair and replacement is dependent on the particular technique and type of valve prosthesis. Repair, preserving the native valve theoretically has the highest chance of preserving the biophysical characteristics of the valve and the surrounding anatomy of the heart but data are lacking to support this. Prosthetic valve replacements sacrifice precise biophysical mirroring specific to a particular heart for simplicity in the form of a sewing ring.

Tricuspid Valve Repair

While early studies showed discordance with the apparent technical ease of tricuspid valve repair and the expected mortality rate, additional studies have found that this may be attributable to the more severe underlying cardiac pathology that is present in tricuspid valve disease *(134)*. For example, late survival in patients who have had primary tricuspid reconstruction is only 20% after 15 years *(135)*. The higher rate of tricuspid valve repair can also be attributable to undetected right heart disease in the setting of left heart failure; reoperation for right heart failure following left heart surgery has a high operative mortality and poor long-term survival *(6, 19)*.

The number of devices and techniques available for tricuspid valve repair are limited. Among these techniques include simple suture annuloplasty (De Vega repair), bicuspidization annuloplasty, and prosthetic annuloplasty. Simple suture repair, while accessible from a technical and anatomic standpoint, is limited by a significant rate of tricuspid repair failure with a 34% chance of recurrent regurgitation and 10% chance of reoperation *(20, 136, 137)*.

The De Vega repair is often used as a primary technique for reducing moderate tricuspid annular dilation. This repair involves plication of the annulus around the anterior and posterior leaflets and is the most common type of repair used for tricuspid valve surgery *(32, 33, 138–142)*. The high recurrence rate, especially with severe tricuspid dilation and pulmonary hypertension, limits its use; in these situations, the use of a ring repair is recommended *(136, 143–145)*. Recurrent tricuspid valve disease following primary suture repair is significantly greater compared to ring procedures, and the use of De Vega repair is falling out of favor. In one study, the recurrence rate of tricuspid regurgitation following De Vega repair was 45% compared to 6% with ring repair *(146)*. Long-term recurrent disease after 3 years was over 55% in those with De Vega repair compared to less than 6% with ring repair *(143, 144)*.

The use of a flexible prosthetic band for tricuspid valve annuloplasty has recently gained some support *(147)*. In one study, 53 patients with tricuspid valve regurgitation underwent primary repair of the tricuspid valve. Four patients died in the immediate postoperative period, but overall NYHA class decreased from an average of 2.7 to 1.4 (p <0.0001) and symptomatic right heart failure improved dramatically.

Despite the evidence described above, some forms of suture annuloplasty still have their advocates *(50)*. In fact, in certain clinical settings such as in patients with severe endocarditis techniques such as bicuspidization (as described for Ebstein's anomaly) may be useful by avoiding severe TR in cases where valvulectomy may be contemplated *(148)*. Mid-term results at 3 years have suggested that bicuspidization is effective at reducing tricuspid regurgitation with results similar to patients who receive ring annuloplasty, perhaps making it an attractive option in situations where prosthetic rings are not as available.

Tricuspid Valve Replacement

Long-term results with tricuspid valve replacement are limited. One study followed 42 patients over a 17-year period that underwent isolated tricuspid valve replacement or combined tricuspid with mitral or aortic valve replacement *(13)*. One third of patients had a mechanical valve; the remainder had a bioprosthetic implant. They found that over a quarter of patients died in the immediate postoperative period. Ten-year survival was 37% and 10-year event-free survival was 31%. These long-term survival curves were strongly affected by the underlying etiology of the valve disease. Patients with congenital disease had a 53% 10-year survival; those with underlying rheumatic disease had a 41% survival. These results are in line with those reported by other investigators *(3, 25, 27, 149–151)*. Theories to explain the higher failure rate with TV replacement surgery include changes in flow dynamics and pressure changes from the rigid circular frame of prosthetic valves which may lead to septal distortion with subsequent remodeling and decompensation by the remainder of the ventricle and heart, and the lower pressures of the right heart that may be affected by these physiologic parameters increasing the sensitivity to seemingly minor biophysical characteristics of various heart valves *(13, 91)*.

The tricuspid valve may also be amenable to replacement using a mitral valve homograft. Though initial studies, especially from experimental models involving animals, indicated a disproportionately high failure rate, additional studies regarding the anatomic changes following transplantation with adjustment of postsurgical management have significantly improved morbidity and mortality *(152)*. This procedure remains somewhat obscure and uncommon due to the lack of standardization of technique and anatomic distortion of the homograft related to difference between the two valves. The most common complications following homograft valve replacement include papillary muscle rupture, chordal rupture, dehiscence of leaflet suture, homograft mismatch, and late failure due to stenosis or, less commonly, regurgitation *(153, 154)*.

McGrath indicates that tricuspid valve procedures are approximately 6% of all valvular operations *(135)*. The rate of postoperative regurgitation is nearly 15% when considering all tricuspid procedures, while the rate of reoperation for replacement of the valve is nearly 8%. Other studies cite early mortality and reoperation rates between 10 and 30%. Five-year survival is 50—70% while overall 10-year survival is 40% *(27, 28, 91, 92, 155–158)*. The primary cause of death in the early postoperative period is right heart failure due to ventricular dysfunction. Preoperative indicators of this type of failure include preoperative right heart failure, limited functional capacity, length of time on bypass, and the presence of additional valvular disease. Late postoperative mortality is influenced by preoperative fluid status, length of aortic cross-clamping, pulmonary artery pressures, tricuspid valve size, advanced age, and prior operation *(13)*.

Numerous studies have indicated that there is no difference in survival or outcome between mechanical heart valves or bioprosthetic valves *(26, 27, 149, 159–163)*. Bioprosthetic valves are preferred by some surgeons due to the lower pressures and stresses in the right heart. Studies seem to favor larger prostheses when bioprosthetic valves are used. Mechanical heart valves are limited by the requirement for lifelong anticoagulation with all of its attendant complications and risks and the incidence of thromboembolic events. Bileaflet valves are preferred when mechanical heart valves are used due to their improved biophysical characteristics, improved flow dynamics, decreased shear stress, and improved durability. Bioprosthetic valves have a durability of 7 years on average *(27)*.

Pulmonary Valve Repair and Replacement

The most common long-term complication of primary pulmonary valve repair is moderate to severe pulmonary regurgitation (37%). Over time this leads to volume overload of the right ventricle causing right ventricular dilation. Secondary effects include tricuspid regurgitation, right atrial dilation, arrhythmias, and right ventricular dysfunction. At one time it was felt that pulmonary regurgitation would be well tolerated long term, but current thinking tends toward intervention before these complications occur.

Long-term results of pulmonary valve replacement are generally favorable. A recent study documented a 20-year actuarial survival of 92.3% overall, and a 15-year valve-related event-free ratio of 85.7% for bioprosthetic and 66.7% for mechanical valve replacements *(164)*. Another recent report showed a 22% incidence of late prosthetic valve dysfunction, a freedom from valve explantation at 5 years of 78–92% depending on valve prosthesis type *(165)*. Longer term data and larger series are lacking.

SUMMARY

Surgery for tricuspid and pulmonary valve disease, which often occurs in the setting of other cardiac disease and prior cardiac surgeries, is less common than for mitral and aortic pathology. As a result of these factors, operative and long-term outcomes are variable. Surgical decision making, in collaboration with cardiologists and cardiac anesthesiologists, must consider and address often complex preoperative, procedural, and postoperative factors to achieve the optimal outcome for the individual patient.

REFERENCES

1. Waller BF, Howard J, Fess S. Pathology of tricuspid valve stenosis and pure tricuspid regurgitation – Part III. Clin Cardiol 1995;18(4):225–30.
2. Peterffy A, Szentkiralyi I, Galajda Z. Tricuspid valve repair: indication and type of repair. J Thorac Cardiovasc Surg 2007;134(1):266–7; author reply 267.
3. Filsoufi F, et al. Long-term outcomes of tricuspid valve replacement in the current era. Ann Thorac Surg 2005;80(3):845–50.
4. Shatapathy P, Aggarwal BK, Kamath SG. Tricuspid valve repair: a rational alternative. J Heart Valve Dis 2000;9(2):276–82.
5. Schoevaerdts JC, et al. Tricuspid valve surgery. J Cardiovasc Surg (Torino) 1977;18(4):397–9.
6. Tang GH, et al. Tricuspid valve repair with an annuloplasty ring results in improved long-term outcomes. Circulation 2006;114(Suppl 1):577–81.
7. Bonow RO, et al. ACC/AHA 2006 guidelines for the management of patients with valvular heart disease: a report of the American College of Cardiology/American Heart Association Task Force on Practice Guidelines (writing Committee to revise the 1998 guidelines for the management of patients with valvular heart disease) developed in collaboration

with the Society of Cardiovascular Anesthesiologists endorsed by the Society for Cardiovascular Angiography and Interventions and the Society of Thoracic Surgeons. J Am Coll Cardiol 2006;48(3):e1–148.

8. Borges AC, et al. Dynamic three-dimensional transesophageal echocardiography using a computed tomographic imaging probe – clinical potential and limitation. Int J Card Imaging 1995;11(4):247–54.

9. Meloni L, et al. Intraoperative echocardiography by a new miniaturized epicardial probe: preliminary findings. Echocardiography 1993; 10(4):351–8.

10. Kin N. [Intraoperative transesophageal echocardiography]. Kyobu Geka 2007;60(Suppl 8):674–9.

11. Lee KK, et al. Off-pump tricuspid valve replacement for severe infective endocarditis. Ann Thorac Surg 2007;84(1):309–11.

12. Smith ST, et al. Transthoracic and transesophageal echocardiography in the diagnosis and surgical management of right atrial myxoma. Chest 1991;100(2):575–6.

13. Iscan ZH, et al. What to expect after tricuspid valve replacement? Long-term results. Eur J Cardiothorac Surg 2007;32(2):296–300.

14. Bossone E, et al. Valve surgery in octogenarians: in-hospital and long-term outcomes. Can J Cardiol 2007;23(3): 223–7.

15. Chang BC, et al. Long-term clinical results of tricuspid valve replacement. Ann Thorac Surg 2006;81(4):1317–23; discussion 1323–4.

16. Shah PM, Raney AA. Tricuspid valve disease. Curr Probl Cardiol 2008;33(2):47–84.

17. Kratz JM, et al. Trends and results in tricuspid valve surgery. Chest 1985;88(6):837–40.

18. Bajzer CT, et al. Tricuspid valve surgery and intraoperative echocardiography: factors affecting survival, clinical outcome, and echocardiographic success. J Am Coll Cardiol 1998;32(4):1023–31.

19. Staab ME, Nishimura RA, Dearani JA. Isolated tricuspid valve surgery for severe tricuspid regurgitation following prior left heart valve surgery: analysis of outcome in 34 patients. J Heart Valve Dis 1999;8(5):567–74.

20. De Paulis R, et al. The De Vega tricuspid annuloplasty. Perioperative mortality and long term follow-up. J Cardiovasc Surg (Torino) 1990;31(4):512–17.

21. Czer LS, et al. Tricuspid valve repair. Operative and follow-up evaluation by Doppler color flow mapping. J Thorac Cardiovasc Surg 1989;98(1):101–10; discussion 110–1.

22. Holper K, et al. Surgery for tricuspid insufficiency: long-term follow-up after De Vega annuloplasty. Thorac Cardiovasc Surg 1993;41(1):1–8.

23. Solomon NA, et al. Tricuspid valve replacement: bioprosthetic or mechanical valve? Asian Cardiovasc Thorac Ann 2004;12(2):143–8.

24. Rizzoli G, et al. Biological or mechanical prostheses in tricuspid position? A meta-analysis of intra-institutional results. Ann Thorac Surg 2004;77(5):1607–14.

25. Kaplan M, et al. Prosthetic replacement of tricuspid valve: bioprosthetic or mechanical. Ann Thorac Surg 2002;73(2):467–73.

26. Del Campo C, Sherman JR. Tricuspid valve replacement: results comparing mechanical and biological prostheses. Ann Thorac Surg 2000;69(4):1295.

27. Ratnatunga CP, et al. Tricuspid valve replacement: UK Heart Valve Registry mid-term results comparing mechanical and biological prostheses. Ann Thorac Surg 1998;66(6):1940–7.

28. Singh AK, et al. Follow-up assessment of St. Jude Medical prosthetic valve in the tricuspid position: clinical and hemodynamic results. Ann Thorac Surg 1984;37(4):324–7.

29. Unger F, et al. Standards and concepts in valve surgery. J Cardiovasc Surg (Torino) 2000;41(4):585–93.

30. Hecart J, et al. Technique for tricuspid annuloplasty with a flexible linear reducer: medium-term results. J Thorac Cardiovasc Surg 1980;79(5):689–92.

31. Kay JH, Maselli-Campagna G, Tsuji KK. Surgical treatment of tricuspid insufficiency. Ann Surg 1965;162:53–8.

32. de Vega NG, de Rabago G, Castillon L. Triple replacement of the tricuspid valve. Ann Chir Thorac Cardiovasc 1973;12(1):61–2.

33. De Vega NG, et al. A new tricuspid repair. Short-term clinical results in 23 cases. J Cardiovasc Surg (Torino) 1973;Spec No:384–6.

34. Paone SA. Mastery of Cardiothoracic Surgery. Lippincott-Raven Publishers, Philadelphia PA and New York, NY 1998; pp. 356–7.

35. Choudhary SK, et al. Mitral valve repair in a predominantly rheumatic population. Long-term results. Tex Heart Inst J 2001;28(1):8–15.

36. Duebener LF, et al. Mitral-valve repair without annuloplasty rings: results after repair of anterior leaflet versus posterior-leaflet defects using polytetrafluoroethylene sutures for chordal replacement. Eur J Cardiothorac Surg 2000;17(3):206–12.

37. Aoyagi S, et al. Long-term results of mitral valve repair for non-rheumatic mitral regurgitation. Cardiovasc Surg 1995;3(4):387–92.

38. Kalil RA, et al. Late outcome of unsupported annuloplasty for rheumatic mitral regurgitation. J Am Coll Cardiol 1993;22(7):1915–20.
39. Hashimoto K, Arai T, Kurosawa H. Technical considerations and intermediate-term results with modified DeVega tricuspid annuloplasty. Cardiovasc Surg 1993;1(5):573–6.
40. Rabago G, et al. The new De Vega technique in tricuspid annuloplasty (results in 150 patients). J Cardiovasc Surg (Torino) 1980;21(2):231–8.
41. Zegdi R, et al. Long-term results of mitral valve repair in active endocarditis. Circulation 2005;111(19):2532–6.
42. Mavroudis C, Backer CL. Surgical management of severe truncal insufficiency: experience with truncal valve remodeling techniques. Ann Thorac Surg 2001;72(2):396–400.
43. Talwar S, et al. Mitral valve repair in children with rheumatic heart disease. J Thorac Cardiovasc Surg 2005;129(4):875–9.
44. Maisano F, et al. Annular-to-leaflet mismatch and the need for reductive annuloplasty in patients undergoing mitral repair for chronic mitral regurgitation due to mitral valve prolapse. Am J Cardiol 2007;99(10):1434–9.
45. Duran CM, et al. The vanishing tricuspid annuloplasty. A new concept. J Thorac Cardiovasc Surg 1992;104(3):796–801.
46. Gatti G, Pacilli P, Pugliese P. Tricuspid valve annuloplasty using a partial flexible ring: mid-term follow-up. Ital Heart J 2003;4(2):121–4.
47. Maazouzi W, et al. The incomplete ring with modulated flexibility: a new concept of mitral annuloplasty. Surg Technol Int 2002;10:151–5.
48. Timek TA, et al. Will a partial posterior annuloplasty ring prevent acute ischemic mitral regurgitation? Circulation 2002;106(12 suppl 1):I33–9.
49. Grondin P, et al. Carpentier's annulus and De Vegas annuloplasty. The end of the tricuspid challenge. J Thorac Cardiovasc Surg 1975;70(5):852–61.
50. Ghanta RK, et al. Suture bicuspidization of the tricuspid valve versus ring annuloplasty for repair of functional tricuspid regurgitation: midterm results of 237 consecutive patients. J Thorac Cardiovasc Surg 2007;133(1):117–26.
51. Fundaro P, et al. Mitral valve repair: is there still a place for suture annuloplasty? Asian Cardiovasc Thorac Ann 2007;15(4):351–8.
52. Revuelta JM, Garcia-Rinaldi M, Duran CM. Tricuspid commissurotomy. Ann Thorac Surg 1985;39(5):489–91.
53. Choudhary SK, et al. Open mitral commissurotomy in the current era: indications, technique, and results. Ann Thorac Surg 2003;75(1):41–6.
54. Colonna D, et al. [Indications and results of tricuspid commissurotomy]. Coeur Med Interne 1969;8(2):209–20.
55. Gueron M, et al. Isolated tricuspid valvular stenosis. The pathology and merits of surgical treatment. J Thorac Cardiovasc Surg 1972;63(5):760–4.
56. Duran CM, Tricuspid valve surgery revisited. J Card Surg 1994;9(2):242–7.
57. Cobanoglu A, Starr A. Tricuspid valve surgery: indications, methods, and results. Cardiovasc Clin 1986;16(2):375–87.
58. Kouchoukos NT, Stephenson LW. Indications for and results of tricuspid valve replacement. Adv Cardiol 1976;17:199–206.
59. Ellis LB. Indications for surgery in patients with acquired valvular disease. Cardiovasc Clin 1971;3(2):61–9.
60. Chen JM, et al. Early and medium-term results for repair of Ebstein anomaly. J Thorac Cardiovasc Surg 2004;127(4):990–8; discussion 998–9.
61. Knott-Craig CJ, et al. Repair of Ebstein's anomaly in the symptomatic neonate: an evolution of technique with 7-year follow-up. Ann Thorac Surg 2002;73:1786–93.
62. Mehrizi A, Folger GM Jr, Puri P. Ebstein malformation of the tricuspid valve associated with ventricular septal defect. Bull Johns Hopkins Hosp 1965;116:89–94.
63. Danielson GK, Fuster V. Surgical repair of Ebstein's anomaly. Ann Surg 1982;196(4):499–504.
64. Katz NM, Pallas RS. Traumatic rupture of the tricuspid valve: repair by chordal replacements and annuloplasty. J Thorac Cardiovasc Surg 1986;91(2):310–4.
65. Revuelta JM, Garcia-Rinaldi R, Duran CM. Conservative repair of the mitral and tricuspid valves: eight years experience with Duran flexible ring annuloplasty. Bol Asoc Med P R 1984;76(10):429–41.
66. Fujiwara K, et al. Successful repair of traumatic tricuspid valve regurgitation. Jpn J Thorac Cardiovasc Surg 2005;53(5):259–62.
67. Kleikamp G, et al. Tricuspid valve regurgitation following blunt thoracic trauma. Chest 1992;102(4):1294–6.
68. Filsoufi F, Carpentier A. Principles of reconstructive surgery in degenerative mitral valve disease. Semin Thorac Cardiovasc Surg 2007;19(2):103–10.
69. Tomaru T, et al. Postinflammatory mitral and aortic valve prolapse: a clinical and pathological study. Circulation 1987;76(1):68–76.
70. Oliveira DB, et al. Chordal rupture. I: aetiology and natural history. Br Heart J 1983;50(4):312–7.

71. Baxley WA, et al. Hemodynamics in ruptured chordae tendineae and chronic rheumatic mitral regurgitation. Circulation 1973;48(6):1288–94.
72. Kim HK, et al. Determinants of the severity of functional tricuspid regurgitation. Am J Cardiol 2006;98(2):236–42.
73. Grinberg AR, et al. Rupture of mitral chorda tendinea following blunt chest trauma. Clin Cardiol 1998;21(4):300–1.
74. Ansari A, Cruz W. Case in point. Acute regurgitation due to ruptured mitral chordae tendineae. Hosp Pract (Minneap) 1997;32(5):236.
75. Sanders CA, et al. Etiology and differential diagnosis of acute mitral regurgitation. Prog Cardiovasc Dis 1971;14(2):129–52.
76. Musci M, et al. Surgical treatment of right-sided active infective endocarditis with or without involvement of the left heart: 20-year single center experience. Eur J Cardiothorac Surg 2007;32(1):118–25.
77. Ferguson E, Reardon MJ, Letsou GV. The surgical management of bacterial valvular endocarditis. Curr Opin Cardiol 2000;15(2):82–5.
78. Chan P, Ogilby JD, Segal B. Tricuspid valve endocarditis. Am Heart J 1989;117(5):1140–6.
79. De Simone R, et al. [Role of transesophageal echocardiography in tricuspid valve repair]. Cardiologia 1994;39(12 suppl 1):87–101.
80. Drexler M, et al. Assessment of successful valve reconstruction by intraoperative transesophageal echocardiography (TEE). Int J Card Imaging 1986;2(1):21–30.
81. Allen MD, et al. Tricuspid valve repair for tricuspid valve endocarditis: tricuspid valve "recycling". Ann Thorac Surg 1991;51(4):593–8.
82. Wait JH, Mustard WT. Excision of the septal leaflet of the atrioventricular tricuspid valve: an experimental study. J Thorac Cardiovasc Surg 1965;49:968–73.
83. Evora PR, et al. Surgical excision of the vegetation as treatment of tricuspid valve endocarditis. Cardiology 1988;75(4):287–8.
84. Renzulli A, et al. Surgery for tricuspid valve endocarditis: a selective approach. Heart Vessels 1999;14(4):163–9.
85. Boudjemline Y, et al. Steps toward the percutaneous replacement of atrioventricular valves an experimental study. J Am Coll Cardiol 2005;46(2):360–5.
86. Bartlett HL, et al. Early outcomes of tricuspid valve replacement in young children. Circulation 2007;115(3):319–25.
87. Maleszka A, Kleikamp G, Koerfer R. Tricuspid valve replacement: clinical long-term results for acquired isolated tricuspid valve regurgitation. J Heart Valve Dis 2004;13(6):957–61.
88. Arcidiacono G, Corvi A, Severi T. Functional analysis of bioprosthetic heart valves. J Biomech 2005;38(7):1483–90.
89. Kunadian B, et al. Should the tricuspid valve be replaced with a mechanical or biological valve? Interact Cardiovasc Thorac Surg 2007;6(4):551–7.
90. Sako EY. Newer concepts in the surgical treatment of valvular heart disease. Curr Cardiol Rep 2004;6(2):100–5.
91. Dalrymple-Hay MJ, et al. Tricuspid valve replacement: bioprostheses are preferable. J Heart Valve Dis 1999;8(6):644–8.
92. Rizzoli G, et al. Prosthetic replacement of the tricuspid valve: biological or mechanical? Ann Thorac Surg 1998;66(6):S62–7.
93. Okada Y, et al. Long-term echocardiographic follow-up of patients with a tricuspid bioprosthesis. ASAIO Trans 1990;36(3):M535–7.
94. De Smet JM, et al. Long-term durability of three mechanical valves. Ann Thorac Surg 2004;78(1):384; author reply 384–5.
95. Bonow RO, et al. ACC/AHA Guidelines for the management of patients with valvular heart disease. Executive summary. A report of the American College of Cardiology/American Heart Association Task Force on practice guidelines (Committee on management of patients with valvular heart disease). J Heart Valve Dis 1998;7(6):672–707.
96. Butchart EG, et al. Better anticoagulation control improves survival after valve replacement. J Thorac Cardiovasc Surg 2002;123(4):715–23.
97. Ezekowitz MD. Anticoagulation management of valve replacement patients. J Heart Valve Dis 2002;11(Suppl 1):S56–60.
98. Spandorfer J. The management of anticoagulation before and after procedures. Med Clin North Am 2001;85(5):1109–16, v.
99. Reiss N, et al. Mechanical valve replacement in congenital heart defects in the era of international normalized ratio self-management. ASAIO J 2005;51(5):530–2.
100. Warnes CA, et al. ACC/AHA 2008 Guidelines for the management of adults with congenital heart disease. A report of the American College of Cardiology/American Heart Association Task Force on practice guidelines (Writing committee to develop guidelines on the management of adults with congenital heart disease). Circulation 2008;118:2395–451.
101. Lurz P, Bonhoeffer B. Percutaneous implantation of pulmonary valves for treatment of right ventricular outflow tract dysfunction. Cardiol Young 2008;18(3):260–7.

102. Cesnjevar R, et al. Late pulmonary valve replacement after correction of Fallot's tetralogy. Thorac Cardiovasc Surg 2004;52(1):23–8.
103. Borowski A, et al. Severe pulmonary regurgitation late after total repair of tetralogy of Fallot: surgical considerations. Pediatr Cardiol 2004;25(5):466–71.
104. Discigil B, et al. Late pulmonary valve replacement after repair of tetralogy of Fallot. J Thorac Cardiovasc Surg 2001;121(2):344–51.
105. Therrien J, et al. Optimal timing for pulmonary valve replacement in adults after tetralogy of Fallot repair. Am J Cardiol 2005;95(6):779–82.
106. Warner KG, et al. Expanding the indications for pulmonary valve replacement after repair of tetralogy of fallot. Ann Thorac Surg 2003;76(4):1066–71; discussion 1071–2.
107. Sinzobahamvya N, et al. Compared fate of small-diameter Contegras and homografts in the pulmonary position. Eur J Cardiothorac Surg 2007;32(2):209–14.
108. Schoof PH, et al. Pulmonary root replacement with the Freestyle stentless aortic xenograft in growing pigs. Ann Thorac Surg 1998;65(6):1726–9.
109. Carrel T. Bovine valved jugular vein (Contegra) to reconstruct the right ventricular outflow tract. Expert Rev Med Devices 2004;1(1):11–9.
110. Grigg LE, et al. Transesophageal Doppler echocardiography in obstructive hypertrophic cardiomyopathy: clarification of pathophysiology and importance in intraoperative decision making. J Am Coll Cardiol 1992;20(1):42–52.
111. Williams GA, Labovitz AJ. Doppler hemodynamic evaluation of prosthetic (Starr-Edwards and Bjork-Shiley) and bioprosthetic (Hancock and Carpentier-Edwards) cardiac valves. Am J Cardiol 1985;56(4):325–32.
112. Rosti L, et al. Pulmonary valve replacement: a role for mechanical prostheses? Ann Thorac Surg 1998;65(3):889–90.
113. Urrea MS, et al. Ross operation using a bovine bioprosthetic valve with autologous pericardial conduit in the pulmonary position. Tex Heart Inst J 1993;20(4):271–4.
114. Yankah C, Hetzer R. Valve selection and choice in surgery of endocarditis. J Card Surg 1989;4(4):324–30.
115. Fleming WH, et al. Valve replacement in the right side of the heart in children: long-term follow-up. Ann Thorac Surg 1989;48(3):404–8.
116. Hazekamp MG. A mechanical prosthesis for pulmonary valve replacement? Eur J Cardiothorac Surg 2006;30(1):33–4.
117. Waterbolk TW, et al. Pulmonary valve replacement with a mechanical prosthesis. Promising results of 28 procedures in patients with congenital heart disease. Eur J Cardiothorac Surg 2006;30(1):28–32.
118. Prasongsukarn K, Jamieson WR, Lichtenstein SV. Performance of bioprostheses and mechanical prostheses in age group 61–70 years. J Heart Valve Dis 2005;14(4):501–8, 510–1; discussion 509.
119. Chiappini B, Barrea C, Rubay J. Right ventricular outflow tract reconstruction with contegra monocuspid transannular patch in tetralogy of Fallot. Ann Thorac Surg 2007;83(1):185–7.
120. Jun TG, et al. Homologous monocuspid valve patch in right ventricular outflow tract reconstruction. J Cardiovasc Surg (Torino) 2001;42(1):17–21.
121. Bigras JL, et al. Short-term effect of monocuspid valves on pulmonary insufficiency and clinical outcome after surgical repair of tetralogy of Fallot. J Thorac Cardiovasc Surg 1996;112(1):33–7.
122. Fantidis P, et al. A new physiologic correction technique for re-establishment of pulmonary circulation. Experimental surgical development. Scand J Thorac Cardiovasc Surg 1989;23(2):155–64.
123. Sievers HH, et al. Superior function of a bicuspid over a monocuspid patch for reconstruction of a hypoplastic pulmonary root in pigs. J Thorac Cardiovasc Surg 1993;105(4):580–90.
124. Forbess JM, et al. Cryopreserved homografts in the pulmonary position: determinants of durability. Ann Thorac Surg 2001;71(1):54–9; discussion 59–60.
125. Brown JW, et al. Valved bovine jugular vein conduits for right ventricular outflow tract reconstruction in children: an attractive alternative to pulmonary homograft. Ann Thorac Surg 2006;82(3):909–16.
126. Morales DLS, et al. Encouraging results for the Contegra conduit in the problematic right ventricle–to–pulmonary artery connection. J Thorac Cardiovasc Surg 2006;132:665–71.
127. Sierra J, et al. Right ventricular outflow tract reconstruction: what conduit to use? Homograft or Contegra? Ann Thorac Surg 2007;84(2):610–1.
128. Kanter KR, et al. Results with the freestyle porcine aortic root for right ventricular outflow tract reconstruction in children. Ann Thorac Surg 2003;76(6):1889–94.
129. Chard RB, et al. Use of the Medtronic Freestyle valve as a right ventricular to pulmonary artery conduit. Ann Thorac Surg 2001;71:S361–4.
130. Lodge AJ, et al. A novel bioresorbable film reduces adhesions after infant cardiac surgery. Ann Thorac Surg 2008;86:614–21.
131. Lurz P, et al. Percutaneous pulmonary valve implantation: impact of evolving technology and learning curve on clinical outcome. Circulation 2008;117(15):1964–72.

132. Diab KA, Cao QL, Hijazi ZM. Device closure of congenital ventricular septal defects. Congenit Heart Dis 2007;2(2):92–103.

133. McKay R, Ross DN. Primary repair and autotransplantation of cardiac valves. Annu Rev Med 1993;44:181–8.

134. Kay JH. Surgical treatment of tricuspid regurgitation. Ann Thorac Surg 1992;53(6):1132–3.

135. McGrath LB, et al. Determination of the need for tricuspid valve replacement: value of preoperative right ventricular angiocardiography. J Invasive Cardiol 1991;3(1):35–40.

136. McCarthy PM, et al. Tricuspid valve repair: durability and risk factors for failure. J Thorac Cardiovasc Surg 2004;127(3):674–85.

137. Fukuda S, et al. Determinants of recurrent or residual functional tricuspid regurgitation after tricuspid annuloplasty. Circulation 2006;114(Suppl 1):I582–7.

138. De Vega NG. Selective, adjustable and permanent annuloplasty. An original technic for the treatment of tricuspid insufficiency. Rev Esp Cardiol 1972;25(6):555–6.

139. Chidambaram M, et al. Long-term results of DeVega tricuspid annuloplasty. Ann Thorac Surg 1987;43(2):185–8.

140. Abe T, et al. [Surgical management of acquired tricuspid valve disease–the effects and comparison of tricuspid annuloplasty (De Vega) and tricuspid valve replacement]. Kokyu To Junkan 1989;37(7):757–63.

141. Morishita A, et al. Long-term results after De Vega's tricuspid annuloplasty. J Cardiovasc Surg (Torino) 2002;43(6):773–7.

142. Rivera JM, et al. Which physical factors determine tricuspid regurgitation jet area in the clinical setting? Am J Cardiol 1993;72(17):1305–9.

143. Yada I, et al. Preoperative evaluation and surgical treatment for tricuspid regurgitation associated with acquired valvular heart disease. The Kay-Boyd method vs the Carpentier-Edwards ring method. J Cardiovasc Surg (Torino) 1990;31(6):771–7.

144. Konishi Y, et al. [Tricuspid annuloplasty – De Vega's and Carpentier's method]. Kyobu Geka 1983;36(4):263–7.

145. Rivera JM, et al. Quantification of tricuspid regurgitation by means of the proximal flow convergence method: a clinical study. Am Heart J 1994;127(5):1354–62.

146. Matsuyama K, et al. De Vega annuloplasty and Carpentier-Edwards ring annuloplasty for secondary tricuspid regurgitation. J Heart Valve Dis 2001;10(4):520–4.

147. Gatti G, et al. Tricuspid valve annuloplasty with a flexible prosthetic band. Interact Cardiovasc Thorac Surg 2007;6(6):731–5.

148. Isidro AB, et al. Bicuspidization of the tricuspid valve for the treatment of posterior leaflet endocarditis: a case report. Heart Surg Forum 2007;10(2):E129–30.

149. Kawano H, et al. Tricuspid valve replacement with the St. Jude Medical valve: 19 years of experience. Eur J Cardiothorac Surg 2000;18(5):565–9.

150. Carrier M, et al. Tricuspid valve replacement: an analysis of 25 years of experience at a single center. Ann Thorac Surg 2003;75(1):47–50.

151. Chang YY, et al. Long-term clinical results of tricuspid valve replacement. Ann Thorac Surg 2006;81:1317–24.

152. Tamura H, et al. [A case report of surgical treatment of prosthetic valve endocarditis in tricuspid position]. Nippon Kyobu Geka Gakkai Zasshi 1990;38(12):2469–73.

153. Bolger AP, Gatzoulis MA. Towards defining heart failure in adults with congenital heart disease. Int J Cardiol 2004;97(Suppl 1):15–23.

154. Kumar AS, et al. Homograft mitral valve replacement: five years' results. J Thorac Cardiovasc Surg 2000;120(3):450–8.

155. Nakano K, et al. Tricuspid valve replacement with bioprostheses: long-term results and causes of valve dysfunction. Ann Thorac Surg 2001;71(1):105–9.

156. Glower DD, et al. In-hospital and long-term outcome after porcine tricuspid valve replacement. J Thorac Cardiovasc Surg 1995;109(5):877–83; discussion 883–4.

157. Van Nooten GJ, et al. Tricuspid valve replacement: postoperative and long-term results. J Thorac Cardiovasc Surg 1995;110(3):672–9.

158. Niwaya K, et al. [Tricuspid valvular regurgitation due to infective endocarditis with ventricular septal defect]. Kyobu Geka 1988;41(12):983–7.

159. Munro AI, et al. Tricuspid valve replacement: porcine bioprostheses and mechanical prostheses. Ann Thorac Surg 1995;60(Suppl 2):S470–3.

160. Scully HE, Armstrong CS. Tricuspid valve replacement. Fifteen years of experience with mechanical prostheses and bioprostheses. J Thorac Cardiovasc Surg 1995;109(6):1035–41.

161. Nakano K, et al. Tricuspid valve replacement with the bileaflet St. Jude Medical valve prosthesis. J Thorac Cardiovasc Surg 1994;108(5):888–92.

162. Katsumata T, Westaby S. Mitral homograft replacement of the tricuspid valve for endocarditis. Ann Thorac Surg 1997;63(5):1480–2.

163. McKay R, Sono J, Arnold RM. Tricuspid valve replacement using an unstented pulmonary homograft. Ann Thorac Surg 1988;46(1):58–62.

164. Tokunaga S, et al. Isolated pulmonary valve replacement: analysis of 27 years of experience. J Artif Organs 2008;11(3):130–3.

165. Fiore AC, et al. Pulmonary valve replacement: a comparison of three biological valves. Ann Thorac Surg 2008;85(5):1712–8; discussion 1718.

166. Douglas JM. Mitral valve replacement. In Atlas of Cardiothoracic Surgery Sabiston DC (Ed.). Philadelphia: Saunders; 1995, p. 388

167. Dearani JA, et al. Surgical treatment of Ebstein's malformation: state of the art in 2006. Cardiol Young 2006;16(Suppl 3):12–20.

16 Medical Therapy of Valvular Heart Disease

Sahil A. Parikh and Patrick T. O'Gara

CONTENTS

INTRODUCTION

The management of patients with valvular heart disease (VHD) requires an integrated understanding of pathophysiology and natural history. While surgical intervention is often required, medical treatment may in some circumstances retard the progression of valvular and ventricular dysfunction and reduce associated complications. Patients with VHD commonly require treatment for other cardiovascular disorders, such as coronary artery disease (CAD), hypertension (HTN), dyslipidemia, peripheral arterial disease (PAD), and venous thromboembolic (VTE) disease. Management of atrial fibrillation (AF) is especially relevant for patients with mitral valve disease, heart failure, or prior valve replacement or repair surgery. In this chapter, we will review general considerations for the medical management of patients with VHD and then discuss individual valve lesions with a focus on specific pathophysiologic principles and recommendations for non-surgical treatment. The chapter is intended to supplement the more detailed discussion of each valve lesion, which appears elsewhere in the text.

GENERAL CONSIDERATIONS

Atrial Fibrillation

Atrial fibrillation (AF) is the most common arrhythmia encountered in patients with valvular heart disease, especially those with mitral valve disease. Its onset is often accompanied by clinical decompensation and mandates prompt intervention, with aggressive rate control, appropriate use of anticoagulation, and early consideration of cardioversion, as per current guidelines (*1, 2*). The occurrence of AF during longitudinal patient follow-up should also prompt reconsideration of the indications for surgery. On occasion, AF or an associated thromboembolic complication is the first manifestation of VHD. AF is also a common complication of valve surgery, particularly mitral valve surgery. Its prevention and management in the early post-operative setting are the focus of institutional critical care

From: *Contemporary Cardiology: Valvular Heart Disease*
Edited by: Andrew Wang, Thomas M. Bashore, DOI 10.1007/978-1-59745-411-7_16
© Humana Press, a part of Springer Science+Business Media, LLC 2009

pathways. Prophylactic beta-adrenoreceptor blockade or amiodarone is recommended, but variably effective (2). Catheter-based or surgical treatment of AF at the time of mitral valve surgery has become standard for patients with paroxysmal or persistent AF (3). Patients with permanent AF and/or large and diseased left atria are less likely to benefit from these interventions. Anticoagulation with vitamin K antagonists (VKA) for prevention of stroke or systemic embolus is critical (1, 4). Among patients with native valve disease, those with MS are at highest risk of thromboembolic complications after AF onset. Despite a relatively lower risk of stroke, patients with isolated mitral regurgitation (MR) and those with aortic or tricuspid valve disease are also provided VKA therapy. AF with either valve repair or bioprosthetic replacement is an indication for anticoagulation. The use of low-molecular weight heparin preparations as a "bridge" to therapeutic warfarin anticoagulation, commonly employed to reduce length of stay after surgery or to avoid hospitalization in the ambulatory setting, has not been rigorously assessed. Whether anticoagulation can be safely discontinued in post-operative AF patients without mechanical prostheses after restoration of sinus rhythm must be assessed on an individual basis. The recommended goal for the intensity of anticoagulation for AF patients with native valve disease or previous valve repair is an INR of 2.5, range 2.0–3.0 (1, 4). The INR goals for patients with prosthetic heart valves vary and will be discussed later in the chapter. Low-dose aspirin (75–100 mg daily) is generally considered safe for the treatment of concomitant CAD. The addition of clopidogrel, when indicated for management of an intra-coronary stent, is problematic. In this setting, a bare metal stent may be preferred. It may also be necessary to restrict exposure to dual anti-platelet therapy (aspirin and clopidogrel) to the first 4 weeks after PCI, with continuation of aspirin and warfarin thereafter (5). No randomized, prospective data are available to provide guidance on this very difficult issue, especially for elderly patients.

Infective Endocarditis (IE) Prophylaxis

Transient bacteremia from daily activities including tooth brushing and flossing has long been implicated as a potential cause of IE, particularly in patients with pre-existing valve or congenital heart disease. However, no prospective data regarding either the absolute risk of IE from dental procedures or the efficacy of IE prophylaxis administered prior to dental work exist. The American Heart Association has recently revised its recommendations for IE prophylaxis (6). The current guidelines have narrowed substantially the primary (Class IIa, Level of Evidence C) indications for antimicrobial prophylaxis. Emphasis is placed on the use of prophylactic antibiotics in patients who are felt to be at highest risk of adverse outcomes from IE. Susceptible patients include those with a history of IE, prosthetic valve, various types of native or repaired congenital heart disease, or valvulopathy after cardiac transplantation (Table 1). Antimicrobial regimens for IE prophylaxis prior to dental procedures are listed in Table 2. The use of prophylactic antiobiotics solely to prevent IE is not recommended for patients who undergo GU or GI tract procedures. Concomitant infections should be treated as appropriate.

Rheumatic Fever Prophylaxis

Rheumatic fever (RF) remains an important cause of VHD, particularly in the developing world. The causative organism for rheumatic carditis is the Group A beta-hemolytic streptococcus. The M-protein, a capsular antigen, induces an auto-immune response in vulnerable hosts and results in pancarditis with valvulopathy. The diagnosis of acute RF is established by use of the 2001 WHO criteria (7). Primary detection and treatment of Group A beta-hemolytic streptococcal infection is the principle method for prevention of acute RF (Table 3). Secondary RF prevention must be continued for several years after the index infection, even following interim valve repair or replacement surgery (Table 4).

Table 1
Cardiac Conditions Associated with Highest Risk of Adverse Outcome from Endocarditis for Which Prophylaxis Before Dental Procedures Is Recommended

- Prosthetic cardiac valve
- Previous infective endocarditis (IE)
- Congenital heart disease (CHD)*
  - Unrepaired cyanotic CHD, including palliative shunts and conduits
  - Completely repaired congenital heart defect with prosthetic material or device, whether placed by surgery or by catheter intervention, during the first 6 months after the procedure[†]
  - Repaired CHD with residual defects at the site or adjacent to the site of a prosthetic patch or prosthetic device (which inhibit endothelialization)
- Cardiac transplantation recipients who develop cardiac valvulopathy

*Except for the conditions listed above, antibiotic prophylaxis is no longer recommended for any other form of CHD.

[†]Prophylaxis during this time frame is recommended because endothelialization of prosthetic material usually occurs within 6 months of the procedure, after which prophylaxis is not necessary.

Adapted from Wilson et al. (6).

Table 2
Regimens for IE Prophylaxis Before Dental Procedures

Situation	Agent	Regimen for adult*	Regimen for children*
Oral	Amoxicillin	2.0 g	50 mg/kg
Unable to take oral medications	Ampicillin	2.0 g IM or IV	50 mg/kg IM or IV
Penicillin-allergic	Clindamycin or	600 mg	20 mg/kg
	Cefalexin or cephadroxil or	2.0 g	50 mg/kg
	Azithromycin or clarithromycin	500 mg	15 mg/kg
Penicillin-allergic and unable to take oral medications	Clindamycin or	600 mg IV	20 mg/kg IV
	Cefazolin	1.0 g IM or IV	25 mg/kg IM or IV

*Administered 30–60 minutes before procedure; IM = intramuscular; IV = intravenous
From Wilson et al. (6).

MEDICAL THERAPY FOR LEFT-SIDED NATIVE VALVE DISEASE

Aortic Stenosis

GENERAL CONSIDERATIONS

The obstruction to LV outflow imposed by valvular aortic stenosis (AS) results in pressure overload with concentric hypertrophy. Diastolic dysfunction and myocardial oxygen supply–demand imbalance ensue, followed later in the natural history of the disease by afterload mismatch and systolic pump dysfunction. Pathophysiologic deterioration may be accelerated by the superimposition of systemic hypertension, epicardial CAD, and/or AF, problems which occur commonly among older patients. Systemic hypertension and valvulo-arterial impedance may in part explain the adverse natural history experienced by some patients with low output/low gradient severe AS despite normal

Table 3
Primary Prevention of Rheumatic Fever

Agent	Dose	Mode	Duration
Benzathine penicillin G	Patients 27 kg (60 lb) or less: 600,000 U Patients greater than 27 kg (60 lb): 1,200,000 U	Intramuscular	Once
Or Penicillin V (phenoxymethyl penicillin)	Childeren: 250 mg two to three times daily Adolescents and adults: 500 mg two to three times daily	Oral	10 days
For individuals allergic to penicillin Erythromycin Estolate	20–40 mg per kg per day, two to four times daily (maximum 1 g per day)	Oral	10 days
Or Ethylsuccinate	40 mg per kg per day, two to four times daily (maximum 1 g per days)	Oral	10 days
Or Azithromycin	500 mg on first day, 250 mg per day for the next 4 days	Oral	5 days

From Guidelines for the Diagnosis of Rheumatic Fever *(25)*.

Table 4
Secondary Prevention of Rheumatic Fever

Agent	Dose	Mode
Benzathine penicillin G	1 200 000 U every 4 week (every 3 week for high-risk* patients such as those with residual carditis)	Intramuscular
Or Penicillin V	250 mg twice daily	Oral
Or Sulfadiazine	0.5 g once daily for patients 27 g (60 lb) or less; 1.0 g once daily for patients greater than 27 kg (60 lb)	Oral
For individuals allergic to penicillin and sulfadiazine Erythromycin	250 mg twice daily	Oral

From Guidelines for the Diagnosis of Rheumatic Fever *(25)*.

EF. Symptom onset is an indication for surgery, performance of which should not be delayed in the non-acute setting in the hope that medical therapy may delay its need *(1)*. Medical therapy is palliative, with the possible exception of the use of statin medications to delay the progression of the disease.

MEDICAL MANAGEMENT OF DECOMPENSATED SEVERE AS

Medical interventions are largely supportive until surgery is feasible. Medical management of patients with severe AS and LV dysfunction, heart failure, or shock, should be guided by invasive monitoring of pulmonary artery (PA) and pulmonary capillary wedge (PCW) pressures, cardiac output (CO), and systemic vascular resistance (SVR). Diuresis may alleviate pulmonary congestion, but patients with severe AS have preload-dependent physiology, and overdiuresis may cause a precipitous fall in blood pressure. For patients in cardiogenic shock, mean arterial pressure should be preserved with inotropic support until urgent AVR can be performed. Vasodilators may produce a rapid reduction in afterload and hemodynamic instability, and their use should be restricted to carefully selected patients. In this regard, recent data suggest that the judicious use of sodium nitroprusside in selected AS patients with ejection fraction < 0.35 and AVA ≤ 1.0 cm^2 can increase cardiac output and improve hemodynamic status *(8, 9)*. The use of percutaneous aortic balloon valvuloplasty (PABV) as a bridge to AVR in patients with severe heart failure or shock is controversial and no longer widely practiced *(1)*.

HYPERTENSION AND CORONARY ARTERY DISEASE

Management of hypertension and CAD in patients with AS and normal LV systolic function generally follows the treatment guidelines for these conditions, including aggressive risk factor reduction. Caution is advised when increasing the doses of anti-hypertensive medications in patients with severe AS to avoid abrupt falls in blood pressure. This concern is less applicable among patients with only mild or moderate AS. Low-dose diuretics, beta-adrenoreceptor blockers, angiotensin-converting enzyme inhibitors, and angiotensin receptor blockers are generally well tolerated. Patients with CAD and AS must be instructed carefully in the use of nitroglycerin for the treatment of angina. It is advisable for the patient to take his/her first dose under clinical supervision.

ATRIAL FIBRILLATION

The atrial contribution to LV filling in patients with AS becomes increasingly important as the disease progresses. The loss of AV synchrony can result in marked hemodynamic deterioration in susceptible patients. Onset of AF should prompt reconsideration of the indications for surgery in patients with AS followed longitudinally. Expeditious restoration of sinus rhythm is advised. When cardioversion fails, rate control is essential. Anticoagulation should be provided in the absence of contraindications.

PROGRESSION OF AS

The pathogenesis of degenerative aortic valve disease shares many features in common with that of atherosclerosis, including the important roles played by endothelial dysfunction, inflammation, atherothrombosis, and smooth muscle cell transformation. Several retrospective, observational studies suggested that statin therapy might reduce the rate of progression of AS. An randomized trial with atorvastatin, performed in patients with advanced disease, was disappointing *(10)*. A more recent non-randomized study using rosuvastatin in patients with relatively less severe AS was more encouraging *(11)* (Fig. 1). However, a larger randomized trial of combination simvastatin and ezetimibe in patients with moderate AS showed no effect on valve related outcomes *(11 A)*. There are no prospective data available for other preventive therapies, such as medications targeted against the renin–angiotensin–aldosterone system (RAAS). At present, it is appropriate to treat AS patients with dyslipidemia in accordance with existing primary and secondary prevention guidelines until further data emerge.

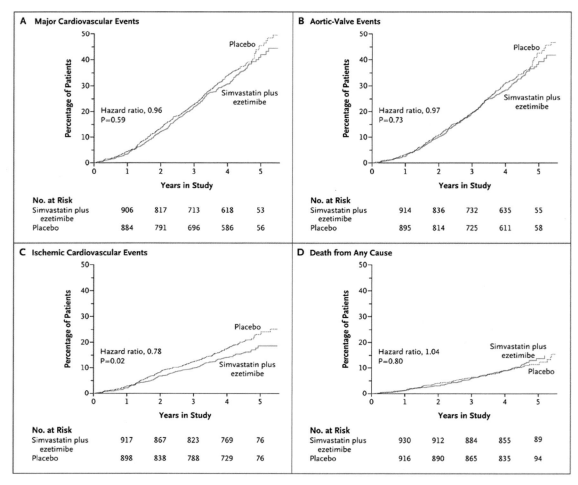

Fig. 1. Kaplan-Meier Curves for Primary and Secondary Outcomes and Death. The primary outcome was a composite of major cardiovascular events, including death from cardiovascular causes, aortic-valve replacement, nonfatal myocardial infarction, hospitalization for unstable angina pectoris, heart failure, coronary-artery bypass grafting, percutaneous coronary intervention, and nonhemorrhagic stroke (Panel A). Secondary outcomes were events related to aortic-valve stenosis (Panel B) and ischemic cardiovascular events (Panel C). There was no difference between the study groups in overall mortality (Panel D).

Aortic Regurgitation

GENERAL CONSIDERATIONS

Aortic regurgitation results in progressive LV volume overload, cavity dilation, and increased wall stress. AR, in contrast to MR, is a state of excess preload and afterload. Medical therapy is aimed at increasing effective forward stroke volume and decreasing regurgitant fraction. In the acute setting, the LV operates on the steep portion of its pressure–volume relationship, such that for any increase in volume there is a precipitous and exponential increase in pressure. Patients are invariably tachycardiac with signs of low output. The diastolic murmur is misleadingly soft and of short duration, features indicative of the rapid rate of rise of LV diastolic pressure. In chronic AR, the LV is allowed to compensate over time and operates on a relatively flat portion of its diastolic pressure–volume relationship such that there is a lesser rise in pressure for any given increase in volume. The LV can remain compensated for variable and often prolonged periods of time. Diastolic blood pressure is low and signs of diastolic runoff are prominent, including a long, blowing diastolic murmur and bounding peripheral pulses. Medical therapy to prolong this compensated phase has been the subject of several small-scale studies, which have reported disparate results. Many patients with chronic severe AR are hypertensive (i.e., systolic blood pressure >140 mm Hg) and are candidates for anti-hypertensive drug therapy.

ACUTE SEVERE AR

Acute severe AR has a high mortality rate. Death can result from sudden aggravation of pulmonary edema with cardiac arrest, ventricular arrhythmias, or cardiogenic shock. Type A dissection with acute AR can result in pericardial tamponade, rupture, and sudden death. Urgent or sometimes emergent surgical intervention is required, depending on the cause. Medical management should not delay surgery; the goal of therapy is stabilization in anticipation of operative repair (1).

Congestive heart failure and cardiogenic shock are the principle targets of treatment. There is an accepted role for intravenous vasodilator therapy in patients with acute severe AR. Sodium nitroprusside, an agent which reduces both preload and afterload, is the gold standard. Diuretics are needed to reduce pulmonary congestion. Beta-adrenoreceptor blockers are contraindicated in the absence of an acute aortic dissection. Any reduction in heart rate could significantly imperil cardiac output and allow for a further increase in diastolic regurgitant volume. Thiocyanate levels should be monitored if nitroprusside is used for more than 24 h (12). Hydralazine has also been demonstrated to be useful in the acute setting, but is used less frequently. Inotropic agents such as dopamine or dobutamine may be required and can augment forward cardiac output in the short term. Endotracheal intubation and mechanical ventilation may be necessary. Intra-aortic balloon counterpulsation is contraindicated. Antibiotics are provided for management of IE, though surgery in this setting should not be delayed once heart failure intervenes.

CHRONIC SEVERE AR

Hypertension is a risk factor for progressive LV dysfunction in AR. Spagnuolo et al. demonstrated that hypertension was a predictor of adverse outcomes in patients with rheumatic AR (13). The treatment of hypertension in patients with chronic, severe AR has been widely accepted, although specific guidelines are lacking, other than to treat to currently recommended JNC-7 targets (13). While therapy with vasodilator agents has been shown to be beneficial in acute AR, oral agents such as hydralazine (14), nifedipine (15, 16), felodipine (17), and ACE inhibitors (18, 19) have demonstrated mixed results in the chronic setting. An early randomized study in patients with asymptomatic, chronic, severe AR comparing long-acting nifedipine with digoxin suggested that nifedipine could extend the compensated phase of AR and delay the need for surgery (16). In a more recent randomized trial, however, neither nifedipine nor enalapril proved different than placebo for this indication (20) (Fig. 2). In current practice, vasodilators are indicated to treat hypertension in patients with AR, regardless of the severity of the valve lesion, and to manage systolic heart failure in patients who are not considered candidates for surgery (1). Blood pressure targets should be lower (e.g., 120 mm Hg systolic) for patients with concomitant root or ascending aortic pathology, as may occur in patients with bicuspid aortic valve disease.

Mitral Stenosis

GENERAL CONSIDERATIONS

LV inflow obstruction due to mitral valve stenosis (MS) results in inadequate LV filling and LA hypertension. Rheumatic carditis is the most common cause of isolated MS. Less frequently encountered causes include severe mitral annular calcification with extension onto the leaflets, left atrial

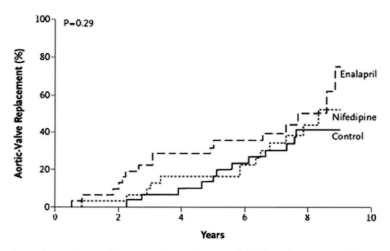

Fig. 2. Probability of aortic valve replacement in patients with chronic severe AR treated with enalapril, nifedipine, or control *(20)*.

myxoma, and congenital valve disease. Rheumatic fever prophylaxis, management of AF, and provision of anticoagulation are essential aspects of patient care.

ACUTE, DECOMPENSATED MS

In all patients with MS and acute pulmonary edema, reversible precipitants, such as anemia, sepsis, volume overload, and thyrotoxicosis, should be sought and treated promptly. New onset rapid atrial fibrillation is often the inciting event. In patients with mild or moderate MS, medical stabilization will suffice without the need for mechanical intervention. Patients with severe MS will require intervention, without which their prognosis is poor *(21)*. Interventional therapy might consist of percutaneous mitral balloon valvuloplasty (PMBV), surgical mitral valve commissurotomy, or mitral valve replacement (MVR), the indications for which are reviewed elsewhere.

Medical therapy is directed at slowing the heart rate (whether sinus or AF) and alleviation of pulmonary and systemic venous congestion. Beta-blockers or rate-slowing calcium blockers are the preferred agents for rate control and can be administered intravenously, if needed. Anticoagulation should be provided for AF and continued indefinitely, unless contraindications are present, such as pregnancy or active bleeding. Cardioversion may be required in the acute setting to restore hemodynamic stability more quickly, though most patients respond to rate control and diuresis. Loop diuretics are given as per usual treatment protocols for pulmonary edema.

CHRONIC MS

Long-term management of patients with MS includes clinical and echocardiographic surveillance, with careful attention to the emergence of AF, heart failure symptoms, or signs of pulmonary artery hypertension. Success rates for cardioversion of AF in the non-acute setting are dependent on the duration of the arrhythmia and LA size. Anti-arrhythmic medications may be less effective in patients with MS than in those with non-valvular AF because of rheumatic involvement of the LA myocardium and persistence of LA hypertension. Symptom onset is an indication for mechanical therapy in patients with moderate or severe MS (valve area ≤ 1.5 cm^2).

Mitral Regurgitation

GENERAL CONSIDERATIONS

In acute severe MR, LA pressure rises dramatically. The unprepared, non-dilated, and relatively non-compliant LA operates on the steep portion of its pressure–volume relationship and marked elevations of pressure with giant "v" waves are the rule. LV size is not increased and systolic function may be normal, hyperdynamic, or subnormal, depending on the cause. In chronic MR, the LV dilates to ensure an adequate stroke volume and net forward cardiac output. End-diastolic volume increases and the ventricle operates on a relatively flat portion of its diastolic pressure–volume relationship. In contrast to chronic AR, afterload is not increased in chronic MR and ejection phase indices of systolic function are preserved until late in the natural history of the disease. The left atrium dilates and becomes more compliant, acting as a low-impedance sink into which the LV can empty. This condition is well tolerated for years and poses a challenge during clinical follow-up for recognition of the early signs of LV decompensation.

ACUTE SEVERE MR

Medical therapy for acute severe MR depends in part on etiology. For example, antibiotics are necessary for treatment of IE, and anti-ischemic measures and surgery are critical for patients with post-MI papillary muscle rupture. Patients tend to have labile hemodynamics and invasive monitoring of both systemic and PA pressures is often required. Pre and afterload reduction with intravenous vasodilators, as tolerated by the systemic blood pressure, is a mainstay of therapy in the acute setting. Sodium nitroprusside is preferred. An inotrope such as dobutamine or dopamine may also be required for support of cardiac output and mean arterial pressure. Intra-aortic balloon counterpulsation can be particularly helpful by improving forward cardiac output, decreasing regurgitant volume, and decreasing LV end-diastolic pressure. It should be instituted promptly for patients with shock. Loop diuretics decrease LV filling pressures and alleviate the symptoms and signs of pulmonary edema. Surgical planning should not be delayed by these interventions, but operation may have to await improvement in vital organ function in selected patients (1). While there are reports attesting to the efficacy of PCI for management of severe MR following acute MI, surgical correction is usually needed despite successful coronary reperfusion. PCI as stand alone therapy is not appropriate when papillary muscle rupture is present.

CHRONIC MR

There is no role for vasodilator therapy in the management of normotensive patients with chronic, non-ischemic MR, and normal left ventricular systolic function. Chronic MR is a state of low afterload and there is no long-term experience with attempts to lower it further. Although a few small scale studies have suggested benefit with vasodilators in this setting, the aggregate data have not met threshold for consistent benefit. Indications for vasodilator therapy in the chronic setting would include hypertension or LV systolic dysfunction in patients not considered candidates for surgery (1). Beta-adrenoreceptor blockers are also appropriate in the latter setting. Patients with ischemic MR should be treated aggressively with measures directed at secondary prevention of recurrent ischemia or infarction, arrhythmias, and LV remodeling. The latter should include bi-ventricular pacing (with or without defibrillator capability) in appropriately selected patients with wide QRS duration and LV dyssynchrony.

TRICUSPID VALVE DISEASE

The medical treatment of chronic tricuspid valve (TV) disease is generally targeted to the management of volume overload with loop diuretics and anticoagulation for AF. Native TV stenosis is extremely rare in the modern era; its associated symptoms and signs are typically dwarfed by concomitant left-sided valve disease. Tricuspid regurgitation (TR) is most often secondary in nature and develops in response to pulmonary artery hypertension and right ventricular/annular dilatation. Primary TR can occur with carcinoid heart disease, Ebstein's anomaly, IE, myxomatous degeneration, blunt chest wall trauma, and as a complication of RV endomyocardial biopsy. Spironolactone may be particularly helpful in patients with long-standing TR and right-sided volume overload, not only as a potassium sparing agent, but also to counteract high circulating levels of aldosterone. Octreotide is indicated for treatment of metastatic carcinoid (22). A major goal of therapy in patients with secondary TR is to lower PA pressures by the appropriate treatment of left-heart or primary pulmonary vascular disease. TV repair at the time of mitral valve surgery has become commonplace, as dictated by the severity of TR and/or the size of the TV annulus, though indications are not standardized (1). Acute severe TR is usually well tolerated when pulmonary vascular resistance is normal and may not require specific therapy. Surgery may be indicated for selected patients with TV IE not curable with antibiotic therapy.

PULMONIC VALVE DISEASE

There is no specific medical therapy for congenital pulmonic stenosis. Guidelines for balloon valvuloplasty and surgery are predicated on severity of the valve lesion, symptoms, and RV function (1). Similarly, there is little effective medical therapy for pulmonic regurgitation (PR), except treatment directed at lowering elevated PA pressures. Primary PR may be congenital, or occur with IE. Secondary PR is a complication of childhood repair of Tetralogy of Fallot or balloon valvuloplasty for congenital PS (25). It may also develop as a consequence of long-standing pulmonary hypertension of any cause. Mixed PS/PR may occur with carcinoid disease. Longitudinal attention must be paid to RV size and function. The need for diuretic therapy should prompt consideration of the indications for surgery (1).

PROSTHETIC HEART VALVES

General Considerations

The choice of heart valve replacement, when repair is not feasible, is predicated on several factors, chief among which are the attendant risks of thromboembolism and anticoagulation with a mechanical prosthesis vs. the expected durability of a bioprosthesis. Management after heart valve replacement surgery focuses on anticoagulation when indicated, prevention of infective endocarditis, and recognition and treatment of mechanical complications such as hemolytic anemia, prosthetic valve thrombosis, or structural valve degeneration.

Antithrombotic Therapy

All patients with mechanical valves require vitamin K antagonist (VKA) therapy, the intensity of which varies as a function of valve type, position, and number, as well as the presence of any one or more patient risk factors for thromboembolism including AF, LV systolic dysfunction, a history of a prior thromboembolic event, and evidence of a hypercoagulable state (1, 4, 23) (Table 5). The combination of aspirin and clopidogrel is not a substitute for VKA therapy. Low-dose aspirin (81 mg daily)

Table 5
Recommended Anticoagulation for Prosthetic Valves

Valve type	Anticoagulation with prosthetic valves		ASA[2]
	VKA[1]		
	INR 2.0–3.0	INR 2.5–3.5	75–100 mg
Mechanical			
First 3 months (aortic and mitral)		⊕	⊕
After 3 months			
Aortic valve (St. Jude, Hall-Medtronic)	⊕		±
Aortic valve + risk factor[3]		⊕	⊕
Mitral valve ± risk factor[3]		⊕	⊕
Bioprosthetic			
First 3 months (aortic and mitral)[4]		⊕	⊕
After 3 months			
No risk factors (aortic and mitral)[3]			⊕
Aortic valve + risk factor[3]	⊕		⊕
Mitral valve + risk factor[3]		⊕	⊕

[1]VKA = vitamin K antagonist.

[2]ASA = aspirin.

[3]Risk factors for thromboembolism: AF, history of stroke or TIA or systemic embolus, hypercoagulable state, mechanical prosthesis in mitral position, >1 prosthesis, and thrombogenic prosthesis (Starr–Edwards, Bjork–Shiley).

[4]Many institutions have abandoned the use of VKA therapy for the first 3 months in patients with an aortic bioprosthesis and no risk factors, including peri-operative AF.

Adapted from Bonow et al. *(1)* and O'Donoghue et al. *(26)*.

is added to full dose VKA therapy for patients with coronary or peripheral arterial disease, and after thromboembolism despite a therapeutic INR, if the aggregate risk of hemorrhage is deemed acceptable *(1, 4, 23)*. Treatment to a higher INR goal is an alternative strategy for management of patients with thromboembolism despite a therapeutic INR. In some instances, both approaches are necessary. Practice patterns vary. Consensus guidelines from the American College of Cardiology/American Heart Association (ACC/AHA), American College of Chest Physicians (ACCP), and European Society of Cardiology (ESC) differ on the routine addition of aspirin to VKA therapy in patients with mechanical valves *(1, 4, 23)*. Clopidogrel is reserved for patients with true aspirin allergy. Most surgical centers have abandoned the use of a short course (3 months) of VKA therapy after bioprosthetic AVR in patients without other risk factors for thromboembolism. Such patients are managed with aspirin alone despite the lack of data attesting to its efficacy in this and other settings in which a bioprosthesis is used. As is recommended for all patients after mechanical heart valve replacement, patients with a mitral bioprosthesis are managed with heparin as soon after operation as is deemed safe and until the INR reaches the therapeutic range, after which VKA therapy is continued for at least the first three post-operative months. Both intravenous unfractionated heparin and low-molecular weight heparin have been used peri-operatively as a bridge to therapeutic VKA therapy *(24)*. Institutional practices vary widely regarding the choice of heparin and the intensity of anticoagulant effect deemed safe in the early post-operative period. VKA therapy is indicated indefinitely for patients with a mitral bioprosthesis and risk factors for thromboembolism; aspirin monotherapy is recommended after the first 3 months in patients without risk factors.

Management of Anticoagulant Therapy During Invasive Procedures

Interruption of VKA therapy for the performance of invasive procedures requires a collaborative decision between the cardiologist and proceduralist, dentist, or surgeon (Table 6). For minor procedures such as cataract removal, tooth extraction, or cardiac device implantation, it is preferable to proceed without any interruption or after 1 or 2 days of lower dose therapy and an INR of approximately 2.0, with resumption of full dose therapy thereafter *(4)*. For major procedures which carry a higher risk of serious bleeding, VKA therapy is usually stopped 4 days beforehand. Bridging therapy with either intravenous UFH or subcutaneous LMWH, once the INR falls below a threshold value (e.g., 2.5), is predicated on the perceived risk of thromboembolism during this treatment gap. The gradient of risk varies as a function of prosthesis and patient characteristics referenced above. Higher risk patients, such as those with a mechanical mitral valve, AF, and a history of stroke, should be treated with heparin before and after surgery, whereas lower risk patients, such as those with a St. Jude bileaflet mechanical valve in the aortic position, sinus rhythm, normal LV function, and no history of stroke, can be managed without a heparin bridge. Low-molecular weight heparin is used more frequently than intravenous unfractionated heparin in such circumstances; randomized trials comparing these agents for this indication are lacking. Heparin and VKA therapy are resumed post-operatively as soon as they are deemed safe and continued together until the INR is therapeutic.

Table 6
Management of Peri-Procedural Anticoagulation in Patients with Valve Replacements

Management of anticoagulation peri-procedure	
Minor procedure (e.g., dental work, cataract, skin biopsy, Moh's procedure)	Continue VKA as per prior schedule or taper/stop anticoagulation for 1–2 days before procedure and proceed with INR ~ 2.0.
Major procedure without patient risk factors* for thromboembolism (e.g., hip surgery, prostatectomy, laparotomy, thoracotomy)	Discontinue VKA 72–96 h before surgery. Resume VKA the night of surgery if bleeding controlled.
Major procedures with risk factors for thromboembolism*	Discontinue VKA 72–96 h before surgery. Begin intravenous unfractionated heparin by continuous infusion or subcutaneous low-molecular weight heparin once INR falls below 2.5. Stop intravenous unfractionated heparin 6 h before surgery or low-molecular weight heparin 12 h before surgery. Resume heparin and VKA post-operatively after bleeding controlled (usually on day 1) and continue both until INR > 2.5. Decision regarding safety of resuming heparin must be individualized.

* Risk factors for thromboembolism:
AF, history of stroke or TIA or systemic embolus, hypercoagulable state, mechanical prosthesis in mitral position, > 1 prosthesis, thrombogenic prosthesis (Starr–Edwards, Bjork–Shiley). VKA, vitamin K antagonist.
Adapted from Bonow et al. *(1)* and O'Donoghue et al. *(26)*.

Management of Elevated INRs and Bleeding

Treatment of an elevated INR depends on the severity of the hypoprothrombinemia and the presence or threat of active bleeding *(4)*. Evaluation should include a search for potential causes such as incorrect dose, assay error, change in vitamin K1 intake or absorption, or initiation of medications that can interfere with VKA metabolism or function. For patients whose INR is elevated but less than 5.0, VKA therapy is held for one or two doses, INR monitoring is performed more frequently, and the weekly cumulative dose is reduced by 10–20% once the INR returns to a therapeutic range. For patients with an INR of 5.0–9.0 who are not bleeding, VKA therapy is held and oral vitamin K provided in a dose of 1.0–2.5 mg. The INR should decrease toward the therapeutic range in 24 h. Larger doses of vitamin K (5–10 mg) are required when the INR exceeds 9.0. The oral route of vitamin K administration is preferred in the absence of serious or life-threatening bleeding, as the response to subcutaneous vitamin K is more variable and anaphylactic reactions have been reported with intravenous treatment. Serious or life-threatening bleeding requires prompt reversal of the INR with fresh frozen plasma or Factor VIIa concentrate. In these circumstances, vitamin K is given intravenously as a slow infusion of 10 mg. When high doses of vitamin K are employed, there will be a relative period of hypercoagulabilty thereafter, often extending over several days.

Management of Anticoagulant Therapy in Pregnancy

The management of anticoagulant therapy in pregnancy, a state of relative hypercoagulability, is fraught with hazard. The aggregate risks of hemorrhage and thromboembolism, for both mother and fetus, as well as the superimposition of VKA-related embryopathy, must be carefully considered by patient, partner, and all members of the health care team. Treatment must be individualized. Many practitioners advocate the withdrawal of VKA therapy during the first trimester or at least during weeks 6–12, the period during which the risk of embryopathy is highest, especially when the daily dose of warfarin exceeds 5 mg (1, 4). VKA therapy should also be stopped at week 36 (or 2–3 weeks before term) in anticipation of labor and delivery to avoid fetal hemorrhage (1, 4, 23). VKAs can be considered for use between weeks 12 and 36, with a target INR of 3.0 (range 2.5–3.5). In high-risk circumstances, low-dose aspirin can be added after week 12. Other practitioners and patients choose to avoid VKA therapy throughout the entire duration of pregnancy. If unfractionated heparin is given continuously by intravenous infusion, the dose should be adjusted to maintain the aPTT at 2–2.5 times control. Unfractionated heparin can be given subcutaneously and the dose adjusted according to the mid-interval aPTT. Despite a paucity of data, many practitioners prefer weight-adjusted subcutaneous low-molecular weight heparin, aiming for a 4-h post-dose anti-Xa level of 0.7–1.2 U/ml (4). It is important to realize that the dose will vary over the course of pregnancy in relation to weight. Low-molecular weight heparin should not be used if anti-Xa levels cannot be assayed (1). VKAs are not excreted in breast milk and can be resumed as soon as possible after delivery, using a heparin bridge.

Prosthetic Valve Thrombosis

Thrombosis of a mechanical heart valve can have devastating consequences and hence early clinical recognition is critical (Fig. 3). Suspicion should be raised by symptoms of heart failure, thromboembolism, and/or low cardiac output, coupled with a decrease in the intensity of the mechanical valve closure sounds, new and pathologic murmurs, and documentation of inadequate anticoagulation. Thrombosis is more common in the mitral and tricuspid positions than in the aortic position. Evaluation with TTE/TEE can help guide management decisions. Confirmation of abnormal leaflet or disc excursion in the presence of an occluding thrombus can also be obtained rapidly with cardiac fluoroscopy. Although differentiation from pannus formation can be difficult, the clinical context usually allows accurate diagnosis. Emergency re-operation is recommended for patients with left-sided prosthetic valve thrombosis (PVT) and shock or NYHA Class III–IV symptoms (1). Surgery is also recommended for patients with left-sided PVT and a large thrombus burden (>0.8 cm^2). Fibrinolytic

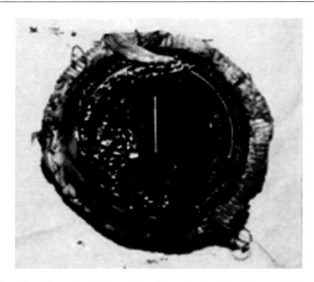

Fig. 3. Prosthetic valve thrombosis in a bileaflet mitral valve. From Goldsmith et al. *(27)*.

therapy with tPA (100 mg in accelerated fashion), SK, or UK, which carries a risk of 10–15% for death or cerebral embolic complications with left-sided PVT, can be considered for patients with NYHA Class I–II symptoms and small clot burdens, or for sicker patients with larger clot burdens when surgery is either not available or inadvisable *(1)*. Fibrinolytic therapy is also recommended for patients with right-sided PVT *(1)*. Some patients with no or minimal symptoms and small clot burdens can be managed with intravenous unfractionated heparin (UFH) and then converted to fibrinolytic therapy if unsuccessful. Any course of fibrinolytic therapy is followed at the appropriate interval by a continuous infusion of UFH during the transition to VKA therapy targeted to a higher INR with or without aspirin. Serial TTE studies are useful to assess the response to treatment.

Hemolytic Anemia

The development of a non-immune hemolytic anemia after valve replacement or repair surgery is usually attributable to a regurgitant, paravalvular leak with red cell destruction. Diagnosis is based on a high index of suspicion, coupled with laboratory evidence of hemolysis, including the characteristic changes in RBC morphology, elevated indirect bilirubin and LDH, a high reticulocyte count, and depressed serum haptoglobin. Re-operative surgery or catheter closure of the defect is indicated when heart failure, a persistent transfusion requirement, or poor quality of life intervene. Empiric medical measures include iron and folic acid replacement therapy and beta-adrenoreceptor blockers. It is important to exclude prosthetic valve endocarditis as a cause.

Antibiotic Prophylaxis to Prevent Infective Endocarditis

Antibiotic prophylaxis is indicated (Class I) to prevent infective endocarditis in all patients with prosthetic heart valves prior to dental procedures that involve manipulation of gingival tissue or the peri-apical region of teeth or perforation of the oral mucosa. Antibiotic prophylaxis may be considered (Class IIb) for selected GI or GU procedures associated with bacteremia *(6)*.

CONCLUSION

The medical treatment of patients with VHD is closely linked to an established schedule of clinical and echocardiographic follow-up, as dictated by the specific valve lesion and its anticipated natural history. There are at present no specific medical therapies available to arrest the progression of native valve disease. VKA therapy is critical to the management of patients with native valve disease or bioprosthetic substitutes and risk factors for thromboembolism, and is indicated for all patients with mechanical valve replacements. Concomitant medical treatment of co-existent disease, particularly CAD, hypertension, and diabetes, is usually unaffected by the presence of VHD, except in the instance of symptomatic, severe AS or advanced LV systolic dysfunction.

REFERENCES

1. Bonow R, Carabello B, Chatterjee K, et al. ACC/AHA 2006 Guidelines for the Management of Patients with Valvular Heart Disease: a report of the American College of Cardiology/American Heart Association Task Force on Practice Guidelines (Writing Committee to Develop Guidelines for the Management of Patients with Valvular Heart Disease). J Am Coll Cardiol 2006;48(3):e1–148.
2. Fuster V, Ryden LE, Cannom DS, et al. ACC/AHA/ESC 2006 Guidelines for the Management of Patients with Atrial Fibrillation: a report of the American College of Cardiology/American Heart Association Task Force on Practice Guidelines and the European Society of Cardiology Committee for Practice Guidelines (Writing Committee to Revise the 2001 Guidelines for the Management of Patients with Atrial Fibrillation): developed in collaboration with the European Heart Rhythm Association and the Heart Rhythm Society. Circulation 2006 Aug 15; 114(7):e257–354.
3. Stulak JM, Sundt TM III, Dearani JA, Daly RC, Orsulak TA, Schaff HV. Ten-year experience with the Cox-maze procedure for atrial fibrillation: how do we define success? Ann Thorac Surg 2007 Apr;83(4):1319–24.
4. Salem DN, Stein PD, Al-Ahmad A, et al. Anti-thrombotic therapy in valvular heart disease-native and prosthetic. The seventh ACCP conference on anti-thrombotic and thrombolytic therapy. Chest 2004;126(suppl);457S–82S.
5. Smith SC, Feldman TE, Hirshfeld JW, et al. ACC/AHA/SCAI 2005 guideline update for percutaneous coronary intervention. Available at http://www.acc.org
6. Wilson W, Taubert KA, Gewitz M, et al. Prevention of infective rndocarditis. guidelines from the American Heart Association. A guideline from the American Heart Association Rheumatic Fever, Endocarditis, and Kawasaki Disease Committee, Council on Cardiovascular Disease in the Young, and the Council on Clinical Cardiology, Council on Cardiovascular Surgery and Anesthesia, and the Quality of Care and Outcomes Research Interdisciplinary Working Group. Circulation 2007;116:1736–54.
7. WHO. Rheumatic fever and rheumatic heart disease: report of a WHO Expert Consultation, Geneva. 29 October–1 November, 2001.
8. Awan NA, DeMaria AN, Miller RR, et al. Beneficial effects of nitroprusside administration on left ventricular dysfunction and myocardial ischemia in severe aortic stenosis. Am Heart J 1981 Apr;101(4):386–94.
9. Khot UN, Novaro GM, Popovic ZB, et al. Nitroprusside in critically ill patients with left ventricular dysfunction and aortic stenosis. N Engl J Med 2003;348:1756–63.
10. Cowell SJ, Newby DE, Prescott RJ, et al. A randomized trial of intensive lipid-lowering therapy in calcific aortic stenosis. N Engl J Med 2005 Jun 9;352(23):2389–97.
11. Moura LM, Ramos SF, Zamorano JL, et al. Rosuvastatin affecting aortic valve endothelium to slow the progression of aortic stenosis. J Am Coll Cardiol 2007 Feb 6;49(5):554–61.
11a. Roseboro AB, Pedersen TR, Boman K et al. Intensive lipid lowering with simvastatin and ezetimibe in aortic stenosis. N Engl J Med 2008;359:1343–56.
12. Nessim SJ, Richardson RM. Dialysis for thiocyanate intoxication: a case report and review of the literature. ASAIO J. 2006 Jul–Aug;52(4):479–81.
13. The Seventh Report of the Joint National Committee on Prevention, Detection, Evaluation, and Treatment of High Blood Pressure (JNC 7). Available at http://www.nhlbi.nih.gov/guidelines/hypertension/
14. Greenberg B, Massie B, Bristow JD, et al. Long-term vasodilator therapy of chronic aortic insufficiency. A randomized double-blinded, placebo-controlled clinical trial. Circulation 1988 Jul;78(1):92–103.
15. Scognamiglio R, Fasoli G, Ponchia A, et al. Long-term nifedipine unloading therapy in asymptomatic patients with chronic severe aortic regurgitation. J Am Coll Cardiol 1990 Aug;16(2):424–9.
16. Scognamiglio R, Rahimtoola SH, Fasoli G, et al. Nifedipine in asymptomatic patients with severe aortic regurgitation and normal left ventricular function. N Engl J Med 1994 Sep 15;331(11):689–94.

17. Sondergaard L, Aldershvile J, Hildebrandt P, et al. Vasodilatation with felodipine in chronic asymptomatic aortic regurgitation. Am Heart J 2000 Apr;139(4):667–74.
18. Schon HR, Dorn R, Barthel P, et al. Effects of 12 months quinapril therapy in asymptomatic patients with chronic aortic regurgitation. J Heart Valve Dis 1994 Sep;3(5):500–9.
19. Lin M, Chiang HT, Lin SL, et al. Vasodilator therapy in chronic asymptomatic aortic regurgitation: enalapril versus hydralazine therapy. J Am Coll Cardiol 1994 Oct;24(4):1046–53.
20. Evangelista A, Tornos P, Sambola A, et al. Long-term vasodilator therapy in patients with severe aortic regurgitation. N Engl J Med 2005 Sep 29;353(13):1342–9.
21. Olesen KH. The natural history of 271 patients with mitral stenosis under medical treatment. Br Heart J 1962;24:349–57.
22. Melen-Mucha G, Lawnicka H, Kierszniewska-Stepien D, Komorowski J, Stepien H. The place of somatostatin analogs in the diagnosis and treatment of the neuoroendocrine glands tumors. Recent Pat Anticancer Drug Discov. 2006; 1(2):237–54.
23. The Task Force on Management of Valvular Heart Disease of the European Society of Cardiology. Guidelines on the management of valvular heart disease. Euro Heart J 2007;28:230–68.
24. Kulik A, Rubens FD, Wells PS, et al. Early postoperative anticoagulation after mechanical valve replacement: a systematic review. Ann Thorac Surg 2006 Feb;81(2):770–81.
25. Guidelines for the Diagnosis of Rheumatic Fever. Jones Criteria, 1992 update. Special Writing Group of the Committee on Rheumatic Fever, Endocarditis, and Kawasaki Disease of the Council on Cardiovascular Disease in the Young of the American Heart Association. JAMA 1992 Oct 21;268(15):2069–73.
26. O'Donoghue M, Malhotra R, Baggish A, et al. Cardiology. In: Sabatine M, Ed. Pocket Medicine (3rd ed). Philadelphia, PA: Lippincott, Williams and Wilkins; 2007.
27. Goldsmith I, Turpie AGG, Lip GYH. ABC of antithrombotic therapy: valvular heart disease and prosthetic heart valves. BMJ 2002 Nov 23;325:1228–31.

17 Percutaneous Valve Replacement

John G. Webb and Lukas Altwegg

CONTENTS

INTRODUCTION

The concept of an expandable stented valve prosthesis was first reported in an animal model by Andersen in 1992 (Fig. 1) *(1)*. Subsequently a number of groups pursued various approaches to percutaneous valve replacement *(2–9)*. Clinical implantation of a catheter-delivered stented valve in a pulmonary conduit was first reported by Bonhoeffer in 2000 *(10)*. This was followed successfully by implantation of an aortic prosthesis by Cribier in 2002 *(11)*. The demonstration of feasibility has been followed by rapid evolution of transcatheter procedures.

PULMONARY VALVE

Although the first percutaneous pulmonary valve implantation was described in 2000 *(12, 13)* as of early 2007 approximately 200 pulmonary implants had been performed *(10, 14)*. In fact the great majority of these implants are not into the native pulmonary artery, but rather into stenotic surgical conduits connecting the right ventricle to the pulmonary artery. While conduits are tubular and the diameter often ideally suited to stent implantation, the native pulmonary annulus is typically too large in diameter and the anatomy poorly suited to accommodate currently available pulmonary implants.

Right ventricular outflow tract disease in patients with congenital heart disease is commonly an indication for surgical implantation of a conduit. Currently such conduits generally incorporate a homograft or xenograft valve. With time, stenosis of the conduit or regurgitation of the valve commonly develops. Progressive right heart dilation and failure often requires reoperation to replace the conduit and valve *(15)*. Percutaneous balloon dilatation or stenting has played an important role in the management of conduit stenosis. Percutaneous valve implantation offers the additional possibility of addressing regurgitation.

From: *Contemporary Cardiology: Valvular Heart Disease*
Edited by: Andrew Wang, Thomas M. Bashore, DOI 10.1007/978-1-59745-411-7_17
© Humana Press, a part of Springer Science+Business Media, LLC 2009

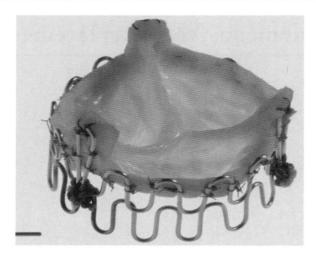

Fig. 1. The Andersen valve.

Pulmonary valve implantation has, for the most part, been performed under general anesthesia. Vascular access is gained from the femoral or internal jugular vein. The prototypic Melody™ valve (Medtronic Inc) is constructed from a platinum–iridium stent into which is sewn a bovine jugular venous valve (Fig. 2). The stent is manually crimped onto a valvuloplasty balloon. The valve delivery catheter incorporates a retractable sheath to cover the crimped stent and improve deliverability. The balloon utilized is a balloon-in-balloon catheter (BIB, Numed Inc) in which the inner balloon is initially inflated to fix the stent following which the outer balloon is inflated to fully expand the stent (Fig. 3). Because the bovine jugular valve is a low-pressure and very compliant structure it can remain functional even in a relatively small diameter conduit. However, because of the diameter of the bovine

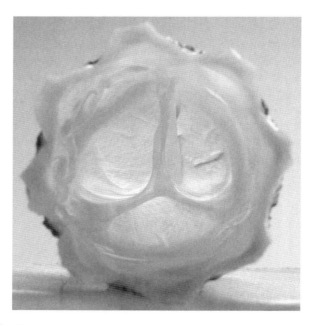

Fig. 2. The Melody bovine jugular valve (courtesy Medtronic Inc.).

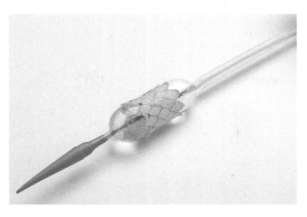

Fig. 3. Melody valve mounted on a balloon catheter (courtesy Medtronic Inc.).

jugular vein the valve is typically suitable only for conduits with a diameter of 22 mm or less. This size limitation excludes the majority of patients with large pulmonary trunks *(7)*.

Pulmonary conduit valve implantation has been shown to result in an improvement in right heart pressures, gradients, and volumes as well as left ventricular function and exercise tolerance. Success rates are very high, morbidity low, and mortality rare in elective patients *(10, 12, 14, 16)*. Homograft rupture during valve implantation is very rare. A relatively small risk of ectopic coronary artery compression can be minimized by pre-implantation screening. Stent fracture has been relatively common with an incidence of 21% at intermediate term follow-up *(10)*. Stent fracture is most often managed conservatively. While loss of integrity may occur implantation of a new valve within an old one appears feasible and may delay the need for surgical conduit replacement. Future modification of the current stent may lessen the frequency of stent fracture.

Recently the Cribier–Edwards aortic stent valve has also been utilized in the pulmonary position with good success (Fig. 4) *(17)*. In contrast to the bovine jugular valve, the use of pericardial tissue to form leaflets facilitates the manufacture of multiple valve sizes and the stent design may benefit from greater resistance to fracture. Potential disadvantages include the accuracy required when positioning this relatively short stent and the delivery system which is not yet optimized for use in the pulmonary position.

AORTIC VALVE

Aortic stenosis is the commonest lesion for which aortic valve surgery is performed. Aortic stenosis has a prolonged and relatively benign latent period. Once symptoms develop survival averages only a few years and the benefits of medical management are limited *(18)*. In contrast aortic valve replacement surgery appears to offer benefit in terms of both survival and symptoms. Current guidelines specify aortic stenosis in combination with symptoms, a left ventricular ejection fraction <50% or concomitant coronary bypass, aortic or heart valve surgery as class I indications for surgical valve replacement *(18)*.

Aortic valve replacement can be performed at very low risk with excellent and durable results. However, many patients with severe aortic stenosis have significant comorbidities that increase the risks of open heart surgery with thoracotomy and cardiopulmonary bypass. According to the Society of Thoracic Surgeons Database (1998–2001) surgical aortic valve replacement carries a rate of serious complication or mortality of 16.8%. Medicare data document an operative mortality of 8.8% *(19)*. Operative risk is increased in the setting of comorbidities *(20–24)*.

The prevalence of aortic stenosis increases with advanced age. Community data document a prevalence of moderate or severe aortic stenosis of 0.6% in patients aged 55–64, 1.4% between the ages

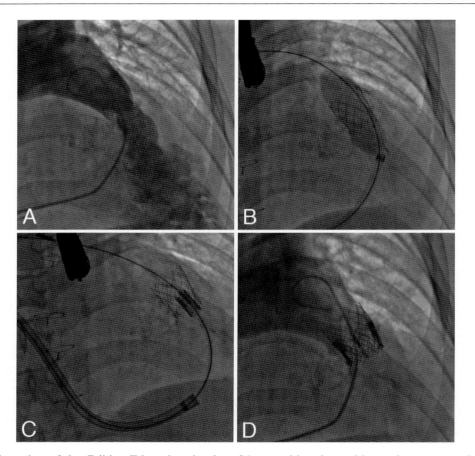

Fig. 4. Implantation of the Cribier–Edwards valve in a 24-year-old patient with a pulmonary conduit, **A**. The stenotic homograft right ventricular to pulmonary arterial conduit, **B**. The conduit has been stented open, **C**. A Cribier–Edwards valve is positioned within the previously placed stent and conduit, **D**. The implanted valve is competent.

of 65 and 74, to 4.6% in patients $\geq$ 75 *(25)*. Patients with symptomatic aortic stenosis are very often elderly and are particularly likely to be managed medically due to surgical risks that either they, or their physicians, consider unacceptable *(25, 26)*. The limitations of current surgery have prompted interest in less invasive options. Early enthusiasm for balloon valvuloplasty was quickly tempered as the limitations became apparent. Symptomatic benefit is marginal and the benefit is not durable *(27–29)*.

BALLOON-EXPANDABLE AORTIC VALVE

The prototype balloon-expandable Cribier–Edwards™ valve (Edwards Lifesciences Inc) is constructed of a stainless steel frame (Fig. 5). A tissue valve constructed of equine pericardial leaflets is sewn to the stent frame. The bottom one-third of the stent is covered with a fabric sealing cuff intended to form a seal against the aortic annulus. Currently this valve is available in two sizes measuring 23 or 26 mm in external diameter with respective lengths of just over 14 and 16 mm. The valves are supplied sterile and a mechanical crimping device is utilized to compress the stent onto a standard balloon catheter.

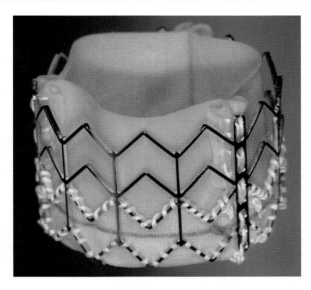

Fig. 5. The Cribier–Edwards balloon-expandable aortic valve (courtesy Edwards Lifesciences Inc.).

Currently three approaches to transcatheter aortic valve replacement utilizing balloon-expandable stents are utilized: transvenous, transarterial, and transapical.

Transvenous Procedure

An antegrade transvenous approach was initially utilized due to the large profile of the stent-based prosthesis *(30)*. The femoral vein is accessed percutaneously. Transseptal puncture and dilation allows access to the left atrium. A flotation balloon is passed from the left atrium, through the mitral valve and into the left ventricle. A wire is advanced through the aortic valve and around the aortic arch to the descending aorta. At this point a snare catheter is utilized to exteriorize the wire through the contralateral femoral artery. This leaves a large wire loop entering one femoral vein and exiting the opposite femoral artery. The prosthesis is mounted onto a valvuloplasty balloon and then passed through the femoral vein, the interatrial septum, mitral valve, and then to the aortic valve. Tensioning the two ends of the exteriorized wire facilitates passage of the prosthesis through the heart. Burst pacing is utilized to stabilize balloon position during prosthesis deployment.

The transvenous antegrade approach to the aortic valve does have advantages. The femoral vein is larger and more compliant than the femoral artery and can relatively easily accommodate a large profile catheter; it rarely requires repair and hemostasis is easily achieved. Crossing the stenotic native aortic valve with a large profile prosthesis is more easily accomplished from the funnel-like ventricular approach than from the aortic aspect.

There are also a number of disadvantages associated with the transvenous approach. Transseptal puncture has an inherent risk of tamponade. Catheter passage through the left heart may result in mitral insufficiency, arrhythmias, hemodynamic instability, or serious mitral injury. The procedure is complex and difficult to reproduce. Although initial experience with the transvenous approach demonstrated the feasibility of percutaneous valve replacement this procedure has been supplanted by the transarterial approach.

Transarterial

A few early attempts at transarterial retrograde access to the aortic valve were met with difficulty due to arterial access with large sheaths and catheters, passage of the large diameter prostheses around the aortic arch, and difficulty in crossing the stenotic aortic valve from the retrograde direction. Initial attempts utilizing balloon-expandable valves crimped onto standard valvuloplasty balloons were only sporadically successful *(31, 32)*.

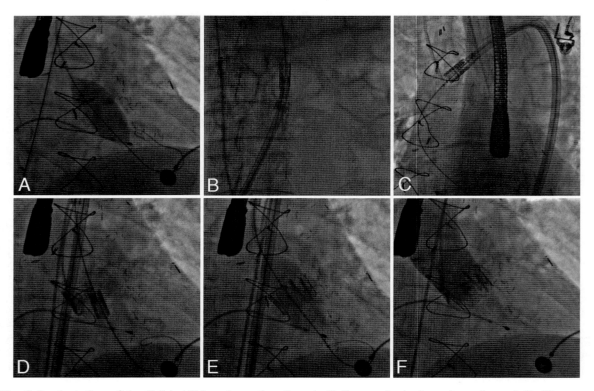

Fig. 6. Implantation of the Cribier–Edwards aortic valve, **A**. Balloon valvuloplasty is performed, **B**. The stent valve is mounted on a balloon catheter and advance out of a femorally placed sheath into the abdominal aorta, **C**. The stent is advanced through the aortic arch and native valve with the assistance of a deflectable delivery catheter, **D**. The stent is positioned within the native valve, **E**. The stent valve is expanded displacing the native valve, **F**. The prosthetic valve is seen to be well positioned with no regurgitation following implantation.

Subsequently a more reliable transarterial approach was developed *(33)*. The currently available Cribier–Edwards valve requires insertion of a 22 or 24 F sheath, depending on the size of the prosthesis. The procedure utilizes a steerable, deflectable guiding catheter (RetroFlex, Edwards Lifesciences Inc) along with specially designed dilators and sheaths (Fig. 6).

Initial results were more favorable than had previously been seen with the transvenous approach *(33)*. Subsequently we reported our experience in the first 50 patients undergoing transarterial balloon-expandable valve implantation due to "inoperability" *(34)*. Valve implantation was successful in 86% of patients with an intra-procedural mortality of 2%. Mortality at 30 days was 12%, comparing favorably to a logistic Euroscore estimate of 28% in this high-risk group. With experience, procedural success increased from 76% in the first 25 patients to 96% in the second half of this experience and 30-day mortality fell from 16 to 8%. Valve replacement was associated with an increase in echocardiographic valve area from 0.6 ± 0.2 to 1.7 ± 0.4 cm^2 (Fig. 7). There were significant improvements in left ventricular ejection fraction, mitral regurgitation, and functional class which were maintained

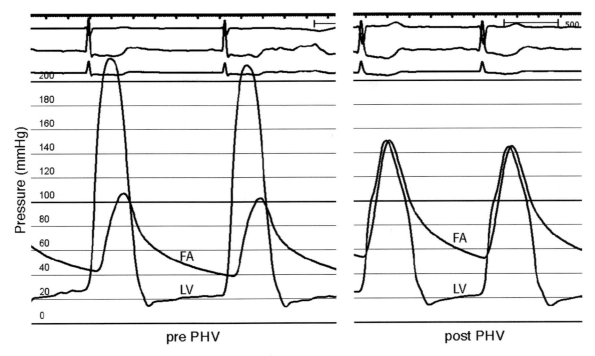

Fig. 7. Left ventricular aortic gradient. *Left*: Aortic stenosis. *Right*: Percutaneous valve.

at 1 year. Structural valve deterioration was not observed with a median follow-up of almost 1 year and over 2 years in some patients. Our subsequent experience with almost 100 patients confirms this early experience as do, as yet unpublished, data from the European/ Canadian REVIVE trial with 63 patients and the REVIVE-II trial in the United States with 67 patients.

Transapical Approach

Although the transfemoral arterial procedure has proven successful, some patients are poorly suited to this approach due to femoral, iliac or aortic size, tortuosity, or atheroma. Our group utilized direct balloon catheter implantation of experimental prostheses through the left ventricular apex in early experimental studies of percutaneous valve implantation *(4)*. Subsequently this approach was extensively trialed in animals *(35)*. Early attempts at human application were performed through a median sternotomy with cardiopulmonary bypass *(36)*. Subsequently we described transapical implantation through an intercostal thoracotomy without cardiopulmonary bypass *(37, 38)*. This approach has now been widely applied with demonstrated reproducibility (Fig. 8) *(36, 39, 40)*.

This procedure is performed in an operating room or catheterization laboratory setting with fluoroscopy and echocardiographic guidance typically by a combined team of interventional cardiologists and cardiac surgeons. Under general anesthesia the pleural space overlying the apex is entered via a small anterolateral thoracotomy. The pericardium over the apex of the left ventricle is opened. Temporary epicardial ventricular pacing wires are placed, as during valvuloplasty and prosthesis deployment, rapid pacing is applied to minimize transaortic flow and cardiac motion *(41)*. The thin portion of the left ventricular apex is identified and punctured with an arterial needle. A large 24–34 French sheath is placed from the apex into the left ventricular cavity. Aortic balloon valvuloplasty is typically performed. Fluoroscopy, aortic root angiography, and TEE are used to aid positioning. Hemostasis is secured with pledgeted sutures and a chest tube is placed.

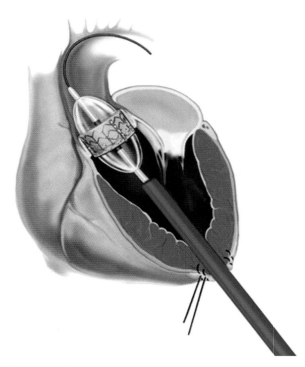

Fig. 8. Transapical sheath placement through a thoracotomy allows access for a catheter-mounted stent valve (courtesy Edwards Lifesciences Inc.).

Advantages of this approach include the avoidance of problems related to arterial access. The aortic valve is more easily crossed antegrade and the relatively short distance from the access site to the aortic valve may facilitate positioning. Disadvantages include the need for a thoracotomy and chest tube drainage resulting in respiratory compromise, a possibility of mitral injury, apical injury, and need for apical repair and hemostasis. To date experience with this procedure is limited. As of early 2007, 136 procedures had been performed in 6 centers in Canada, Europe, and the United States with a 30 day mortality of 18% in a high-risk cohort (Source: Edwards Lifesciences Inc., unpublished data).

SELF-EXPANDING AORTIC VALVE

The self-expanding CoreValve™ device (CoreValve Inc) incorporates a self-expanding stent laser cut from a tube of nitinol (Fig. 9). This nickel–titanium alloy is soft and compliant at low temperature allowing compression within a relatively low-profile delivery sheath. At body temperature the alloy will assume its predetermined configuration becoming rigid and structurally strong when the restraining sheath is retracted (Fig. 10). The lower portion of the stent has a high radial force and is positioned within the aortic annulus. The middle portion of the stent contains the biologic valve and is tapered to avoid interference with the coronary arteries. The upper portion of the stent is flared to fix the stent against the wall of the ascending aorta. A bovine or porcine pericardial valve is sutured to the frame. Currently the valve is available in two sizes depending on the diameter of the ascending aorta (<35 or <45 mm) with one aortic annular diameter (23 mm). The stent measures 50 mm in length. Initially the delivery system was 24 F, but subsequently evolved to 21 F and more recently to 18 F.

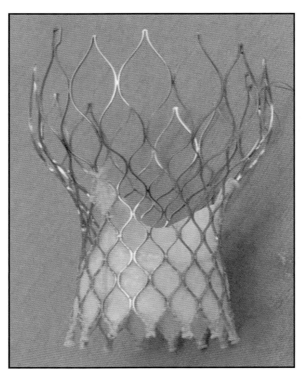

Fig. 9. The CoreValve self-expanding aortic valve with its upper flared portion designed to anchor within the ascending aorta (courtesy CoreValve Inc.).

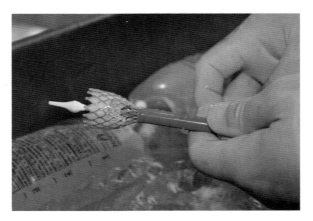

Fig. 10. The CoreValve self-expanding aortic valve partially released from its constraining sheath (courtesy of Raoul Bonan MD).

CoreValve Procedure

The CoreValve procedure has been termed "revalving." Initial procedures required a surgical cutdown on the femoral artery but as device size has fallen the feasibility of percutaneous access and closure has been reported *(42)*.

Initial procedures were performed with a 24 F catheter which required a cutdown with a complex delivery mechanism. Valve implantation required femoral–femoral cardiopulmonary support due to obstruction to transvalvular flow during release of the valve. Initial experience demonstrated the feasibility of the procedure. Subsequently Grube et al. reported their single center experience *(43, 44)*. The valve was successfully implanted in 88% of 25 patients with major in-hospital adverse events in 32% and in-hospital mortality in 20%. Thrombocytopenia proved problematic. This was thought possibly related to cardiopulmonary bypass and ameliorated with the use of clopidogrel and more recent experience suggests this is less of a concern. As of early 2007 over 168 CoreValve procedures have been performed *(42, 45, 46)*. Unpublished data are available on 83 cases performed with the current generation 18F system with a reported procedural success of 89% and 30-day mortality of 16% as compared to a logistic Euroscore estimate of 20% (Source: CoreValve Inc., unpublished data).

NEWER VALVES

Multiple additional valves are currently under development. At this time human aortic implants have been performed with at least three devices. The Panigua valve is a prototypic balloon-expandable stent valve. The Direct Flow™ valve utilizes a hollow tubular frame which is filled with a fluid material which solidifies forming a rigid structure. The Sadra™ valve combines self-expanding properties with the ability to shorten and simultaneously expand or lengthen and constrict the prosthesis allowing repositioning when necessary. Experience remains preliminary.

PROCEDURAL ISSUES

Vascular Access

Transarterial access is usually achieved via the femoral artery. The large diameter of currently available prosthesis is a major limiting factor. First generation valves were typically 7–8 mm in diameter, requiring the use of a 22–24 French sheath. While an elastic, disease-free femoral artery may be easily able to accommodate such a sheath with an external diameter of 8–9 mm many patients have atherosclerosis, tortuosity, or calcification which renders this problematic. Careful angiographic and often CT screening of the femoral and iliac arteries is required to assess suitability. Currently the majority of patients are potential candidates for transarterial valve replacement and as device size is reduced this will become less of an issue.

Imaging During Valve Implantation

Accurate positioning of the prosthetic valve is obviously critical. In the early percutaneous experience, operators sought to position the midpoint of the prosthetic valve adjacent to the major leaflet calcification. Aortography is routinely utilized to assist positioning. Transesophageal echocardiography is variably utilized due to the requirement for anesthetic and difficulty imaging the prosthetic valve prior to implantation. We utilize echocardiography routinely and find it useful for positioning, particularly when calcification is limited. Additional value comes from the ability to rapidly assess left ventricular function and filling, pericardial fluid, and paravalvular insufficiency.

Device Stabilization During Deployment

Unpredictable movement can compromise precise positioning of transcatheter valves. A number of methods have been utilized to transvalvular flow and cardiac motion during valve deployment *(43, 47–57)*. Adenosine-induced atrio-ventricular block *(50, 57)*, temporary ventricular fibrillation, and temporary obstruction of right heart flow have been proposed. However, only two methods have been utilized to date.

Burst pacing is relatively reliable and reproducible *(58)*. Pacing-induced atrio-ventricular asynchrony, left ventricular dyskinesis, compromised ventricular filling, reduction in stroke volume, and cardiac output are possible mechanisms. Typically less than 15 s of rapid pacing is required for balloon-expandable valve deployment and rapid pacing is generally, but not always, well tolerated (Fig. 11) *(33)*.

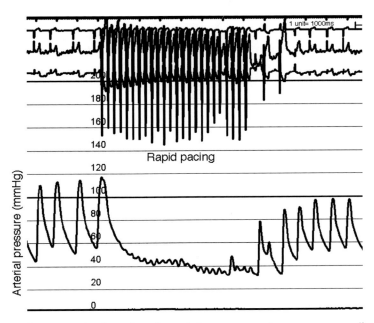

Fig. 11. Burst pacing produces transiently reduced arterial pressure, pulse pressure, cardiac output, and cardiac motion.

Both femoral arterial–venous bypass and left atrial–arterial bypass (TandemHeart™) have been utilized to reduce transvalvular phasic flow during CoreValve implantation *(42–44, 46)*. Although circulatory support may be advantageous in hemodynamically unstable patients, the invasiveness and complexity of routine circulatory support is problematic. More recently, as the mechanism of CoreValve deployment has evolved it appears that cardiopulmonary support may not routinely be necessary with this procedure *(42, 46)*.

Paravalvular Insufficiency

With current transcatheter valves some degree of paravalvular insufficiency is commonly found if sought with sufficient diligence. Moderate leaks are not uncommon and severe leaks may occur. This appears true with both current balloon-expandable and self-expanding valves. Transesophageal echocardiography is currently the most sensitive means of detecting paravalvular jets. Early experience with balloon-expandable valves suggested that severe insufficiency was relatively common and problematic *(3, 11)*. Subsequent experience demonstrated that routine oversizing, aggressive balloon dilation, and optimal positioning of the sealing cuff reduced the clinical significance of paravalvular regurgitation. Furthermore mild paravalvular leaks did not appear to have major clinical consequences *(33, 34)*. Hemolysis, common with mitral paravalvular leaks, is uncommonly seen with aortic leaks presumably to the lesser diastolic gradient between the aorta and the left ventricle. Nevertheless more effective sealing mechanisms, more accurate positioning, better sizing, and patient screening will be needed to reduce concerns surrounding paravalvular regurgitation and further surveillance will be required.

Coronary Obstruction

There are several potential mechanisms of coronary obstruction. Embolization of friable valvular debris could occur, although this has not been recognized to date. Occlusion of a coronary ostium by a prosthetic sealing cuff has been a concern; however, it is unlikely that a current sealing cuff positioned in the aortic annulus would extend to the level of the coronary ostia. In any event the diameter of the stent is typically less than that of the aorta at the level of the sinus of Valsalva. However, it does appear that a prosthetic valve can displace a bulky native coronary leaflet over a coronary ostium (41). Echocardiographic, fluoroscopic, angiographic, and CT screening may be useful for preventing this problem.

Stroke

Prior experience with balloon valvuloplasty found that stroke was relatively uncommon despite heavy aortic valve calcification (29, 59). It has been suggested that the thin valvular endothelium remains relatively intact during valvuloplasty, thereby reducing the potential for embolization of calcific debris. However, stroke may also occur due to ascending aortic atheroembolism, thromboembolism from catheters or wires, intravascular air, hypotension, or bleeding due to anticoagulation.

In our experience with balloon-expandable valve implantation the incidence of clinically detected stroke with both the transarterial and the transapical procedure has been approximately 4% to date (34, 60). It is reasonable to assume that the incidence of subclinical cerebral embolism and undetected stroke may be higher. In the REVIVAL study the incidence of stroke or TIA was reportedly 9%, presumably in part due to the inclusion of milder events (such as TIAs) and study mandated routine neurologic screening. Similarly the incidence of stroke in the largest CoreValve experience to date was 10% (46). Hopefully this incidence will decline with procedural and equipment enhancements.

Patient Selection

Transcatheter aortic valve implantation is still a procedure for which broader experience is needed prior to broad application. Currently this procedure is appropriate only for patients poorly suited to conventional surgery. Specific exclusions are few (Table 1). An annulus that is too small or too large for available prosthesis is an obvious exclusion. Currently available valves are suitable for an annulus diameter of 18–26 mm. The CoreValve device is also specific as to the diameter of the ascending aorta due to its additional fixation at that location. Transarterial procedures require arterial access adequate for the sheath size required for the specific-sized prosthesis. We exclude patients in whom a reasonable quality and duration of life is unlikely even should valve implantation be successful, a not uncommon issue in patients with multiple comorbidities.

Learning Curve

Transcatheter aortic valve implantation is a relatively complex procedure and the stakes are high. Technical errors are not well tolerated and mortality may be the consequence. Outcomes clearly improve with improvements in equipment, techniques, and experience (Fig. 12) (34, 46). Consequently

Table 1
Screening for Transcatheter Valve Implantation

Questions to be answered	Evaluation	Comments
Should the patient have conventional AVR?	Surgical consult	Estimated operative mortality $< 20\%$ Acceptable morbidity
What is the annulus diameter?	Echo (maybe CT?)	Valves are specific to a range of diameters
Is percutaneous access adequate?	Ilio-femoral catheter, CT, or MR angiogram	Assess lumen diameter, tortuosity and calcification
Is the aortic root adequate?	Ascending catheter, CT or MR angiogram	Assess abnormal root, potential for coronary obstruction
Is there LV dysfunction?	Echo or LV angiogram	Increases risk of ischemia during implantation
Is there the potential for ischemia?	Coronary angiogram	Is there increased risk of ischemia during implantation? Is revascularization required?
Is there anemia or a clotting disorder?	Hb, platelets, PTT	There is a risk of blood loss from access sites
Is there renal dysfunction?	Cr	Contrast nephropathy and transient hypotension can occur
Are there anesthetic concerns?	Anesthetic consult	Intubation and ventilation may be utilized
Are expectations realistic?	History, family support, comorbidities	Do comorbidities permit a reasonable quality and duration of life?

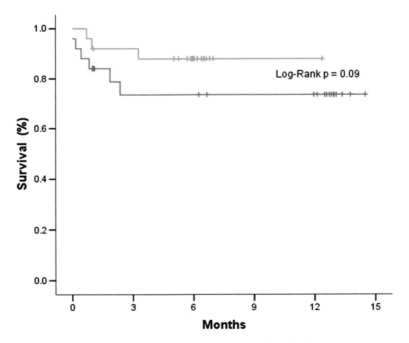

Fig. 12. Evidence for a learning curve and improving outcomes. Survival in the first-in-man transarterial balloon-expandable aortic valve experience in patients declined conventional surgery. Kaplan–Meier survival curve. First 25 patients vs. second 25 patients. Logistic Euroscore 26 and 30%, respectively.

cautious dissemination appears prudent. Formal educational programs and proctoring are desirable. Virtual reality simulators have been developed and appear helpful. Regional centers of expertise may be desirable to optimize patient selection and results.

Long-Term Follow-Up

Early experience demonstrated an acute improvement in left ventricular systolic function *(42, 61)*. Longer term follow-up has confirmed that this is sustained and associated with a sustained improvement in mitral insufficiency and functional class *(34)*. In vitro valve testing of currently available devices anticipate durability in excess of 10 years and structural valve deterioration has not been reported. However, only one report has documented late survival beyond 1 year in a significant number of patients *(34)* (Fig. 12) and follow-up beyond 3 years has only been reported in a few patients to date *(31, 34)*.

Design of Clinical Trials

Percutaneous valve implantation in pulmonary conduits is rapidly becoming standard practice where this is available. The small number of patients and limited options available to these patients mean that we will likely be reliant on registry evaluation for some time. Transcatheter aortic valve implantation is more complex and associated with greater risk. Acquired aortic stenosis is common and the availability of a proven surgical alternative argues for rigorous comparison of these therapies *(62, 63)*. A randomized comparison of transarterial aortic valve implantation versus standard of care is currently underway in the United States and Canada and will hopefully further clarify the role of this therapeutic approach.

SUMMARY

Transcatheter valve replacement is in its infancy and continues to evolve rapidly. As technology, techniques, and expertise evolve it appears likely that this new therapeutic modality will join surgical valve replacement as a routine option for patients with valve disease.

REFERENCES

1. Andersen HR, Knudsen LL, Hasenkam JM. Transluminal implantation of artificial heart valves. Description of a new expandable aortic valve and initial results with implantation by catheter technique in closed chest pigs. Eur Heart J 1992;13:704–708.
2. Andersen HR, Knudsen LL, Hasenkam JM. Transluminal implantation of artificial heart valves. Description of a new expandable aortic valve and initial results with implantation by catheter technique in closed chest pigs. Eur Heart J 1992;13:704–708.
3. Cribier A, Eltchaninoff H, Bash A, Borenstein N, Tron C, Bauer F, Derumeaux G, Anselme F, Laborde F, Leon MB. Trans-catheter implantation of balloon-expandable prosthetic heart valves. Early results in an animal model. Circulation 2001;104(Suppl 2):I552.
4. Stone GW, Webb JG, Cox D, Brodie B, Qureshi M, Dulas D, Kalynych A, Turco M, Schultheiss HP, Rutherford B, Krucoff MW, Gibbons R, Lansky AJ, Pop R, Mehran R, Jones D. Primary angioplasty in acute myocardial infarction with distal protection of the microcirculation: principal results from the prospective, randomized EMERALD trial. J Am Coll Cardiol 2004;43(5):285A.
5. Sochman J, Peregrin JH, Pavcnik D, Timmermans H, Rosch J. Percutaneous transcatheter aortic disc valve prosthesis implantation: a feasibility study. Cardiovasc Intervent Radiol 2000;23:384–388.
6. Lutter G, Kuklinski D, Berg G, Von Samson P, Martin J, Handke M, Uhrmeister P, Beyersdorf F. Percutaneous aortic valve replacement: an experimental study. J Thorac Cardiovasc Surg 2002;123:768–776.

7. Boudjemline Y, Agnoletti G, Bonnet D, et al. Percutaneous pulmonary valve replacement in a large right ventricular outflow tract: an experimental study. J Am Coll Cardiog 2004;43:1082–1087.

8. Boudjemline Y, Bonhoeffer P. Percutaneous implantation of a valve in the descending aorta in lambs. Eur Heart J 2002;23:1045–1049.

9. Vassiliades TA Jr, Block PC, Cohn LH, Adams DH, Borer JS, Feldman T, Holmes DR, Laskey WK, Lytle BW, Mack MJ, Williams DO. The clinical development of percutaneous heart valve technology: a position statement of the Society of Thoracic Surgeons (STS), the American Association for Thoracic Surgery (AATS), and the Society of Cardiovascular Angiography and Intervention (SCAI). Cathet Cardiovasc Interv 2005; 65:73–79.

10. Nordmeyer J, Khambadkone S, Coats L, Schievano S, Lurz P, Parenzan G, Taylor AM, Lock JE, Bonhoeffer P. Risk stratification, systematic classification and anticipatory management strategies for stent fracture after percutaneous pulmonary valve implantation. Circulation 2007;115:1392–1397.

11. Cribier A, Eltchaninoff H, Bash A, Borenstein N, Tron C, Bauer F, Derumeaux G, Anselme F, Laborde F, Leon MB. Percutaneous transcatheter implantation of an aortic valve prosthesis for calcific aortic stenosis: first human case description. Circulation 2002;106:3006–3008.

12. Bonhoeffer P, Boudjemline Y, Saliba Z, Hausse AO, Aggoun Y, Bonnet D, Sidi D, Kachaner J. Transcatheter implantation of a bovine valve in pulmonary position: a lamb study. Circulation 2000;102:813–816.

13. Bonhoeffer P, Boudjemline Y, Saliba Z, Merckx J, Aggoun Y, Bonnet D, Acar P, Le Bidois J, Sidi D, Kachaner J. Percutaneous replacement of pulmonary valve in a right-ventricle to pulmonary-artery prosthetic conduit with valve dysfunction. Lancet 2000;356:1403–1405.

14. Bonhoeffer P, Boudjemline Y, Qureshi SA, Le Bidois J, Iserin L, Acar P, Merckx J, Kachaner J, Sidi D. Percutaneous insertion of the pulmonary valve. J Am Coll Cardiol 2002;39:1664–1669.

15. Bouzas B, Kilner PJ, Gatzoulis MA. Pulmonary regurgitation: not a benign lesion. Eur Heart J 2005;26:433–439.

16. Boudjemline Y, Bonhoeffer P. Percutaneous implantation of a valve in the descending aorta in lambs. Eur Heart J 2002;23:1045–1049.

17. Garay F, Webb J, Hijazi ZM. Percutaneous replacement of pulmonary valve using the Edwards-Cribier percutaneous heart valve: first report in a human patient. Cathet Cardiovasc Interv 2006;67:659–662.

18. Bonow RO, Carabello BA, Kanu C, de Leon AC, Jr, Faxon DP, Freed MD, Gaasch WH, Lytle BW, Nishimura RA, O'Gara PT, O'Rourke RA, Otto CM, Shah PM, Shanewise JS, Smith SC, Jr, Jacobs AK, Adams CD, Anderson JL, Antman EM, Faxon DP, Fuster V, Halperin JL, Hiratzka LF, Hunt SA, Lytle BW, Nishimura R, Page RL, Riegel B. ACC/AHA 2006 guidelines for the management of patients with valvular heart disease: a report of the American College of Cardiology/American Heart Association Task Force on practice guidelines. Circulation 2006;114:e84–231.

19. Goodney PP, O'Connor GT, Wennberg DE, Birkmeyer JD. Do hospitals with low mortality rates in coronary artery bypass also perform well in valve replacement? Ann Thorac Surg 2003;76:1131–1136.

20. Sundt TM, Bailey MS, Moon MR, Mendeloff EN, Huddleston CB, Pasque MK, Barner HB, Gay WB, Jr. Quality of life after aortic valve replacement at the age of > 80 years. Circulation 2000;102(19 Suppl 3):III70–74.

21. Mullany CJ. Aortic valve surgery in the elderly. Cardiol Rev 2000;8:333–339.

22. Mortasawi A, Gehle S, Schroder T, Ennker IC, Rosendahl U, Dalladaku F, Bauer S, Albert A, Ennker J. [Aortic valve replacement in 80 – and over 80-year-old patients. Short-term and long-term results]. Z Gerontol Geriatr 2000;33:438–446.

23. Bloomstein LZ, Gielchinsky I, Berstein AD, Parsonnet V, Saunders C, Karanam R, Graves B. Aortic valve replacement in geriatric patients: determinants of in-hospital mortality. Ann Thorac Surg 2001;71:597–600.

24. Kolh P, Kerzmann A, Lahaye L, Gerard P, Limet R. Cardiac surgery in octogenarians; peri-operative outcome and long-term results. Eur Heart J 2001;22:1235–1243.

25. Nkomo VT, Gardin JM, Skelton TN, Gottdiener JS, Scott CG, Enriquez-Sarano M. Burden of valvular heart diseases: a population-based study. Lancet 2006;368:1005–1011.

26. Iung B, Baron G, Butchart EG, Delahaye F, Gohlke-Barwolf C, Levang OW, Tornos P, Vanoverschelde JL, Vermeer F, Boersma E, Ravaud P, Vahanian A. A prospective survey of patients with valvular heart disease in Europe: The Euro Heart Valve Survey on Valvular Disease. Eur Heart J 2003;24:1231–1243.

27. Otto CM, Mickel MC, Kennedy JW, Alderman EL, Bashore TM, Block PC, Brinker JA, Diver D, Ferguson J, Holmes DR Jr. Three-year outcome after balloon aortic valvuloplasty: insights into prognosis of valvular aortic stenosis. Circulation 1994;89:642–650.

28. Lieberman EB, Bashore TM, Hermiller JB, Wilson JS, Pieper KS, Keeler GP, Pierce CH, Kisslo KB, Harrison JK, Davidson CJ. Balloon aortic valvuloplasty in adults: failure of procedure to improve long-term survival. J Am Coll Cardiol 1995;26:1522–1528.

29. Feldman T. Core curriculum for interventional cardiology: percutaneous valvuloplasty. Catheter Cardiovasc Interv 2003;60:48–56.

30. Cribier A, Eltchaninoff H, Bash A, Borenstein N, Tron C, Bauer F, Derumeaux G, Anselme F, Laborde F, Leon MB. Percutaneous transcatheter implantation of an aortic valve prosthesis for calcific aortic stenosis: first human case description. Circulation 2002;106(24):3006–3008.

31. Cribier A, Eltchaninoff H, Tron C, Bauer F, Gerber L. Percutaneous implantation of aortic valve prosthesis in patients with calcific aortic stenosis: technical advances, clinical results and future strategies. J Invasive Cardiol 2006;19:S88–S96.

32. Hanzel GS, Harrity PJ, Schreiber TL, O'Neill WW. Retrograde percutaneous aortic valve implantation for critical aortic stenosis. Catheter Cardiovasc Interv 2005;64(3):322–326.

33. Webb JG, Chandavimol M, Thompson CR, Ricci DR, Carere RG, Munt BI, Buller CE, Pasupati S, Lichtenstein S. Percutaneous aortic valve implantation retrograde from the femoral artery. Circulation 2006;113(6):842–850.

34. Webb JG, Pasupati SJ, Humphries K, Thompson C, Altwegg L, Moss R, Sinhal A, Carere RG, Munt B, Ricci D, Ye J, Cheung A, Lichtenstein SV. Percutaneous transarterial aortic valve replacement in selected high risk patients with aortic stenosis. Circulation 2007;116:755–763.

35. Walther T, Dewey T, Wimmer-Greinecker G, Doss M, Hambrecht R, Schuler G, Mohr FW, Mack M. Transapical approach for sutureless stent-fixed aortic valve implantation: experimental results. Eur J Cardiothorac Surg 2007;29:703–708.

36. Walter T, Mohr FW. Aortic valve surgery: time to be open-minded and to rethink. Euro J Cardiothorac Surg 2007;31:4–6.

37. Ye J, Cheung A, Lichtenstein SV, Carere RG, Thompson CR, Pasupati S, Webb JG. Transapical aortic valve implantation in man. J Thorac Cardiovasc Surg 2006;131:1194–1196.

38. Ye J, Cheung A, Lichtenstein SV, Pasupati S, Carere R, Thompson C, Sinhal A, Webb JG. Six-month outcome of transapical transcatheter aortic valve implantation in the initial seven patients. Eur J Cardiothorac Surg 2007;31:16–21.

39. Huber CH, von Segesser LK. Direct access valve replacement (DAVR) – are we entering a new era in cardiac surgery? Eur J Cardio-thorac Surg 2006;29:380–385.

40. Antunes MJ. Off-pump aortic valve replacement with catheter-mounted valved stents. Is the future already here? Eur J Cardiothorac Surg 2007;31:1–3.

41. Webb JG, Chandavimol M, Thompson C, Ricci DR, Carere R, Munt B, Buller CE, Pasupati S, Lichtenstein S. Percutaneous aortic valve implantation retrograde from the femoral artery. Circulation 2006;113:842–850.

42. Berry C, Asgar A, Lamarche Y, Marcheix B, Couture P, Basmadjian A, Ducharme A, Laborde JC, Cartier R, Bonan R. Novel therapeutic aspects of percutaneous aortic valve replacement with the 21F CoreValve Revalving System. Cathet Cardiovasc Interv 2007;70:610–616.

43. Grube E, Laborde JC, Zickmann B, Gerckens U, Felderhoff T, Sauren B, Bootsveld A, Buellesfeld L, Iversen S. First report on a human percutaneous transluminal implantation of a self-expanding valve prosthesis for interventional treatment of aortic valve stenosis. Catheter Cardiovasc Interv 2005;66:465–469.

44. Grube E, Laborde JC, Gerckens U, Felderhoff T, Sauren B, Buellesfeld L, Mueller R, Menichelli M, Schmidt T, Zickmann B, Iversen S, Stone GW. Percutaneous implantation of the CoreValve self-expanding valve prosthesis in high-risk patients with aortic valve disease: the Siegburg first-in-man study. Circulation 2006;114(15): 1616–1624.

45. Berry C, Cartier R, Bonan R. Fatal ischemic stroke related to nonpermissive peripheral artery access for percutaneous aortic valve replacement. Cathet Cardiovasc Interv 2007;69:56–63.

46. Grube E, Schuler G, Buellesfeld L, Gerckens U, Linke A, Wenaweser P, Sauren B, Mohr FW, Zickmann B, Ivesen S. Felderhoff T, Cartier R, Bonan R. Percutaneous aortic valve replacement for severe aortic stenosis in high-risk patients using the second and current third generation self-expanding CoreValve prosthesis: device success and 30 day outcome. J Am Coll Cardiol 2007;50:69–76.

47. Baker AB, Bookallil MJ, Lloyd G. Intentional asystole during endoluminal thoracic aortic surgery without cardiopulmonary bypass. B J Anesth 1997;78:444–448.

48. Dorros G, Cohn JM. Adenosine-induced transient cardiac asystole enhances precise deployment of stent-grafts in the thoracic and abdominal aorta. J Endovasc Surg 1996;3:270–272.

49. Daehnert I, Rotzsh C, Wiener M, Schneider P. Rapid right atrial pacing is an alternative to adenosine in catheter interventional procedures for congenital heart. Heart 2004;90:1047–1050.

50. De Giovanni JV, Edgar RA, Cranston A. Adenosine induced transient cardiac standstill in catheter interventional procedures for congenital heart disease. Heart 1998;80:330–333.

51. Webb JG, Daly PA. Attempted balloon catheter obstruction of pulmonary arterial outflow in ventricular septal rupture. Cathet Cardiovasc Diagn 1990;19:246–247.

52. Cribier A, Eltchaninoff H, Bash A, Borenstein N, Tron C, Bauer F, Derumeaux G, Anselme F, Laborde F, Leon MB. Percutaneous transcatheter implantation of an aortic valve prosthesis for calcific aortic stenosis. Circulation 2002;106:3006–3008.

53. Ing FF. Improving control and delivery of coils and stents and management of malpositioned coils and stents. Prog Pediatr Cardiol 2001;14:13–25.

54. Berdjis F, Moore JW. Balloon occlusion technique for closure of patent ductus arteriosus. Am Heart J 1997;133:601–604.
55. Kohn RA, Marin ML, Hollier L, et al. Induction of ventricular fibrillation to facilitate endovascular stent graft repair of thoracic aortic aneurysms. Anesthesiology 1998;88:534–536.
56. Kohn RA, Moskowitz DM, Marin ML, et al. Safety and efficacy of high dose adenosine induced asystole during endovascular AAA repair. J Endovasc Ther 2000;7:292–296.
57. Hashimoto T, Young WL, Aagaard BD, et al. Adenosine-induced ventricular asystole to induce transient profound systemic hypotension in patients undergoing endovascular therapy: dose-response characteristics. Anesthesiology 2000;93:998–1001.
58. Webb JG, Pasupati S, Achtem L, Thompson CR. Rapid pacing to facilitate transcatheter prosthetic heart valve implantation. Catheter Cardiovasc Interv 2006;68:199–204.
59. O'Neill WW. Predictors of long-term survival after percutaneous aortic valvuloplasty: report of the Mansfield Scientific Balloon Aortic Valvuloplasty Registry. J Am Coll Cardiol 1991;17(1):193–198.
60. Lichtenstein SV, Cheung A, Ye J, Thompson CR, Carere RG, Pasupati S, Webb JG. Transapical transcatheter aortic valve implantation in man. Circulation 2006;114:591–596.
61. Bauer F, Eltchaninoff H, Tron C, et al. Acute improvement in global and regional left ventricular systolic function after percutaneous heart valve implantation in patients with symptomatic aortic stenosis. Circulation 2004;110:1473–1476.
62. Zuckerman BD, Sapirstein W, Swain JA. The FDA role in the development of percutaneous heart valve technology. Eurointervention 2006;1(Suppl A):A75–A78.
63. Vassiliades TA, Jr, Block PC, Cohn LH, Adams DH, Borer JS, Feldman T, Holmes DR, Laskey WK, Lytle BW, Mack MJ, Williams DO. The clinical development of percutaneous heart valve technology: a position statement of the Society of Thoracic Surgeons (STS), the American Association for Thoracic Surgery (AATS), and the Society for Cardiovascular Angiography and Interventions (SCAI) Endorsed by the American College of Cardiology Foundation (ACCF) and the American Heart Association (AHA). J Am Coll Cardiol 2005;45:1554–1560.

18 Percutaneous Balloon Valvuloplasty and Mitral Valve Repair

Ted Feldman

Percutaneous therapies for valvular heart disease were employed as early as the 1950s, using a wire valvulotome to treat pulmonic stenosis. The contemporary era of catheter therapy for valve lesions began with the introduction of balloon mitral valvotomy by Inoue in 1982. Descriptions of balloon aortic valvuloplasty (BAV) and balloon mitral valvotomy (BMV) using a variety of techniques followed over the ensuing decade. During that time and until recently, treatment for regurgitant lesions and the potential to replace valves percutaneously were distant concepts.

Balloon valvotomy has matured and reached its plateau, while new mitral valve repair therapies for mitral regurgitation (MR) and aortic valve replacement approaches are developing rapidly. This chapter will review in detail the techniques of BAV and BMV. In addition there will be a detailed discussion of percutaneous mitral valve repair technologies and approaches.

Despite the limitations of balloon therapy for stenotic lesions, there are still well-defined roles for both BMV and BAV. BMV is the preferred therapy for most patients with mitral stenosis, while BAV is an effective palliative therapy in highly selected high-risk patients with aortic valve stenosis.

BALLOON AORTIC VALVULOPLASTY (BAV)

Aortic valve replacement surgery has been the gold-standard therapy for symptomatic aortic stenosis for decades. It is arguably the most successful procedure developed in cardiac surgery. Symptoms are relieved and the vast majority of patients' survival is improved by this intervention. Despite the success of aortic valve replacement surgery, there remains a large cohort of patients for whom no referral is made for surgical evaluation. In the EuroHeart Survey, over one-third of patients with critical aortic stenosis were not referred to surgeons, and in preliminary reports in the United States, this may be as many as two-thirds of the critical aortic stenosis population *(1)*. A substantial proportion of these patients are elderly and have multiple comorbid conditions making them unattractive for aortic valve replacement surgery *(2)*. From this group, there is a clear subgroup of patients for whom palliative treatment with BAV is useful *(3, 4)*.

BAV has been limited by restenosis, which occurs almost ubiquitously with the procedure *(5)*. The vast majority of patients have echocardiographic restenosis within 6–12 months after BAV, but they

From: *Contemporary Cardiology: Valvular Heart Disease*
Edited by: Andrew Wang, Thomas M. Bashore, DOI 10.1007/978-1-59745-411-7_18
© Humana Press, a part of Springer Science+Business Media, LLC 2009

also experience clinical improvement for 1 to 1-1/2 years. Thus, BAV is useful for palliation in symptomatic patients who are unattractive for valve surgery.

The AHA–ACC guidelines for therapy in valvular heart disease recommend that BAV is a class IIB indication as a bridge to surgery or in patients for whom comorbid conditions preclude surgery (6). Thus, the usefulness and efficacy of this procedure is less well established by evidence or opinion than class IIA procedures, where the weight of evidence is in favor of their usefulness or efficacy. In my opinion, BAV is useful in a variety of clinical situations and is underutilized (Table 1) (3).

Table 1
Clinical Situations Where Balloon Aortic Valvuloplasty (BAV) May Be Useful

Congenital aortic stenosis
Rheumatic aortic stenosis
Cardiogenic shock
Bridge to surgery in high-risk patients for surgical valve replacement
Palliation in patients with serious comorbid conditions and/or advanced age
Prior to non-cardiac surgical procedures
Trial of therapy for low-gradient aortic stenosis with poor left ventricular
    function
Treatment of restenosis after prior BAV

It is useful to consider limitations of aortic valve replacement surgery in the elderly to better frame the utility of BAV. Survival is not clearly improved in elderly, high-risk patients by aortic valve replacement surgery. Mack et al. have reported a 1-year mortality of almost 50% in patients from the upper decile of STS risk undergoing aortic valve replacement, which is similar to the natural history of the disease. Prolonged hospital stay beyond 2 weeks is common in this population (7). The incidence of stroke and transient ischemic attack is as high as 15% (8). Less than half of these patients are discharged to home and most spend 2–4 months in a rehabilitation facility (9). From the Medicare database, which does not solely focus on the very elderly, the re-admission after aortic valve replacement within 30 days was almost 20% for indications of predominantly heart failure, arrhythmias, and wound infections (10). In speaking with elderly patients with aortic stenosis, few fear mortality from procedures. Rather, they fear disability. More than mortality, they are concerned with loss of quality of life, stroke, or confinement to a nursing home or rehabilitation facility. Thus, balloon aortic valvuloplasty is an attractive alternative for the symptomatic ambulatory elderly who are higher risk for aortic valve replacement surgery. It also has an important place as a bridge to surgery for patients who are acutely ill, often in shock, with aortic valve stenosis. In these patients, immediate hemodynamic salvage with BAV may allow them to recover sufficiently to have a less eventful elective valve replacement. An additional group in whom BAV is useful is those with low cardiac output and low ejection fractions. In this group of patients, aortic valve replacement surgery has excellent results for the patients in whom left ventricular function recovers after valve replacement. Unfortunately, if cardiomyopathy is the primary problem, with correction of the aortic valve stenosis there is no improvement in left ventricular function, and surgical mortality is extremely high. Thus, BAV may be used as a trial of therapy. If there is no improvement in left ventricular function with relief of the aortic stenosis via a balloon procedure, the patient may be spared aortic valve replacement surgery. Alternatively, if there is substantial recovery of left ventricular function, then aortic valve replacement may be pursed with greater confidence for a good outcome.

There are two techniques for BAV. The most common approach is via the retrograde transfemoral arterial route (11). Alternatively, an antegrade approach using transseptal access is possible and has some advantages (12).

Evaluation for coronary disease is ordinarily performed before the valve area is measured. In patients with elevated creatinine or renal failure, it is often wise to forego coronary arteriography, recognizing that the risk of infarction during these procedures is relatively small, and that since relief of symptoms is the only objective, in the absence of angina there is no special reason to treat coronary disease even when it is detected.

Retrograde BAV

The retrograde technique for BAV involves securing femoral arterial excess for placement of a large-caliber sheath for retrograde passage of the balloon, venous access for right heart pressure and cardiac output measurement, and an additional venous access for temporary pacing during the balloon inflations. Fluoroscopic guidance to puncture in the middle-third of the femoral head is critically important. A puncture in one of the distal femoral branch vessels limits the ability to place a large enough sheath and adds substantially to the potential for vascular complications or transfusions resulting from large sheath placement. After placement of a 5- or 6-French sheath, femoral arteriography is mandatory to assess the iliofemoral access for the sheath and balloon. If a puncture is made in the superficial femoral artery or profunda femoris, options include puncturing the contralateral femoral artery or using suture closure for the initial puncture and re-puncturing at a higher location on the same side. If contralateral puncture is chosen, arteriography from the initial puncture site will clearly define the optimum puncture location to ensure common femoral artery cannulation with the 11- or 12-French arterial sheath. After a 5- or 6-French sheath is successfully placed in the common femoral artery, preclosure using a suture closure device greatly facilitates sheath removal and diminishes the requirement for transfusions resulting from femoral bleeding from these large bore access sheaths (13). Heparin is administered to achieve an activated clotting time of at least 250s after all the sheaths have been placed.

An initial hemodynamic assessment is made. It is critical to obtain central aortic present as the comparator for left ventricular pressure for gradient measurement, since pulse amplification in the peripheral vessels can falsely diminish the gradient substantially and result in errors large enough to change clinical judgments about patient selection. It is my practice to use table-mounted, rather than manifold-mounted, transducers for gradient measurement. The amount of drift in the pressures is substantially less with the table-mounted transducers, and it is easier to re-zero them repeatedly during a procedure to ensure that hemodynamic measurements are accurate.

After the gradient has been assessed and cardiac output measured to determine the valve area, the left ventricular catheter is used to deliver an extra-stiff guidewire to the left ventricle (Fig. 1). An exchange length guidewire is used for the remainder of the procedure, and it is important to place a large curve at the end of the wire. A 3-mm J wire can be curled over the end of a hemostat or the rounded edge of a scissors to give it a "ram's horn" configuration. This curve will sit in the left ventricular apex and diminish the chance for ventricular apical perforation during passage of the balloons. The exchange wire is placed in the ventricle, the left ventricular diagnostic catheter removed, and then the valvuloplasty balloon advanced to the left ventricle. The balloon is difficult to inflate using a large syringe, which is necessary due to the large inflation volume of these balloons. Accordingly, the large syringe can be attached to a high-pressure stopcock with a 10-cc syringe from the other luer port. After full inflation of the balloon is achieved with the large syringe, the stopcock then can be turned to allow the smaller syringe to "boost" the inflation and achieve maximal distention of the balloon. This maximal balloon inflation in conjunction with rapid left ventricular pacing is necessary to adequately transmit dilatation force to the valve. Without rapid left ventricular pacing, the balloon tends to squirt back and forth in the valve due to the force of systole, and it is extremely difficult to deliver and adequate inflation under those circumstances. A 5-French temporary right ventricular pacemaker can be used to pace at least between 200 and 220 beats with burst mode pacing per minute during the balloon inflation, which eliminates this problem of balloon movement or "watermelon seeding." Ventricular

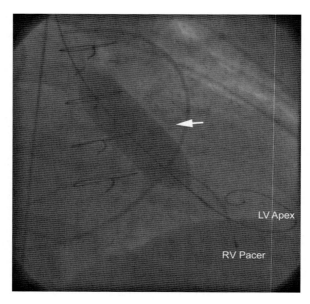

Fig. 1. Retrograde BAV. A stiff guidewire has been passed retrograde into the left ventricle (LV). A temporary pacemaker has been placed in the right ventricular (RV) apex for rapid pacing during balloon inflations. The balloon straddles the aortic valve. Calcifications are denoted by the *arrow*.

fibrillation occurs in a remarkably small proportion of patients, but must be anticipated. There is a need for coordination between the primary operator and the staff who are operating the pacemaker. An assistant who coordinates the onset and offset of pacing is useful to make this part of the procedure as smooth as possible.

It is important to see that the balloon locks into the valve during balloon inflation. It continues to move easily throughout the inflation, it is probably undersized, or is not adequately dilating the valve. At the over-sized end of the balloon size spectrum, if the patient begins to complain of chest pain or angina, it is possible that the aortic annulus is being stretched or even torn. This is a clear stopping point for the inflation. Of course, it is possible that coronary compromise has occurred, which needs to be investigated if chest pain is persistent or associated with ECG changes.

After successful balloon inflation, the balloon catheter is withdrawn over the wire from the sheath. In some cases, the re-wrap of the balloon is very poor and the balloon will get stuck in the sheath. In this instance it is easiest to remove the sheath and balloon as a unit over the exchange wire and then pass a new sheath. A pigtail catheter can then be exchanged over the long, stiff wire for an assessment of the post-BAV result. While it is ideal to repeat cardiac output measurements at the conclusion of the procedure, numerous investigations have shown that while statistically significant, the rise in cardiac output seen after these procedures is usually small in magnitude. A reasonable assessment of the result can be achieved with baseline cardiac output used in the Gorlin calculation of the valve area.

If the result appears satisfactory, the sheath is removed over a wire using the initially placed preclosure sutures. In the event that the result is inadequate, a larger balloon can be used if the arterial sheath will accommodate it or if the patient's femoral artery is larger enough for a larger sheath and larger balloon. The vast majority of the patients can be treated initially with a 20, 22, or 23 mm balloon. Routine use of 25 mm balloons for the initial inflations will result in aortic insufficiency more frequently than the smaller balloons. With 20 and 22 mm balloons, clinically important aortic insufficiency is rare. If the foot of the aortic pressure waveform has not decreased after balloon dilatation, even if aortic insufficiency has resulted it is not likely to be clinically important. Routine aortography either before or after BAV imposes a large contrast load and yields almost no useful clinical information.

Antegrade Technique for BAV

An alternative to retrograde BAV is antegrade transseptal aortic valvuloplasty *(12)*. In contrast to the retrograde technique, femoral venous access is used and the aortic valve is accessed via transseptal puncture. After venous puncture it is my practice to use a single 6-French suture closure device to preclose the venous sheath site *(14)*. A 6-French sheath or 8-French dilator is placed before suture closure, and then the suture device is placed. A wire is replaced via the suture device and a 14-French sheath exchanged for the suture delivery device in the femoral accesssite. Transseptal puncture is accomplished using standard methods. After verification of left atrial placement of the Mullins sheath, heparin is administrated to achieve an activated clotting time of at least 250s. A single lumen balloon catheter can be passed through the Mullins sheath and used to cross the mitral valve. This catheter can then be used as the left ventricular site for transaortic valve gradient measurement with a pigtail introduced from the femoral artery into the ascending aorta for central aortic pressure. After hemodynamic assessments are completed, the balloon catheter is advanced into the left ventricular apex until it curves around and floats toward the outflow tract and aortic valve. In some cases, it necessary to create a 3 cm radius curve on the end of the soft J-tipped guidewire to facilitate passage of the balloon catheter around the left ventricular apex. At that point, it is often also necessary to use a Wholey-type wire to cross the aortic valve antegrade. Once the balloon catheter is in the aorta it can be advanced into the aortic arch and then descending aorta. It is critical to maintain a loop in the left ventricle throughout the procedure (Fig. 2). At this point a 0.032 inch exchange length extra-stiff guidewire is advanced from the venous access through the single lumen balloon catheter to transverse the septal puncture, left ventricle, and into the descending aorta. A gooseneck snare is then introduced via the femoral artery and used to snare and secure the 0.032 inch guidewire in the descending aorta. While it is possible to exteriorize the extra-stiff wire via the femoral arterial sheath this step is not needed for the antegrade BAV procedure, and it is more convenient to snare the support wire in the descending aorta and simply leave the snare in place to support passage of the balloon catheter antegrade.

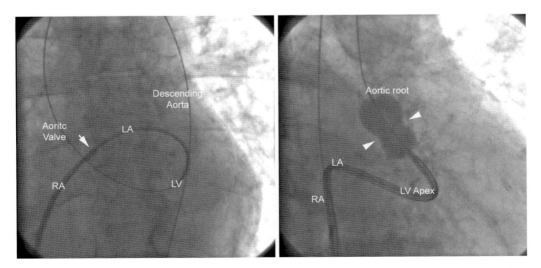

Fig. 2. Antegrade BAV. The *left panel* (PA view) shows the course of the guidewire. Via transseptal puncture, a giudewire has been passed from the right atrium (RA) to left atrium (LA) and across the mitral valve into the left ventricle (LV), across the aortic valve and into the descending aorta. This creates a wire loop through the circulation. The wire is snared in the distal aorta to provide the stability needed to pass the balloon antegrade across the aortic valve. The *arrow* indicates the tip of the transspetal sheath in the LA. The *right panel* (RAO view) shows the inflated balloon. The center of the balloon is indented by the calcified leaflets (*arrowheads*).

A 26 mm Inoue balloon can then be advanced over the wire, across the atrial septum, and then looped through the left ventricle into the aortic root. The distal part of the balloon is inflated and withdrawn. It will lock firmly against the aortic valve and then the remainder of the balloon can be inflated (Fig. 2). The inflation–deflation cycle is relatively rapid and the balloon can be withdrawn back into the left atrium by simultaneously pulling on the balloon and advancing the wire. This will re-establish the wire loop in the left ventricle, and get the balloon out of the valve as quickly as possible so that obstruction of outflow is relieved and the patient's blood pressure can recover.

In most women, a single 24 or 25 mm inflation can be used, and in most men a 25 or 26 mm inflation. This is in contrast to conventional balloons which are pressure driven. The Inoue balloon is volume driven and the character of the inflation is apparently different. Aortic insufficiency with these sized balloon inflations is infrequent and a single inflation seems to be as effective as multiple inflations. In fact multiple inflations may lead to left ventricular depression, and some patients will not recover left ventricular function after a second or third balloon inflation. The Inoue balloon is fundamentally different than a conventional balloon used for retrograde valvuloplasty. The balloon almost completely occludes outflow so the degree of hypotension may be more profound than in retrograde valvuloplasty. If pressure recovery is not adequate immediately after balloon inflation, 100 or 200 mcg boluses of epinephrine may be given to help restore the circulation.

After the balloon has been withdrawn into the left atrium, it can be elongated using the stretching metal tube that is part of the usual Inoue balloon procedure and removed from the femoral venous sheath. The Mullins sheath with the dilator in place is placed over the wire after withdrawal of the balloon catheter. After the Mullins sheath has been advanced into the left atrium the dilator is removed, the sheath flushed, and then a pigtail passed over the wire through the Mullins sheath and over the wire loop until it is at least in the aortic arch or the proximal descending aorta. This leaves the extra-stiff guidewire looped through the circulation and still secured by a snare in the descending aorta. At this point, it is critical to pass a pigtail catheter from the venous limb over the wire loop through the atria, the left ventricle, and at least into the aortic arch. This "plastic cover" over the guidewire protects the mitral valve from being cut by the wire as it is removed. At this point, the snare can be released from the distal end of the wire in the descending aorta. The wire can be pulled back until it is completely within the pigtail catheter. At this point, the pigtail catheter can be withdrawn until it sits within the left ventricular cavity for final gradient measurement.

The sheaths are removed as soon as the activated clotting time falls below 180s if manual compression is to be used. It is possible to "preclose" the puncture using percutaneous suture closure (Perclose). This approach is successful in almost 90% of the cases (13).

If manual compression is to be used it is important to use a FemoStop (RADI Medical, Uppsala, Sweden) or clamp for at least 30–60 min after manual compression has been completed since this large puncture has a strong tendency to rebleed. Patients who are not in critical condition before the procedure are able to leave the hospital on the morning following aortic valvuloplasty. It is important to obtain a postprocedure echocardiogram prior to hospital discharge so that serial comparisons can be made.

Long-term follow-up requires no more than surveillance for recurrent symptoms and periodic echocardiographic examinations to monitor the transaortic valve pressure gradient. An important consideration in follow-up is the status of other valve lesions. When the aortic valve is successfully opened, afterload reduction will often result in improvement in the mitral regurgitation that is often seen in these patients.

Among patients who have recurrence of the stenosis, repeat valvuloplasty may be accomplished with a high expectation for success. I rarely offer repeat procedures to patients who re-stenose quickly, within 6–8 months following the initial procedure. For those who achieve a year or more of clinical benefit, repeat procedures can be performed even three or four times, though the resultant valve areas are usually no better than the first procedure and aortic insufficiency may become limiting.

The aortic valve area usually increases between 80 and 100% after valvuloplasty. The transvalvular pressure gradient declines by more than 50%. Postdilatation valve area ranges between 0.7 and 1.1 cm^2. An increase in valve area, from 0.5 cm^2 to greater than 0.7 cm^2, will be associated with dramatic clinical improvement in most patients. Predilatation valve areas greater than 0.5 cm^2 may ultimately yield postdilatation valve areas of 1 cm^2 or more. It is notable that prosthetic aortic valves have an area between 0.9 and 1.2 cm^2 especially in small women with small aortic annuli.

The greatest limitation of balloon aortic valvuloplasty is the almost inevitable occurrence of restenosis following dilatation. The majority of patients have anatomic and symptomatic restenosis between 6 and 18 months after the procedure. Survival is not clearly improved with aortic valvuloplasty. The mechanism of restenosis may be related to the mechanism of relief of aortic stenosis. The majority of these elderly patients have calcific tri-leaflet aortic stenosis with calcification and thickening of the valve cusps and no commissural fusion. The calcium deposits are acellular and nodular. Histologically the nodules are encased densely in fibrous tissue. This explains the striking lack of embolization during this procedure. After balloon dilatation small fractures or cracks may be seen in the calcified nodules. This allows increased leaflet mobility due to the presence of many "hinge points" or fissures. The restenosis process probably involves regrowth of granulation tissue, fibrosis, and possibly true ossification of these fissures. This active process of restenosis follows a time course that is consistent with new scar formation. Recently, external radiation therapy has shown some promise to delay restenosis after BAV (15). The RADAR pilot trial suggests external beam radiation following valve dilatation is a treatment for restenosis, inhibiting scar as in keloid or ectopic ossification following hip arthroplasty. Restenosis in the RADAR study was 20% at 12 months in a population with average age 89 years suggesting utility in elderly patients. A larger trial using radiation is underway.

BALLOON MITRAL VALVULOPLASTY (BMV)

Mitral stenosis is almost synonymous with rheumatic valvular disease. Non-rheumatic etiology is only occasionally encountered. Congenital mitral stenosis may still be found in a rare patient. Calcific mitral stenosis is appearing with increasing frequency, especially among patients on chronic hemodialysis or those with severe mitral annular calcification. Mitral annular calcium may encroach on the body of the mitral leaflets with resultant restriction in their motion, and hemodynamically important mitral valve obstruction can result. Calcific stenosis is distinctly different from rheumatic mitral stenosis, since there is no commissural fusion. In the absence of commissural fusion, BMV is not very successful.

The typical symptom of the disease is dyspnea on exertion. Common misdiagnoses are chronic asthma or repeated episodes of hospitalization for pneumonia, upper respiratory infections, or congestive heart failure. Dyspnea is manifest as exercise intolerance and dyspnea develops in almost all patients with mitral stenosis. Acute rheumatic fever is a pancarditis and the myocardium is also involved. Low normal or depressed left ventricular performance is common and may contribute to the symptoms.

Many patients with mitral stenosis seem to be asymptomatic. Patients may gradually decrease their activity level to avoid symptoms. When the symptomatic status of the patient is not clear, exercise testing is often a useful method to ascertain the degree of exercise limitation. Dobutamine stress is often substituted for exercise and yields similar diagnostic results (16).

Echocardiographic Evaluation and Patient Selection

Transthoracic echocardiography is essential for assessment of the suitability of the valve for BMV. An echo scoring system characterizes four morphologic features of valve deformity (17). Leaflet mobility, leaflet thickening, calcification, and subvalvular involvement are all assessed on a scale

Table 2
Echocardiographic Scoring System for Mitral Valve Deformity

Leaflet mobility
Highly mobile valve with restriction of only the leaflet tips
Mid-portion and base of leaflets have reduced mobility
Valve leaflets move forward in diastole mainly at the base
No or minimal forward movement of the leaflets in diastole

Valvular thickening
Leaflets near normal (4–5 mm)
Mid-leaflet thickening, marked thickening of the margins
Thickening extends through the entire leaflets (5–8 mm)
Marked thickening of all leaflet tissues (>8–10 mm)

Subvalvular Thickening
Minimal thickening of chordal structures just below the valve
Thickening of chordae extending up to one-third of chordal length
Thickening extending to the distal third of the chordae
Extensive thickening and shortening of all chordae extending down to the papillary muscle

Valvular Calcification
A single area of increased echo brightness
Scattered areas of brightness confined to leaflet margins
Brightness extending into the mid-portion of leaflets
Extensive brightness through most of the leaflet tissue

where 1 is minimal deformity and 4 is severe deformity (Table 2). The scoring system is subjective, but remains useful to describe echo findings in these patients. Scores of 8 or less have been associated with excellent long-term results. Echocardiographic scores greater than 12 are associated with significantly poorer long-term outcomes with intermediate results with echocardiographic scores between 9 and 12. Symmetric commissural fusion is associated with better results than asymmetric fusion (18). A short-axis transthoracic echocardiogram is used to assess the symmetry of commissural fusion. When there is calcification in both commissures, the results are less good than when there is symmetrical commissural fusion without calcification (19).

Coronary arteriography prior to BMV should be done for patients with chest pain, evidence of ischemia by any method, diminished left ventricular function, history of coronary artery disease, any man over the age of 35, and women over the age of 35 with any risk factors or who are postmenopause.

Screening transesophageal echocardiography is a critical part of preparation for all patients undergoing balloon valvuloplasty. Patients with left atrial thrombus present a special challenge (20). When a left atrial thrombus is detected, anticoagulation therapy may be continued for 2–4 months with either new or more aggressive anticoagulant therapy. About 80% of thrombi will resolve after 2 months (21). Those patients with large mobile thrombi might best be referred for valve replacement to minimize the risk of stroke. Intense left atrial smoke by itself is not a contraindication.

BMV is the therapy of choice for patients with symptomatic, predominant mitral stenosis. Class I indications include patients who have New York Heart Association functional class II through IV with a mitral valve area of less than 1.5 cm^2, favorable valve morphology, absence of left atrial thrombus, and the absence of moderate or severe MR (6). BMV for asymptomatic patients is useful for those who have mitral valve area <1.5 cm^2 and who have a pulmonary artery systolic pressure of greater than 50 mmHg at rest or 60 mmHg with exercise. Patients who fall under symptomatic classes III to IV with a diminished valve area, a calcified valve, and who are at high risk for mitral valve replacement surgery are good candidates for valvuloplasty. Asymptomatic patients with a valve area <1.5 cm² and new atrial fibrillation have a class IIb indication for BMV and derive less certain benefit than those previously mentioned categories. Classes III to IV patients with a valve area <1.5 cm², a calcified valve with morphology not ideal for commissurotomy, and low surgical risk similarly have a class IIb indication.

BMV Techniques

Many techniques have been described to accomplish catheter commissurotomy for mitral stenosis. Inoue et al. *(22)* first described a single balloon approach in 1984. Subsequently, conventional single, double, and monorail balloons have been utilized for this procedure. Dilatation is usually performed via an antegrade approach using transseptal puncture but most of these balloon devices have also been passed retrograde throughout the arterial system and back into the left atrium. Cribier *(23)* described the use of a metal commissurotome. This is effectively a surgical Tubbs dilator adapted for percutaneous use, but has never been available in the United Sates.

The most commonly used device for catheter mitral valvuloplasty worldwide is the Inoue balloon catheter *(24)*. This is a single balloon that inflates in three stages (Fig. 3). After the balloon is passed into the left atrium, the front portion is inflated, and then the balloon is passed across the mitral valve. This is accomplished with the aid of a wire stylette, which has a preformed anterior curve. After the balloon has traversed the mitral valve and is demonstrated to be free from chordal entanglement, it is pulled back until it engages the stenotic mitral orifice. With further inflation, the proximal portion of the balloon inflates. As the balloon is completely inflated, the middle section opens, applying pressure to the commissures and causing a commissurotomy *(25)*. The balloon may be inflated with increasing volumes of contrast with resultant increase in diameter. After each balloon inflation, the pressure gradient is measured and MR assessed by hemodynamics, echocardiographic visualization, or by repeat ventriculography. Successive inflations at larger balloon diameters can be performed in a stepwise fashion until either a minimum gradient is achieved or MR begins to increase.

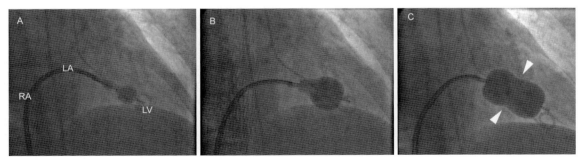

Fig. 3. BMV balloon inflation. In **A**, the balloon has been passed across the mitral valve via transseptal puncture, and partially inflated in the left ventricle (LV). **B**, the balloon is further inflated and pulled back to engage the mitral leaflets. **C**, after full inflation the center of the valve "cracks" the fused mitral commissures (*arrowheads*).

The procedure may also be accomplished using conventional balloons *(26)*. Typically, two balloons of 15–20 mm diameter are used together. Two wires must be passed through the transseptal puncture. The wires are looped in the ventricular apex or passed into the aorta to provide stability for advancing the balloons into the mitral orifice. The balloon catheters for this approach are longer than the Inoue balloon and either the balloon catheter tips or the guidewire may cause ventricular apical perforation. One advantage of the Inoue approach is that the balloon is passed into the left ventricle without the use of a guidewire. Ventricular perforation is thus a rare complication of the Inoue technique. It is also possible to pass balloons retrograde from the aorta through the left ventricle and across the mitral valve *(27)*. This approach avoids transseptal puncture, but requires large-caliber bilateral femoral arterial access. A double-balloon commissurotomy may also be accomplished using a single wire with a monorail balloon advanced initially and then a second over the wire balloon to follow the first on the same wire *(28)*.

Acute Results and Complications of Balloon Mitral Valvuloplasty

The mechanism of percutaneous commissurotomy is splitting of the fused commissures by balloon inflation. A single commissure is split in 40–60% of patients and bilateral commissural splitting is seen in the remainder. Occasional patients have a fibro-elastic valve that will not yield. The hemodynamic results of BMV have been consistent for all methods. There is an immediate decline in left atrial pressure, transmitral pressure gradient, and an associated rise in the cardiac output and mitral valve area *(29)*. In older patients, coexistent coronary disease or hypertensive heart disease may cause increased left ventricular diastolic pressure. These patients may have persistently elevated left atrial pressure after successful BMV. The interpretation of postprocedure hemodynamics in these patients can be difficult and symptoms may not resolve completely when these conditions coexist. The mitral valve area increases from about 1.0 cm^2 to between 1.8 and 2.2 cm^2. Pulmonary hypertension usually improves by 10–25% immediately *(30)*. When significant declines in left atrial pressure occur immediately, patients usually have marked improvement in their dyspnea. Further decreases in pulmonary pressure typically require weeks or months to occur. Severe pulmonary hypertension does not usually resolve completely. Atrial fibrillation resolves in only 20–25% of patients. This may be due to rheumatic involvement of the atria as the underlying mechanism of the arrhythmia rather than atrial stretch.

The techniques for BMV involve transseptal puncture with creation of an iatrogenic atrial septal defect *(31)*. While color flow Doppler studies demonstrate shunt flow in almost all patients immediately after valvuloplasty, most atrial septal defects close spontaneously within a few weeks or months. Less than 2% of patients have atrial septal shunting with shunt ratios >1.5 to 1. Persistent shunting is most likely to occur when left atrial decompression has not been successful and elevated left atrial pressure maintains shunt flow.

Complications of BMV

One of the most serious complications is an increase in MR. About 2.5% of patients require mitral valve replacement during the initial hospitalization for severe MR *(32)*. As many as one-third have some detectable increase in MR. Hospital death is infrequent and occurs in less than 1% of patients. Transient ischemic attack or stroke as a consequence of embolization from the left atrial appendage during the procedure has almost been eliminated with routine use of preprocedure screening transesophageal echocardiography. The incidence now appears to be similar to that of most other catheterization procedures. Cardiac perforation as a consequence of transseptal puncture or perforation with a balloon device or wire occurs in about 1% of patients in most series.

Late Results of BMV

Overall results consistently show overall event-free survival rates after 5 years of about 70% for patients in the United States *(29)*. In addition to patients with pliable mitral valves, these overall results include patients with significant valve deformity and older age patients who might otherwise be considered better candidates for valve replacement, and also a subgroup of patients who are elderly and debilitated with comorbid features that make them unattractive for valve surgery of any kind. All these subgroups have results that are significantly different from each other. The ideal younger patients for

BMV with echo scores ≤8 have a 5-year event-free survival rate of about 80%, while those with more severe degrees of valve deformity can be expected to have about 60% event-free survival rate. For the more elderly and debilitated group, palliation is the objective therapy and their long-term event-free survival is less good.

Published comparisons of surgery and balloon therapy are difficult to evaluate. Nonrandomized reports of surgical commissurotomy patients do not include follow-up of patients who were converted intraoperatively from intended commissurotomy to mitral valve replacement. Randomized trials remain the only credible way to compare the various approaches to mitral commissurotomy. Randomized comparisons of balloon versus open surgical commissurotomy have consistently demonstrated the two approaches to be equivalent *(33–34)*. The hemodynamics and valve area results have been reported in detail by Reyes et al. *(33)* with follow-up for 10 years after commissurotomy. Commissurotomy yields similar acute and long-term results to open surgical commissurotomy.

Some patients will present with mitral stenosis during pregnancy *(35)*. Pregnancy causes hemodynamic changes that provoke symptoms, and catheter commissurotomy is the procedure of choice in this setting. When a patient's clinical condition allows, balloon dilatation is best performed after the end of the first trimester so that fetal organogenesis is relatively complete and the risks of radiation exposure are minimized for the fetus. Using echocardiographic assistance to evaluate both improvement in valve area and the development of MR during the procedure, it is possible to accomplish commissurotomy with fluoroscopic time under 4 or 5 min. Some operators have completed the procedure using echocardiographic guidance without fluoroscopy. The potential for severe MR is no different in a pregnant patient and so a very conservative approach to balloon dilatation is important, with relief of hemodynamic overload for the short term as the major goal of therapy.

PERCUTANEOUS MITRAL VALVE REPAIR THERAPIES

Over the last few years a variety of catheter-based, percutaneous approaches to valve repair for MR have been developed. These technologies are all based on existing surgical procedures, though some of the predicate surgical techniques are not in wide use by surgeons. Percutaneous mitral repair approaches include coronary sinus annuloplasty, direct annuloplasty, and leaflet repair. There are also approaches that combine annular remodeling with chamber remodeling (Table 3).

Table 3
**Percutaneous Mitral Valve Repair
Approaches**

Coronary sinus annuloplasty
Direct annuloplasty
Leaflet repair
Combined chamber and annulus remodeling

Coronary Sinus Annuloplasty

The most frequent surgical therapy has been annuloplasty with an implanted ring, either as a stand-alone treatment for MR or in conjunction with mitral leaflet repair. A simplified interventional approach to simulate surgical annuloplasty has been using device placement in the coronary sinus to deform the mitral annulus and diminish the annular circumference. This approach relies on the anatomic relationship of the mitral annulus and the coronary sinus. Anchors or stents can be placed in the distal coronary sinus and the coronary sinus ostium, with a connector which constrains the coronary sinus and reduces the circumference of the mitral annulus.

The Monarc device (Edwards Lifesciences Inc., Orange, CA) has been implanted in more than 80 patients outside the United States. The coronary sinus and anterior interventricular vein are cannulated via the right internal jugular vein with deployment of distal and proximal self-expanding stent anchors which are separated by a connecting bridge element. The connecting bridge is a coiled spring, held in an open position by a biodegradable material in the spring interstices. Tension on the coronary sinus and mitral annulus develops as the spring shortens over 3–6 weeks. This device is in phase I clinical trials, with results presented on only the first few patients treated. In the first few patients treated, bridge fractures between the two anchors occurred in three of the four implanted patients (detected at days 22, 28, and 81 after device implantation), which were not associated with clinical sequelae other than worsening MR *(36)*. After a redesign of the bridge element, additional procedures have been performed without fractures or other device failures. Importantly, since the device acts slowly on the mitral annulus, reductions in MR can only be determined after weeks to months.

Another coronary sinus device is the Carillon mitral contour system (Cardiac Dimensions, Kirkland, WA). It is a nitinol wire shaping ribbon between proximal and distal anchors *(37–39)*. Tension is applied to the wire element between the two anchors to constrain the coronary sinus, reducing annular circumference. The device is delivered via a transjugular puncture with a 9-French guiding catheter. During deployment it is progressively shortened and the reduction in MR is measured using echocardiography. This device has been inserted successfully in patients both outside and inside the United States and has already undergone a device redesign to improve coronary sinus anchoring.

The percutaneous transvenous mitral annuloplasty (PTMA) system (Viacor, Wilmington, MA) is another coronary sinus shape deforming device. PTMA was invented by cardiac surgeons and consists of a 7-French multi-lumen PTFE catheter, within which are inserted variable stiffness rods. The rods deform the shape of the mid-portion of the coronary sinus which diminishes the septal to lateral dimension of the mitral annulus and reduces the severity of MR in animal models *(40)*. After the optimal number and stiffness of rods have been inserted in a temporary diagnostic catheter, a permanent version of the device is implanted. Importantly, the system shape and stiffness can be adjusted over time by addition or substitution of rods, depending on the patient response and changes in the severity of MR. A small series of temporary implants were inserted in the operating room to establish proof of concept.

Another similar coronary sinus approach is the percutaneous septal-sinus shortening procedure. An anchor is placed in the coronary sinus and a cord traversing the left atrium is attached to an anchor in the fossa ovalis. The cord is tensioned to diminish the mitral annulus septal–lateral dimension *(41)*. This system is in the process of initiating first-in-man clinical trials.

There may be important limitations associated with coronary sinus annuloplasty. The coronary sinus does not directly parallel the mitral annulus in many patients, and is often about a centimeter above the annulus plane *(42)*. The coronary sinus crosses over branches of the circumflex coronary artery in about half of the patients. In some cases these devices cause important circumflex artery compression and ischemia, necessitating either repositioning or removal of the device. Early experience is showing this to be less of a problem than originally anticipated.

The potential for erosion and thrombosis of the coronary sinus can only be ascertained after increased clinical experience with these devices. The coronary sinus has become a frequently utilized anatomic space over the past several years and it would be important to maintain access for lead placements during procedures such as resynchronization therapy.

Direct Mitral Annuloplasty

Direct approaches to the mitral annulus are being developed to address the potential limitations of indirect annuloplasty via the coronary sinus. The Mitralign device (Mitralign, Tewksbury, MA) uses anchor pledgits placed directly into the mitral annulus and a "drawstring" to cinch the annulus. This is similar to surgical plication annuloplasty initially described in 1977 *(43)*. Good surgical results with suture annuloplasty have been reported recently *(44, 45)*. A 20% reduction of the posterior annulus circumference can normalize the septal–lateral dimension and eliminate ischemic MR *(46)*. The Mitralign annuloplasty system places anchors directly into the mitral annulus from the left ventricular side and tethers them with a plication suture. Retrograde left ventricular catheterization using standard guiding catheter shapes is used for left ventricular access to the peri-annular space below the posterior mitral leaflet. Clinical studies with the Mitralign device are being planned.

Leaflet Repair

Direct leaflet repair has been accomplished using a surgical approach pioneered by Alfieri in the early 1990s *(47, 48)*. Suturing of the free leaflet edges of the mid-part of the line of coaptation results in a double orifice mitral valve. This edge-to-edge, or "bow tie" repair, can be successful as an isolated surgical approach in patients with regurgitation localized to the mid-segments of the anterior or posterior leaflets, in the absence of a grossly dilated annulus. The edge-to-edge repair, often combined with an annuloplasty ring, obliterates the gap in coaptation caused by the redundant leaflets.

Surgical edge-to-edge repair has had mixed clinical results *(49–50)*. It has been used as a "bailout" procedure in cases of both functional and degenerative MR when more conventional surgical approaches had suboptimal outcomes. A report of isolated edge-to-edge surgical repair in patients with optimal leaflet morphology had a 5-year 90% freedom from reoperation and MR >2+, and after 12 years, almost 80% freedom from reoperation and MR >2+ *(51)*. This demonstrates that isolated surgical edge-to-edge repair can be durable in selected patients.

The edge-to-edge repair has been duplicated using percutaneous clip *(52–56)*. After transseptal puncture, a MitraClip™ (Evalve, SanFranciso, CA) is delivered to the left atrium via a 24-French guide catheter, and positioned in the mid-left atrial cavity above the mitral orifice (Fig. 4). The clip must be aligned in the center of the valve orifice, with the clip arms perpendicular to the line of coaptation. The process of steering the guide catheter into optimal position is accomplished using steering knobs on the guide catheter and clip delivery catheter, utilizing both fluoroscopic and transesophageal echocardiographic guidance. When the clip is centered above the origin of the regurgitant jet, along the line of leaflet coaptation, the clip is opened. The open clip arms are passed through the mitral orifice; the open arms minimize the chance for chordal entanglement. After the clip is passed into the left ventricle, below the mitral leaflets, it is pulled back, the leaflets are grasped, and the clip arms are closed to create a double orifice. The device can be repositioned if control of the MR is not adequate, and removed if it appears to be unsuccessful. A second clip can also be placed if a first clip appears inadequate in decreasing the magnitude of MR.

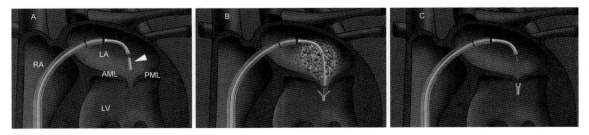

Fig. 4. Evalve clip for mitral leaflet repair. (**A**) the clip *(arrowhead)* is introduced into the left atrium (LA) using a 24-French guide catheter. (**B**) It is centered over the mitral orifice, and the opened clip arms are passed across the mitral leaflets (AML, anterior mitral leaflet; PML, posterior mitral leaflet) into the left ventricle (LV). (**C**) The clip is withdrawn and the leaflets grasped. If the MR is reduces adequately, the clip is released.

This device approach has been successfully used in a phase I clinical trial in the United States, and results at 12 months have been reported *(57, 58)*. Surgical candidates with moderately severe or severe MR and cardiac symptoms or no symptoms with signs of LV dysfunction were included in the EVEREST-I clinical trial (Endovascular Valve Edge-to-edge REpair STudy). Patients fulfilled the AHA-ACC guidelines criteria for surgical treatment of MR *(6)* and echocardiograms were evaluated using the American Society for Echocardiography methods for assessment of MR severity *(59)*. Mitral leaflet morphology and MR jet origin must be suited to this approach. The regurgitant jet must arise from the central two-thirds of the line of coaptation. Leaflet coaptation length and depth must be ≥ 2 mm and ≤ 11 mm, respectively. When flail segments are present, the flail gap must be <10 mm and the flail width <15 mm. These rigorous clinical and morphologic criteria effectively exclude patients with severe annular dilatation. Less than 20% of echocardiograms evaluated by the core lab are considered appropriate for treatment with the Mitraclip device.

Over 100 patients were enrolled in this Phase I trial and in the run-in portion of the subsequent EVEREST-II trial *(see below)* with >6 months follow-up in about 80 patients. Compared to results from the most recent STS database, patients referred for this percutaneous procedure were significantly older; median age was 71 years for the clip procedure compared to 59 years for surgical repairs. Clips were successfully implanted in 90% and there were no intra-procedural major complications. Acute procedure success, defined as successful clip placement with reduction in MR severity to $\leq 2+$, was $>70\%$. Major adverse events within 30 days included partial clip detachment without embolization in 8% of patients, all of whom underwent successful elective valve surgery, and a postprocedure stroke in one patient, which resolved in 1 month. Average length of hospital stay was less than 2 days. When a clip was placed and the results were suboptimal, mitral leaflet repair using standard surgical techniques has been possible as late as 18 months after the index interventional procedure *(60)*. Two-year freedom from death, mitral valve surgery, or recurrent MR $>2+$ has been 80% among patients discharged with successful clip therapy *(58)*.

The encouraging success of the Evalve clip procedure, both safety and effectiveness, has led to a randomized trial comparing this device with mitral valve surgery in the United States. EVEREST-II is currently randomizing patients to percutaneous repair versus a standard surgical approach (2:1 allocation), with clinical and echocardiographic safety and efficacy endpoints. Importantly, there has never been a prospective, echocardiography core lab evaluated, intention-to-treat trial of mitral valve repair therapy in the surgical literature. The EVEREST-II trial will be important not only in the assessment of a new percutaneous mitral valve therapy, but also in defining the contemporary results of surgery for mitral valve disease.

Annulus and Left Ventricular Chamber Remodeling

This percutaneous technology is based on a novel surgical device. The Coapsys surgical system (Myocor, Maple Grove, MN) places pads on either side of the left ventricle with a cord passing through the left ventricular cavity to apply tension to the mitral annulus and the basal left ventricular chamber *(61)*. This off-pump surgical procedure is a direct approach to achieve both left ventricular remodeling and an associated mitral annuloplasty. Initial results of the Coapsys surgical system implanted during coronary revascularization in patients with ischemic MR have shown sustained reductions in MR and improved ventricular chamber dimensions for as long as 1 year after the procedure. A percutaneous transpericardial method to simulate this surgical procedure (iCoapsys) is under development in preclinical models *(62)*.

Development of Percutaneous Mitral Repair Devices

It has been demonstrated that asymptomatic patients with severe MR have a poor prognosis compared to those with less-severe MR *(63)*. There is a compelling need for a clinical trial to demonstrate that early mitral valve therapy might benefit these patients. The lower morbidity of percutaneous therapies may be well suited for such an asymptomatic, lower risk population. Alternatively, there is evidence to indicate favorable outcomes with "watchful waiting" in this patient group; thus, a randomized clinical trial versus either medical or surgical therapy would be critical to evaluate the utility of any therapy in this patient population (64). Indirect or direct annuloplasty approaches are better suited to patients with functional MR due to heart failure or coronary ischemia. This population is often not treated surgically, and comparisons with medical therapy may be more appropriate.

There have been no prior randomized trials or prospective, intention-to-treat reports on surgical approaches for MR. Percutaneous therapy is fundamentally different (65). Outcomes measurement after percutaneous therapy is not easily comparable to surgery. The most common endpoint in long-term surgical reports is freedom from reoperation. The combined endpoint of freedom from death, reoperation, and recurrent MR has not been used. Surgical outcomes have never been reported using the intention-to-treat principle. Core lab evaluation of baseline echocardiograms, use of American Society for Echocardiography criteria for grading severity of MR, or prospective echocardiographic follow-up are being introduced with percutaneous device trials, but are not part of the development of traditional surgical therapies.

REFERENCES

1. Lung B, Baron G, Butchart EG, Delahaye F, Gohlke-Barwolf C, Levang OW, Tornos P, Vanoverschelde JL, Vermeer F, Boersma E, Ravaud P, Vahanian A. A prospective survey of patients with valvular heart disease in Europe: The Euro Heart Survey on Valvular Heart Disease. Eur Heart J. 2003;24:1231–1243.

2. Varadarajan P, Kapoor N, Bansal RC, Pai RG. Clinical profile and natural history of 453 nonsurgically managed patients with severe aortic stenosis. Ann Thorac Surg. 2006;82:2111–2115.

3. Feldman T. Balloon aortic valvuloplasty appropriate for elderly patients. J Interventional Cardiol. 2006;19:276–279.

4. Hara H, Pedersen WR, Ladich E, Mooney M, Virmani R, Nakamura M, Feldman T, Schwartz RS. Percutaneous balloon aortic valvuloplasty revisited: time for a renaissance? Circulation. Mar 2007;115:e334–e338.

5. Feldman T, Glagov S, Carroll JD. Restenosis following successful balloon valvuloplasty; bone formation in aortic valve leaflets. Cathet Cardiovasc Diag. 1993;29:1–7.

6. Bonow O, Carabello B, Chaterjee K, DeLeon AC, Jr, Faxon DP, Freed MD, Gaasch WH, Lytle BW, Nishimura RA, O'Gara PT, O'Rourke RA, Otto CM, Shah PM, Shanewise J. ACC/AHA 2006 guidelines for the management of patients with valvular heart disease. Executive summary. Circulation. 2006;114:450–527. American Heart Association Web Site. Available at: http://www.americanheart.org

7. Kolh P, Kerzmann A, Lahaye L, Gerard P, Limet R. Cardiac surgery in octogenarians: peri-operative outcome and long-term results. Eur Heart J. 2001;22:1235–1243.

8. Alexander KP, Anstrom KJ, Muhlbaier LH, Grosswald RD, Smith PK, Jones RH, Peterson ED. Outcomes of cardiac surgery in patients age 80 years: results from the National Cardiovascular Network. J Am Coll Cardiol. Mar 2000;35:731–738.

9. Sharony R, Grossi EA, Saunders PC, Schwartz CF, Ribakove GH, Culliford AT, Ursomanno P, Baumann FG, Galloway AC, Colvin SB. Minimally invasive aortic valve surgery in the elderly: a case-control study. Circulation. 2003;108(Suppl 1):II43–1147.

10. Goodney PP, Stukel TA, Lucas FL, Finlayson EV, Birkmeyer JD. Hospital volume, length of stay, and readmission rates in high-risk surgery. Ann Surg. 2003;238(2):161–167.

11. Feldman T. Core Curriculum for interventional cardiology: percutaneous valvuloplasty. Cathet Cardiovasc Intervent. 2003;60:48–56.

12. Sakata Y, Sayed Y, Salinger MH, Feldman T. Percutaneous balloon aortic valvuloplasty: antegrade transseptal vs. conventional retrogradetransarterial approach. Cathet Cardiovasc Intervent. 2005;64:314–321.

13. Solomon LW, Fusman B, Jolly N, Kim A, Feldman T. Percutaneous suture closure for management of large French size arterial puncture in aortic valvuloplasty. J Invasive Cardiol. 2001;13:592–596.

14. Mylonas I, Sakata Y, Salinger MH, Sanborn T, Feldman T. The use of percutaneous suture-mediated closure for the management of 14 French Femoral Venous Access. J Invasive Cardiol. 2006;18:299–302. Website Available at: http://www.invasivecardiology.com/jic/displayArticle.cfm?articleID=article5852

15. Pedersen WR, Mooney MR, Schwartz RS, et al. Radiation following Percutaneous balloon aortic valvuloplasty to prevent restenosis (RADAR Pilot): one year follow-up. Circulation. Oct. 25 2005;112(17):Supplement II–520.

16. Hecker SL, Zabalgoitia M, Ashline P, Oneschuk L, O'Rourke RA. Comparison of exercise and dobutamine stress echocardiography in assessing mitral stenosis. Am J Cardiol. 1997;80:1374–1377.

17. Wilkins GT, Weyman AE, Abascal VM, Block PC, Palacios IF. Percutaneous balloon dilatation of the mitral valve: an analysis of echocardiographic variables related to outcome and the mechanism of dilatation. Br Heart J. 1988;60:299–308.

18. Fatkin O, Roy P, Morgan JJ, Feneley MP. Percutaneous balloon mitral valvotomy with the Inoue single-balloon catheter: commissural morphology as a determinant of outcome. J Am Coll Cardiol. 1993;21:390–397.

19. Levin TN, Feldman T, Bednarz J, Carroll JD, Lang RM. Transesophageal echocardiographic evaluation of mitral valve morphology to predict outcome after balloon mitral valvotomy. Am J Cardiol.1994;73:707–710.

20. Tessler P, Mercier LA, Burelle O, Bonan R. Results of percutaneous mitral commissurotomy in patients with a left atrial appendage thrombus detected by transesophageal echocardiography. J Am Soc Echocardiogr. 1994;7:394–399.

21. Jaber WA, Prior DL, Thamilarasan M, Grimm RA, Thomas JD, Klein AL, Asher CR. Efficacy of anticoagulation in resolving left atrial and left atrial appendage thrombi: a transesophageal echocardiographic study. Am Heart J. 2000;140:150–156.

22. Inoue K, Owaki T, Nakamura T, Kitamura F, Miyamoto N. Clinical application of transvenous mitral commissurotomy by a new balloon catheter. J Thorac Cardiovasc Surg. 1984;87:394–402.

23. Cribier A, Rath PC, Letac B. Percutaneous mitral valvotomy with a metal dilatator. Lancet. 1997;349:1667.

24. Feldman T, Herrmann HC, Inoue K. Technique of percutaneous transvenous mitral commissurotomy using the Inoue balloon catheter. Cathet Cardiovasc Diagn. 1994;2(Supp 1):26–34.

25. Feldman T, Carroll JD, Herrmann HC, Holmes DR, Bashore TM, Isner JM, Dorros G, Tobis JM. Effect of balloon size and stepwise inflation technique on the acute results of Inoue mitral commissurotomy: Inoue balloon catheter investigators. Cathet Cardiovasc Diagn. 1993;28:199–205.

26. Al Zaibag M, Ribeiro PA, Al Kasab S, Al Fagih MR. Percutaneous double-balloon mitral valvotomy for rheumatic mitral-valve stenosis. Lancet. 1986;1:757–761.

27. Stefanadis CI, Stratos CG, Lambrou SG, Toutouzas PK. Retrograde nontransseptal balloon mitral valvuloplasty: immediate results and intermediate long-term outcome in 441 cases-a multicenter experience. J Am Coll Cardiol. 1998;32:1009–1016.

28. Bonhoeffer P, Piechaud JF, Sidi D, Yonga G, Jowi C, Joshi M, Mugo M, Kachaner J, Parenzan L. Mitral dilatation with the multi-track system: an alternative approach. Cathet Cardiovasc Diagn. 1995;36:189–193.

29. Feldman T. Hemodynamic results, clinical outcome and complications of Inoue balloon mitral valvotomy. Cathet Cardiovasc Diagn. 1994;2(Supp 1):2–7.

30. Ribeiro PA, al Zaibag M, Abdullah M. Pulmonary artery pressure and pulmonary vascular resistance before and after mitral balloon valvotomy in 100 patients with severe mitral valve stenosis. Am Heart J. 1993;125:1110–1114.

31. Levin N, Feldman T, Carroll JD. Effect of atrial septal occlusion on mitral area after Inoue balloon valvotomy. Cathet Cardiovasc Diagn. 1994;33:308–314.

32. National Heart, Lung and Blood Institute Balloon Valvuloplasty Registry. Complications and mortality of percutaneous balloon mitral commissurotomy: a report from the National Heart, Lung and Blood Institute Balloon Valvuloplasty Registry. Circulation. 1992;85:2014–2024.

33. Reyes VP, Raju BS, Wynne J, Stephenson LW, Raju R, Fromm BS, Rajagopal P, Mehta P, Singh S, Rao DP. Percutaneous balloon valvuloplasty compared with open surgical commissurotomy for mitral stenosis. N Engl J Med. 1994;331:961–967.

34. Ben Farhat M, Ayari M, Maatouk F, Betbout F, Garnra H, Jarra M, Tiss M, Hammami S, Thaalbi R, Addad F. Percutaneous balloon versus surgical closed and open mitral commissurotomy: seven year follow-up results of a randomized trial. Circulation. 1998;97:245–250.

35. Lung B, Cormier B, Elias J, Michel PL, Nallet O, Porte JM, Sananes S, Uzan S, Vahanian A, Acar J. Usefulness of percutaneous balloon commissurotomy for mitral stenosis during pregnancy. Am J Cardiol. 1994;73:398–400.

36. Webb JG, Harnek J, Munt BI, Kimblad PO, Chandavimol M, Thompson CR, Solem JO. Percutaneous transvenous mitral annuloplasty: initial human experience with device implantation in the coronary sinus. Circulation. 2006;113:851–855.

37. Byrne MJ, Power JM, Alferness CA, Reuter DG, Kaye DM. Percutaneous mitral annular reduction. A novel approach to the management of heart failure associated mitral regurgitation. Circulation. 2003;108:1795–1799.

38. Maniu CV, Patel JB, Reuter DG, Meyer DM, Edwards WD, Rihal CS, Redfield MM. Acute and chronic reduction of functional mitral regurgitation in experimental heart failure by percutaneous mitral annuloplasty. J Am Coll Cardiol. 2004;44:1652–1661.

39. Byrne MJ, Kaye DM, Mathis M, Reuter DG, Alferness CA, Power JM. Percutaneous mitral annular reduction provides continued benefit in an ovine model of dilated cardiomyopathy. Circulation. 2004;110:3088–3092.

40. Liddicoat JR, Mac Neill BD, Gillinov AM, Cohn WE, Chin CH, Prado AD, Pandian NG, Oesterle SN. Percutaneous mitral valve repair: a feasibility study in an ovine model of acute ischemic mitral regurgitation. Catheter Cardiovasc Interv. 2003;60:410–416.

41. Rogers JH, Macoviak JA, Rahdert DA, Takeda PA, Palacios IF, Low RI. Percutaneous septal sinus shortening: a novel procedure for the treatment of functional mitral regurgitation. Circulation. 2006;113:2329–2334.

42. Maselli D, Guarracino F, Chiaramonti F, Mangia F, Borelli G, Minzioni G. Percutaneous mitral annuloplasty: an anatomic study of human coronary sinus and its relation with mitral valve annulus and coronary arteries. Circulation. 2006;114:377–380.

43. Burr LH, Krayenbuhl C, Sutton MS. The mitral plication suture: a new technique of mitral valve repair. J Thorac Cardiovasc Surg. 1977;73:589–595.

44. Nagy ZL, Bodi A, Vazily M, Szerafin T, Horvath A, Peterffy A. Five-year experience with a suture annuloplasty for mitral valve repair. Scand Cardiovasc J. 2000;34:528–532.

45. AybekT, Risteski P, Miskovic A, Simon A, Dogan S, Abdel-Rahman U, Moritz A. Seven years' experience with suture anuloplasty for mitral valve repair. J Thorac Cardiovasc Surg. 2006;101:99–106.

46. Tibayan FA, Rodriguez F, Liang D, Daughters GT, Ingels NB Jr, Miller DC. Paneth suture annuloplasty abolishes acute ischemic mitral regurgitation but preserves annular and leaflet dynamics. Circulation. 2003;108(Suppl 1):II128–133.

47. Alfieri O, Elefteriades JA, Chapolini RJ, Steckel R, Allen WJ, Reed SW, Shreck S. Novel suture device for beating-heart mitral leaflet approximation. Ann Thorac Surg. 2002;74:1488–1493.

48. Alfieri O, Maisano F, DeBonis M, Stefano PL, Torracca L, Oppizzi M, LaCanna G: The edge-to-edge technique in mitral valve repair: a simple solution for complex problems. J Thorac Cardiovasc Surg. 2001;122:674–681.

49. Bhudia SK, McCarthy PM, Smedira NG, Lam BK, Rajeswaran J, Blackstone EH. Edge-to-edge (Alfieri) mitral repair: results in diverse clinical settings. Ann Thorac Surg. 2004;77:1598–1606.

50. Kherani AR, Cheema FH, Casher J, Fal JM, Mutrie CJ, Chen JM, Morgan JA, Vigilance DW, Garrido MJ, Smith CR, Oz MC. Edge-to-edge mitral valve repair: the Columbia Presbyterian experience. Ann Thorac Surg. 2004;78(1):73–76.

51. Maisano F, Vigano G, Blasio A, Columbo A, Calabrese C, Alfieri O. Surgical isolated edge-to-edge mitral repair without annuloplasty – clinical proof of principle for an endovascular approach. EuroIntervention. 2006;2:181–186.

52. St. Goar FG, James FI, Komtebedde J, Foster E, Oz MC, Fogarty TJ, Feldman T, Block PC. Endovascular edge-to-edge mitral valve repair: short-term results in a porcine model. Circulation. 2003;108:1990–1993.

53. Fann JI, St. Goar FG, Komtebedde J, Oz MC, Block PC, Foster E, Feldman T, Burdon TA. Off-pump edge-to-edge mitral valve technique using a mechanical clip in a chronic model. Circulation. 2003;108:Supp IV – 493.

54. St. Goar FG, Fann JI, Feldman TE, Block PC, Herrmann HC. Percutaneous mitral valve repair with the edge-to-edge technique. In Herrman HC (Ed): Contemporary Cardiology: Interventional Cardiology-Percutaneous Noncoronary Intervention. Humana Press, Totowa, NJ; 2005, pp. 87–95.

55. Herrmann HC, Feldman T. Percutaneous mitral valve edge-to-edge repair with the Evalve Mitraclip system: rationale and phase I results. EuroIntervention. 2006;Supplement A: A36–39.

56. Feldman T, Alfieri O, St. Goar F. Percutaneous leaflet repair for mitral regurgitation using the Evalve edge-to-edge clip technique. In Hijazi Z, Bonhoeffoer P, Feldman T, Ruiz C (Eds): Transcatheter Valve Repair. Martin Dunitz & Parthenon Publishing/Taylor & Francis Medical Books, London; 2006, pp. 275–284.

57. Feldman T, Wasserman HS, Herrmann HC, Gray W, Block PC, Whiltlow PL, St. Goar F, Rodriguez L, Silvestry F, Schwartz A, Sanborn TA, Condado JA, Foster E. Percutaneous mitral valve repair using the edge-to-edge technique: six-month results of the EVEREST Phase I Clinical Trial. J Am Coll Cardiol. 2005;46:2134–2140.

58. Feldman T, Wasserman HS, Herrmann HC, Whitlow PL, Block PC, Gray WA, Foster E, St Goar F. Edge-to-edge mitral valve repair using the Evalve MitraClip: one year results of the EVEREST phase I clinical trial. Am J Cardiol. 2005;96:Supp 49H.

59. Zoghbi WA, Enriquez-Sarano M, Foster E, Grayburn PA, Kraft CD, Levine RA, Nihoyannopoulos P, Otto CM, Quinones MA, Rakowski H, Stewart WJ, Waggoner A, Weissman NJ. Recommendations for evaluation of the severity of native valvular regurgitation with two-dimensional and Doppler echocardiography. J Am Soc Echocardiogr. 2003;16:777–802.

60. Dang NC, Aboodi MS, Sakaguchi T, Wasserman HS, Argenziano M, Cosgrove DM, Rosengart TK, Feldman T, Block PC, Oz MC. Surgical revision after percutaneous mitral valve repair with a clip: initial multicenter experience. Ann Thorac Surg. 2005;80:2338–2342.

61. Grossi EA, Saunders PC, Woo J, Gangahar DM, Laschinger JC, Kress DC, Caskey MP, Schwartz CF, Wudel J. Intraoperative effects of the Coapsys annuloplasty system in a randomized evaluation (RESTOR-MV) of functional ischemic mitral regurgitation. Ann Thorac Surg. 2005;80:1706–1711.

62. Pedersen WR, Block P, Feldman T. The iCoapsys repair system for the percutaneous treatment of functional mitral insufficiency. EuroIntervention. 2006;Supplement A: A44–48.

63. Enriquez-Sarano M, Avierinos JF, Messika-Zeitoun D, Detaint D, Capps M, Nkomo V, Scott C, Schaff HV, Tajik AJ. Quantitative determinants of the outcome of asymptomatic mitral regurgitation. N Engl J Med. 2005;352;9:875–883.

64. Rosenhek R, Rader F, Klaar U, Gabriel H, Krejc M, DKalbeck D, Schemper M, Maurer G, Baumgartner H. Outcome of watchful waiting in asymptomatic severe mitral regurgitation. Circulation. 2006;113:2238–2244.

65. Feldman T. Percutaneous valve repair and replacement: challenges encountered, challenges met, challenges ahead. Circulation. 2006;113:771–772.

19 Post-operative Care of the Patient Undergoing Valve Surgery

Aslan T. Turer, Thomas R. Gehrig, and J. Kevin Harrison

CONTENTS

There are few naturally occurring medical illnesses that rival the acuity and severity of illness which can complicate the post-operative course following cardiac valvular surgery. Some complications are potentially predictable, while others are not. Fortunately, improved surgical and anesthetic techniques have decreased the frequency of many of these adverse events.

Cardiologists may receive little training with respect to post-operative evaluation and management of patients following valvular heart surgery. Nevertheless, they are asked to provide guidance to patients considering such surgery and are asked to assist in the management of individuals when complications do arise. Understanding the risks of valvular surgery is important in guiding the patient pre-operatively and in assisting in their post-operative recovery. The purpose of this chapter is to discuss the post-operative cardiac and extra-cardiac complications frequently encountered following cardiac surgery.

POST-OPERATIVE HEMODYNAMICS IN THE VALVULAR PATIENT

The hemodynamic management of the cardiac surgical patient may be challenging in the immediate post-operative period. This is because of simultaneous changes in ventricular preload, afterload, and contractility which are acute in onset and may be significant in magnitude.

From: *Contemporary Cardiology: Valvular Heart Disease*
Edited by: Andrew Wang, Thomas M. Bashore, DOI 10.1007/978-1-59745-411-7_19
© Humana Press, a part of Springer Science+Business Media, LLC 2009

Certain goals of post-operative care are relatively straightforward. In general, a cardiac index of ≥ 2.0 L/min/m^2 is targeted assuming this is needed to maintain adequate systemic perfusion. At the same time attempts are made to minimize myocardial oxygen demand by reducing afterload and avoiding excessive tachycardia. Goal-directed therapy for cardiac output and systemic perfusion has been validated for patients undergoing heart surgery *(1, 2)* similar to other acutely ill patients. Common causes of low output are outlined in Table 1. Echocardiography (chest wall or transesophageal) and invasive hemodynamic monitoring can be invaluable at this stage in the diagnosis and management of these individuals who are clinically doing poorly.

Table 1
Common Etiologies of Low Cardiac Output in the Perioperative Period

- Hypovolemia
    Intra and extravascular volume shifts
    Active bleeding
- Excessive ventricular afterload
    Severe hypertension
    Hypothermia
    Vasoconstrictor infusions
    LV cavity dilation
- Left ventricular dysfunction
    Pre-existing cardiomyopathy
    Transient myocardial stunning from cardioplegic arrest
    Iatrogenic dysfunction from inadequate intra-operative cardioprotection
    Active myocardial ischemia/infarction
    Diastolic dysfunction
- Right ventricular dysfunction
    Pre-existing RV dysfunction
    RV ischemia/infarction
    Inadequate cardioprotection
    Pulmonary hypertension
- Dynamic left ventricular outflow tract obstruction
    Hypovolemia
    Catecholamine excess (endogenous or exogenous)
    LV cavity obliteration
    Systolic anterior motion of anterior mitral valve leaflet
- Tamponade
- Arrhythmias
    Bradycardia or heart block
    Tachycardia (e.g., atrial fibrillation)
    Loss of AV synchrony

Left Ventricular (LV) Dysfunction

Both LV and right ventricular (RV) dysfunction are commonly encountered in the perioperative period. In some cases, the ventricular dysfunction may not have been recognized prior to surgery or has developed during surgery. Acquired myocardial dysfunction from a period of global ischemia–reperfusion following surgery is frequent, but an abnormal LV ejection fraction usually normalizes by 24–48 hours *(Fig. 1) (3, 4)*. Patients with pre-existing LV dysfunction have a higher operative risk *(5)* and a variable improvement in myocardial function following correction of their underlying

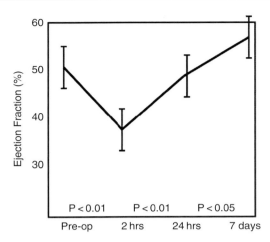

Fig. 1. The LV ejection fraction tends to drop acutely after surgery but generally recovers by post-operative day 1–2. Modified from *(4)*, used with permission.

valvular pathology. Regardless of the etiology of LV dysfunction, the fundamentals of post-operative hemodynamic support remain the same.

The myocardial stunning observed after cardioplegic arrest frequently requires supportive agents aimed primarily at improving contractility. Table 2 outlines the usual drugs used, their major hemodynamic effects, starting doses, and maintenance dosages. Intravenous epinephrine is often the drug of choice in this setting. Despite minimal increases in heart rate, epinephrine infusions at 0.02 and 0.04 μg/kg/min have been shown to increase cardiac index by 0.7 and 1.2 L/min/m^2, respectively *(6)*. Doses in excess of this, however, may result in significant increases in heart rate and arrhythmias *(7)* and should be avoided. Dopamine, once the first-line agent for weaning from bypass, is occasionally still used for this purpose, though at doses resulting in similar increases in contractility as epinephrine, there is significantly more tachycardia seen with dopamine *(8)*. Conversely, despite being both inotropic and lusitropic, phosphodiesterase inhibitors, such as milrinone, appear to minimally increase myocardial oxygen consumption *(9)*. As such, there is an established role for these drugs in the treatment of post-operative LV dysfunction. Furthermore, as a vasodilator this drug may be particularly useful in cases of coincidental high systemic (SVR) and/or pulmonary vascular resistance (PVR).

Besides maintaining an adequate cardiac output, left ventricular filling or preload also must be optimized. The systemic vasodilation associated with surgery and post-operative blood loss may lead to a reduced LV preload. Additionally, LV preload may be low from poor RV systolic function or impaired RV filling (e.g., from positive pressure ventilation and an elevated end-expiratory thoracic pressure). In these cases supplemental crystalloid or colloid infusions may be required to improve cardiac output. Monitoring the central venous pressure (CVP) and the pulmonary capillary wedge pressure (PCWP) may be useful in this regard.

Finally, ventricular afterload conditions following valve surgery are often markedly different from pre-operatively. Urine output and serum creatinine measurements often serve as surrogates for tissue perfusion. An increase in LV wall stress, whether due to a dilated, volume-overloaded ventricle or due to increased peripheral vascular resistance (e.g., from vasoconstriction, hypothermia, or systemic hypertension), may worsen cardiac output. In these situations, vasodilation is key, and aggressive diuresis may be required if the PCWP is elevated. Nitroprusside, nitroglycerine, or a phosphodiesterase inhibitor may be useful in this setting.

Increased afterload may also result from the mechanical effects of the valve procedure. Examples include prosthetic valve systolic pressure gradients following AVR *(10)*, a new subvalvular LV

Table 2
Drugs and Their Hemodynamic Effects and Usual Dosages

Drug type	Hemodynamic effect					Receptor	Starting dose	Maintenance dose
	HR	SBP	PCWP	SVR	CO			
Vasopressors								
Dopamine								
<3	+2	0	0	0	0	$D > \beta_1$	3–10 mg/kg/min	to 20 mg/kg
3–10	+2	+1	+1	0	+1	$\beta_1 > \beta_2 > D$		
>10	+2	+2	+2	+1	+1	$\alpha > \beta_1 >> \beta_2$		
Dobutamine								
<0.05	+3	0	0	0 to 1	+3	$\beta_1 >> \beta_2$	1 µg/min	10 µg/min
0.05–0.15	+3	+1	+2	+1	+3	$\beta_1 > \alpha > \beta_2$		
>0.15	+3	+2	+2	+3	+2	$\alpha > \beta_2$		
Norepinephrine	+2	+3	+3	+3.5	0	$\alpha >>> \beta_1$	2 µg/min	30 µg/min
Phenylephrine	0	+2	+2	+	0	α	100 µg/min	40–60 µg/min
Vasopressin	0	+1	+1	+1	0 to +1	Hormonal	0.01 U/min	0.04 U/min
Inotropes								
Dobutamine								
2–10	+1	+1	−1	+1	+1	$\beta_1 > \beta_2 > \alpha$	1 µg/kg/min	20 µg/kg/min
10–20	+1	0 to −1	−1	0 to −1	+2			
Isoproterenol	+3	−2	−2	−3	+3	$\beta_1 >>> \beta_2$	0.01 µg/kg/min	0.3 µg/kg/min
Milrinone	+1	0	−1	−2	+1	PDEI	0.25 µg/kg/min	0.75 µg/kg/min
Vasodilators								
Nitroglycerin	0	−1	−2	−1	0 to −1	NO agonist	5 µg/min	200 µg/min
Nitroprusside	0	−2	−1	−2	−1 to 1	NO agonist	0.5 µg/kg/min	10 µg/kg/min

Relative effects are noted. HR = heart rate, SBP = systemic blood pressure, PCWP = pulmonary capillary wedge pressure, SVR = systemic vascular resistance, CO = cardiac output. PDEI = phosphodiesterase inhibitor, NO = nitric oxide.

outflow tract obstruction, and removal of the low-pressure "pop-off" circuit after correction of mitral regurgitation.

Special Issues After Aortic Valve Surgery

Aortic regurgitation (AR) results in both afterload and preload increase on the LV. In patients undergoing aortic valve replacement (AVR) for AR, the loss of the regurgitant volume will result in a smaller LV. This lowers afterload by reducing wall stress for any given systolic blood pressure. The prosthetic valve may impose a new afterload burden in the form of a new transvalvular systolic pressure gradient, however.

For these reasons, careful attention must be paid to the status of both the ventricle as well as the systemic vascular resistance (SVR). The post-operative ventricle of chronic AR is able to handle relatively large amounts of volume without increasing LV filling pressure. Maintaining adequate preload and contractility is especially important when ventricular function is impaired prior to surgery and a new prosthetic valve systolic pressure gradient exists. The SVR may be low, normal, or elevated post-operatively in these patients, and appropriate therapy for reduced organ perfusion often requires determination of the PCWP and SVR.

In contrast to chronic AI, the hallmark of the ventricle with aortic valve stenosis is its relatively poor LV compliance due to concentric hypertrophy. Intrinsic systolic function is usually preserved, and with removal of the outflow tract obstruction, LV systolic emptying increases still further following AVR *(11, 12)*, although at times this improvement may be delayed and occur only later *(13)*. Diastolic dysfunction is common. Additionally, compared to AR patients, AS patients are generally older and have a high prevalence of coincidental coronary artery disease *(14)*, which may increase the negative effects on diastolic function observed.

Managing AS patients after AVR patients therefore differs from AR patients. Since contractility is often normal or supra-normal after relief of the afterload burden at the level of the aortic valve *(11, 12, 15–17)*, inotropic support will usually only transiently needed in the post-operative period. Indeed, these inotropic agents may *worsen* the patient's hemodynamics by decreasing diastolic filling time, inducing poorly tolerated arrhythmias, or provoking otherwise latent LV outflow tract or mid-cavitary LV obstruction. Conversely, at times, beta-blockers (or calcium channel blockers) may be useful at this stage to increase diastolic filling time and blunt the hyperdynamic ventricular response. Similarly, preload must be maintained to allow adequate LV stroke volume and avoid excessive reflexive tachycardia. The poorly compliant hypertrophied AS ventricle may, however, be very preload sensitive with abrupt rises in LV filling pressures with even small increases in volume. As such, PCWP and the patient's oxygenation status should be monitored frequently as pulmonary edema and respiratory decompensation may occur especially quickly with a small amount of fluid excess.

Special Issues After Mitral Valve Surgery

Generally speaking, in isolated mitral valve stenosis (MS) the ventricle is relatively "protected" from pressure and volume overload, and, as such, systolic function and LV dimension remain grossly preserved. This contrasts with chronic mitral regurgitation (MR) where the volume load on the left ventricle leads to LV dilation and eccentric hypertrophy similar to that observed in AR. The reduced afterload that occurs in MR, however, increases the measured ejection fraction (EF). Ventricular impairment may become obvious only after the MR is repaired or the mitral valve replaced. When mixed regurgitant and stenotic pathophysiology coexist, the post-operative hemodynamics and LV performance immediately following mitral valve procedures will be largely determined by the predominant lesion valvular pathology that existed prior to surgery.

Subtle systolic dysfunction is often present even in patients with pure MS *(18–20)* (possibly due to rheumatic pancarditis). Diastolic dysfunction may also be present depending on the age of the patient and other coexisting medical conditions, such as hypertension or CAD. The major problem, in MS, however, tends to be right ventricular function. Pulmonary hypertension of some degree will invariably be present before MVR because of the elevated left atrial pressures and a variable amount of transpulmonary pressure gradient. Some of the pulmonary hypertension will be acutely reduced following MVR due to the loss of the diastolic pressure gradient into the LV. Often some fixed, or only partially reversible, pulmonary hypertension is present resulting in an increased measured PVR. In addition, the temporal course of the reversible component of existing transpulmonary gradient is widely variable and may not be resolved until months after surgery.

Severe pulmonary hypertension associated with MS poses a significant negative influence on post-operative recovery, especially when coupled with resultant right ventricular dysfunction. These factors are associated with increased short-term post-operative mortality *(21–23)*. Management of this condition targets both pulmonary vasodilation and augmentation of right ventricular systolic function. The MS patient with pulmonary hypertension will often be significantly volume overloaded pre-operatively. Thus, intravenous diuretics in addition to augmenting RV function prove beneficial post-op. This treatment combination is in distinction to other forms of acute RV failure where RV preload must be maintained at a high level to provide an adequate RV functional contribution to the cardiac output.

The status of the LV in MR differs dramatically from that found in pure MS. Whereas LV dysfunction is not a typical feature of the post-operative course in MS, it is a common occurrence in patients undergoing MVR for mitral regurgitation. Even among patients with grossly normal LV function going into MR surgery, LV dysfunction and low cardiac output frequently occur afterward. This is largely because of increased left ventricular wall stress (higher afterload) that occurs post-op with loss of the MR. These conditions may lead to a consequent drop in stroke volume and forward flow. While overall mechanical efficiency improves, LV ejection fraction drops and both wall stress and mean ejection pressure increase early on after mitral surgery *(15)*. Afterload reducing drugs, such as IV vasodilators and ACE inhibitors, are important for maintaining adequate cardiac output following surgery in these individuals. Additionally, inotropic agents may be needed to help increase contractility or afterload reduction with mechanical devices, such as an intra-aortic balloon pump, is required, especially in cases of coincidental LV systolic dysfunction associated with hypotension. In many of these cases, milrinone may prove particularly useful to provide both afterload reduction and positive inotropy. The frequency of severe LV dysfunction following mitral surgery has decreased owing to improved surgical techniques favoring MV repair over replacement, as well as chordal preservation, and to a better appreciation for the need to operate on these patients at an earlier time in their disease course.

Dynamic Left Ventricular Outflow Tract (LVOT) Obstruction

Dynamic obstruction of the LVOT is an important consideration in the post-operative period when the ventricle is hyperdynamic and the cardiac output is low. It is important to diagnose this complication promptly, as the appropriate management is opposite to that of ventricular systolic dysfunction. Echocardiography is paramount to the diagnosis, as physical examination may be challenging in the noisy post-operative ICU environment.

Unmasking latent LV obstruction may occur even in a patient with a normal ventricle (i.e., not associated with hypertrophic cardiomyopathy). Excess endogenous or exogenous catecholamines, hypovolemia, and left ventricular hypertrophy may interact to lead to LVOT obstruction *(24–29)*. This combination of factors is commonly encountered in the perioperative setting. A new subvalvular LVOT gradient may particularly be seen following aortic valve replacement and has been postulated to be related to a hyperdynamic, hypertrophied, and relatively underfilled LV which no longer has the after-load burden at the level of the aortic valve *(10)*. The characteristics of this gradient by ECHO appear to be similar to that typically seen in hypertrophic obstructive cardiomyopathy and are associated with an adverse prognosis *(10)*.

Mitral valve repair may also be associated with LVOT obstruction. The incidence of this complication had been reported to be as high as 6–14% *(30)* prior to the identification of echocardiographic predictors and the introduction of the sliding annuloplasty *(31, 32)*. When, during repair, the coaptation point of the mitral leaflets is moved anteriorly toward the septum, the anterior leaflet may then become sufficiently long and redundant to obstruct the LVOT during ventricular systole. This is especially true when the posterior leaflet is excessively elongated. This anatomy has been identified as an anatomic risk factor for LVOT obstruction following MV repair procedures *(33, 34)*.

The treatment of acquired outflow tract obstruction, regardless of cause, is similar. Positive inotropes should be discontinued and, when necessary, negative inotropes (e.g., beta-blockers, calcium channel blockers) administered. Assessment of ventricular volume should be performed by echocardiography and hypovolemia addressed with volume infusions. Filling pressures often must be monitored since diastolic dysfunction and poor ventricular compliance commonly coexist.

Right Ventricular Dysfunction and Pulmonary Hypertension

Although refractory RV failure is rare *(35)*, less severe degrees of right-sided cardiac dysfunction are very common following cardiac surgery *(36, 37)*. Given the difficulty in accurately quantifying right ventricular function, the exact incidence and magnitude of post-operative RV dysfunction are difficult to discern. Among patients evaluated for post-cardiotomy low output, significant RV dysfunction is present in over 40% *(38)*. Acute, severe RV dysfunction after cardiac surgery is associated with significant mortality although the amount of data published on this subject is not large *(38, 39)*.

To date, there are no widely accepted risk factors predicting the development of clinically significant RV dysfunction after surgery. The RV is traditionally regarded as being relatively resistant to hypoxic injury, but intra-operatively it can be susceptible to ischemia due to oxygen supply–demand mismatch, air embolism down the right coronary artery, or poor cardioprotection afforded from retrograde cardioplegia administration (although this last factor is considered contentious). Importantly, positive pressure ventilation and PEEP can impair RV function by decreasing RV preload and increasing left atrial pressures at the same time. Latent and unrecognized RV dysfunction may also have been present before surgery.

There are two main groups of patients in whom right ventricular dysfunction is most commonly encountered. Patients with severe LV dysfunction may also have right ventricular dysfunction as a result of the cardiomyopathic process or secondary to high left-sided filling pressures and pulmonary hypertension. Although valve repair or replacement in this setting may decrease left atrial pressures, RV performance might not improve as rapidly, especially when other perioperative insults to the RV occur. The short-term mortality of patients with simultaneous left and right ventricular dysfunction undergoing cardiac surgery has been reported to be in excess of 70% *(40)*.

The other patients who commonly experience morbidity from RV dysfunction are those with mitral valve disease, especially those with MS. In most cases, LV systolic function is preserved. Long-standing MS may result in a mixed form of pulmonary hypertension, part of which is due to high LA pressures, and which improves with MVR. Particular difficulty arises in managing those patients with coexisting high PVR and associated high pre-operative RV end-diastolic pressures indicative of a failing RV. The additional effects of post-cardiotomy RV dysfunction and positive pressure ventilation often can contribute to severe hemodynamic compromise and low cardiac output post-operatively.

RV dysfunction should be suspected when cardiac output is low despite an adequate (or high) CVP, and especially in those patients who are known to be at high risk for this condition. It is important to recognize that although PA pressures will typically be elevated (reflecting the underlying pulmonary hypertension), they may be relatively normal when the RV is unable to overcome the afterload of a high PVR. An echocardiogram should be performed in suspected cases. It is also critical to visually exclude extrinsic compression of the RA or RV by pericardial hematoma or fluid, as this will similarly increase the CVP measurement and drop cardiac output. The echocardiogram of RV failure demonstrates RV free wall hypocontractility and cavity dilation. New tricuspid regurgitation (TR) may also be evident.

Treatment of RV dysfunction requires increasing RV contractility while decreasing pulmonary vascular resistance. RV preload (as measured by the CVP) will generally already be high. In cases of isolated RV dysfunction (such as with RV infarction), volume administration may be required to target a CVP goal of 15–20 mmHg in order to maintain systemic cardiac output. In most cases of RV dysfunction seen after valve surgery, administration of significant amounts of volume is not possible, either because of coexisting LV dysfunction or significant pre-operative volume overload. Furthermore, excessive pressure/volume overload of the RV may further reduce systolic function and may negatively impact left ventricular filling by causing a posterior, leftward septal shift.

RV contractility may be augmented using the same agents that are used for the LV failure *(41)*. The optimal agent will depend on the magnitude of pulmonary hypertension, as well as the systemic blood pressure. Beta-agonists, such as epinephrine or dobutamine, are useful to improve RV systolic and diastolic functions and may be necessary when LV function is also impaired or when the patient is hypotensive. If systemic pressure is adequate, the phosphodiesterase inhibitors are good agents as they vasodilate both the peripheral and pulmonary vasculatures while simultaneously increasing inotropy of both ventricles *(42–44)*. The use of nitrates to lower pulmonary vascular resistance is generally limited by their lowering of right ventricular preload and potential for creating systemic hypotension. Vasopressin may also be considered to support systemic blood pressures since it causes minimal increases in PVR *(45)*.

Selective pulmonary vasodilators, such as inhaled nitric oxide (iNO) (20–40 parts per million) *(46, 47)* and intravenous prostaglandin E$_1$ *(47,48)*, will all cause a significant drop in PVR. Although these agents are useful, they have limitations. iNO can only be administered through a ventilator and tachyphylaxis will occur, both of which mean it is impractical for anything more than short-term post-operative administration. Although intravenous prostaglandin E$_1$ has little effect on the systemic blood pressure at low doses, higher doses cause systemic hypotension.

Tamponade

Mediastinal or pericardial bleeding is common and may occur at graft anastamoses and other incisions in the myocardium, such as at the cannula insertion sites. Early in the post-operative course, functioning mediastinal chest tubes generally drain post-operative bleeding from around the heart. Therefore, in most cases, early take-back procedures, which complicate between 2 and 6% of cardiac surgeries *(49–51)*, are for excessive bleeding which does not result in tamponade. Nonetheless, this diagnosis must be considered for any patient with progressive hypotension, a drop in cardiac output, and an increase in the CVP. Tamponade may also occur if the mediastinal tube becomes clotted or in cases of loculated or posterior effusions. It is important to recognize that these post-procedural effusions may localized and not circumferential *(52–56)*. As such, they may not always demonstrate the classic equalization of diastolic pressures despite causing hemodynamic compromise *(52, 53, 56)*. This can be especially true if, rather than free fluid, there is thrombus. Thrombus may also compromise the left atrium or pulmonary venous inflow, leading to a reduction in cardiac output.

Late tamponade occurs more commonly than the acute form and complicates 0.2–1.1% of cardiac surgeries *(57–60)*. It appears to be more common after valve procedures than routine CABG, probably because of greater use of anticoagulation in patients with valvular disease *(50, 54, 55, 60)*. Late tamponade typically occurs 1–2 weeks post-operatively, with the highest incidence occurring around days 8–10 *(57)*. The etiology of these effusions is usually related to unrecognized, persistent bleeding or pericardial inflammation (post-cardiotomy syndrome) and, as such, they are generally bloody *(61)*. An elevated sedimentation rate may help make the diagnosis when the effusion is several weeks out from the surgery.

Only symptomatic pericardial effusions require drainage. In fact, most patients (up to 75%) will have some pericardial fluid after surgery, but these usually do not require percutaneous or surgical drainage as they eventually resolve on their own without causing hemodynamic compromise *(62, 63)*. More than two-thirds of these pericardial effusions are small in size but may be moderate (30%) or even large (<2%) and still remain asymptomatic *(54, 63)*. Some physicians recommend treatment with non-steroidal anti-inflammatory agents for patients with moderate-to-large post-operative pericardial effusions not requiring mechanical drainage although the efficacy of this approach has never been systematically studied. Systemic corticosteroids are typically reserved for those patients with severe inflammatory symptoms, including fever, once infectious causes have been evaluated and excluded. Most of these patients, including those with large effusions, will not progress to tamponade *(60, 62, 63)*. Those patients without high-risk echocardiographic and clinical features can be followed expectantly *(60)*. Post-cardiotomy effusions are a risk factor for later developing constriction, however *(64, 65)*.

PERIOPERATIVE MYOCARDIAL INJURY

The pathogenesis of myocardial damage in the perioperative setting is multifactorial and complex. Although typically referred to as perioperative myocardial "infarction" (MI), the mechanisms behind MI are largely distinct from those of the typical acute coronary syndrome. The operating room environment is marked by alternating anti- and pro-coagulation, a prolonged period of ischemia with brisk reperfusion, profound temperature swings, and significant volume shifts. Myocardial injury after cardiac surgery is likely the result of these unique extremes of physiology to which the heart is exposed during the procedure.

Intra-operative Mechanisms

There are a several intra-operative time periods when the myocardium appears most vulnerable for MI. Subendocardial ischemia, especially when coincidental coronary disease or ventricular hypertrophy exists, may occur from increases in myocardial workload. Maintaining coronary perfusion pressure while avoiding large increases in afterload and heart rate (especially with use of beta-blockers) is of major importance from the time of induction of anesthesia until the patient is on cardiopulmonary bypass. Cardioprotection during periods of cardiac arrest plays a vital role in protecting against MI and early myocardial dysfunction. The duration of the aortic cross-clamp and the total cardiopulmonary bypass time, as well as the adequacy of cardioplegia are all key intra-operative variables linked to MI. Following cross-clamp removal and de-airing of the heart, air emboli may occur. With the patient supine on the operating table this usually results in inferior wall ischemia as the result of the right coronary artery's anterior takeoff from the aorta. Although this may usually be treated by acutely increasing systemic perfusion pressures, myocardial damage can result. Although uncommon, MI may also be related to surgical technique. Examples include an aortic valve prosthesis sewn superior to the true aortic annulus causing occlusion to coronary blood flow or *hyper*acute (i.e., intra-operative) graft loss in patients who are undergoing coincidental CABG surgery.

Post-operative Mechanisms

Myocardial injury may occur in the post-operative phase, as well. The mechanisms are again diverse. Following major vascular (i.e., non-cardiac) surgery, there is a high rate of myocardial infarction (up to 25%) *(66–69)* after the first few post-operative days. Since this risk does not appear to be reduced by revascularization, post-op MI in this setting has been attributed to the pro-thrombotic milieu following major surgery and myocardial oxygen supply–demand mismatch and thus is more in line with the traditional notion of acute coronary syndrome (ACS). Most of the observed myocardial damage appears very early in the post-operative period. Studies have shown that cardiac biomarkers peak within 12 hours of surgery *(70)*. Since most patients will normalize their shorter half-life cardiac markers (e.g., CK, CK-MB) by 24–48 hours *(71, 72)*, late elevations or bimodal peaks in biomarkers should be considered particularly abnormal and are suggestive of recurrent myocardial ischemia or graft loss *(73, 74)*.

Some valve patients undergo simultaneous coronary revascularization. The rate of early graft loss has been reported to be between 3 and 12% at 30 days *(75, 76)*, but a significant proportion of these will be lost prior to discharge *(73, 74, 77–79)*. It is important to recognize that the patient may not be symptomatic from acute graft closure. Technical issues at the time of graft placement are certainly of central importance, but randomized trial data have shown that immediate post-operative use of aspirin reduces the risk of early graft occlusion, suggesting a role of early thrombosis in this process as well *(80)*.

Lastly, post-operative management should focus on the rate–pressure product to minimize myocardial oxygen demand. Elevated blood pressure in the immediate post-operative setting is more of an issue during the recovery phase. More challenging can be the management of tachyarrhythmias, such as rapid atrial fibrillation, which are common and may cause hypotension, myocardial ischemia, and/or congestive heart failure in the days and weeks following surgery. In these cases, careful attention must be paid to heart rate and, when appropriate, rhythm control.

Incidence and Diagnosis

A precise estimate of the rate of occurrence of MI has been hindered by the lack of a standard definition of what constitutes a MI and what is the "expected" amount of myocardial injury following cardiac surgery. Furthermore, the reported estimates are almost exclusively based on post-operative CABG data and may not be applicable to the valve population, where both the cross-clamp times and amount of myocardial manipulation are typically much greater. The limited data which do exist suggest that cardiac biomarkers are more frequently elevated following valve procedures than in CABG cases *(72)*. Nonetheless, several large randomized trials of CABG surgery have suggested a rate of MI around 10% *(81, 82)*. These studies defined MI based on an arbitrary cutoff value of CK-MB measurement (usually 5–10-fold above the upper limit of the reference range) within the first few days following surgery, with or without ECG changes *(81–84)*.

The ECG alone is not a sensitive tool to diagnose MI. The development of new, fixed Q waves (a diagnostic criteria of the traditional Minnesota code) is a poorly sensitive measure of infarction post-operatively *(85–87)*, especially in the subendocardium, where a substantial fraction of MIs are known to occur. Additionally, post-operative pericarditis, ventricular pacing, and even just the physical barriers to placing ECG leads in standard and reproducible locations from dressings and chest tubes further limit the reliability of ECG-based MI diagnosis.

Although impractical for routine use in suspected cases of MI, myocardial imaging has been useful. By SPECT nuclear imaging, the incidence of new perfusion defects following cardiac surgery ranges from 10 to 25% *(87–89)*. Although new perfusion defects are relatively specific for infarct,

SPECT suffers in this setting for lacking the sensitivity to detect small defects that are often patchy and subendocardial. Therefore, the estimates of infarct occurrence by nuclear imaging are likely to be an underestimation of the true incidence. More recently, cardiac MRI has been employed to study this question. New areas of hyperenhancement (which correlate to infarcted regions on gross pathology) have been reported in about 40% of patients based on follow-up imaging after CABG *(90)*. Cardiac MRI has demonstrated that most new infarcts after surgery are scattered, small, and frequently subendocardial (Fig. 2) *(90–92)*. The frequency and distribution of infarcts following cardiac surgery for valve procedures are yet to be studied using this modality.

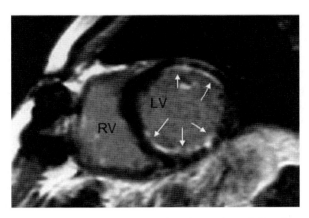

Fig. 2. Contrast-enhanced cardiac MRI in basal short axis of a patient following cardiac surgery. New areas of scattered subendocardial hyperenhancement typical of perioperative myocardial injury are clearly shown by *arrow*. From *(90)*, used with permission.

Prognosis After MI

Higher levels of biomarker release are consistently associated with higher odds of death over the short *(93, 94)* and intermediate terms *(95)*. Furthermore, there is evidence that MI holds its negative prognostic importance over the long term and that the magnitude in the biomarker level increase correlates with a progressive increase in mortality at the first *(93, 96)* and third years *(96)*. Also, MI is associated with a more than twofold increase in the development of heart failure and subsequent readmission to the hospital after surgery *(97)*.

ATRIAL FIBRILLATION

Atrial fibrillation (AF) and atrial flutter are very common (25–40%) after cardiac surgery, as the post-operative milieu is replete with pro-arrhythmogenic stimuli *(98–101)*. As such, the mechanism of post-operative atrial arrhythmias is multifactorial. There are physical manipulations of the heart which also play a role in the process, most notably at the right atrial and pulmonary vein cannulation sites. Supporting this idea is the fact that the rates of AF are higher following valve procedures (upward of 40%) *(102)* than after isolated CABG surgery. While longer ischemic times and the degree of cardiac manipulation are greater in valve surgery, all the causes are unclear. Post-operative AF is also seen after off-pump CABG (where there is no pump time or atrial cannulation) in more than 20% of cases *(103)*. Post-operative AF also complicates recovery from non-cardiac thoracic surgery, where there is usually no cardiac handling at all (an incidence of at least 20%) *(104, 105)*. There are likely additional humoral contributors to the post-operative development of atrial fibrillation, e.g., mediators of inflammation, catecholamine surges, and electrolyte disturbances along with anemia and the use of inotropic agents.

Prophylactic Measures

AF is associated with morbidity, slower post-operative recovery, increased length of hospitalization, and resource utilization in the post-operative period. A number (>60 to date) of studies have investigated prophylactic measures to prevent post-operative AF. These have been summarized by the Cochrane Collaboration which examined the effect of pure beta-blockers and the antiarrythmics, sotalol and amiodarone, on the incidence of post-operative AF *(106)*.

In aggregate, pre-operative beta-blockers have been shown to reduce the incidence of AF compared with placebo from 31 to 18%. Similarly, amiodarone (33 vs. 21%) and sotalol (40 vs. 21%) also lower the risk for post-operative AF compared with placebo. The PAPABEAR study, which included a significant proportion of patients undergoing combined valve or combined valve–CABG procedures, confirmed the benefit of amiodarone (loaded pre-operatively) in this population and appeared to support the efficacy of this drug even on a background of beta-blocker use *(102)*. It should be emphasized that this study involved primarily elective cardiac surgery patients, where amiodarone loading for a week pre-operatively could be accomplished. This is not always possible with the way medicine is practiced in the United States.

In addition to antiarrhythmics, the use of steroids, presumably targeting the "inflammatory" component of AF, has also been evaluated. Most recently, among 241 patients undergoing cardiac surgery, including valve procedures, perioperative hydrocortisone administration was shown to decrease the incidence of AF from 48 to 30% *(107)*. These findings have been confirmed in a meta-analysis, where steroids were associated with a 45% lower risk of developing atrial fibrillation *(108)*. Importantly, there is no apparent increase in pneumonia or mediastinitis seen with this therapy.

In summary, there is ample evidence that the incidence of post-operative AF can be lowered with prophylactic medical therapy. Barring contraindications, every patient undergoing cardiac surgery should be treated with a beta-blocker and consideration should be given to pre-procedural amiodarone loading. Importantly, this decrease in AF attributed to these prophylactic measures translated into a decreased risk of stroke and appeared to be associated with lower resource utilization *(109)*.

Treatment

The decision of whether to treat post-operative AF should take into account several factors, including (1) the absolute burden of the arrhythmia and its hemodynamic consequences; (2) whether or not symptoms are present; (3) coexisting conditions which make systemic embolization more likely, such as the presence of a mechanical prosthesis; and (4) the patient's risk for becoming *bradycardic* with therapies aimed at controlling the tachycardia. In addition, it is often not possible to resolve the arrhythmia when adrenergic agents are being given at the same time (a common situation post-operatively).

Short paroxysms of AF, especially if asymptomatic, are best treated with AV nodal blockade, using either a beta-blocker or calcium channel blocker. Often, however, the paroxysms of AF will last more than a few minutes or are poorly controlled by nodal agents. In these instances, the patient may be symptomatic, especially in cases where the pre-existing valvular disease has led to left ventricular hypertrophy or dilation, and treatments aimed at restoring normal sinus rhythm should be considered.

If the patient is hemodynamically unstable or severely symptomatic, emergent direct current cardioversion (DCCV) is required. If AF has been persistent but present for less than 48 hours, elective DCCV can be done, usually without the need for a pre-procedural transesophageal echocardiogram. Several important caveats should be noted, however. First, if the patient is having paroxysmal AF interspersed with periods of sinus rhythm, DCCV will be ineffective and should not be performed and antiarrhythmic drug therapy should be considered. If the patient has been in AF for more than 48 hours without systemic anticoagulation, a transesophageal echocardiogram should be performed prior

DCCV to rule out the presence of a left atrial appendage thrombus since there is a risk of systemic embolization following DCCV. Consideration should be given to *at least* a brief period of full systemic anticoagulation in patients who require DCCV and who convert to sinus rhythm. The risk of systemic embolization and stroke is highest in the first 10 days *after* conversion, and the first 48–72 hours in particular *(110)*. Lastly, if DCCV fails to convert the patient to sinus (or the rhythm subsequently relapses back to AF) and the clinician feels sinus rhythm is important to achieve, anticoagulation and drug loading should again be considered before DCCV is repeated.

Amiodarone

Amiodarone is the drug of choice for pharmacologic conversion of post-operative AF or to improve the success rates of subsequent DCCV. Success rates of maintaining sinus rhythm in patients with chronic or paroxysmal (i.e., non-post-operative) AF are higher with amiodarone than with other antiarrhythmic drugs, but there are no studies comparing these drugs head-to-head for post-operative AF treatment. Amiodarone benefits from having an intravenous formulation that allows it to be loaded more rapidly than other agents. This is also an advantage in the post-operative patient who cannot readily take oral medications or when gastrointestinal absorption unpredictable. Amiodarone, unlike many other antiarrhythmic agents, does not rely on renal elimination. It, therefore, is often the only reasonable antiarrhythmic drug in those post-operative patients with impaired renal function.

The typical oral loading dose of amiodarone is 5 g in the setting of atrial arrhythmias. The total dose required when administered intravenously is usually estimated to be half of the total oral dose, because the bioavailability of amiodarone from the gut is widely variable at 20–80% *(111)*. It should be recognized that oral amiodarone will often cause nausea and GI upset and the dose may need to be decreased, the dosing intervals increased, or the route of administration changed, so the patient can tolerate the loading phase of the drug. Some advocate loading with both the IV form and the oral form for the first 24 hours, then changing to the oral form after the first day.

Amiodarone affects a number of cardiomyocyte channels and is not easily classifiable in the traditional Vaughn-Williams system. Because it has both calcium channel and beta-blocking properties, bradycardia and precipitation of heart failure can occur. As a potassium channel blocker, it can prolong the QT interval, and serial ECGs should be obtained to watch for this. On balance, however, amiodarone is less likely to cause polymorphic ventricular tachycardia than other Class III agents, perhaps because of its ability to simultaneously block sodium channels.

Sotalol

As mentioned previously, sotalol has been studied in the perioperative period as prophylaxis against developing AF. In this role it appears more effective than typical beta-blockers and appears similar in efficacy compared with amiodarone *(112)*. It can also be used to treat post-operative AF (i.e., not in a prophylactic role) but several limitations exist. First, no intravenous formulation of this drug is available; the drug loading must be done orally. The drug may have antiarrhythmic effects earlier, but sotalol is usually not considered fully loaded until about five doses. Next, it must be recognized that sotalol is actually a racemic mixture of D- and L-enantiomers with two very different effects. The beta-blocking properties of the drug reside with the L-enantiomer, so chronotropic and dromotropic incompetence, as well as depressed myocardial contractility, may occur. The D-enantiomer is a Vaughn-Williams Class III antiarrhythmic with potassium channel blocking properties. As such, the ECG should be scrutinized daily for prolongation of the QT interval, and electrolytes meticulously supplemented, as hypomagnesemia and hypokalemia will themselves prolong the QT interval, putting the patient at increased risk for polymorphic ventricular tachycardia. Sotalol is renally eliminated and should not be used in patients with renal insufficiency. Lastly, based on the SWORD trial, there are some safety concerns with this drug, so sotalol should be used with caution in patients with ischemic cardiomyopathy *(113)*.

Ibutilide

Ibutilide, an intravenous Class III antiarrhythmic, has been studied in the context of post-surgical AF and may be considered in patients with persistent AF as a substitute for or adjunct to DCCV *(114)*. Success rates with the drug *alone* have been reported at more than 50%. As with other agents of its class, magnesium and potassium levels should be corrected before its administration and co-administration with other antiarrhythmics avoided, as the rates of proarrhythmia are high. The published rates of polymorphic ventricular tachycardia are between 3.6 and 8.3%, with about 2% of patients requiring defibrillation *(115–117)*. The drug acts rapidly and most patients who convert will do so within 30–60 minutes. Despite this, late proarrhythmia has been reported and patients therefore need to remain on continuous monitoring for at least 4 hours after receiving ibutilide. Ibutilide is hepatically metabolized and does not require dose reduction with renal insufficiency. Its pro-arrhythmic nature makes it difficult to use when other antiarrhythmics are being given at the same time.

Other Antiarrhythmic Agents and Follow-Up

At times other antiarrhythmic agents may be considered, including intravenous procainamide, oral procainamide, oral propafenone, or oral dofetilide. In all of these situations, removal of agents that may be triggering AF should be done first. Many will resolve the AF once time has passed, so some do prefer to simply rate control initially (if that is done, then the patient must be placed on adequate anticoagulation). If drugs have been used to resolve the AF, and it is a new arrhythmia post-operatively, then it is often possible to discontinue the drug about 6 weeks after surgery. If rate control only has been chosen, then DCCV can usually be done at this 6 week anniversary.

DISORDERS OF CARDIAC CONDUCTION

The reported incidence of new conduction disorders following cardiac surgery is wide, ranging from <5 to >50%. This statistic is largely dependent on the definition of what constitutes a conduction defect and the timing of the ECG assessment relative to surgery. The most common abnormalities appear to be new right bundle branch block (RBBB) and first-degree atrioventricular (AV) block *(118)*. These results form a combination of factors, including myocardial ischemia, incomplete cardioprotection during cardioplegia, perioperative beta-blockade, and, in the case of valve surgery, direct surgical injury to the conduction system.

Temporary Pacing

Epicardial pacing wires are routinely placed in the operating room to provide backup pacing in case post-operative bradycardia appears. Bipolar leads are generally used and placed on both the RA and RV (rarely the LA and/or LV). AV sequential pacing is preferred with pacing rate set to between 80 and 100 bpm because that rate appears to optimize cardiac output without compromising ventricular filling or myocardial metabolism *(119, 120)*. It is important to carefully document pacing thresholds daily after surgery. In order to minimize current outputs, but still maintain a margin for safety, outputs are usually set at twice the capture threshold.

There are several causes of failure to capture (which are generally the same as the causes of failure to sense), but the majority of cases are caused by increased resistance at the myocardial/lead interface caused by fibrosis or swelling *(121)*. Atrial and ventricular pacing thresholds are generally stable for the first four post-operative days, but increase abruptly thereafter *(122)*. It has been reported that after 5 days, more than 60% of right atrial and more than 80% of left atrial leads will no longer capture *(123)*. Outside of their capacity to provide backup pacing, on occasion, epicardial wires can be useful in the diagnosis and management of post-operative arrhythmias, as well. In order to obtain an atrial ECG, the bipolar pacing leads should be attached to the right and left arm leads of the ECG recorder. Lead 1 will then record electrical activity in the proximity of the pacing wire and will allow for greater discrimination of atrioventricular relationships and activation sequence.

Some idea of AV nodal function can be obtained by using the epicardial wires to pace the atrium at progressively faster rates and assess the rate at which the AV node begins to block. Epicardial wires can also be used to prevent and treat post-operative arrhythmias in certain cases. Biatrial pacing has been shown to be effective in preventing post-operative AF in a number of studies *(123, 124)*. Outside of a prophylactic role, atrial wires may be used to overdrive suppress ectopic or re-entrant arrhythmias and can also be used to "burst pace" the atrium out of atrial flutter *(121)*. Similarly, in cases of pause-dependent polymorphic ventricular tachycardia, which may be seen post-operatively when QT-prolonging drugs, ischemia, bradycardia, and/or electrolytic disorders act to increase cardiac repolarization periods, pacing the heart at a rate above the intrinsic rate (thus shortening the QT interval) may reduce ventricular ectopy while the underlying cause of QT prolongation is being simultaneously addressed.

Need for Permanent Pacing

Often, new post-operative conduction disorders will disappear prior to discharge, but, in certain cases, implantation of a permanent pacemaker (PPM) is required. When complete heart block is present during the first post-operative day and persists for more than 48 hours, it is unlikely to resolve within the next 1–2 weeks and pre-discharge PPM must be considered *(125)*. Most patients who develop third-degree heart block will do so immediately after surgery, although some patients will do so later. Patients who only display heart block *after* the first 48 hours post-operatively are very likely to have resolution by the time of hospital discharge *(125)*, and waiting before PPM placement in this group is reasonable unless the temporary pacing wires are failing. Data suggest that patients who require PPM for post-surgical complete heart block have a high rate of long-term pacer dependency, regardless if the escape complexes were narrow (70%) or wide (82%) *(126)*.

It is important to recognize that high-degree (i.e., complete) heart block, although the most common, is not the only reason patients may require long-term pacing after surgery. Occasionally, post-operatively sinus or AV node function will be sufficiently impaired that the patient will be left with bradycardia or a second-degree block with an inadequate ventricular response rate and PPM becomes necessary. Additionally, pacing may be necessary in patients with sick sinus syndrome. Occasionally patients with post-operative AF will have paroxysms of arrhythmia with long sinus node recovery times or sinus bradycardia after spontaneous conversion to normal rhythm. This may also be aggravated by SA and AV nodal blocking drugs used to treat the bouts of tachycardia. It becomes vital, therefore, to meticulously inspect the period of conversion to sinus rhythm from AF to ensure the patient is not having significant pauses or bradycardic episodes.

The need for PPM following isolated CABG, approximately 0.5–1%, is much lower than after valve procedures (about 3–6%). The largest series published to date reported a 2.4% need for PPM in a general cardiac surgery population of more than 10,000 patients operated on from 1990 to 1995. Eight factors, validated in an additional 2,200+ patients, appeared important in predicting the need for post-operative PPM (Table 3) *(127)*. Not surprisingly, valve procedures, especially when the tricuspid

Table 3
Predictors of Need for Permanent Pacing After Cardiac
Surgery

Risk factor	Odds ratio (95% CI)
Valve surgery	
• Aortic	5.8 (3.9–8.7)
• Mitral	4.9 (3.1–7.8)
• Tricuspid	8.0 (5.5–11.9)
• Double valve	8.9 (5.5–14.6)
• Triple valve	7.5 (2.9–19.3)
Repeat surgery	2.4 (1.8–3.3)
Age over 75	3.0 (2.0–4.4)
Ablative arrhythmia surgery	4.2 (1.9–9.5)
MV annular reconstruction	2.4 (1.4–4.2)
Use of cold blood cardioplegia	2.0 (1.2–3.6)
Pre-operative renal failure	1.6 (1.0–2.6)
Active endocarditis	1.7 (0.9–3.0)

From *(127)* with permission.

valve or multiple valves were being replaced, were associated with the highest odds of requiring a permanent pacemaker following surgery.

Additionally, several risk factors for PPM have been identified specifically among patients undergoing AVR *(128)*. The presence of a pre-existing bundle branch block was more common in those that require PPM, most likely because of the proximity of the aortic valve to the conduction system and AV node. Likewise, calcification of the aortic annulus, which may require debridement in the region of the membranous septum in order to facilitate prosthetic valve placement, was also associated with the need for post-operative PPM for similar reasons.

RENAL FAILURE

Acute renal failure (ARF) is one of the most common complications following cardiac surgery. The exact rates of kidney injury are difficult to summarize because of considerable heterogeneity in the characterization of the condition. By defining ARF by a serum creatinine rise of more than 1 mg/dL over baseline, the incidence has been reported at about 8% *(129)*, while a more liberal >50% rise in serum creatinine definition has yielded rates of up to 30% *(130–132)*. Despite these semantic differences, there is a clearly higher incidence of ARF following valve, and especially combined CABG/valve procedures, than with bypass surgery alone. Relative to CABG alone, a more than twofold increase in incidence of ARF following valve and almost fourfold increase following combined procedures have been reported *(133, 134)*. Not surprisingly, the rates of renal failure requiring dialysis after surgery are similarly higher after valve (1.7%) or combined (3.3%) procedures, compared with isolated CABG alone (<1%).

The clinical feature and time course of post-cardiac surgery ARF have been categorized into three major types by Myers and Moran *(135)*. Type A ARF is the most common and is marked by a sharp drop in creatinine clearance immediately after surgery, followed by complete resolution after the creatinine peaks around post-operative day 4. Type B ARF occurs as a result of coincidental poor cardiac output delaying renal recovery after surgery. This form again displays an abrupt drop in renal function with complete, albeit delayed, recovery. Finally, Type C ARF occurs as a result of superimposed, successive renal insults after surgery and tends to lead to irreversible renal dysfunction. This occurs, for instance, in cases of systemic inflammatory response syndrome (SIRS) complicating pre-existent ARF (Fig. 3).

Although in most cases ARF improves, perioperative renal injury is important because it has been clearly associated with increased mortality. Even minimal changes in creatinine clearance have been associated with a higher risk for death following surgery, and this risk increases dramatically with the severity of injury. Most studies suggest a 15–30% rate of short-term death after cardiac surgery-related ARF, with an even higher rate of death (60–70%) if dialysis is required *(136)*. Beyond the immediate post-operative period, ARF after CPB also influences survival adversely over the long term as well *(137, 138)*.

The need to identify patients at high risk for post-operative ARF led to the development of the Cleveland Clinic Foundation Scoring System which takes into account *pre*-operative factors in its prediction model *(134)*. Patients are assigned a score from 0 to 17 and a graded risk of ARF can then be assigned, ranging from 0.4% in the lowest risk group to over 21% in the highest. In addition to pre-operative clinical factors, there is also a growing interest in identifying pre-existing genetic factors which may predispose to post-surgical renal insufficiency, such as the ACE gene insertion/deletion and inflammatory gene polymorphisms *(139)*.

Although good pre-procedural predictive tools are available, the operating room is a very dynamic environment and a significant portion of the risk will not be ascertainable before surgery. Intra-operative hemodynamic factors such as hypotension, reduced cardiac output, and low bypass flow rates are important intra-operative variables. Exposure to the CPB circuit itself has been associated with a higher risk of renal insufficiency than that seen in off-pump cases *(103, 140)*. CPB causes a dramatic increase in circulating inflammatory mediators and usually results in significant hemolysis with consequent free hemoglobin release both of which may also be involved in renal injury. Vaso-constrictor infusions, LV dysfunction, and intravascular volume depletion are important factors in the development of ARF in the post-operative phase. Overall, the pathogenesis of renal injury is usually complex and appears to reflect the summation of a number of pre-, intra-, and post-operative factors (Table 4).

NEUROLOGICAL COMPLICATIONS

Some of the most feared complications of cardiac surgery are neurological. There are two main types of adverse neurological outcomes: stroke, a relatively infrequent event, and cognitive dysfunction, which is by far more common.

Stroke

Post-operative stroke is a potentially devastating complication of cardiac surgery. It is associated with significant prolongation of hospitalization and costs. Mortality is increased dramatically follow-ing this event, and most patients will experience severe acute and long-term disability *(141, 142)*.

The incidence of stroke following cardiac surgery varies, depending on procedure type and patient features. Isolated CABG surgery appears to have a lower rate of stroke (approximately 1.5–4%) than valvular procedures (and particularly aortic valve procedures), especially when combined with coronary revascularization *(142, 143)*. Furthermore, clinically silent cerebral ischemic lesions defined by post-operative MRI have been noted in more than 40% of patients undergoing AVR *(144–147)*, sug-gesting this group of patients is particularly at risk for ischemic neurological complications. A similar risk of silent cerebral infarcts has not been noted for mitral valve procedures *(145)*.

The prevalence and clinical importance of stroke have stimulated interest in predicting this com-plication pre-operatively, though the data are primarily related to CABG alone. The Multicenter Study of Perioperative Ischemic Research Group *(148,149)* identified seven variables as predictive

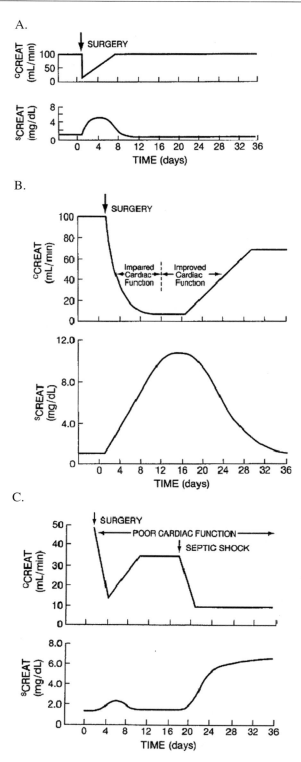

Fig. 3. Clinical courses of the three major categories of acute renal failure after cardiac surgery. **(A)** Type A is marked by improvement over the course of days, with complete resolution. **(B)** Immediate recovery of renal function is delayed by impaired cardiac output but returns to baseline over weeks in Type B. **(C)** Superimposed renal insults lead to severe renal dysfunction in Type C ARF. From *(135)*, reprinted with permission.

Table 4
Risk Factors for Acute Renal Failure After Cardiac Surgery

- Pre-operative
  - Female gender
  - Congestive heart failure/LV dysfunction
  - Pre-operative intra-aortic balloon pump
  - Emergency surgery
  - COPD
  - Diabetes mellitus
  - Redo surgery
  - Valve or combined procedures
  - Pre-existing renal insufficiency
  - Exposure to nephrotoxins (e.g., intravenous contrast media)
  - Genetic factors
- Intra-operative
  - Hypotension/flow pump flows
  - Embolic events
  - Nephrotoxins (e.g., pre-operative antibiotics, free hemoglobin)
  - Exposure to CPB circuit
- Post-operative
  - Systemic inflammation
  - LV dysfunction
  - Hypotension
  - Vasoconstrictors

of post-operative stroke or TIA after multivariate analysis among 2,107 patients undergoing CABG surgery. Smaller cohort studies of CABG patients undergoing concomitant intracardiac left-sided procedures have identified these types of procedures as a significant risk factor for stroke (Table 5).

Intra-operative factors which contribute to the risk of stroke have also been identified. Hypotension, especially in the presence of significant carotid stenosis, can be particularly detrimental to cerebral perfusion. Second, much of the risk for stroke has been attributed to macroembolism from the atheromatous debris from the ascending aorta and arch (150–152) as a consequence of repeated aortic manipulation during surgery. Additionally, the high-velocity jet of blood as it leaves the aortic cannula has been termed the "sand-blasting effect" and has been ascribed a role in the pathogenesis of systemic embolization. Opened cardiac chambers and cardioplegic arrest introduce significant amounts of air into the heart, which may cause cerebral air emboli once the aortic cross-clamp has been removed. Off-pump CABG surgery is associated with a much lower risk of stroke (103, 153, 154). These procedures are associated with relatively minimal aortic manipulations, no cardioplegia or opening of cardiac chambers, and no exposure to the CPB circuit.

There is also a *late* risk of stroke (Fig. 4) (143). This probably occurs as a consequence of post-operative atrial fibrillation and from a generalized pro-inflammatory and pro-thrombotic environment linked to surgical trauma and exposure to the bypass circuit (155).

Neurocognitive Deficits

The risk of post-operative cognitive dysfunction (POCD) has been an area of active study over the last decade and is estimated to occur in 30–50%. POCD has been linked to poorer quality of life scores after surgery which, in turn, has the potential to negatively impact the overall clinical and subjective benefits seen with cardiac surgery (156).

Table 5
Predictors of Neurological Complications After Cardiac Surgery

Stroke
- Age
- Use of cardiopulmonary bypass
- Aortic atheroma
- Intracardiac procedures, especially aortic valve surgery and combined with revascularization
- History of hypertension
- Coincidental pulmonary disease
- Diabetes mellitus
- Pre-operative intra-aortic balloon pump
- History of cerebrovascular disease
- Intra-operative hypotension
- Unstable angina
- Redo surgery
- Post-operative atrial fibrillation
- Pro-inflammatory genetic polymorphisms

Cognitive decline
- Age
- Lower level of education
- Poor LV function
- Prolonged ICU stay
- Higher baseline test scores
- Pro-inflammatory genetic polymorphisms
- Rapid rewarming from hypothermia
- Low intra-operative mean arterial pressures
- Pre-existing disabling neurological illness
- Living alone

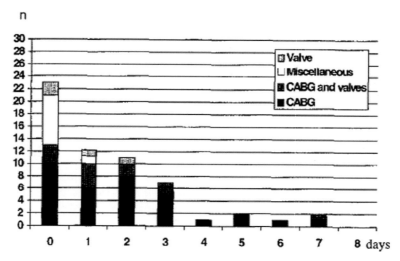

Fig. 4. Occurrence of stroke following cardiac surgery. There is an early preponderance of events, but a significant fraction only becomes evident on later post-operative days. From *(143)*, used with permission.

Short-term POCD risk factors, in distinction to stroke, appear to be less related to intra-operative factors and more closely linked to patient-specific pre-operative factors (Table 5) *(157–161)*. In general, POCD does not appear to be related to atheromatous disease of the aorta *(162)* or the carotids *(159)* or the appearance of new lesions on MRI *(146, 147)*. There is also little evidence that off-pump procedures reduce the risk *(163)*. Although about half of patients will have improvement in their cognition function by 6 months, the finding of POCD clearly identifies a patient at risk for further long-term impairment. Newman et al. identified age, level of education, and baseline test scores as predictive of cognitive function at 5 years *(161)*.

PULMONARY COMPLICATIONS

Pulmonary function usually declines after cardiac surgery because of distortion of the chest wall anatomy from the thoracotomy and various intra-parenchymal insults to the lung. Although respiratory insufficiency is common after cardiac surgery, its incidence is difficult to quantify exactly because of its heterogeneity in timing and etiology. Like many other complications in the post-operative period, respiratory failure represents the accumulation of intra- and post-operative factors interacting with pre-existing patient comorbidities.

Although there is no absolute threshold to exclude a patient from cardiac surgery, pre-operative assessment, including pulmonary function tests, can be useful as a guide. In general, FEV_1 values <1.0 L increase the risk for prolonged ventilatory failure post-operatively, especially when sternotomy incisions and mitral valve replacement are required. There is also natural decline in pulmonary function and reserve with age. Similarly, pre-existing lung disease, whether it be from obstructive (e.g., emphysema) or restrictive (e.g., obesity) causes, and ongoing tobacco abuse are major risks for pulmonary complications *(164, 165)*. Smoking cessation should be mandatory for all patients contemplating such procedures with the hope that this reduces the risk.

In the operating room there are several situations which may lead to post-operative pulmonary complications. Once the patient is placed on cardiopulmonary bypass, the lungs no longer inflate, predisposing them to atelectasis and post-operative pneumonias. Second, the bypass circuit stimulates a vigorous immune response, and subsequent re-exposure of the pulmonary capillaries, which have been bypassed during the course of surgery, to large volumes of activated blood may result in an inflammatory reaction in the lung. This life-threatening complication is, fortunately, uncommon (0.4–3%) *(166–169)*.

An additional intra-operative mechanism for respiratory compromise is transient phrenic nerve injury, which may result in unilateral or bilateral diaphragmatic paralysis. The incidence of this complication is reported at 10–60% *(170–172)*. It may occur as a result of direct injury (i.e., through inadvertent severing or disruption of the blood supply to the nerve) *(170, 173)*, but has also been associated with topical slush used to provide myocardial cooling *(170, 171)* and with pre-existing COPD *(174, 175)*. Longer term diaphragmatic paralysis is important because it is associated with prolonged need for mechanical ventilation *(170, 175)*, as well as persistent dyspnea and poorer quality of life after hospital discharge *(171, 176)*.

Pleural effusions are extremely common after surgery and usually are controlled initially with appropriately placed chest tubes. Recurrent large pleural effusions after chest tube removal cause respiratory compromise late in the course of recovery and may prompt readmission after the post-operative hospital discharge. Post-operative pleural effusions are usually bloody or serosanguinous, but occasionally a chylothorax may occur from accidental trauma to the thoracic duct.

Respiratory compromise from cardiac causes leading to pulmonary edema is also commonly encountered in the post-operative period. Patients with pre-existing LV dysfunction (either systolic or diastolic) are particularly at risk for this complication.

Finally, acute pulmonary embolism must be considered in any patient with respiratory failure in the post-operative period. The incidence of pulmonary embolism after cardiac surgery is generally felt to be low (<1%) *(177, 178)*. Saphenous vein harvesting and femoral arterial or venous cannulations (e.g., from pre-operative cardiac catheterization, intra-aortic balloon pumps, or percutaneous venous inflow cannula placement) all predispose toward developing deep venous thrombosis at a very high rate (17–48%) *(179–181)*. It is, therefore, important to maintain an index of suspicious for pulmonary embolism.

HEMATOLOGIC DISORDERS

The physiologic stress of cardiac surgery, exposure to the cardiopulmonary bypass circuit, significant intravascular volume shifts, bleeding, and coagulation issues all can lead to profound changes in the all three of the major cellular components of the hematologic system.

Anemia

Some degree of anemia is routine after cardiac surgery and has many causes. There is some hemolysis which occurs as the erythrocytes pass through the filters and roller pumps of the bypass machine. This may be a particular issue following extended pump times. The bypass pump also requires between 1.3 and 1.8 L of priming volume, which will lead to immediate intravascular volume expansion and hemodilution. Although this has been mitigated somewhat with the introduction of autologous priming (whereby ultra-filtration is used to withdraw some of the priming crystalloid volume off during surgery), the dilutional effects of crystalloids administered by priming, numerous simultaneous intravenous infusions, and with cardioplegic solutions can be profound.

Blood loss from intra-operative surgical site bleeding is routine but is minimized by autotransfusion systems which reclaim red blood cells lost in the operating field. These units of blood are then given back to the patient before the end of surgery. Nonetheless, site bleeding is an inevitable source of blood loss in the intra-operative and immediate post-operative periods. Once out of the operating room, chest- and mediastinal tube drainage must be carefully monitored. Excessive or prolonged drainage will generally prompt an explorative take-back procedure to identify the source of bleeding. Unfortunately, this is not a rare occurrence, complicating as many as 6% of cardiac surgeries *(49–51, 182, 183)*. The risk factors for post-operative blood loss have been summarized by the Society of Thoracic Surgeons (Table 6) based on the available published evidence *(184)*.

Ultimately, the decision of whether to transfuse should take into account the severity and tempo of the post-surgical anemia. Although the decision to transfuse must be individualized to each patient, the Societies of Thoracic Surgeons and Cardiovascular Anesthesiologists have published joint guidelines regarding the indications for post-operative blood transfusion *(184)*. While acknowledging the relative dearth of high-quality data in this field directly, the growing concern regarding the association between transfusion and mortality in the setting of both acute coronary syndromes, as well as cardiac surgery, coupled with the lack of clear efficacy of arbitrary transfusion triggers led the taskforce to conclude transfusion to be reasonable at hemoglobin levels of 7 g/dL or less.

Leukocytosis

Leukocytosis is also very common after surgery and generally represents an acute phase response to the stress of the operative environment. In general, the leukocytosis, which may be profound initially, improves on serial measurements. Persistent elevations in the white blood cell count after surgery (or a rebound elevation after an initial decline) should be assumed to be caused by infection until

Table 6
Factors Associated with Risk for Post-operative Blood Transfusions

- Advanced age (over 70 years old)
- Female gender
- Low pre-operative RBC volume
  - Baseline anemia
  - Small body size
- Pre-operative antithrombotic or antiplatelet drugs
  - Aspirin
  - Clopidogrel
  - Low-molecular weight heparins
  - Glycoprotein IIb/IIIa inhibitors
  - Direct thrombin inhibitors
  - Thrombolytics
- Procedural characteristics
  - Prolonged bypass time
  - Redo operations
  - Profound hypothermia
  - Valvular/combined procedures
  - Emergency surgery
- Congestive heart failure or LV dysfunction
- Renal insufficiency
- Insulin-dependent diabetes mellitus

Adapted from *(184)*.

proven otherwise. Blood cultures should be obtained and the initiation of broad spectrum antibiotics considered, depending on the index of suspicion. Alternative diagnoses, such as systemic inflammatory response syndrome, drug reaction, and post-pericardiotomy syndrome may also feature persistent leukocytosis. Additionally, corticosteroids may be administered intra-operatively for a variety of conditions, including transfusion reactions, suspected anaphylaxis, or during cases of deep hypothermic circulatory arrest and may easily be overlooked as a cause. Steroids will cause a demargination of leukocytes which may persist for days after administration.

Thrombocytopenia

Thrombocytopenia is very common after cardiac surgery. Typically, the platelet count will drop by half over the first 2–3 days post-operatively, and this is mainly due to the acute hemodilution and platelet consumption from the cardiopulmonary bypass circuit. The platelet count will start to recover shortly after surgery, and any failure to see such an improvement should raise alarm that another, potentially serious etiology is at play. Septicemia and the systemic inflammatory response syndrome can feature thrombocytopenia as a component, but these entities will almost invariably be associated with other manifestations (such as fever or multi-organ failure) that will alert clinicians to their presence.

Heparin-induced thrombocytopenia (HIT) is one of the most devastating potential complications of the post-operative period. It is usually associated with exposure to unfractionated heparin although low-molecular weight heparins can also be implicated. It is marked by significant thrombocytopenia (median platelet count of 60×10^9/L) which may, at times, be severe; 10% of cases may have a platelet count nadir under 20×10^9/L. Typically, the platelet count will drop 5–10 days following surgery (Fig. 5), as heparin exposure continues.

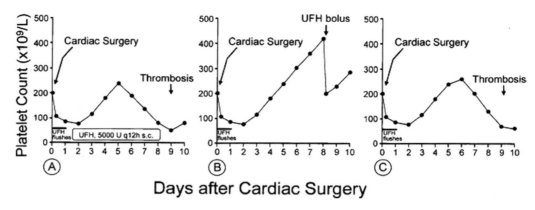

Fig. 5. Typical time course of heparin-induced thrombocytopenia following cardiac surgery. **(A)** Initial exposure to large doses of heparin in surgery, with continued exposure on subsequent hospital days in the form of heparin flushes or through sub-cutaneous routes leads to drops in platelet counts 5–10 days from surgery. **(B)** Rapid onset HIT following repeat heparin bolus dosing. **(C)** Delayed onset HIT following heparin dosing in cardiac surgery is thought to be due to high titers of HIT antibodies which can cause thrombosis without heparin re-exposure. This form of HIT is, fortunately, rare. From *(186)*, used with permission.

With the low platelet counts, the propensity toward both arterial and venous thromboses, rather than bleeding, is the hallmark of this syndrome. The pathogenesis of HIT is the formation of antibodies (usually IgG) against platelet factor 4 and heparin molecules. The resulting antibody–antigen complexes bind to Fc receptors on the platelet surface. This causes their activation and, consequently, thrombosis. Approximately 50–70% of patients with clinical HIT will go on to develop overt heparin-induced thrombocytopenia with thrombosis (HITT) *(185, 186)*.

It is important to recognize that the presence of HIT antibodies is common both before and, especially, after cardiac surgery, and the diagnosis of HIT should be reserved for those patients with clinical and laboratory evidence of this condition and not solely based on this laboratory value. The incidence of heparin–platelet factor 4 antibodies *before* cardiac surgery has been reported at between 5 and 19% *(187–189)* and may be due to prior exposure to heparin from previous procedures or hospitalizations. After cardiac surgery employing cardiopulmonary bypass, which routinely exposes patients to heparin boluses in excess of 25,000–30,000 units, between 25 and 50% of patients will develop HIT antibodies *(187, 190)*. The reported incidence of clinical HIT following cardiac surgery is between 2 and 2.5% *(186, 191, 192)*. Therefore, while post-operative HIT antibody presence is not rare, the rate of clinical HIT is much lower than the rate of seroconversion.

When HIT is suspected based on the tempo or pattern of thrombocytopenia after surgery, it is vital to stop all heparin products, including low-molecular weight heparins and heparin flushes, and alternative anticoagulants should be sought. Direct thrombin inhibitors, such as lepirudin, bivalirudin, or argatroban, should be used if the clinical suspicion is present before the HIT panel results are available. Management of suspected or confirmed cases of HIT should be done in conjunction with hematology consultation. A multi-disciplinary approach to this condition is important because the complications are common *(185, 189, 193)* and the overall mortality rate is very high (25–40%) *(193–195)*. A period of warfarin use after the event is generally recommended.

INFECTIOUS COMPLICATIONS

Nosocomial infections are, unfortunately, common following surgeries in general, and patients who have had cardiac valve surgeries are especially predisposed to these complications because of the length of time they spend convalescing in the hospital following their procedures and the number of invasive lines and catheters used to monitor their post-operative progress. Pneumonias and urinary tract infections are the most commonly encountered post-operative infections and a likely source of fever in this patient population. In the febrile patient, wound infections and evidence for bacteremia must be investigated as these are associated with significant complications and high mortality.

Wound incisions need to be checked daily to ensure a localized cellulitis is not developing. Sternal wound infections, which occur in up to 10–20% of sternotomies *(196, 197)*, may be categorized as superficial or deep. Superficial sternal infections are by far more common than deep (i.e., mediastinitis), which are seen in 1–2% *(197–199)*. These deep infections are associated with very high rates of morbidity, and the mortality associated with them is between 10 and 15% *(196, 200, 201)*.

The risk factors for sternal wound infections have been intensely assessed *(196, 197, 200–204)*. Age, obesity, diabetes mellitus, smoking, peripheral vascular disease, COPD, and heart failure have been repeatedly shown to be pre-operative predispositions for this condition. Prolonged mechanical ventilation and the need for re-exploration surgeries are post-operative factors associated with an increased likelihood of sternal infections, as are intra-procedural variables, such as the use of internal mammary artery grafts (especially bilateral) and the duration of surgery. Valve procedures per se do not appear to be associated with an increased risk for sternal wound infections after adjusting for total operative time *(197)*. Use of minimally invasive, i.e., right lateral thoracotomy or "Port-Access," procedures has been consistently associated with a lower risk for sternal complications *(205–208)*, although patient selection and surgical proficiency may confound this relationship. Some of these less invasive approaches still sacrifice the right internal thoracic artery, however.

Nosocomial bacteremia is another major infectious complication of particular importance following cardiac valvular surgery. The overall rate of bacteremia following cardiac surgery is approximately 3% *(209)*. Although gram-negative bloodstream infections may occur (usually associated with urinary catheters or mechanical ventilation), gram-positive bacteremia, especially the staphylococci, is especially serious for this patient population. At experienced centers the incidence of staphylococcal bacteremia is less than 1% after cardiac surgery *(209)*, but valvular procedures increase this risk *(210)*. Bacteremia following valvular heart surgery is associated with a very high rate (50%) of prosthetic valve endocarditis *(211, 212)*. Prosthetic valve endocarditis, in turn, is associated with considerable morbidity and mortality *(213–215)*. It is important, therefore, to (1) remove all indwelling catheters as soon as possible in the post-operative phase to minimize potential portals of entry and (2) to maintain a high index of suspicion for this complication and consider TEE early in suspected cases.

CONCLUSIONS

The post-operative environment following valvular heart surgery is a complex and dynamic one. The challenges of managing these individuals reflect the complex interaction between the extremes of physiology that occur during cardiac surgery, as well as the pathophysiology reflective of the underlying valve disease, co-existent non-cardiac medical illnesses, and individual host responses. Managing the valvular heart disease patient after surgery can be particularly challenging as they are generally more predisposed to a variety of complications compared with patients undergoing CABG. Anticipation of potential complications and awareness of an individual patient's risk factors help physicians and patients in their decisions regarding whether to undergo valve surgery and, in those individuals who do ultimately undergo heart valve surgery, improve outcomes.

REFERENCES

1. Polonen P, Ruokonen E, Hippelainen M, Poyhonen M, Takala J. A prospective, randomized study of goal-oriented hemodynamic therapy in cardiac surgical patients. *Anesthesia and Analgesia.* 2000;90:1052–1059.
2. Goepfert MS, Reuter DA, Akyol D, Lamm P, Kilger E, Goetz AE. Goal-directed fluid management reduces vasopressor and catecholamine use in cardiac surgery patients. *Intensive Care Medicine.* 2007;33:96–103.
3. Breisblatt WM, Stein KL, Wolfe CJ, Follansbee WP, Capozzi J, Armitage JM, Hardesty RL. Acute myocardial dysfunction and recovery: a common occurrence after coronary bypass surgery. *Journal of the American College of Cardiology.* 1990;15:1261–1269.
4. Roberts AJ, Spies SM, Sanders JH, Moran JM, Wilkinson CJ, Lichtenthal PR, White RL, Michaelis LL. Serial assessment of left ventricular performance following coronary artery bypass grafting. Early postoperative results with myocardial protection afforded by multidose hypothermic potassium crystalloid cardioplegia. *The Journal of Thoracic and Cardiovascular Surgery.* 1981;81:69–84.
5. Sharony R, Grossi EA, Saunders PC, Schwartz CF, Ciuffo GB, Baumann FG, Delianides J, Applebaum RM, Ribakove GH, Culliford AT, Galloway AC, Colvin SB. Aortic valve replacement in patients with impaired ventricular function. *The Annals of Thoracic Surgery.* 2003;75:1808–1814.
6. Leenen FH, Chan YK, Smith DL, Reeves RA. Epinephrine and left ventricular function in humans: effects of beta-1 vs nonselective beta-blockade. *Clinical Pharmacology and Therapeutics.* 1988;43:519–528.
7. Sung BH, Robinson C, Thadani U, Lee R, Wilson MF. Effects of 1-epinephrine on hemodynamics and cardiac function in coronary disease: dose-response studies. *Clinical Pharmacology and Therapeutics.* 1988;43:308–316.
8. Steen PA, Tinker JH, Pluth JR, Barnh, rst DA, Tarhan S. Efficacy of dopamine, dobutamine, and epinephrine during emergence from cardiopulmonary bypass in man. *Circulation.* 1978;57:378–384.
9. Griffin MJ, Hines RL. Management of perioperative ventricular dysfunction. *Journal of Cardiothoracic and Vascular Anesthesia.* 2001;15:90–106.
10. Aurigemma G, Battista S, Orsinelli D, Sweeney A, Pape L, Cuenoud H. Abnormal left ventricular intracavitary flow acceleration in patients undergoing aortic valve replacement for aortic stenosis. A marker for high postoperative morbidity and mortality. *Circulation.* 1992;86:926–936.
11. Connolly HM, Oh JK, Schaff HV, Roger VL, Osborn SL, Hodge DO, Tajik AJ. Severe aortic stenosis with low transvalvular gradient and severe left ventricular dysfunction:result of aortic valve replacement in 52 patients. *Circulation.* 2000;101:1940–1946.
12. Vaquette B, Corbineau H, Laurent M, Lelong B, Langanay T, de Place C, Froger-Bompas C, Leclercq C, Daubert C, Leguerrier A. Valve replacement in patients with critical aortic stenosis and depressed left ventricular function: predictors of operative risk, left ventricular function recovery, and long term outcome. *Heart (British Cardiac Society).* 2005;91:1324–1329.
13. Robiolio PA, Rigolin VH, Hearne SE, Baker WA, Kisslo KB, Pierce CH, Bashore TM, Harrison JK. Left ventricular performance improves late after aortic valve replacement in patients with aortic stenosis and reduced ejection fraction. *The American Journal of Cardiology.* 1995;76:612–615.
14. Kvidal P, Bergstrom R, Horte LG, Stahle E. Observed and relative survival after aortic valve replacement. *Journal of the American College of Cardiology.* 2000;35:747–756.
15. Harpole DH, Jr., Gall SA, Jr., Wolfe WG, Rankin JS, Jones RH. Effects of valve replacement on ventricular mechanics in mitral regurgitation and aortic stenosis. *The Annals of Thoracic Surgery.* 1996;62:756–761.
16. Harpole DH, Davidson CJ, Skelton TN, Kisslo KB, Jones RH, Bashore TM. Changes in left ventricular systolic performance immediately after percutaneous aortic balloon valvuloplasty. *The American Journal of Cardiology.* 1990;65:1213–1218.
17. Harpole DH, Davidson CJ, Skelton TN, Kisslo KB, Jones RH, Bashore TM. Early and late changes in left ventricular systolic performance after percutaneous aortic balloon valvuloplasty. *The American Journal of Cardiology.* 1990;66:327–332.
18. Gaasch WH, Folland ED. Left ventricular function in rheumatic mitral stenosis. *European Heart Journal.* 1991;12 Suppl B:66–69.
19. Gash AK, Carabello BA, Cepin D, Spann JF. Left ventricular ejection performance and systolic muscle function in patients with mitral stenosis. *Circulation.* 1983;67:148–154.
20. Ibrahim MM. Left ventricular function in rheumatic mitral stenosis. Clinical echocardiographic study. *British Heart Journal.* 1979;42:514–520.
21. Vincens JJ, Temizer D, Post JR, Edmunds LH, Jr., Herrmann HC. Long-term outcome of cardiac surgery in patients with mitral stenosis and severe pulmonary hypertension. *Circulation.* 1995;92:II137–142.
22. Cesnjevar RA, Feyrer R, Walther F, Mahmoud FO, Lindemann Y, von der Emde J. High-risk mitral valve replacement in severe pulmonary hypertension – 30 years experience. *European Journal of Cardiothoracic Surgery.* 1998;13:344–351;discussion 351–342.

23. Cevese PG, Gallucci V, Valfre C, Giacomin A, Mazzucco A, Casarotto D. Pulmonary hypertension in mitral valve surgery. *The Journal of Cardiovascular Surgery*. 1980;21:7–10.
24. Luria D, Klutstein MW, Rosenmann D, Shaheen J, Sergey S, Tzivoni D. Prevalence and significance of left ventricular outflow gradient during dobutamine echocardiography. *European Heart Journal*. 1999;20:386–392.
25. Auer J, Berent R, Weber T, Lamm G, Eber B. Catecholamine therapy inducing dynamic left ventricular outflow tract obstruction. *International Journal of Cardiology*. 2005;101:325–328.
26. Mingo S, Benedicto A, Jimenez MC, Perez MA, Montero M. Dynamic left ventricular outflow tract obstruction secondary to catecholamine excess in a normal ventricle. *International Journal of Cardiology*. 2006;112:393–396.
27. Come PC, Bulkley BH, Goodman ZD, Hutchins GM, Pitt B, Fortuin NJ. Hypercontractile cardiac states simulating hypertrophic cardiomyopathy. *Circulation*. 1977;55:901–908.
28. Yalcin F, Muderrisoglu H, Korkmaz ME, Ozin B, Baltali M, Yigit F. The effect of dobutamine stress on left ventricular outflow tract gradients in hypertensive patients with basal septal hypertrophy. *Angiology*. 2004;55:295–301.
29. Roldan FJ, Vargas-Barron J, Espinola-Zavaleta N, Keirns C, Romero-Cardenas A. Severe dynamic obstruction of the left ventricular outflow tract induced by dobutamine. *Echocardiography (Mount Kisco, NY)*. 2000;17:37–40.
30. Grossi EA, Galloway AC, Parish MA, Asai T, Gindea AJ, Harty S, Kronzon I, Spencer FC, Colvin SB. Experience with twenty-eight cases of systolic anterior motion after mitral valve reconstruction by the Carpentier technique. *The Journal of Thoracic and Cardiovascular Surgery*. 1992;103:466–470.
31. Freeman WK, Schaff HV, Khandheria BK, Oh JK, Orszulak TA, Abel MD, Seward JB, Tajik AJ. Intraoperative evaluation of mitral valve regurgitation and repair by transesophageal echocardiography: incidence and significance of systolic anterior motion. *Journal of the American College of Cardiology*. 1992;20:599–609.
32. Jebara VA, Mihaileanu S, Acar C, Brizard C, Grare P, Latremouille C, Chauvaud S, Fabiani JN, Deloche A, Carpentier A. Left ventricular outflow tract obstruction after mitral valve repair. Results of the sliding leaflet technique. *Circulation*. 1993;88:II30–34.
33. Maslow AD, Regan MM, Haering JM, Johnson RG, Levine RA. Echocardiographic predictors of left ventricular outflow tract obstruction and systolic anterior motion of the mitral valve after mitral valve reconstruction for myxomatous valve disease. *Journal of the American College of Cardiology*. 1999;34:2096–2104.
34. Maslow AD, Singh A. Mitral valve repair: to slide or not to slide-precardiopulmonary bypass echocardiogram examination. *Journal of Cardiothoracic and Vascular Anesthesia*. 2006;20:842–846.
35. Kaul TK, Fields BL. Postoperative acute refractory right ventricular failure: incidence, pathogenesis, management and prognosis. *Cardiovascular Surgery (London, England)*. 2000;8:1–9.
36. Wranne B, Pinto FJ, Hammarstrom E, St Goar FG, Puryear J, Popp RL. Abnormal right heart filling after cardiac surgery: time course and mechanisms. *British Heart Journal*. 1991;66:435–442.
37. Michaux I, Filipovic M, Skarvan K, Schneiter S, Schumann R, Zerkowski HR, Bernet F, Seeberger MD. Effects of on-pump vs. off-pump coronary artery bypass graft surgery on right ventricular function. *The Journal of Thoracic and Cardiovascular Surgery*. 2006;131:1281–1288.
38. Davila-Roman VG, Waggoner AD, Hopkins WE, Barzilai B. Right ventricular dysfunction in low output syndrome after cardiac operations: assessment by transesophageal echocardiography. *The Annals of Thoracic Surgery*. 1995;60:1081–1086.
39. Reichert CL, Visser CA, van den Brink RB, Koolen JJ, van Wezel HB, Moulijn AC, Dunning AJ. Prognostic value of biventricular function in hypotensive patients after cardiac surgery as assessed by transesophageal echocardiography. *Journal of Cardiothoracic and Vascular Anesthesia*. 1992;6:429–432.
40. Maslow AD, Regan MM, Panzica P, Heindel S, Mashikian J, Comunale ME. Precardiopulmonary bypass right ventricular function is associated with poor outcome after coronary artery bypass grafting in patients with severe left ventricular systolic dysfunction. *Anesthesia and Analgesia*. 2002;95:1507–1518, table of contents.
41. Maslow AD, Regan MM, Schwartz C, Bert A, Singh A. Inotropes improve right heart function in patients undergoing aortic valve replacement for aortic stenosis. *Anesthesia and Analgesia*. 2004;98:891–902, table of contents.
42. Feneck RO. Intravenous milrinone following cardiac surgery: II. Influence of baseline hemodynamics and patient factors on therapeutic response. The European Milrinone Multicentre Trial Group. *Journal of Cardiothoracic and Vascular Anesthesia*. 1992;6:563–567.
43. Feneck RO. Intravenous milrinone following cardiac surgery: I. Effects of bolus infusion followed by variable dose maintenance infusion. The European Milrinone Multicentre Trial Group. *Journal of Cardiothoracic and Vascular Anesthesia*. 1992;6:554–562.
44. Doolan LA, Jones EF, Kalman J, Buxton BF, Tonkin AM. A placebo-controlled trial verifying the efficacy of milrinone in weaning high-risk patients from cardiopulmonary bypass. *Journal of Cardiothoracic and Vascular Anesthesia*. 1997;11:37–41.
45. Tayama E, Ueda T, Shojima T, Akasu K, Oda T, Fukunaga S, Akashi H, Aoyagi S. Arginine vasopressin is an ideal drug after cardiac surgery for the management of low systemic vascular resistant hypotension concomitant with pulmonary hypertension. *Interactive Cardiovascular and Thoracic Surgery*. 2007.

46. Solina A, Papp D, Ginsberg S, Krause T, Grubb W, Scholz P, Pena LL, Cody R. A comparison of inhaled nitric oxide and milrinone for the treatment of pulmonary hypertension in adult cardiac surgery patients. *Journal of Cardiothoracic and Vascular Anesthesia*. 2000;14:12–17.

47. Schmid ER, Burki C, Engel MH, Schmidlin D, Tornic M, Seifert B. Inhaled nitric oxide versus intravenous vasodilators in severe pulmonary hypertension after cardiac surgery. *Anesthesia and Analgesia*. 1999;89:1108–1115.

48. Camara ML, Aris A, Alvarez J, Padro JM, Caralps JM. Hemodynamic effects of prostaglandin E1 and isoproterenol early after cardiac operations for mitral stenosis. *The Journal of Thoracic and Cardiovascular Surgery*. 1992;103:1177–1185.

49. Karthik S, Grayson AD, McCarron EE, Pullan DM, Desmond MJ. Reexploration for bleeding after coronary artery bypass surgery: risk factors, outcomes, and the effect of time delay. *The Annals of Thoracic Surgery*. 2004;78:527–534; discussion 534.

50. Moulton MJ, Creswell LL, Mackey ME, Cox JL, Rosenbloom M. Reexploration for bleeding is a risk factor for adverse outcomes after cardiac operations. *The Journal of Thoracic and Cardiovascular Surgery*. 1996;111:1037–1046.

51. Munoz JJ, Birkmeyer NJ, Dacey LJ, Birkmeyer JD, Charlesworth DC, Johnson ER, Lahey SJ, Norotsky M, Quinn RD, Westbrook BM, O'Connor GT. Trends in rates of reexploration for hemorrhage after coronary artery bypass surgery. Northern New England Cardiovascular Disease Study Group. *The Annals of Thoracic Surgery*. 1999;68: 1321–1325.

52. Chuttani K, Pandian NG, Mohanty PK, Rosenfield K, Schwartz SL, Udelson JE, Simonetti J, Kusay BS, Caldeira ME. Left ventricular diastolic collapse. An echocardiographic sign of regional cardiac tamponade. *Circulation*. 1991;83:1999–2006.

53. Chuttani K, Tischler MD, Pandian NG, Lee RT, Mohanty PK. Diagnosis of cardiac tamponade after cardiac surgery: relative value of clinical, echocardiographic, and hemodynamic signs. *American Heart Journal*. 1994;127: 913–918.

54. Pepi M, Muratori M, Barbier P, Doria E, Arena V, Berti M, Celeste F, Guazzi M, Tamborini G. Pericardial effusion after cardiac surgery: incidence, site, size, and haemodynamic consequences. *British Heart Journal*. 1994;72:327–331.

55. Kuvin JT, Harati NA, Pandian NG, Bojar RM, Khabbaz KR. Postoperative cardiac tamponade in the modern surgical era. *The Annals of Thoracic Surgery*. 2002;74:1148–1153.

56. Russo AM, O'Connor WH, Waxman HL. Atypical presentations and echocardiographic findings in patients with cardiac tamponade occurring early and late after cardiac surgery. *Chest*. 1993;104:71–78.

57. Solem JO, Kugelberg J, Stahl E, Olin C. Late cardiac tamponade following open-heart surgery. Diagnosis and treatment. *Scandinavian Journal of Thoracic and Cardiovascular Surgery*. 1986;20:129–131.

58. Aksoyek A, Tutun U, Ulus T, Ihsan Parlar A, Budak B, Temurturkan M, Katircioglu SF, Cobanoglu A. Surgical drainage of late cardiac tamponade following open heart surgery. *The Thoracic and Cardiovascular Surgeon*. 2005;53:285–290.

59. Yilmaz AT, Arslan M, Demirklic U, Kuralay E, Ozal E, Bingol H, Oz BS, Tatar H, Ozturk OY. Late posterior cardiac tamponade after open heart surgery. *The Journal of Cardiovascular Surgery*. 1996;37:615–620.

60. Meurin P, Weber H, Renaud N, Larrazet F, Tabet JY, Demolis P, Ben Driss A. Evolution of the postoperative pericardial effusion after day 15: the problem of the late tamponade. *Chest*. 2004;125:2182–2187.

61. Matsuyama K, Matsumoto M, Sugita T, Nishizawa J, Yoshioka T, Tokuda Y, Ueda Y. Clinical characteristics of patients with constrictive pericarditis after coronary bypass surgery. *Japanese Circulation Journal*. 2001;65:480–482.

62. Ikaheimo MJ, Huikuri HV, Airaksinen KE, Korhonen UR, Linnaluoto MK, Tarkka MR, Takkunen JT. Pericardial effusion after cardiac surgery: incidence, relation to the type of surgery, antithrombotic therapy, and early coronary bypass graft patency. *American Heart Journal*. 1988;116:97–102.

63. Weitzman LB, Tinker WP, Kronzon I, Cohen ML, Glassman E, Spencer FC. The incidence and natural history of pericardial effusion after cardiac surgery – an echocardiographic study. *Circulation*. 1984;69:506–511.

64. Ribeiro P, Sapsford R, Evans T, Parcharidis G, Oakley C. Constrictive pericarditis as a complication of coronary artery bypass surgery. *British Heart Journal*. 1984;51:205–210.

65. Killian DM, Furiasse JG, Scanlon PJ, Loeb HS, Sullivan HJ. Constrictive pericarditis after cardiac surgery. *American Heart Journal*. 1989;118:563–568.

66. Fleisher LA, Newman MF, St Aubin LB, Cropp AB, Billing CB, Bonney S, Mackey WC, Poldermans D, Corbalan R, Pereira AH, Coriat P. Efficacy of zoniporide, an Na/H exchange ion inhibitor, for reducing perioperative cardiovascular events in vascular surgery patients. *Journal of Cardiothoracic and Vascular Anesthesia*. 2005;19:570–576.

67. Landesberg G, Shatz V, Akopnik I, Wolf YG, Mayer M, Berlatzky Y, Weissman C, Mosseri M. Association of cardiac troponin, CK-MB, and postoperative myocardial ischemia with long-term survival after major vascular surgery. *Journal of the American College of Cardiology*. 2003;42:1547–1554.

68. Lopez-Jimenez F, Goldman L, Sacks DB, Thomas EJ, Johnson PA, Cook EF, Lee TH. Prognostic value of cardiac troponin T after noncardiac surgery: 6-month follow-up data. *Journal of the American College of Cardiology*. 1997;29:1241–1245.

69. McFalls EO, Ward HB, Moritz TE, Goldman S, Krupski WC, Littooy F, Pierpont G, Santilli S, Rapp J, Hattler B, Shunk K, Jaenicke C, Thottapurathu L, Ellis N, Reda DJ, Henderson WG. Coronary-artery revascularization before elective major vascular surgery. *The New England Journal of Medicine*. 2004;351:2795–2804.

70. Ramsay J, Shernan S, Fitch J, Finnegan P, Todaro T, Filloon T, Nussmeier NA. Increased creatine kinase MB level predicts postoperative mortality after cardiac surgery independent of new Q waves. *The Journal of Thoracic and Cardiovascular Surgery*. 2005;129:300–306.

71. Griesmacher A, Grimm M, Schreiner W, Muller MM. Diagnosis of perioperative myocardial infarction by considering relationship of postoperative electrocardiogram changes and enzyme increases after coronary bypass operation. *Clinical Chemistry*. 1990;36:883–887.

72. Swaanenburg JC, Loef BG, Volmer M, Boonstra PW, Grandjean JG, Mariani MA, Epema AH. Creatine kinase MB, troponin I, troponin T release patterns after coronary artery bypass grafting with or without cardiopulmonary bypass and after aortic and mitral valve surgery. *Clinical Chemistry*. 2001;47:584–587.

73. Thielmann M, Massoudy P, Schmermund A, Neuhauser M, Marggraf G, Kamler M, Herold U, Aleksic I, Mann K, Haude M, Heusch G, Erbel R, Jakob H. Diagnostic discrimination between graft-related and non-graft-related perioperative myocardial infarction with cardiac troponin I after coronary artery bypass surgery. *European Heart Journal*. 2005;26:2440–2447.

74. Thielmann M, Massoudy P, Marggraf G, Knipp S, Schmermund A, Piotrowski J, Erbel R, Jakob H. Role of troponin I, myoglobin, and creatine kinase for the detection of early graft failure following coronary artery bypass grafting. *European Journal of Cardiothoracic Surgery*. 2004;26:102–109.

75. Bourassa MG. Fate of venous grafts: the past, the present and the future. *Journal of the American College of Cardiology*. 1991;17:1081–1083.

76. Fitzgibbon GM, Kafka HP, Leach AJ, Keon WJ, Hooper GD, Burton JR. Coronary bypass graft fate and patient outcome: angiographic follow-up of 5,065 grafts related to survival and reoperation in 1,388 patients during 25 years. *Journal of the American College of Cardiology*. 1996;28:616–626.

77. Goldman S, Zadina K, Moritz T, Ovitt T, Sethi G, Copeland JG, Thottapurathu L, Krasnicka B, Ellis N, Anderson RJ, Henderson W. Long-term patency of saphenous vein and left internal mammary artery grafts after coronary artery bypass surgery: results from a Department of Veterans Affairs Cooperative Study. *Journal of the American College of Cardiology*. 2004;44:2149–2156.

78. Holmvang L, Jurlander B, Rasmussen C, Thiis JJ, Grande P, Clemmensen P. Use of biochemical markers of infarction for diagnosing perioperative myocardial infarction and early graft occlusion after coronary artery bypass surgery. *Chest*. 2002;121:103–111.

79. Antona C, Scrofani R, Lemma M, Vanelli P, Mangini A, Danna P, Gelpi G. Assessment of an aortosaphenous vein graft anastomotic device in coronary surgery: clinical experience and early angiographic results. *The Annals of Thoracic Surgery*. 2002;74:2101–2105.

80. Goldman S, Copeland J, Moritz T, Henderson W, Zadina K, Ovitt T, Doherty J, Read R, Chesler E, Sako Y, et al. Improvement in early saphenous vein graft patency after coronary artery bypass surgery with antiplatelet therapy: results of a Veterans Administration Cooperative Study. *Circulation*. 1988;77:1324–1332.

81. Verrier ED, Shernan SK, Taylor KM, Van de Werf F, Newman MF, Chen JC, Carrier M, Haverich A, Malloy KJ, Adams PX, Todaro TG, Mojcik CF, Rollins SA, Levy JH. Terminal complement blockade with pexelizumab during coronary artery bypass graft surgery requiring cardiopulmonary bypass: a randomized trial. *JAMA*. 2004;291:2319–2327.

82. Alexander JH, Hafley G, Harrington RA, Peterson ED, Ferguson TB, Jr., Lorenz TJ, Goyal A, Gibson M, Mack MJ, Gennevois D, Califf RM, Kouchoukos NT. Efficacy and safety of edifoligide, an E2F transcription factor decoy, for prevention of vein graft failure following coronary artery bypass surgery: PREVENT IV: a randomized controlled trial. *JAMA*. 2005;294:2446–2454.

83. van Dijk D, Nierich AP, Jansen EW, Nathoe HM, Suyker WJ, Diephuis JC, van Boven WJ, Borst C, Buskens E, Grobbee DE, Robles De Medina EO, de Jaegere PP. Early outcome after off-pump versus on-pump coronary bypass surgery: results from a randomized study. *Circulation*. 2001;104:1761–1766.

84. Nathoe HM, Moons KG, van Dijk D, Jansen EW, Borst C, de Jaegere PP, Grobbee DE. Risk and determinants of myocardial injury during off-pump coronary artery bypass grafting. *The American Journal of Cardiology*. 2006;97:1482–1486.

85. Olthof H, Middelhof C, Meijne NG, Fiolet JW, Becker AE, Lie KI. The definition of myocardial infarction during aortocoronary bypass surgery. *American Heart Journal*. 1983;106:631–637.

86. Warren SG, Wagner GS, Bethea CF, Roe CR, Oldham HN, Kong Y. Diagnostic and prognostic significance of electrocardiographic and CPK isoenzyme changes following coronary bypass surgery: correlation with findings at one year. *American Heart Journal*. 1977;93:189–196.

87. Burdine JA, DePuey EG, Orzan F, Mathur VS, Hall RJ. Scintigraphic, electrocardiographic, and enzymatic diagnosis of perioperative myocardial infarction in patients undergoing myocardial revascularization. *Journal of Nuclear Medicine*. 1979;20:711–714.

88. Burns RJ, Gladstone PJ, Tremblay PC, Feindel CM, Salter DR, Lipton IH, Ogilvie RR, David TE. Myocardial infarction determined by technetium-99m pyrophosphate single-photon tomography complicating elective coronary artery bypass grafting for angina pectoris. *The American Journal of Cardiology*. 1989;63:1429–1434.

89. Cheng DC, Chung F, Burns RJ, Houston PL, Feindel CM. Postoperative myocardial infarction documented by technetium pyrophosphate scan using single-photon emission computed tomography: significance of intraoperative myocardial ischemia and hemodynamic control. *Anesthesiology*. 1989;71:818–826.

90. Selvanayagam JB, Petersen SE, Francis JM, Robson MD, Kardos A, Neubauer S, Taggart DP. Effects of off-pump versus on-pump coronary surgery on reversible and irreversible myocardial injury: a randomized trial using cardiovascular magnetic resonance imaging and biochemical markers. *Circulation*. 2004;109:345–350.

91. Selvanayagam JB, Pigott D, Balacumaraswami L, Petersen SE, Neubauer S, Taggart DP. Relationship of irreversible myocardial injury to troponin I and creatine kinase-MB elevation after coronary artery bypass surgery: insights from cardiovascular magnetic resonance imaging. *Journal of the American College of Cardiology*. 2005;45:629–631.

92. Steuer J, Bjerner T, Duvernoy O, Jideus L, Johansson L, Ahlstrom H, Stahle E, Lindahl B. Visualisation and quantification of peri-operative myocardial infarction after coronary artery bypass surgery with contrast-enhanced magnetic resonance imaging. *European Heart Journal*. 2004;25:1293–1299.

93. Costa MA, Carere RG, Lichtenstein SV, Foley DP, de Valk V, Lindenboom W, Roose PC, van Geldorp TR, Macaya C, Castanon JL, Fernandez-Avilez F, Gonzales JH, Heyer G, Unger F, Serruys PW. Incidence, predictors, and significance of abnormal cardiac enzyme rise in patients treated with bypass surgery in the arterial revascularization therapies study (ARTS). *Circulation*. 2001;104:2689–2693.

94. Januzzi JL, Lewandrowski K, MacGillivray TE, Newell JB, Kathiresan S, Servoss SJ, Lee-Lewandrowski E. A comparison of cardiac troponin T and creatine kinase-MB for patient evaluation after cardiac surgery. *Journal of the American College of Cardiology*. 2002;39:1518–1523.

95. Klatte K, Chaitman BR, Theroux P, Gavard JA, Stocke K, Boyce S, Bartels C, Keller B, Jessel A. Increased mortality after coronary artery bypass graft surgery is associated with increased levels of postoperative creatine kinase-myocardial band isoenzyme release: results from the GUARDIAN trial. *Journal of the American College of Cardiology*. 2001;38:1070–1077.

96. Croal BL, Hillis GS, Gibson PH, Fazal MT, El-Shafei H, Gibson G, Jeffrey RR, Buchan KG, West D, Cuthbertson BH. Relationship between postoperative cardiac troponin I levels and outcome of cardiac surgery. *Circulation*. 2006;114:1468–1475.

97. Steuer J, Granath F, de Faire U, Ekbom A, Stahle E. Increased risk of heart failure as a consequence of perioperative myocardial injury after coronary artery bypass grafting. *Heart (British Cardiac Society)*. 2005;91:754–758.

98. Frost L, Molgaard H, Christiansen EH, Hjortholm K, Paulsen PK, Thomsen PE. Atrial fibrillation and flutter after coronary artery bypass surgery: epidemiology, risk factors and preventive trials. *International Journal of Cardiology*. 1992;36:253–261.

99. Fuller JA, Adams GG, Buxton B. Atrial fibrillation after coronary artery bypass grafting. Is it a disorder of the elderly? *The Journal of Thoracic and Cardiovascular Surgery*. 1989;97:821–825.

100. Mathew JP, Parks R, Savino JS, Friedman AS, Koch C, Mangano DT, Browner WS. Atrial fibrillation following coronary artery bypass graft surgery: predictors, outcomes, and resource utilization. MultiCenter Study of Perioperative Ischemia Research Group. *JAMA*. 1996;276:300–306.

101. Ommen SR, Odell JA, Stanton MS. Atrial arrhythmias after cardiothoracic surgery. *The New England Journal of Medicine*. 1997;336:1429–1434.

102. Mitchell LB, Exner DV, Wyse DG, Connolly CJ, Prystai GD, Bayes AJ, Kidd WT, Kieser T, Burgess JJ, Ferland A, MacAdams CL, Maitland A. Prophylactic oral amiodarone for the prevention of arrhythmias that begin early after revascularization, valve replacement, or repair: PAPABEAR: a randomized controlled trial. *JAMA*. 2005;294: 3093–3100.

103. Mack MJ, Pfister A, Bachand D, Emery R, Magee MJ, Connolly M, Subramanian V. Comparison of coronary bypass surgery with and without cardiopulmonary bypass in patients with multivessel disease. *The Journal of Thoracic and Cardiovascular Surgery*. 2004;127:167–173.

104. Curtis JJ, Parker BM, McKenney CA, Wagner-Mann CC, Walls JT, Demmy TL, Schmaltz RA. Incidence and predictors of supraventricular dysrhythmias after pulmonary resection. *The Annals of Thoracic Surgery*. 1998;66:1766–1771.

105. Rena O, Papalia E, Oliaro A, Casadio C, Ruffini E, Filosso PL, Sacerdote C, Maggi G. Supraventricular arrhythmias after resection surgery of the lung. *European Journal of Cardiothoracic Surgery*. 2001;20:688–693.

106. Crystal E, Garfinkle MS, Connolly SS, Ginger TT, Sleik K, Yusuf SS. Interventions for preventing post-operative atrial fibrillation in patients undergoing heart surgery. *Cochrane Database of Systematic Reviews (Online)*. 2004:CD003611.

107. Halonen J, Halonen P, Jarvinen O, Taskinen P, Auvinen T, Tarkka M, Hippelainen M, Juvonen T, Hartikainen J, Hakala T. Corticosteroids for the prevention of atrial fibrillation after cardiac surgery: a randomized controlled trial. *JAMA*. 2007;297:1562–1567.

108. Baker WL, White CM, Kluger J, Denowitz A, Konecny CP, Coleman CI. Effect of perioperative corticosteroid use on the incidence of postcardiothoracic surgery atrial fibrillation and length of stay. *Heart Rhythm*. 2007; 4:461–468.

109. Aasbo JD, Lawrence AT, Krishnan K, Kim MH, Trohman RG. Amiodarone prophylaxis reduces major cardiovascular morbidity and length of stay after cardiac surgery: a meta-analysis. *Annals of Internal Medicine*. 2005; 143:327–336.

110. Berger M, Schweitzer P. Timing of thromboembolic events after electrical cardioversion of atrial fibrillation or flutter: a retrospective analysis. *The American Journal of Cardiology*. 1998;82:1545–1547, A1548.

111. Freedman MD, Somberg JC. Pharmacology and pharmacokinetics of amiodarone. *Journal of Clinical Pharmacology*. 1991;31:1061–1069.

112. Wurdeman RL, Mooss AN, Mohiuddin SM, Lenz TL. Amiodarone vs. sotalol as prophylaxis against atrial fibrillation/flutter after heart surgery: a meta-analysis. *Chest*. 2002;121:1203–1210.

113. Waldo AL, Camm AJ, deRuyter H, Friedman PL, MacNeil DJ, Pauls JF, Pitt B, Pratt CM, Schwartz PJ, Veltri EP. Effect of d-sotalol on mortality in patients with left ventricular dysfunction after recent and remote myocardial infarction. The SWORD Investigators. Survival with oral d-sotalol. *Lancet*. 1996;348:7–12.

114. Howard PA. Ibutilide: an antiarrhythmic agent for the treatment of atrial fibrillation or flutter. *The Annals of Pharmacotherapy*. 1999;33:38–47.

115. Foster RH, Wilde MI, Markham A. Ibutilide. A review of its pharmacological properties and clinical potential in the acute management of atrial flutter and fibrillation. *Drugs*. 1997;54:312–330.

116. Stambler BS, Wood MA, Ellenbogen KA, Perry KT, Wakefield LK, VanderLugt JT. Efficacy and safety of repeated intravenous doses of ibutilide for rapid conversion of atrial flutter or fibrillation. Ibutilide Repeat Dose Study Investigators. *Circulation*. 1996;94:1613–1621.

117. Kowey PR, VanderLugt JT, Luderer JR. Safety and risk/benefit analysis of ibutilide for acute conversion of atrial fibrillation/flutter. *The American Journal of Cardiology*. 1996;78:46–52.

118. Cook DJ, Bailon JM, Douglas TT, Henke KD, Westberg JR, Shirk-Marienau ME, Sundt TM. Changing incidence, type, and natural history of conduction defects after coronary artery bypass grafting. *The Annals of Thoracic Surgery*. 2005;80:1732–1737.

119. Eichhorn EJ, Diehl JT, Konstam MA, Payne DD, Salem DN, Cleveland RJ. Left ventricular inotropic effect of atrial pacing after coronary artery bypass grafting. *The American Journal of Cardiology*. 1989;63:687–692.

120. Hilton JD, Weisel RD, Baird RJ, Goldman BS, Jablonsky G, Pym J, Scully HE, Ivanov J, Mickle DA, Feiglin DH, Morch JE, McLaughlin PR. The hemodynamic and metabolic response to pacing after aortocoronary bypass. *Circulation*. 1981;64:II48–53.

121. Reade MC. Temporary epicardial pacing after cardiac surgery: a practical review. Part 2: selection of epicardial pacing modes and troubleshooting. *Anaesthesia*. 2007;62:364–373.

122. Elmi F, Tullo NG, Khalighi K. Natural history and predictors of temporary epicardial pacemaker wire function in patients after open heart surgery. *Cardiology*. 2002;98:175–180.

123. Daoud EG, Dabir R, Archambeau M, Morady F, Strickberger SA. Randomized, double-blind trial of simultaneous right and left atrial epicardial pacing for prevention of post-open heart surgery atrial fibrillation. *Circulation*. 2000;102:761–765.

124. Archbold RA, Schilling RJ. Atrial pacing for the prevention of atrial fibrillation after coronary artery bypass graft surgery: a review of the literature. *Heart (British Cardiac Society)*. 2004;90:129–133.

125. Kim MH, Deeb GM, Eagle KA, Bruckman D, Pelosi F, Oral H, Sticherling C, Baker RL, Chough SP, Wasmer K, Michaud GF, Knight BP, Strickberger SA, Morady F. Complete atrioventricular block after valvular heart surgery and the timing of pacemaker implantation. *The American Journal of Cardiology*. 2001;87:649–651, A610.

126. Glikson M, Dearani JA, Hyberger LK, Schaff HV, Hammill SC, Hayes DL. Indications, effectiveness, and long-term dependency in permanent pacing after cardiac surgery. *The American Journal of Cardiology*. 1997;80:1309–1313.

127. Gordon RS, Ivanov J, Cohen G, Ralph-Edwards AL. Permanent cardiac pacing after a cardiac operation: predicting the use of permanent pacemakers. *The Annals of Thoracic Surgery*. 1998;66:1698–1704.

128. Erdogan HB, Kayalar N, Ardal H, Omeroglu SN, Kirali K, Guler M, Akinci E, Yakut C. Risk factors for requirement of permanent pacemaker implantation after aortic valve replacement. *Journal of Cardiac Surgery*. 2006;21:211–215; discussion 216–217.

129. Conlon PJ, Stafford-Smith M, White WD, Newman MF, King S, Winn MP, Landolfo K. Acute renal failure following cardiac surgery. *Nephrology Dialysis Transplantation*. 1999;14:1158–1162.

130. Andersson LG, Ekroth R, Bratteby LE, Hallhagen S, Wesslen O. Acute renal failure after coronary surgery – a study of incidence and risk factors in 2009 consecutive patients. *The Thoracic and Cardiovascular Surgeon*. 1993;41:237–241.

131. Mangano CM, Diamondstone LS, Ramsay JG, Aggarwal A, Herskowitz A, Mangano DT. Renal dysfunction after myocardial revascularization: risk factors, adverse outcomes, and hospital resource utilization. The Multicenter Study of Perioperative Ischemia Research Group. *Annals of Internal Medicine*. 1998;128:194–203.

132. Zanardo G, Michielon P, Paccagnella A, Rosi P, Calo M, Salandin V, Da Ros A, Michieletto F, Simini G. Acute renal failure in the patient undergoing cardiac operation. Prevalence, mortality rate, and main risk factors. *The Journal of Thoracic and Cardiovascular Surgery*. 1994;107:1489–1495.

133. Grayson AD, Khater M, Jackson M, Fox MA. Valvular heart operation is an independent risk factor for acute renal failure. *The Annals of Thoracic Surgery*. 2003;75:1829–1835.

134. Thakar CV, Arrigain S, Worley S, Yared JP, Paganini EP. A clinical score to predict acute renal failure after cardiac surgery. *Journal of the American Society of Nephrology*. 2005;16:162–168.

135. Myers BD, Moran SM. Hemodynamically mediated acute renal failure. *The New England Journal of Medicine*. 1986;314:97–105.

136. Rosner MH, Okusa MD. Acute kidney injury associated with cardiac surgery. *Clinical Journal of the American Society of Nephrology*. 2006;1:19–32.

137. Loef BG, Epema AH, Smilde TD, Henning RH, Ebels T, Navis G, Stegeman CA. Immediate postoperative renal function deterioration in cardiac surgical patients predicts in-hospital mortality and long-term survival. *Journal of the American Society of Nephrology*. 2005;16:195–200.

138. Lok CE, Austin PC, Wang H, Tu JV. Impact of renal insufficiency on short- and long-term outcomes after cardiac surgery. *American Heart Journal*. 2004;148:430–438.

139. Stafford-Smith M, Podgoreanu M, Swaminathan M, Phillips-Bute B, Mathew JP, Hauser EH, Winn MP, Milano C, Nielsen DM, Smith M, Morris R, Newman MF, Schwinn DA. Association of genetic polymorphisms with risk of renal injury after coronary bypass graft surgery. *American Journal of Kidney Diseases*. 2005;45:519–530.

140. Hix JK, Thakar CV, Katz EM, Yared JP, Sabik J, Paganini EP. Effect of off-pump coronary artery bypass graft surgery on postoperative acute kidney injury and mortality. *Critical Care Medicine*. 2006;34:2979–2983.

141. Salazar JD, Wityk RJ, Grega MA, Borowicz LM, Doty JR, Petrofski JA, Baumgartner WA. Stroke after cardiac surgery: short- and long-term outcomes. *The Annals of Thoracic Surgery*. 2001;72:1195–1201; discussion 1201–1192.

142. Wolman RL, Nussmeier NA, Aggarwal A, Kanchuger MS, Roach GW, Newman MF, Mangano CM, Marschall KE, Ley C, Boisvert DM, Ozanne GM, Herskowitz A, Graham SH, Mangano DT. Cerebral injury after cardiac surgery: identification of a group at extraordinary risk. Multicenter Study of Perioperative Ischemia Research Group (McSPI) and the Ischemia Research Education Foundation (IREF) Investigators. *Stroke; A Journal of Cerebral Circulation*. 1999;30:514–522.

143. Ahlgren E, Aren C. Cerebral complications after coronary artery bypass and heart valve surgery: risk factors and onset of symptoms. *Journal of Cardiothoracic and Vascular Anesthesia*. 1998;12:270–273.

144. Stolz E, Gerriets T, Kluge A, Klovekorn WP, Kaps M, Bachmann G. Diffusion-weighted magnetic resonance imaging and neurobiochemical markers after aortic valve replacement: implications for future neuroprotective trials? *Stroke; A Journal of Cerebral Circulation*. 2004;35:888–892.

145. Floyd TF, Shah PN, Price CC, Harris F, Ratcliffe SJ, Acker MA, Bavaria JE, Rahmouni H, Kuersten B, Wiegers S, McGarvey ML, Woo JY, Pochettino AA, Melhem ER. Clinically silent cerebral ischemic events after cardiac surgery: their incidence, regional vascular occurrence, and procedural dependence. *The Annals of Thoracic Surgery*. 2006;81:2160–2166.

146. Knipp SC, Matatko N, Schlamann M, Wilhelm H, Thielmann M, Forsting M, Diener HC, Jakob H. Small ischemic brain lesions after cardiac valve replacement detected by diffusion-weighted magnetic resonance imaging: relation to neurocognitive function. *European Journal of Cardiothoracic Surgery*. 2005;28:88–96.

147. Cook DJ, Huston J, 3rd, Trenerry MR, Brown RD, Jr., Zehr KJ, Sundt TM, 3rd. Postcardiac surgical cognitive impairment in the aged using diffusion-weighted magnetic resonance imaging. *The Annals of Thoracic Surgery*. 2007;83:1389–1395.

148. Newman MF, Wolman R, Kanchuger M, Marschall K, Mora-Mangano C, Roach G, Smith LR, Aggarwal A, Nussmeier N, Herskowitz A, Mangano DT. Multicenter preoperative stroke risk index for patients undergoing coronary artery bypass graft surgery. Multicenter Study of Perioperative Ischemia (McSPI) Research Group. *Circulation*. 1996;94:II74–80.

149. Roach GW, Kanchuger M, Mangano CM, Newman M, Nussmeier N, Wolman R, Aggarwal A, Marschall K, Graham SH, Ley C. Adverse cerebral outcomes after coronary bypass surgery. Multicenter Study of Perioperative Ischemia Research Group and the Ischemia Research and Education Foundation Investigators. *The New England Journal of Medicine*. 1996;335:1857–1863.

150. Mackensen GB, Ti LK, Phillips-Bute BG, Mathew JP, Newman MF, Grocott HP. Cerebral embolization during cardiac surgery: impact of aortic atheroma burden. *British Journal of Anaesthesia*. 2003;91:656–661.

151. Djaiani G, Fedorko L, Borger M, Mikulis D, Carroll J, Cheng D, Karkouti K, Beattie S, Karski J. Mild to moderate atheromatous disease of the thoracic aorta and new ischemic brain lesions after conventional coronary artery bypass graft surgery. *Stroke; A Journal of Cerebral Circulation*. 2004;35:e356–358.

152. van der Linden J, Bergman P, Hadjinikolaou L. The topography of aortic atherosclerosis enhances its precision as a predictor of stroke. *The Annals of Thoracic Surgery*. 2007;83:2087–2092.

153. Al-Ruzzeh S, Nakamura K, Athanasiou T, Modine T, George S, Yacoub M, Ilsley C, Amrani M. Does off-pump coronary artery bypass (OPCAB) surgery improve the outcome in high-risk patients? a comparative study of 1398 high-risk patients. *European Journal of Cardiothoracic Surgery*. 2003;23:50–55.

154. Demaria RG, Carrier M, Fortier S, Martineau R, Fortier A, Cartier R, Pellerin M, Hebert Y, Bouchard D, Page P, Perrault LP. Reduced mortality and strokes with off-pump coronary artery bypass grafting surgery in octogenarians. *Circulation*. 2002;106:I5–10.

155. Grocott HP, White WD, Morris RW, Podgoreanu MV, Mathew JP, Nielsen DM, Schwinn DA, Newman MF. Genetic polymorphisms and the risk of stroke after cardiac surgery. *Stroke; A Journal of Cerebral Circulation*. 2005;36: 1854–1858.

156. Phillips-Bute B, Mathew JP, Blumenthal JA, Grocott HP, Laskowitz DT, Jones RH, Mark DB, Newman MF. Association of neurocognitive function and quality of life 1 year after coronary artery bypass graft (CABG) surgery. *Psychosomatic Medicine*. 2006;68:369–375.

157. Mathew JP, Podgoreanu MV, Grocott HP, White WD, Morris RW, Stafford-Smith M, Mackensen GB, Rinder CS, Blumenthal JA, Schwinn DA, Newman MF. Genetic variants in P-selectin and C-reactive protein influence susceptibility to cognitive decline after cardiac surgery. *Journal of the American College of Cardiology*. 2007;49:1934–1942.

158. Podgoreanu MV, White WD, Morris RW, Mathew JP, Stafford-Smith M, Welsby IJ, Grocott HP, Milano CA, Newman MF, Schwinn DA. Inflammatory gene polymorphisms and risk of postoperative myocardial infarction after cardiac surgery. *Circulation*. 2006;114:I275–281.

159. Boodhwani M, Rubens FD, Wozny D, Rodriguez R, Alsefaou A, Hendry PJ, Nathan HJ. Predictors of early neurocognitive deficits in low-risk patients undergoing on-pump coronary artery bypass surgery. *Circulation*. 2006; 114:I461–466.

160. Ho PM, Arciniegas DB, Grigsby J, McCarthy M, Jr., McDonald GO, Moritz TE, Shroyer AL, Sethi GK, Henderson WG, London MJ, VillaNueva CB, Grover FL, Hammermeister KE. Predictors of cognitive decline following coronary artery bypass graft surgery. *The Annals of Thoracic Surgery*. 2004;77:597–603; discussion 603.

161. Newman MF, Kirchner JL, Phillips-Bute B, Gaver V, Grocott H, Jones RH, Mark DB, Reves JG, Blumenthal JA. Longitudinal assessment of neurocognitive function after coronary-artery bypass surgery. *The New England Journal of Medicine*. 2001;344:395–402.

162. Bar-Yosef S, Anders M, Mackensen GB, Ti LK, Mathew JP, Phillips-Bute B, Messier RH, Grocott HP. Aortic atheroma burden and cognitive dysfunction after coronary artery bypass graft surgery. *The Annals of Thoracic Surgery*. 2004;78:1556–1562.

163. van Dijk D, Spoor M, Hijman R, Nathoe HM, Borst C, Jansen EW, Grobbee DE, de Jaegere PP, Kalkman CJ. Cognitive and cardiac outcomes 5 years after off-pump vs on-pump coronary artery bypass graft surgery. *JAMA*. 2007;297:701–708.

164. Nashef SA, Roques F, Michel P, Gauducheau E, Lemeshow S, Salamon R. European system for cardiac operative risk evaluation (EuroSCORE). *European Journal of Cardiothoracic Surgery*. 1999;16:9–13.

165. Roques F, Nashef SA, Michel P, Gauducheau E, de Vincentiis C, Baudet E, Cortina J, David M, Faichney A, Gabrielle F, Gams E, Harjula A, Jones MT, Pintor PP, Salamon R, Thulin L. Risk factors and outcome in European cardiac surgery: analysis of the EuroSCORE multinational database of 19030 patients. *European Journal of Cardiothoracic Surgery*. 1999;15:816–822; discussion 822–813.

166. Christenson JT, Aeberhard JM, Badel P, Pepcak F, Maurice J, Simonet F, Velebit V, Schmuziger M. Adult respiratory distress syndrome after cardiac surgery. *Cardiovascular Surgery (London, England)*. 1996;4:15–21.

167. Kaul TK, Fields BL, Riggins LS, Wyatt DA, Jones CR, Nagle D. Adult respiratory distress syndrome following cardiopulmonary bypass: incidence, prophylaxis and management. *The Journal of Cardiovascular Surgery*. 1998; 39:777–781.

168. Messent M, Sullivan K, Keogh BF, Morgan CJ, Evans TW. Adult respiratory distress syndrome following cardiopulmonary bypass: incidence and prediction. *Anaesthesia*. 1992;47:267–268.

169. Milot J, Perron J, Lacasse Y, Letourneau L, Cartier PC, Maltais F. Incidence and predictors of ARDS after cardiac surgery. *Chest*. 2001;119:884–888.

170. Laub GW, Muralidharan S, Chen C, Perritt A, Adkins M, Pollock S, Bailey B, McGrath LB. Phrenic nerve injury. A prospective study. *Chest*. 1991;100:376–379.

171. Dimopoulou I, Daganou M, Dafni U, Karakatsani A, Khoury M, Geroulanos S, Jordanoglou J. Phrenic nerve dysfunction after cardiac operations: electrophysiologic evaluation of risk factors. *Chest*. 1998;113:8–14.

172. Wheeler WE, Rubis LJ, Jones CW, Harrah JD. Etiology and prevention of topical cardiac hypothermia-induced phrenic nerve injury and left lower lobe atelectasis during cardiac surgery. *Chest*. 1985;88:680–683.

173. O'Brien JW, Johnson SH, VanSteyn SJ, Craig DM, Sharpe RE, Mauney MC, Smith PK. Effects of internal mammary artery dissection on phrenic nerve perfusion and function. *The Annals of Thoracic Surgery*. 1991;52:182–188.

174. Cohen A, Katz M, Katz R, Hauptman E, Schachner A. Chronic obstructive pulmonary disease in patients undergoing coronary artery bypass grafting. *The Journal of Thoracic and Cardiovascular Surgery*. 1995;109:574–581.

175. Cohen AJ, Katz MG, Katz R, Mayerfeld D, Hauptman E, Schachner A. Phrenic nerve injury after coronary artery grafting: is it always benign? *The Annals of Thoracic Surgery.* 1997;64:148–153.

176. Katz MG, Katz R, Schachner A, Cohen AJ. Phrenic nerve injury after coronary artery bypass grafting: will it go away? *The Annals of Thoracic Surgery.* 1998;65:32–35.

177. Hashimoto M, Aoki M, Okawa Y, Baba H, Nishimura Y. Massive pulmonary embolism after off-pump coronary artery bypass surgery. *Japanese Journal of Thoracic and Cardiovascular Surgery.* 2006;54:486–489.

178. Shammas NW. Pulmonary embolus after coronary artery bypass surgery: a review of the literature. *Clinical Cardiology.* 2000;23:637–644.

179. Goldhaber SZ, Hirsch DR, MacDougall RC, Polak JF, Creager MA, Cohn LH. Prevention of venous thrombosis after coronary artery bypass surgery (a randomized trial comparing two mechanical prophylaxis strategies). *The American Journal of Cardiology.* 1995;76:993–996.

180. Reis SE, Polak JF, Hirsch DR, Cohn LH, Creager MA, Donovan BC, Goldhaber SZ. Frequency of deep venous thrombosis in asymptomatic patients with coronary artery bypass grafts. *American Heart Journal.* 1991;122:478–482.

181. Ambrosetti M, Salerno M, Zambelli M, Mastropasqua F, Tramarin R, Pedretti RF. Deep vein thrombosis among patients entering cardiac rehabilitation after coronary artery bypass surgery. *Chest.* 2004;125:191–196.

182. Charalambous CP, Zipitis CS, Keenan DJ. Chest reexploration in the intensive care unit after cardiac surgery: a safe alternative to returning to the operating theater. *The Annals of Thoracic Surgery.* 2006;81:191–194.

183. Dacey LJ, Munoz JJ, Baribeau YR, Johnson ER, Lahey SJ, Leavitt BJ, Quinn RD, Nugent WC, Birkmeyer JD, O'Connor GT. Reexploration for hemorrhage following coronary artery bypass grafting: incidence and risk factors. Northern New England Cardiovascular Disease Study Group. *Archives of Surgery.* 1998;133:442–447.

184. Ferraris VA, Ferraris SP, Saha SP, Hessel EA, 2nd, Haan CK, Royston BD, Bridges CR, Higgins RS, Despotis G, Brown JR, Spiess BD, Shore-Lesserson L, Stafford-Smith M, Mazer CD, Bennett-Guerrero E, Hill SE, Body S. Perioperative blood transfusion and blood conservation in cardiac surgery: the Society of Thoracic Surgeons and The Society of Cardiovascular Anesthesiologists clinical practice guideline. *The Annals of Thoracic Surgery.* 2007;83:S27–86.

185. Kuitunen A, Suojaranta-Ylinen R, Raivio P, Kukkonen S, Lassila R. Heparin-induced thrombocytopenia following cardiac surgery is associated with poor outcome. *Journal of Cardiothoracic and Vascular Anesthesia.* 2007;21:18–22.

186. Warkentin TE, Greinacher A. Heparin-induced thrombocytopenia and cardiac surgery. *The Annals of Thoracic Surgery.* 2003;76:2121–2131.

187. Bauer TL, Arepally G, Konkle BA, Mestichelli B, Shapiro SS, Cines DB, Poncz M, McNulty S, Amiral J, Hauck WW, Edie RN, Mannion JD. Prevalence of heparin-associated antibodies without thrombosis in patients undergoing cardiopulmonary bypass surgery. *Circulation.* 1997;95:1242–1246.

188. Bennett-Guerrero E, Slaughter TF, White WD, Welsby IJ, Greenberg CS, El-Moalem H, Ortel TL. Preoperative anti-PF4/heparin antibody level predicts adverse outcome after cardiac surgery. *The Journal of Thoracic and Cardiovascular Surgery.* 2005;130:1567–1572.

189. Kress DC, Aronson S, McDonald ML, Malik MI, Divgi AB, Tector AJ, Downey FX, 3rd, Anderson AJ, Stone M, Clancy C. Positive heparin-platelet factor 4 antibody complex and cardiac surgical outcomes. *The Annals of Thoracic Surgery.* 2007;83:1737–1743.

190. Trossaert M, Gaillard A, Commin PL, Amiral J, Vissac AM, Fressinaud E. High incidence of anti-heparin/platelet factor 4 antibodies after cardiopulmonary bypass surgery. *British Journal of Haematology.* 1998;101:653–655.

191. Warkentin TE, Sheppard JA, Horsewood P, Simpson PJ, Moore JC, Kelton JG. Impact of the patient population on the risk for heparin-induced thrombocytopenia. *Blood.* 2000;96:1703–1708.

192. Walls JT, Curtis JJ, Silver D, Boley TM, Schmaltz RA, Nawarawong W. Heparin-induced thrombocytopenia in open heart surgical patients: sequelae of late recognition. *The Annals of Thoracic Surgery.* 1992;53:787–791.

193. Kerendi F, Thourani VH, Puskas JD, Kilgo PD, Osgood M, Guyton RA, Lattouf OM. Impact of heparin-induced thrombocytopenia on postoperative outcomes after cardiac surgery. *The Annals of Thoracic Surgery.* 2007;84:1548–1553; discussion 1554–1545.

194. Glock Y, Szmil E, Boudjema B, Boccalon H, Fournial G, Cerene AL, Puel P. Cardiovascular surgery and heparin induced thrombocytopenia. *International Angiology.* 1988;7:238–245.

195. Walls JT, Boley TM, Curtis JJ, Silver D. Heparin induced thrombocytopenia in patients undergoing intra-aortic balloon pumping after open heart surgery. *ASAIO Journal.* 1992;38:M574–576.

196. Loop FD, Lytle BW, Cosgrove DM, Mahfood S, McHenry MC, Goormastic M, Stewart RW, Golding LA, Taylor PC. J. Maxwell Chamberlain memorial paper. Sternal wound complications after isolated coronary artery bypass grafting: early and late mortality, morbidity, and cost of care. *The Annals of Thoracic Surgery.* 1990;49:179–186; discussion 186–177.

197. Ridderstolpe L, Gill H, Granfeldt H, Ahlfeldt H, Rutberg H. Superficial and deep sternal wound complications: incidence, risk factors and mortality. *European Journal of Cardiothoracic Surgery.* 2001;20:1168–1175.

198. Baskett RJ, MacDougall CE, Ross DB. Is mediastinitis a preventable complication? A 10-year review. *The Annals of Thoracic Surgery.* 1999;67:462–465.

199. Bitkover CY, Gardlund B. Mediastinitis after cardiovascular operations: a case-control study of risk factors. *The Annals of Thoracic Surgery*. 1998;65:36–40.
200. The Parisian Mediastinitis Study Group. Risk factors for deep sternal wound infection after sternotomy: a prospective, multicenter study. *The Journal of Thoracic and Cardiovascular Surgery*. 1996;111:1200–1207.
201. Borger MA, Rao V, Weisel RD, Ivanov J, Cohen G, Scully HE, David TE. Deep sternal wound infection: risk factors and outcomes. *The Annals of Thoracic Surgery*. 1998;65:1050–1056.
202. L'Ecuyer PB, Murphy D, Little JR, Fraser VJ. The epidemiology of chest and leg wound infections following cardio-thoracic surgery. *Clinical Infectious Diseases*. 1996;22:424–429.
203. Ottino G, De Paulis R, Pansini S, Rocca G, Tallone MV, Comoglio C, Costa P, Orzan F, Morea M. Major sternal wound infection after open-heart surgery: a multivariate analysis of risk factors in 2,579 consecutive operative procedures. *The Annals of Thoracic Surgery*. 1987;44:173–179.
204. Zacharias A, Habib RH. Factors predisposing to median sternotomy complications. Deep vs superficial infection. *Chest*. 1996;110:1173–1178.
205. Liu J, Sidiropoulos A, Konertz W. Minimally invasive aortic valve replacement (AVR) compared to standard AVR. *European Journal of Cardiothoracic Surgery*. 1999;16 Suppl 2:S80–83.
206. Grossi EA, Galloway AC, Ribakove GH, Buttenheim PM, Esposito R, Baumann FG, Colvin SB. Minimally invasive port access surgery reduces operative morbidity for valve replacement in the elderly. *The Heart Surgery Forum*. 1999;2:212–215.
207. Gummert JF, Barten MJ, Hans C, Kluge M, Doll N, Walther T, Hentschel B, Schmitt DV, Mohr FW, Diegeler A. Mediastinitis and cardiac surgery – an updated risk factor analysis in 10,373 consecutive adult patients. *The Thoracic and Cardiovascular Surgeon*. 2002;50:87–91.
208. Schroeyers P, Wellens F, De Geest R, Degrieck I, Van Praet F, Vermeulen Y, Vanermen H. Minimally invasive video-assisted mitral valve surgery: our lessons after a 4-year experience. *The Annals of Thoracic Surgery*. 2001;72:S1050–1054.
209. Shrestha NK, Banbury MK, Weber M, Cwynar RE, Lober C, Procop GW, Karafa MT, Gordon SM. Safety of targeted perioperative mupirocin treatment for preventing infections after cardiac surgery. *The Annals of Thoracic Surgery*. 2006;81:2183–2188.
210. Olsson C, Tammelin A, Thelin S. Staphylococcus aureus bloodstream infection after cardiac surgery: risk factors and outcome. *Infection Control and Hospital Epidemiology*. 2006;27:83–85.
211. El-Ahdab F, Benjamin DK, Jr., Wang A, Cabell CH, Chu VH, Stryjewski ME, Corey GR, Sexton DJ, Reller LB, Fowler VG, Jr. Risk of endocarditis among patients with prosthetic valves and Staphylococcus aureus bacteremia. *The American Journal of Medicine*. 2005;118:225–229.
212. Fang G, Keys TF, Gentry LO, Harris AA, Rivera N, Getz K, Fuchs PC, Gustafson M, Wong ES, Goetz A, Wagener MM, Yu VL. Prosthetic valve endocarditis resulting from nosocomial bacteremia. A prospective, multicenter study. *Annals of Internal Medicine*. 1993;119:560–567.
213. Edwards MB, Ratnatunga CP, Dore CJ, Taylor KM. Thirty-day mortality and long-term survival following surgery for prosthetic endocarditis: a study from the UK heart valve registry. *European Journal of Cardiothoracic Surgery*. 1998;14:156–164.
214. Wang A, Athan E, Pappas PA, Fowler VG, Jr., Olaison L, Pare C, Almirante B, Munoz P, Rizzi M, Naber C, Logar M, Tattevin P, Iarussi DL, Selton-Suty C, Jones SB, Casabe J, Morris A, Corey GR, Cabell CH. Contemporary clinical profile and outcome of prosthetic valve endocarditis. *JAMA*. 2007;297:1354–1361.
215. Akowuah EF, Davies W, Oliver S, Stephens J, Riaz I, Zadik P, Cooper G. Prosthetic valve endocarditis: early and late outcome following medical or surgical treatment. *Heart (British Cardiac Society)*. 2003;89:269–272.

20 Prosthetic Valve Dysfunction

Philippe Pibarot, Jean G. Dumesnil, and Julien Magne

CONTENTS

INTRODUCTION

Approximately 85,000 valve substitutes are implanted in the United States and 275,000 world-wide each year, of which approximately half are mechanical valves and half are bioprosthetic valves. Despite the marked improvements in prosthetic valve design and surgical procedures over the past decades, valve replacement is not a panacea for the patient. Instead, native valve disease is traded for prosthetic valve disease and the outcome of patients undergoing valve replacement is indeed affected by prosthetic valve hemodynamics, durability, and thrombogenicity. Valve-related problems necessitate reoperation or cause death in approximately 50–60% of patients within 10 years after prosthetic valve implantation. This rate is similar for mechanical and bioprosthetic valves. However, the nature and time-related frequency of the specific valve-related complications vary with the type of prosthesis. Mechanical valves have a substantial risk of thromboemboli and thrombotic obstruction and they therefore require chronic anticoagulation therapy, which is in turn associated with an increased risk of hemorrhagic complications. Nonetheless, contemporary mechanical valves have an excellent durability. In contrast, bioprosthetic valves have a low risk of thromboembolism without anticoagulation. However, their durability is limited by calcific or non-calcific tissue deterioration. The purpose of this chapter is to provide an overview of the evaluation, mechanisms, prevention, and treatment of prosthetic valve dysfunction (Table 1).

From: *Contemporary Cardiology: Valvular Heart Disease*
Edited by: Andrew Wang, Thomas M. Bashore, DOI 10.1007/978-1-59745-411-7_20
© Humana Press, a part of Springer Science+Business Media, LLC 2009

Table 1
Prosthetic Valve Dysfunction

Prosthesis–patient mismatch
Prosthetic valve stenosis
    Valve thrombosis or pannus (mechanical valves)
    Mechanical failure (mechanical valves, rare)
    Leaflet calcification or pannus (tissue valves)

Prosthetic valve regurgitation
    Paravalvular regurgitation
    Valve dehiscence
    Transvalvular regurgitation
        Valve thrombosis or pannus (mechanical valves)
        Leaflet tear or perforation (tissue valves)

Thromboembolic complications

Prosthetic valve endocarditis
    Vegetations
    Paravalvular abscess

Hemolytic anemia

PROSTHETIC VALVE DESIGN

The ideal valve substitute should mimic the characteristics of a normal native valve. In particular, it should have excellent hemodynamics, long durability, high thromboresistance, and excellent implantability. Unfortunately, this ideal valve substitute does not exist and each of the currently available prosthetic valves has inherent limitations.

Mechanical Valves

There are three basic types of mechanical valve design: bileaflet, monoleaflet, and ball-cage valves. The ball-cage valves, which consist of a silastic ball with a circular sewing ring and a cage formed by three metal arches, are no longer in use.

MONOLEAFLET VALVES

The monoleaflet or tilting disk valves are composed of a single circular disk within a rigid annulus, with the disk secured by lateral or central metal struts. The opening angle of the disk relative to valve annulus ranges from 60° to 80° resulting in two orifices: one major semi-circular orifice and one minor orifice consisting of two jets separated by a well-defined wake behind the tilted disk *(1)*. The available monoleaflet valves include the Medtronic Hall and Omniscience valves. The Bjork–Shiley is no longer available on the market.

BILEAFLET VALVES

The bileaflet valves are made of two pyrolytic carbon semi-lunar disks attached to a rigid valve ring by small hinges. The opening angle of the leaflets relative to the annulus plane ranges from 75° to 90°, with the open valve consisting of three orifices: a small, slit-like central orifice between the two open leaflets, and two larger semi-circular orifices, laterally *(1)*. The available bileaflet valves include the St. Jude Medical, Carbomedics, On-X, Advantage, ATS, and Mira valves.

Tissue Valves

STENTED BIOPROSTHESES

The traditional design of a bioprosthetic valve consists of three cusps that open to a circular orifice during systole, resembling the anatomy of the native aortic valve. Most commercially produced porcine bioprosthetic valves consist of a whole porcine aortic valve, crosslinked with glutaraldehyde and mounted on a metallic or polymer-supporting stent. The bovine pericardial valves are fabricated from flat sheets of bovine pericardium mounted inside or outside of the stent. Like the porcine valve tissue, the bovine pericardium must also be crosslinked in glutaraldehyde to reduce its antigenicity and stabilize it chemically. The available stented bioprostheses are Carpentier–Edwards Perimount, Epic, Hancock II, Magna, Mitroflow, and Mosaic.

STENTLESS BIOPROSTHESES

In an effort to improve valve hemodynamics and durability while retaining the advantages of a bioprosthetic valve, several types of stentless bioprosthetic valves have been developed. Stentless bioprostheses are manufactured from intact porcine aortic valves or are fabricated from bovine pericardium. These valves may be implanted in the subcoronary position, as an inclusion cylinder, a miniroot or a total root replacement. The available stentless bioprostheses are Freestyle, Toronto SPV, and Prima-Edwards.

EVALUATION OF PROSTHETIC VALVE FUNCTION

Echocardiography is the method of choice to evaluate prosthetic valve function. This evaluation follows the same principles used for the evaluation of native valves with some important caveats. First, imaging of the valve occluder and of transprosthetic flow is limited by reverberations and shadowing caused by the valve components. Second, the fluid dynamics of the mechanical valves may differ substantially from that of the native valve. The flow is eccentric in monoleaflet valves and it is composed of three separate jets in the bileaflet valves with the flow velocity being potentially higher in the central orifice jet than in the two lateral orifice jets. A complete echocardiography includes two-dimensional imaging of the prosthetic valve, measurement of the transprosthetic gradients and EOA, estimation of the degree of regurgitation, evaluation of left ventricular size and systolic function, and calculation of systolic pulmonary arterial pressure.

When measuring the EOA of prosthetic valves, a few specific caveats should be taken into consideration. For aortic prostheses, one should use the standard continuity equation. The substitution of the LV outflow tract (LVOT) diameter for the label prosthesis size in the continuity equation is not a valid method to determine the EOA of aortic prostheses *(2)*. For mitral prostheses, the EOA is calculated by the continuity equation using the stroke volume measured in the LVOT. This method cannot be used in presence of >mild (2+) aortic or mitral regurgitation. It is also important to emphasize that the pressure half time is not valid to estimate the valve EOA of mitral prostheses *(3)*.

Mechanical prostheses have a normal regurgitant volume known as leakage backflow. This "built-in" regurgitation theoretically prevents blood stasis and thrombus formation by a washing mechanism. As opposed to the pathologic regurgitant jets, the normal leakage backflow jets are characterized by being short in duration, narrow, and symmetrical. A small degree of central regurgitation is also often observed in bioprosthetic valves, and more frequently in bovine pericardial valves. In this context, it should be emphasized that echocardiography is a very sensitive technique and will detect even minute amounts of regurgitation.

PROSTHESIS–PATIENT MISMATCH

Definition and Prevalence

The term of valve prosthesis–patient mismatch (PPM) was first proposed in 1978 by Rahimtoola *(4)*. PPM occurs when the EOA of the prosthesis is too small in relation to the patient's body size resulting in abnormally high postoperative gradient and the parameter that is generally used to identify PPM is thus the EOA of the prosthesis indexed for patient's body surface area *(3, 5, 6)*. The rationale behind the normalization of the EOA for body surface area is to account for cardiac output requirements since transvalvular pressure gradients are essentially determined by the EOA and transvalvular flow, which in turn is largely determined by body size. An indexed EOA ≤ 0.85 cm^2/m^2 is generally considered as the threshold for PPM in the aortic position *(7)*. However, it should be pointed out that this definition corresponds to moderate PPM. Severe PPM is considered present when the indexed EOA is ≤ 0.65 cm^2/m^2, whereas PPM is considered not clinically significant when the indexed EOA is >0.85 cm^2/m^2. Moderate PPM may be quite frequent (20–70%) in patients undergoing aortic valve replacement, whereas the prevalence of severe PPM ranges from 2 to 11% depending on the series *(6, 7)*.

Because of the lower pressure regimen, the threshold values for mitral PPM are higher than for aortic PPM. Mitral PPM is considered moderate when the indexed EOA is ≤ 1.2–1.3 cm^2/m^2 and severe when it is ≤ 0.9–1.0 cm^2/m^2 *(3, 8, 9)*. Recent studies report that the incidence of mitral PPM is much higher than previously believed: 30–70% and 5–10% for moderate and severe PPM, respectively *(8, 9)*.

The utilization of the body surface area for the normalization of EOA may potentially overestimate the degree of PPM in obese patients. Future studies are necessary to determine if the indexation of EOA cannot be improved or refined in the case of obese patients.

Clinical Impact

AORTIC PROSTHESIS–PATIENT MISMATCH

There is now a strong body of evidence showing that aortic PPM is an important risk factor with regards to clinical outcomes *(6)*. Indeed, PPM is associated with less improvement in symptoms and functional class *(10)*, lesser regression of left ventricular hypertrophy *(11)*, less improvement in coronary flow reserve *(12)*, and more adverse cardiac events *(10, 13, 14)* after aortic valve replacement (AVR). Moreover, PPM has a significant impact on both short-term *(15)* and long-term mortalities *(14, 16–18)* particularly if LV dysfunction is present. Recent studies have reported a strong interaction between PPM and depressed LV function with regard to occurrence of heart failure as well as to early and late mortality after AVR *(15, 19)*. These findings are consistent with the fact that an increased hemodynamic burden is less well tolerated by a poorly functioning ventricle than by a normal ventricle. Hence, every effort should be made to avoid PPM in the high-risk patients with depressed LV function because these are probably the patients who are the most vulnerable to PPM. Recent studies also reported that the impact of PPM is more pronounced in young patients than in older ones *(20, 21)*. This finding might be related to the fact that younger patients have higher cardiac output requirements and that they are exposed to the risk of PPM for a longer period of time.

MITRAL PROSTHESIS–PATIENT MISMATCH

For a long time, mitral PPM remained quite unexplored and might have been thought to be a relatively rare phenomenon with minimal impact on postoperative outcomes. However, recent studies demonstrate that this is not the case and that mitral PPM is not uncommon and is independently associated with worse hemodynamic and clinical outcomes following mitral valve replacement (MVR) *(8, 9)*. PPM has been shown to be associated with persisting pulmonary hypertension, increased incidence of congestive heart failure, and reduced survival after MVR *(8, 9)*.

Diagnosis

Given that PPM is the most frequent cause of high transprosthetic gradient following aortic valve replacement and mitral valve replacement (MVR), it is important to properly identify this abnormality and to quantify its severity. In particular, a comprehensive algorithm can be used to differentiate PPM from intrinsic prosthetic valve stenosis *(see* Diagnosis in Section Prosthetic Valve Stenosis*)*. This distinction is crucial given that the clinical management of these two conditions is different.

Clinical Management and Prevention

Reoperation may be indicated in the presence of severe PPM if the patient is symptomatic and/or if there is evidence of deteriorating LV systolic dysfunction or pulmonary hypertension that cannot be related to other causes. Asymptomatic patients with PPM should be managed conservatively and followed closely by Doppler echocardiography. Since PPM is a modifiable risk factor, the best way to avoid the PPM-related risk of reoperation is preferably to avoid this problem at the first operation.

PREVENTION OF AORTIC PROSTHESIS–PATIENT MISMATCH

Previous studies demonstrated that the risk of PPM can be predicted at the time of aortic valve replacement with the use of the "projected" indexed EOA that is derived from the normal reference values of EOA provided in the literature for different types and sizes of prostheses *(6, 22)* (Tables 2 and 3). Some studies have also provided robust evidence that the prevention of aortic PPM is feasible *(22, 23)*. Hence, it would appear that there is a significant advantage to systematically calculate the projected indexed EOA of the prosthesis to be inserted and in the case of anticipated PPM, to consider alternate procedures such as insertion of a better performing valve substitute (e.g., newer generation of supra-annular bioprostheses or mechanical valves, stentless bioprostheses, homografts) or insertion of a larger prosthesis by means of aortic root enlargement. The information of the projected indexed EOA can easily be incorporated within the clinical decision making process and utilized in view of the other pertinent clinical factors such as age, level of physical activity, status of LV function, and concomitant procedures. For instance, if one projects moderate PPM in an elderly sedentary patient with normal LV function, it might be estimated that the benefits of doing an alternate procedure to avoid PPM are outweighed by the inherent risks or disadvantages of doing such a procedure. On the other hand, the prevention of PPM becomes an important consideration in a young athletic patient and/or if there is evidence of impaired LV function.

PREVENTION OF MITRAL PROSTHESIS–PATIENT MISMATCH

The prevention of PPM in the mitral position represents a much greater challenge than in the aortic position. Indeed, mitral valve surgery does not allow annular enlargement and the implantation of a

Table 2
Normal Reference Values of Effective Orifice Areas for the Aortic Prostheses

Prosthetic valve size (mm)	19	21	23	25	27	29	References
Stented bioprosthetic valves							
Mosaic	1.1 ± 0.2	1.2 ± 0.3	1.4 ± 0.3	1.7 ± 0.4	1.8 ± 0.4	2.0 ± 0.4	(7)
Hancock II	–	1.2 ± 0.1	1.3 ± 0.2	1.5 ± 0.2	1.6 ± 0.2	1.6 ± 0.2	(7)
Carpentier–Edwards Perimount	1.1 ± 0.3	1.3 ± 0.4	1.50 ± 0.4	1.80 ± 0.4	2.1 ± 0.4	2.2 ± 0.4	(7)
*Carpentier–Edwards Magna	1.3 ± 0.3	1.7 ± 0.3	2.1 ± 0.4	2.3 ± 0.5	–	–	(64, 65)
*Biocor (Epic)	–	1.3 ± 0.3	1.6 ± 0.3	1.8 ± 0.4	–	–	(66)
*Mitroflow	1.1 ± 0.1	1.3 ± 0.1	1.5 ± 0.2	1.8 ± 0.2	–	–	(67)
Stentless bioprosthetic valves							
Medtronic Freestyle	1.2 ± 0.2	1.4 ± 0.2	1.5 ± 0.3	2.0 ± 0.4	2.3 ± 0.5	–	(7)
St. Jude Medical Toronto SPV	–	1.3 ± 0.3	1.5 ± 0.5	1.7 ± 0.8	2.1 ± 0.7	2.7 ± 1.0	(7)
Prima Edwards	–	1.3 ± 0.3	1.6 ± 0.3	1.9 ± 0.4	–	–	(68, 69)
Cryolife O'Brien	–	1.2 ± 0.3	1.6 ± 0.4	1.9 ± 0.4	2.0 ± 0.2	2.2 ± 0.5	(70)
Mechanical valves							(7)
Medtronic-Hall	1.2 ± 0.2	1.3 ± 0.2	–	–	–	–	(7)
Medtronic Advantage	–	1.7 ± 0.2	2.2 ± 0.3	2.8 ± 0.6	3.3 ± 0.7	3.9 ± 0.7	(71)
St. Jude Medical Standard	1.0 ± 0.2	1.4 ± 0.2	1.5 ± 0.5	2.1 ± 0.4	2.7 ± 0.6	3.2 ± 0.3	(7)
St. Jude Medical Regent	1.6 ± 0.4	2.0 ± 0.7	2.2 ± 0.9	2.5 ± 0.9	3.6 ± 1.3	4.4 ± 0.6	(72)
MCRI On-X	1.5 ± 0.2	1.7 ± 0.4	2.0 ± 0.6	2.4 ± 0.8	3.2 ± 0.6	3.2 ± 0.6	(73)
Carbomedics Standard	1.0 ± 0.4	1.5 ± 0.3	1.7 ± 0.3	2.0 ± 0.4	2.5 ± 0.4	2.6 ± 0.4	(7)

Effective orifice area is expressed as mean values available in the literature. *These results are based on a limited number of patients and should thus be interpreted with caution. Further studies are needed to validate these reference values.

Adapted with permission of American Heart Association from (63).

homograft or a stentless prosthesis is technically more demanding and associated with poor long-term durability. Hence, the only alternative at present is the implantation of a prosthesis having a larger EOA for a given annulus size, which unfortunately may not be sufficient to completely avoid PPM in some cases.

PROSTHETIC VALVE STENOSIS

Prevalence and Etiology

Prosthetic valve stenosis is most often encountered with bioprosthetic valves that have been implanted for several years. The degree of bioprosthetic valve calcification increases noticeably after 6 years of implantation and leads to the progressive thickening and stiffening of the valve leaflets.

Table 3
Normal Reference Values of Effective Orifice Areas for the Mitral Prostheses

Prosthetic valve size (mm)	25	27	29	31	33	References
Stented bioprosthetic valves						
Medtronic Mosaic	1.5 ± 0.4	1.7 ± 0.5	1.9 ± 0.5	1.9 ± 0.5	–	(8, 74)
Hancock II	1.5 ± 0.4	1.8 ± 0.5	1.9 ± 0.5	2.6 ± 0.5	2.6 ± 0.7	(9)
*Carpentier–Edwards Perimount	1.6 ± 0.4	1.8 ± 0.4	2.1 ± 0.5	–	–	(8)
Mechanical valves						
St. Jude Medical Standard	1.5 ± 0.3	1.7 ± 0.4	1.8 ± 0.4	2.0 ± 0.5	2.0 ± 0.5	(8)
†MCRI On-X	2.2 ± 0.9	2.2 ± 0.9	2.2 ± 0.9	2.2 ± 0.9	2.2 ± 0.9	(8,73)

Effective orifice area is expressed as mean values available in the literature. *These results are based on a limited number of patients and should thus be interpreted with caution. Further studies are needed to validate these reference values. †The On-X valve has just one size for 27–29 and 31–33 mm prostheses. In addition, the strut and leaflets are identical for all sizes (25–33-mm); only the size of the sewing cuff is different.

Adapted with permission of American Heart Association from (63).

Stenosis of mechanical prostheses may be caused by restriction of occluder motion by thrombus or pannus formation or by narrowed annular area due to pannus ingrowth.

Diagnosis

Doppler echocardiography is the technique of choice to assess prosthetic valve dysfunction. Cinefluoroscopy and computed tomography may also provide important complementary information. The presence of increased mean gradient (>15–20 mmHg for the aortic prostheses and >5–7 mmHg for mitral prostheses) should prompt further evaluation. In particular, it is important to determine if the elevated gradient is due to an intrinsic stenosis of the prosthesis or to PPM. A simple algorithm may be used for this purpose and this algorithm is different depending on whether the evaluation takes place in the intraoperative/early postoperative period or in the late postoperative period.

INTERPRETATION OF HIGH GRADIENT IN THE INTRAOPERATIVE/EARLY POSTOPERATIVE PERIOD

The recording of relatively high transprosthetic gradients in the intraoperative or immediate postoperative period should not be viewed with undue concern. A simple algorithm may be used to assess abnormally high gradients in the intraoperative or early postoperative period (Fig. 1). Given that PPM is the most frequent cause of high gradients, the first step of this algorithm is thus to determine if PPM is present by calculating the projected indexed EOA. It should indeed be noted that the Doppler echocardiographic measurement of LVOT stroke volume and thus of valve EOA in the intraoperative/early postoperative period is often not feasible and/or reliable. The projected indexed EOA is simply calculated by dividing the normal reference EOA for the model and size of prosthesis implanted (*see* Tables 2 and 3) by the patient's body surface area. If the projected indexed EOA is ≤0.85 cm^2/m^2 in the aortic position or ≤1.2 cm^2/m^2 in the mitral position, the abnormally high gradient is likely due to PPM. If, on the other hand, the projected indexed EOA is >0.85 or 1.2 cm^2/m^2, several conditions and technical pitfalls must first be ruled out before concluding to

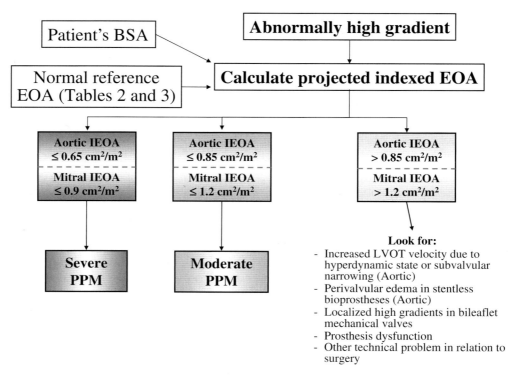

Fig. 1. Interpretation of high transprosthetic gradient in the intraoperative or early postoperative period.

prosthesis dysfunction. One must first determine if the gradient is not partially or principally related to a high flow velocity in the LVOT. In particular, relief of the valvular obstruction in patients operated for aortic stenosis may result in some remodeling and temporary narrowing of the LVOT. The administration of inotropic agents upon coming off cardiopulmonary bypass may also contribute to this phenomenon.

INTERPRETATION OF HIGH GRADIENT IN THE LATE POSTOPERATIVE PERIOD

A more comprehensive algorithm may be used for evaluating abnormally high gradients in the late postoperative period *(6)* (Fig. 2). However, this algorithm should be used only when the hemodynamic condition has settled down and there is, in particular, no high cardiac output state or an abnormally high velocity in the LVOT. The first step is then to compare the measured EOA to the normal reference value of EOA *(see* Tables 2 and 3) for the type and size of prosthesis that has been implanted in the patient (Fig. 2). If the EOA is comparable to its normal reference value, the next step is then to calculate the indexed EOA in order to determine the presence and severity of PPM.

If, on the other hand, the measured EOA is much lower than the normal reference value and, moreover, has decreased over time during follow-up, the diagnosis of prosthetic stenosis should be raised. Causes of such dysfunction include the presence of leaflet calcific degeneration, thrombosis, pannus, or endocarditis. The visualization of an asymmetric transprosthetic jet on Color Doppler and of a restricted leaflet on transthoracic echocardiography (TTE), transesophageal echocardiography (TEE), or cinefluoroscopy (Figs. 4A,B) may help to confirm the presence of dysfunction in mechanical valves. It is also important to keep in mind that both phenomena, i.e., PPM and prosthetic valve stenosis, may often coexist.

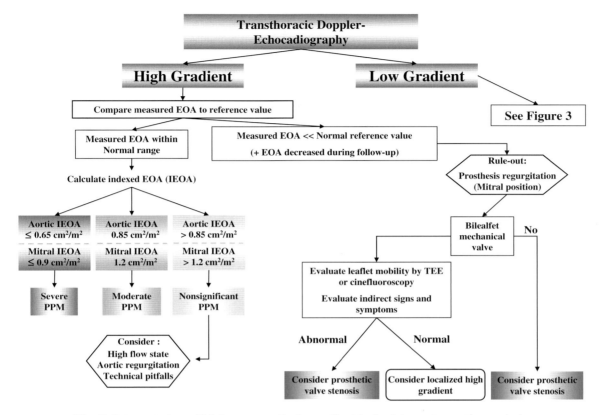

Fig. 2. Interpretation of high transprosthetic gradient in the late postoperative period.

Occasionally, an abnormally high jet velocity corresponding to a localized gradient may be recorded by continuous wave Doppler interrogation through the smaller central slit-like orifice of bileaflet mechanical prosthesis. This phenomenon yields to the measurement of abnormally high gradient and low EOA, thus mimicking the presence of an intrinsic prosthesis dysfunction. The distinction between localized high gradient and prosthetic valve stenosis may be difficult. One should look for other direct (e.g., restricted leaflet motion on TEE or cinefluoroscopy) or indirect (e.g., LV dilation/hypertrophy, LA dilation, pulmonary arterial hypertension) signs to corroborate the presence of intrinsic stenosis.

Role of exercise testing: Exercise stress echocardiography may be helpful in confirming or infirming the presence of hemodynamically significant prosthetic valve stenosis or PPM, especially when there is a discordance between the prosthetic valve hemodynamics measured at resting echocardiography and the patient's symptomatic status. As opposed to normally functioning and well-matched prostheses or to bileaflet mechanical valves with localized high gradient, the presence of valve stenosis or PPM is generally associated with a marked increase in gradients and pulmonary arterial pressure, the occurrence of symptoms, and an impaired exercise capacity on exercise stress echocardiography. An absolute increase in gradient ≥20 mmHg in the aortic position and ≥12 mmHg in the mitral position with a concomitant rise in systolic pulmonary arterial pressure (peak stress value of systolic pulmonary arterial pressure ≥60 mmHg) generally indicates severe prosthesis dysfunction or PPM. Exercise testing is also useful to unmask symptoms in a significant proportion of patients with prosthetic valve dysfunction or PPM who claim to be asymptomatic. This issue is particularly relevant to the elderly patients who may ignore or not report their symptoms or may reduce their level of physical activity to avoid or minimize symptoms.

PARTICULAR SITUATION OF PATIENTS WITH LOW TRANSPROSTHETIC FLOW

The absence of a high transprosthetic gradient does not necessarily imply the absence of PPM or of prosthesis stenosis. In presence of low ejection fraction and low transvalvular flow rate, the gradient may indeed be relatively low despite the presence of severe valve stenosis or mismatch. The measurement of a low gradient in concomitance with a low EOA (EOA < normal reference value) and/or a low indexed EOA (<0.85 cm^2/m^2) should alert the clinician and prompt further evaluation (Fig. 3). Like low-flow, low-gradient native aortic stenosis, dobutamine stress echocardiography may be useful to differentiate a true from a pseudo stenosis or mismatch in patients with prosthetic valves and low cardiac output. In the situation of pseudo stenosis/mismatch, the resting transprosthetic flow rate and thus the force applied on the leaflets are too low to completely open the valve. On dobutamine stress echocardiography, these patients nonetheless have a substantial increase in valve EOA and no or minimal elevation in gradients with increasing flow rate. On the other hand, true stenosis or mismatch is associated with no significant increase in EOA, a marked increase in gradient, and most often the occurrence of indirect signs (LV dysfunction, marked elevation in pulmonary arterial pressure, etc.) and symptoms. It should however be considered that dobutamine stress echocardiography does not allow for the distinction between prosthesis stenosis and prosthesis–patient mismatch. For this purpose, one should apply the algorithm presented in Fig. 2 to the EOA values obtained after normalization of cardiac output on stress echocardiography.

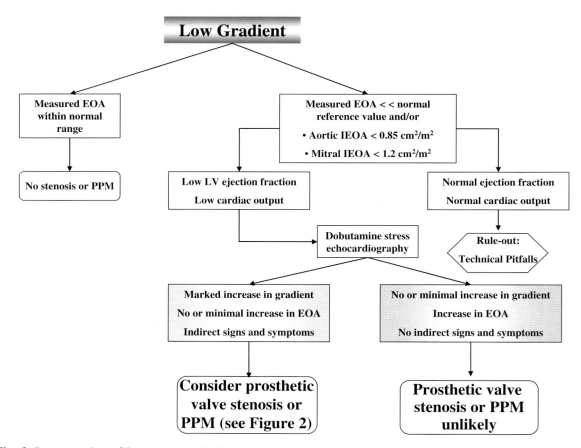

Fig. 3. Interpretation of low transprosthetic gradient in conjunction with small valve effective orifice area and low LV ejection fraction.

INFLUENCE OF PRESSURE RECOVERY

Doppler echocardiography estimates the maximum pressure drop through the prosthesis from the maximum velocity recorded at the tip of the valve leaflets. However, as blood flow velocity decelerates between the valve and the ascending aorta, part of the kinetic energy is reconverted back to static energy (i.e., pressure) due to a phenomenon called pressure recovery, and hence the net gradient between the left ventricle and the ascending aorta is less than the maximum pressure gradient measured by Doppler *(24–26)*. The extent of pressure recovery is determined by the ratio between the valve EOA and the area of the ascending aorta and it generally becomes clinically relevant in patients with smaller aortas, i.e., with an aorta diameter at the sino-tubular junction ≤ 30 mm *(25, 26)*. Patients with a large aneurysm of the ascending aorta have no pressure recovery and therefore a more important energy loss for a given prosthetic valve EOA. Congenital bicuspid aortic stenosis is often associated with dilation of the ascending aorta, which may reduce the extent of pressure recovery and thereby increase the energy loss at the level of the aortic valve/root. In patients with an aortic diameter < 30 mm, it thus becomes appropriate to account for pressure recovery by using the formula proposed by Baumgartner et al. to estimate the net gradient from Doppler measurements *(25)* as well as the simple formula proposed by Garcia et al. to calculate the energy loss coefficient: $ELC = (EOA \times AA/AA - EOA)$, where AA is the cross-sectional area of the aorta measured at the level of the sino-tubular junction *(24)*. Physiologically, the net gradient and the energy loss coefficient are more representative of the actual energy loss caused by the prosthetic valve and thus of the increased burden imposed on the ventricle than the maximum gradient or the EOA and as such, they should be more closely related to symptoms. Not accounting for pressure recovery in patients with small aortas may lead to overestimation of prosthetic valve stenosis by Doppler echocardiography and unwarranted investigations or interventions.

Treatment

Indications for surgery for prosthetic valve stenosis are similar to the indications for native valve stenosis *(27, 28)*. The surgery is indicated for symptomatic severe prosthetic valve stenosis. Asymptomatic patients may be managed conservatively but should be monitored closely by Doppler echocardiography as the valvular obstruction may progress rapidly. Development of LV systolic dysfunction or pulmonary arterial hypertension in patients with prosthetic stenosis provides additional criteria to consider reoperation.

PROSTHETIC VALVE REGURGITATION

Transvalvular Regurgitation

PREVALENCE AND ETIOLOGY

Minor regurgitation is normal in virtually all mechanical valves and in bileaflet valves, three small regurgitant jets can typically be seen throughout diastole. Minor non-clinically relevant regurgitation may also be seen in stented and stentless bioprosthesis but it is usually self-limited and does not progress with time. With mechanical valves, pathologic transvalvular regurgitation is due to incomplete closure of the valve occluder because of pannus or thrombus formation whereas in bioprosthetic valves, it is usually caused by degeneration and/or tear of a valve cusp.

DIAGNOSIS

The approach to detecting and grading prosthetic regurgitation is similar to that of native valves and involves evaluation of several Doppler echocardiographic indices. However, care is needed to separate normal from pathologic prosthetic valve regurgitation. It is also important to localize the origin of the regurgitant jet(s) in order to distinguish paravalvular from transvalvular regurgitation.

PROSTHETIC AORTIC REGURGITATION

Transthoracic echocardiography generally provides a good visualization of the LVOT and of prosthetic aortic regurgitation. The ratio of the height of the regurgitant jet to the LV outflow tract diameter preferably measured in the long-axis view may be used to grade the severity of aortic prosthetic regurgitation. A ratio >60% indicates severe regurgitation. As for native aortic valve regurgitation, it is important to measure LV size and dysfunction to corroborate the severity of the regurgitation. TEE may provide important etiologic information such as flail bioprosthetic cusp, presence of pannus or thrombus interacting with leaflet closure, prosthesis dehiscence, location and size, or paravalvular jets.

PROSTHETIC MITRAL REGURGITATION

Assessment of prosthetic mitral regurgitation by TTE is problematic because of reverberations from the metallic component of the prosthesis and the acoustic shadowing that occult the left atrium (Fig. 4C,D). This problem is more frequent in mechanical than in bioprosthetic valves. The presence of pathologic mitral prosthetic regurgitation should be suspected when the following signs are present: presence of flow convergence downstream of the prosthesis during systole, increased mitral E-wave velocity (>2 m/s) or mean gradient (>5–7 mmHg), unexplained or new worsening of pulmonary arterial hypertension (1, 29, 30). It is important to keep in mind that these indices are sensitive but not specific for the detection of prosthetic mitral regurgitation given that most of them are also often observed in the case of prosthetic mitral stenosis or mismatch (8, 29). TEE should be systematically performed when there is a clinical or TTE suspicion of pathologic mitral regurgitation. Several studies have demonstrated that TEE improves the diagnostic regurgitation of the severity, etiology, and location of prosthetic mitral regurgitation (30) (Fig. 4C,D).

TREATMENT

Indications for surgery for prosthetic regurgitation are similar to the indications for native valve regurgitation (27, 28). Clearly, surgery is indicated for symptomatic severe prosthetic valve regurgitation. Asymptomatic patients and those with mild or moderate regurgitation can often be managed conservatively. Patients with asymptomatic moderate or severe prosthetic regurgitation should be followed carefully with echocardiographic follow-up at least every year. Patients with mild regurgitation can be followed at longer follow-up intervals. As per ACC/AHA guidelines for native valve disease (27), evidence for progression of LV dilation, LV systolic dysfunction, or pulmonary arterial hypertension in patients with prosthetic regurgitation suggests that reoperation may be needed to prevent irreversible LV dysfunction.

Paravalvular Regurgitation

PREVALENCE, ETIOLOGY, AND DIAGNOSIS

Paravalvular regurgitation typically is due to infection, dehiscence of some of the sutures attaching the sewing ring to the annulus, or to fibrosis and calcification of the native annulus leading to inadequate contact between the sewing ring and annulus. The absence of adequate debridement of the aortic or mitral annulus may predispose to a breakdown of the suture line over time with paravalvular leak. Small paravalvular jets of regurgitation are frequently (10–25% of the cases) detected by intraoperative

TEE with all types of prosthesis *(31–33)*. Some will significantly decrease after the injection of protamine before cardiopulmonary bypass weaning and will often resolve in the days, weeks, or months after operation as the healing process evolves. Moderate or severe paravalvular regurgitation is rare (1–2%) and requires returning on cardiopulmonary bypass for immediate correction. Dehiscence of the prosthesis in the late postoperative period is most often related to endocarditis and generally requires emergency surgical treatment.

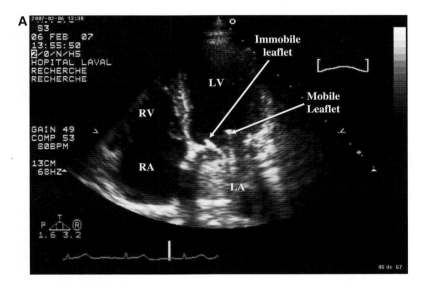

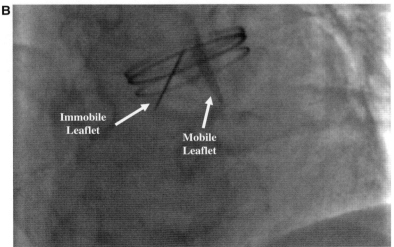

Fig. 4. Pannus causing prosthetic valve stenosis and regurgitation in an On-X mechanical valve implanted in the mitral position. **Panels A** and **B** show the restricted mobility of one of the leaflets on the transthoracic **(Panel A)** and cinefluoroscopic **(Panel B)** views. In the same patient, **Panel C** shows that the transthoracic view markedly underestimates the severity of the prosthetic regurgitation due to acoustic shadowing caused by the metallic components of the prosthesis. Transesophageal echocardiography **(Panel D)** reveals a moderate to severe regurgitation due to incomplete closing of the leaflets.

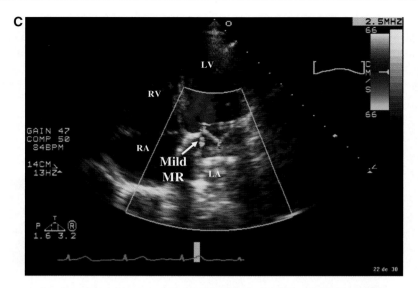

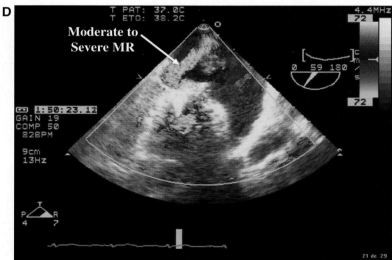

Fig. 4. *(Continued).*

TREATMENT

Follow-up studies suggest a benign long-term prognosis in the patients with mild paravalvular regurgitation identified by intraoperative or early postoperative echocardiography, with progression of regurgitation requiring reoperation in <1% of patients at follow-up >1–2 years *(31, 32)*. Hence, a strategy that includes frequent clinical follow-up appears justified in these patients, with surgical intervention warranted only for those who develop clinical symptoms. In circumstances where there is a paravalvular leak resulting in symptoms, hemolysis or progressive LV dilation and dysfunction, reoperation may well be required.

The paravalvular leaks can be repaired without valve replacement in approximately 50% of the cases *(34)*. Surgical correction of paravalvular leaks can be performed with acceptable mortality and morbidity. In patients with severe paravalvular mitral regurgitation refractory to aggressive medical therapy who are not candidates for surgical intervention, the percutaneous implantation of an Amplatzer septal occluder device offers an alternative therapeutic option *(35)*.

STRUCTURAL VALVE DETERIORATION

Bioprosthetic Valves

EPIDEMIOLOGY

Incidence of Structural Valve Deterioration.   Structural valve deterioration (SVD) in bioprosthetic valves is time-dependent and characterized by calcific or non-calcific tissue degeneration of valve leaflets. SVD is, by far, the most frequent cause of bioprosthetic valves failure. The rate of failure increases over time, particularly after the initial 5–6 years after implantation. With conventional stented bioprostheses, the freedom of structural valve failure is 70–90% at 10 years and 40–70% at 15 years (28, 36–38).

Predictors of Structural Valve Deterioration.   Risk factors previously found to be associated with bioprosthetic SVD include younger age, mitral valve position, renal insufficiency, and hyperparathyroidism (28, 37, 38). Hypertension, LV hypertrophy, poor LV function, and prosthesis size have also been reported as predictors of SVD in bioprostheses implanted in the aortic position (38).

Host-related factors: Bioprosthetic SVD is highly influenced by the age of the patient at the time of implantation (28, 39, 40). Calcification is markedly accelerated in children, adolescents, and young adults. The rate of failure of bioprostheses is approximately 10% at 10 years in elderly patients, but more than 40% at 4 years in most adolescent and preadolescent children (37). Given that the likelihood of structural failure is markedly reduced and that the life expectancy is shorter in the elderly population, bioprosthetic valves are now the valve of choice for patients over 65 years in the case of aortic valve replacement and over 70 years of age in the case of mitral valve replacement (27, 28).

Several studies suggest that freedom from bioprosthetic structural failure is lower in the mitral position than in the aortic position (28, 38). Ruel et al. reported an absolute difference of 14% in the freedom from 15-year reoperation between the bioprostheses implanted in the mitral position versus those implanted in the aortic position (38). This difference is likely related to the higher mechanical stress imposed on the valve leaflets of mitral bioprostheses. Systemic hypertension may also accelerate the SVD of aortic bioprostheses possibly due to the chronically increased diastolic closure stress on the bioprosthesis.

Valve-related factors: Several studies reported that, in general, newer generation bioprosthetic valves are more durable than older ones (28, 37, 38, 40). Some studies also suggested that bovine pericardial valves might be better than porcine valves in terms of hemodynamic performance and durability (41). However, other recent studies showed no appreciable difference in long-term outcomes between pericardial and porcine valves when implanted in the aortic position (42). Hence, there is presently no robust evidence favoring one type of prosthesis over the other in terms of valve durability. Stentless aortic valve bioprostheses have been used for a relatively short period of time. It has been hypothesized that the stentless design may decrease the mechanical stress imposed on the valve cusps and therefore improve the valve durability. The theoretical advantage of mobile commissures and reduced mechanical stress on the cusps may however be hampered by the calcification and stiffening of the aortic wall component of the device that may occur following implantation (43). Recent studies reported a freedom of reoperation due to SVD comprised between 75 and 95% at 10 years (44, 45).

PATHOPHYSIOLOGY

The principal underlying pathologic process leading to SVD is cuspal calcification; secondary tears frequently precipitate regurgitation (Fig. 5A). Calcification can also cause pure stenosis owing to cuspal stiffening. Calcific deposits are usually localized to leaflet tissue (intrinsic calcification), but calcific deposits extrinsic to the cusps may also develop in thrombi or endocarditic vegetations (extrinsic calcification). Although calcification of leaflet tissue is responsible for approximately 75% of bioprosthetic

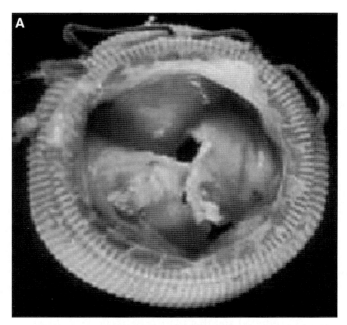

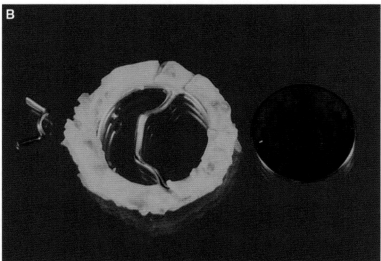

Fig. 5. Prosthetic valves explanted for severe dysfunction. **Panel A**: Leaflet tear secondary to calcific degeneration in a Mosaic porcine bioprosthesis. **Panel B**: Rupture of the outlet strut and leaflet escape in a Bjork–Shiley prosthesis. **Panel C**: Thrombosis on the cage of a Starr–Edwards prosthesis. **Panel D**: Obstructive thrombosis of a Lillehei–Kaster prosthesis. **Panel E**: Pannus ingrowth interacting with leaflet opening in a St. Jude Medical bileaflet valve. Courtesy of Drs Jacques Métras, Christian Couture, and Patrick Mathieu, Hôpital Laval, Québec.

valve failures, progressive collagen damage, independent of calcification, is also a likely important contributor to valve failure *(45–47)*. The SVD of bioprostheses has been considered for the past decades as being a purely degenerative process. However, recent studies suggest that immune and atherosclerotic processes may also contribute to bioprosthetic SVD. Hence, SVD is likely a multifactorial process that involves the interaction between valve and host factors.

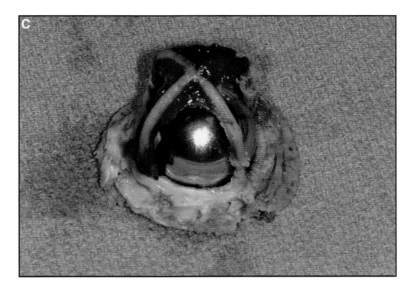

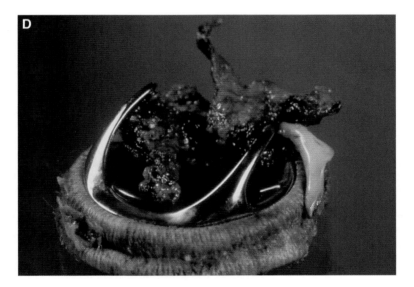

Fig. 5. *(Continued).*

Degenerative Process. The determinants of bioprosthetic valve mineralization include factors related to (1) host metabolism, (2) implant structure and chemistry, and (3) mechanical factors (Fig. 6) *(37)*. The calcification of bioprostheses is, in large part, related to the chemical fixative treatment of porcine or bovine tissue before implantation. Fixative treatment per se induces a calcium influx due to membrane damage, which provides, along with the residual phospholipids of the membranes, an environment prone to calcium crystal nucleation *(37)*. Host factors and mechanical stress then contribute to calcium crystal growth. Different interventions and co-treatment of bioprostheses with anti-calcifying agents have been used by prosthesis manufacturers over the last decades with the hope to reduce the

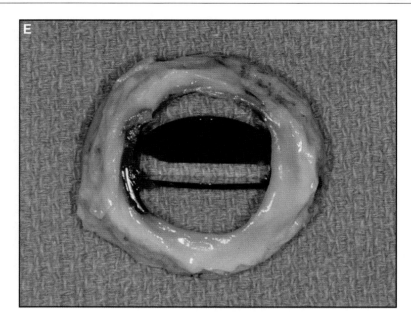

Fig. 5. *(Continued).*

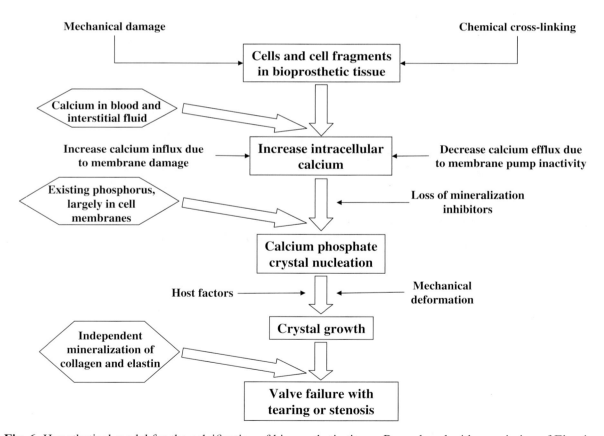

Fig. 6. Hypothetical model for the calcification of bioprosthetic tissue. Reproduced with permission of Elsevier from *(37)*.

incidence of SVD. Although these preimplantation treatments were associated with a major protective effect against cuspal calcification in animal studies, it remains to be confirmed if this effect will persist in the long-term and lead to enhanced valve durability in patients.

Immune Process. To decrease the immunogenicity of bioprosthetic valves, they are fixed in glutaraldehyde, and this process crosslinks and masks the antigens, supposedly making the valves essentially "immunologically inert." However, Manji et al. have recently demonstrated using a young animal model that glutaraldehyde-fixed bioprosthetic valves undergo immune rejection and that inflammation is correlated to calcification (48). In addition, they have also shown that rejection and calcification can be significantly decreased with steroid treatment. These findings suggest that immune rejection process may contribute to the SVD of bioprostheses and may explain the markedly accelerated degeneration observed in younger patients. It is indeed well known that young patients have a more robust immune system than do older people; thus, a possible reason why pediatric patients and young adults "destroy" bioprosthetic valves much more quickly than do elderly patients is that they have an aggressive immune system response to the valve (48).

Atherosclerotic Process. Recent studies have reported an association between bioprosthetic SVD and several atherosclerotic risk factors including hypercholesterolemia, diabetes, metabolic syndrome, and smoking (38, 49–51). A recent histopathologic study of bioprostheses explanted for structural valve failure also documented the presence of foam cells, which is a typical feature of atherosclerosis (52). Moreover, one retrospective study reported that statin therapy is associated with slower progression of SVD (53). These recent findings support the hypothesis that similarly to the native aortic valve, the SVD of bioprostheses may, at least in part, be related to an atherosclerotic process.

PREVENTION AND TREATMENT

Prevention. As opposed to what was previously believed, the data of recent studies (48–51, 53) suggest that the SVD of bioprosthetic valves is not a purely passive degenerative process but that it may also involve some active mechanisms including immune rejection and atherosclerotic processes. This new knowledge raises the possibility that, beyond the pretreatment of the cusp tissue prior to bioprosthesis implantation, the treatment of the patient after implantation could contribute to avoid or delay SVD and thereby enhance valve durability. In particular, a treatment with statins may help to slow the progression of SVD. A randomized trial is needed to confirm the usefulness of such therapy. In addition, the utilization of immuno-suppressive or anti-inflammatory drugs may contribute to reduce the immune response against bioprosthetic tissue, especially in the younger population. The risk-benefit ratio of such a pharmacological treatment would however need to be carefully investigated in future prospective studies. Another option to decrease the immunogenicity of bioprosthetic valves would be to use higher concentration of glutaraldehyde and/or longer exposure duration for the fixation of the bioprosthetic tissues (48). This approach may, however, yield to enhanced calcific degeneration in the longer-term. Other more promising approaches to passivate the immune response against bioprosthetic valves include new treatments of crosslinked xenograft valve tissue, decellularized valves, and "tissue engineered" in vivo recellularized or bioreactor cell-seeded valves based on allograft or xenograft scaffolds.

Treatment. Structural valve deterioration is the most frequent cause of reoperative valve replacement in patients with a bioprosthesis. Other causes of valve explant include thrombosis of the prosthesis, paraprosthetic leak, and prosthetic valve endocarditis.

When a bioprosthesis begins to fail, it should be kept in mind that the failure will be progressive and may accelerate. Advanced NYHA class, presence of LV dysfunction, pulmonary artery hypertension, renal failure, and emergent operation are the most powerful risk factors for operative mortality following reoperation of a failed prosthetic valve *(28, 54)*. These data suggest that, whenever it is possible, the reoperative procedure should be performed early in the disease process before LV function and symptomatic status deteriorate. The operative mortality for good risk elective procedure generally does not exceed 3%.

A recent animal study also demonstrated the feasibility of percutaneous implantation of a stented valve within failed bioprosthetic valves implanted in the tricuspid position in sheep *(55)* (Fig. 7). Percutaneous or transapical "valve-in-valve" implantation may provide a good alternative to standard valve replacement, particularly in the high-risk patients with larger size prostheses. The first two human cases of off-pump transapical valve implantation within failed aortic bioprostheses have been recently performed by the group of the Heart Center in Leipzig in Leipzig, Germany (Drs T Walther and M Borger, personal communication), and by the group of St. Paul's Hospital in Vancouver, Canada (Dr J Webb, personal communication).

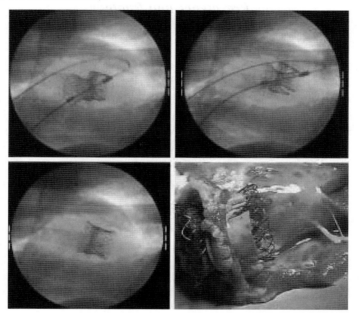

Fig. 7. Percutaneous valve implantation within a bioprosthesis in the tricuspid position in an animal model. Reproduced with permission of the American College of Cardiology from *(55)*.

Mechanical Valves

EPIDEMIOLOGY

Mechanical prosthetic valves have an excellent durability and structural valve deterioration is extremely rare with contemporary valves. Mechanical failure of parts of the prosthetic valve device (e.g., strut fracture, leaflet escape, occluder dysfunction due to lipid adsorption) occurred in some specific valve models in the past. Examples of mechanical failure include ball variance in certain models of caged ball valves, leading to regurgitation or stenosis, wearing of the disc in the Beall valve, and fracture of the strut with certain models of mono- and bileaflet mechanical valves, which could lead to leaflet escape and embolization (Fig. 5B).

PREVENTION AND TREATMENT

Although, primary structural failure is rare in mechanical valves, it is most often a life-threatening event that requires emergency surgery. Several imaging techniques including echocardiography, radiography, fluoroscopy, and computed tomography can be used to localize the embolized leaflet *(56)*. The leaflet may be found in the LV cavity and in this case, the replacement of the failed prosthesis and the removal of the escaped leaflet are performed within the same operation. In the vast majority of the cases (>80%), the leaflet is however found in the descending or abdominal aorta *(57)*. In this situation, the surgery can be performed within a single step as described above or in two steps: a first emergency operation to replace the failed prosthesis and a second operation 3 months later to remove the embolized leaflet. The operative mortality associated with the surgical treatment of a failed mechanical valve with embolized leaflet may be as high as 50% *(57)*. These findings emphasize the need for rigorous evaluation and testing of all new models of mechanical valves.

PROSTHETIC VALVE THROMBOSIS AND PANNUS

Prevalence and Etiology

Prosthetic valve thrombosis is extremely rare in bioprosthetic valves and most often occurs in the early postoperative period. Thrombosis occurs almost exclusively in mechanical valves, leading to predominant stenosis with or without some degree of regurgitation and to thromboembolic events (Fig. 5C,D). Mechanical valve dysfunction may also be related to tissue overgrowth (e.g., pannus) at the annulus blocking normal opening or closing of the valve disk resulting either in stenosis or regurgitation (Fig. 5E).

The risk of valve thrombosis is highest in the tricuspid position with rates as high as 20%, limiting the use of mechanical valves in this position *(58)*. Valve thrombosis is less likely with left-sided heart valves and is almost always due to inadequate anticoagulation therapy. The incidence of obstructive valve thrombosis, i.e., one of the most serious complication after valve replacement, varies between 0.3 and 1.3% patient years in mechanical valve *(59, 60)*.

One of the main mechanisms involved in prosthetic valve thrombosis is the interaction between the plasma components and the surface of the prosthetic material. Early after valve implantation, there is an adsorption of the fibrinogen that may lead to platelets adhesion. Moreover, the turbulent transprosthetic flow associated with mechanical valves may lead to the occurrence of area of stasis, thereby increasing the risk of thrombus formation. Local hypercoagulability mainly due to inadequate anticoagulation may also promote plasma clotting and platelet aggregation and then thrombosis.

Diagnosis

The onset of symptoms may be gradual due to a slowing enlarging thrombus or sudden to limitation of disk motion by thrombosis of the valve hinges. The severity of symptoms highly depends on the degree of valve obstruction caused by the prosthetic valve thrombosis. Whereas non-obstructive valve thrombosis is often asymptomatic and fortuitously diagnosed, severe obstructive thrombosis is generally associated with heart failure, cardiogenic shock and/or cerebral or peripheral embolism.

Prompt echocardiography is essential when a diagnosis of valve thrombosis is suspected, with TEE imaging needed, especially for valves in the mitral position. TEE is a sensitive and accurate tool for the diagnosis of valve thrombosis and for the evaluation of the efficacy of thrombolytic therapy. In particular, it is important to differentiate thrombus from fibrous pannus or vegetation in order to select the appropriate treatment. Although obstructive valve thrombus and pannus may have similar morphology and functional abnormalities, pannus is usually annular and more frequent in the aortic than in the mitral position and most often occurs in patients with adequate anticoagulation. Intermittent or permanent entrapment of preserved subvalvular tissue may also interfere with valve leaflet motion in the mechanical prostheses implanted in the mitral position *(61)*. This complication is rare and is difficult to differentiate from prosthetic valve dysfunction caused by a thrombus or pannus.

The evaluation of the motion and of the opening and closing angles of the leaflets by cinefluoroscopy may be helpful to confirm the presence of prosthetic valve obstruction (Fig. 4B). However, cinefluoroscopy does not permit to detect non-obstructive prosthetic valve thrombosis or to differentiate between thrombus, pannus, or vegetation.

Prevention and Treatment

Non-obstructive Prosthetic Valve Thrombosis

In non-obstructive left-sided prosthetic valve thrombosis confirmed by TTE or TEE, treatment consists of heparin therapy for 1 week with repeat TEE to evaluate treatment efficacy or adjustment of warfarin therapy with addition of low-dose aspirin (100 mg) (Fig. 8) *(60)*. However, if the medical treatment is unsuccessful, surgery should be considered in patients with large (>5–10 mm as determined by TEE) or mobile thrombi, whereas thrombolysis with urokinase, streptokinase, or recombinant tissue plasminogen activator is recommended in other patients *(see* Thrombolytic Treatment Protocols) *(60)*.

Obstructive Prosthetic Valve Thrombosis

Thrombolysis is the first-line treatment for obstructive right-sided valve thrombosis with acceptable complication rates *(62)*. However, in the case of thrombolysis failure, surgery should be envisioned.

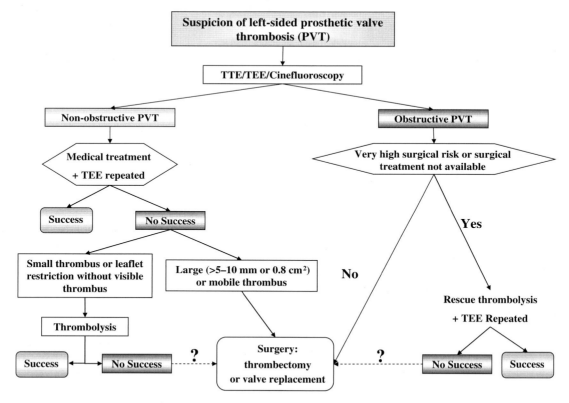

Fig. 8. Management of patients with obstructive left-sided prosthetic valve thrombosis (PVT). TEE, transesophageal echocardiography; TTE, transthoracic echocardiography. Reproduced with permission of the American Heart Association from *(63)*.

Historically, surgical treatment of left-sided obstructive prosthetic valve thrombosis was considered a very high risk procedure with operative mortality comprised between 17 and 50% (60). However, recent advances in surgery, anesthesia, and perioperative care have significantly improved the prognosis of such procedure. In recent series, mortality was 4–5% for patients with NYHA class ≤III, whereas it reached 15–20% in patients with NYHA class IV (60). On the other hand, thrombolysis is associated with a 10–15% mortality rate, 10–15% systemic embolic rate, and 5% hemorrhagic complications rate (36, 60). Hence, surgery is now the first-line therapy for left-sided obstructive valve thrombosis (Fig. 8). The intervention may involve simple thrombectomy or valvular replacement (with bioprosthesis implantation in cases of recurrent thrombosis). Despite the high complication rate, rescue thrombolysis may be preferred in the patients unlikely to survive surgery and in situations where the surgical treatment is not available and the patient cannot be transferred.

THROMBOLYTIC TREATMENT PROTOCOLS

There is no consensus in the literature regarding the most appropriate thrombolytic therapy for prosthetic valve thrombosis. Two types of protocols may be used depending on the hemodynamic status (60). In patients who are hemodynamicaly stable, a long-term protocol is often preferred using either

(1) Urokinase 4500 U/kg/h over a 12 h period or 2000 U/kg/h + heparin over 24 h.
(2) Streptokinase 500,000 IU in 20 min followed by 1,500,000 IU for 10 h without heparin.
(3) Recombinant tissue plasminogen activator (rtPA) 10 mg bolus, 50 mg during the first hour, 20 mg during the second hour, and 20 mg during the third hour.

Table 4
Anticoagulation for Prosthetic Valves

Mechanical valves	
AVR and no risk factor	Long-term warfarin, INR 2.0–3.0
Bileaflet valves	Long-term warfarin, INR 2.5–3.5
Monoleaflet or ball-cage valves	Long-term warfarin, INR 2.5–3.5
AVR + risk factor*	Long-term warfarin, INR 2.5–3.5
MVR	Long-term warfarin, INR 2.5–3.5
Bioprosthesis	Warfarin for 3 months postoperatively, INR 2.0–3.0
Bioprosthesis with no risk factor	Aspirin 80–100 mg/d
Aortic bioprosthesis with risk factor	Long-term warfarin, INR 2.0–3.0
Mitral bioprosthesis with risk factor	Long-term warfarin, INR 2.5–3.5
Embolic events while on anticoagulant therapy	Increase INR to 2.5–3.5, if needed to 3.5–4.5; add aspirin 80–100 mg/d, increase to 325 mg/d if needed
Therapy in patients requiring non-cardiac surgery	
Usual approach	Stop warfarin 72 h before procedure; restart postprocedure after control of active bleeding
High-risk patients†	Stop warfarin 72 h before procedure; start heparin IV when INR falls below 2.0; stop heparin 6 h before procedure; restart heparin within 24 h of procedure and continue until INR ≥ 2.0

*Risk factors: atrial fibrillation, left ventricular dysfunction, previous thromboembolism, hypercoagulable condition.

†High-risk patients are those with recent thromboembolism, Bjork–Shiley valve, AVR with three risk factors or MVR with one risk factor (see above for risk factors).

AVR, aortic valve replacement; INR, international normalized ratio; IV, intravenous; MVR, mitral valve replacement.

Reproduced with permission of Current medicine group (Philadelphia) from (36).

In patients with hemodynamic instability, rescue thrombolysis should be preferred using a short-term protocol consisting of either (1) rtPA 10 mg bolus + 90 mg in 90 mins or (2) streptokinase 1,500,000 U in 60 min without heparin.

The key element for the prevention of prosthetic valve thrombosis is effective anticoagulation treatment. Table 4 summarizes the recommendations for the anticoagulation treatment of patients with prosthetic valves.

CONCLUSION

Many of the prosthetic valve dysfunctions can be prevented, or their impact minimized, with careful medical management and periodic monitoring of valve function. Echocardiographic evaluation allows accurate and precise evaluation of prosthetic valve dysfunction and hemodynamics. Simple algorithm can be applied to differentiate prosthesis–patient mismatch from intrinsic prosthesis dysfunction. Prompt recognition of valve dysfunction allows early treatment, often with repeat surgical intervention. The percutaneous or transapical procedures open new important avenues for the treatment of prosthesis dysfunction.

REFERENCES

1. Otto CM. Prosthetic valves. In: Otto CM (ed.) Valvular Heart Disease. Philadelphia: W. B. Saunders Company, 1999:380–416.
2. Pibarot P, Honos GN, Durand LG, Dumesnil JG. Substitution of left ventricular outflow tract diameter with prosthesis size is inadequate for calculation of the aortic prosthetic valve area by the continuity equation. J Am Soc Echocardiogr 1995;8:511–7.
3. Dumesnil JG, Honos GN, Lemieux M, Beauchemin J. Validation and applications of mitral prosthetic valvular areas calculated by Doppler echocardiography. Am J Cardiol 1990;65:1443–8.
4. Rahimtoola SH. The problem of valve prosthesis-patient mismatch. Circulation 1978;58:20–4.
5. Dumesnil JG, Honos GN, Lemieux M, Beauchemin J. Validation and applications of indexed aortic prosthetic valve areas calculated by Doppler echocardiography. J Am Coll Cardiol 1990;16:637–43.
6. Pibarot P, Dumesnil JG. Prosthesis-patient mismatch: definition, clinical impact, and prevention. Heart 2006;92:1022–9.
7. Pibarot P, Dumesnil JG. Hemodynamic and clinical impact of prosthesis-patient mismatch in the aortic valve position and its prevention. J Am Coll Cardiol 2000;36:1131–41.
8. Magne J, Mathieu P, Dumesnil JG et al. Impact of prosthesis-patient mismatch on survival after mitral valve replacement. Circulation 2007;115:1417–25.
9. Lam BK, Chan V, Hendry P et al. The impact of patient-prosthesis mismatch on late outcomes after mitral valve replacement. J Thorac Cardiovasc Surg 2007;133:1464–73.
10. Ruel M, Rubens FD, Masters RG et al. Late incidence and predictors of persistent or recurrent heart failure in patients with aortic prosthetic valves. J Thorac Cardiovasc Surg 2004;127:149–59.
11. Tasca G, Brunelli F, Cirillo M et al. Impact of valve prosthesis-patient mismatch on left ventricular mass regression following aortic valve replacement. Ann Thorac Surg 2005;79:505–10.
12. Bakhtiary F, Schiemann M, Dzemali O et al. Impact of patient-prosthesis mismatch and aortic valve design on coronary flow reserve after aortic valve replacement. J Am Coll Cardiol 2007;49:790–6.
13. Ruel M, Al-Faleh H, Kulik A, Chan KL, Mesana TG, Burwash IG. Prosthesis-patient mismatch after aortic valve replacement predominantly affects patients with preexisting left ventricular dysfunction: effect on survival, freedom from heart failure, and left ventricular mass regression. J Thorac Cardiovasc Surg 2006;131:1036–44.
14. Tasca G, Mhagna Z, Perotti S et al. Impact of prosthesis-patient mismatch on cardiac events and midterm mortality after aortic valve replacement in patients with pure aortic stenosis. Circulation 2006;113:570–6.
15. Blais C, Dumesnil JG, Baillot R, Simard S, Doyle D, Pibarot P. Impact of prosthesis-patient mismatch on short-term mortality after aortic valve replacement. Circulation 2003;108:983–8.
16. Mohty D, Malouf JF, Girard SE et al. Impact of prosthesis-patient mismatch on long-term survival in patients with small St. Jude medical mechanical prostheses in the aortic position. Circulation 2006;113:420–6.
17. Ruel M, Al-Faleh H, Kulik A, Chan KL, Mesana TG, Burwash IG. Prosthesis-patient mismatch after aortic valve replacement predominantly affects patients with preexisting left ventricular dysfunction: effect on survival, freedom from heart failure, and left ventricular mass regression. J Thorac Cardiovasc Surg 2006;131:1036–44.

18. Walther T, Rastan A, Falk V et al. Patient prosthesis mismatch affects short- and long-term outcomes after aortic valve replacement. Eur J Cardiothorac Surg 2006;30:15–9.

19. Ruel M, Al-Faleh H, Kulik A, Chan KL, Mesana TG, Burwash IG. Prosthesis-patient mismatch after aortic valve replacement predominantly affects patients with preexisting left ventricular dysfunction: effect on survival, freedom from heart failure, and left ventricular mass regression. J Thorac Cardiovasc Surg 2006;131:1036–44.

20. Moon MR, Pasque MK, Munfakh NA et al. Prosthesis-patient mismatch after aortic valve replacement: impact of age and body size on late survival. Ann Thorac Surg 2006;81:481–8.

21. Mohty D, Dumesnil JG, Echahidi N, Mathieu P, Dagenais F, Voisine P, Pibarot P. Impact of prosthesis-patient mismatch on long-term survival after aortic valve replacement: influence of age, obesity, and left ventricular function. J Am Coll Cardiol, 2009;53:39–47.

22. Bleiziffer S, Eichinger WB, Hettich I et al. Prediction of valve prosthesis-patient mismatch prior to aortic valve replacement: which is the best method? Heart 2007;93:615–20.

23. Castro LJ, Arcidi JMJ, Fisher AL, Gaudiani VA. Routine enlargement of the small aortic root: a preventive strategy to minimize mismatch. Ann Thorac Surg 2002;74:31–6.

24. Garcia D, Pibarot P, Dumesnil JG, Sakr F, Durand LG. Assessment of aortic valve stenosis severity: a new index based on the energy loss concept. Circulation 2000;101:765–71.

25. Baumgartner H, Steffenelli T, Niederberger J, Schima H, Maurer G. ”Overestimation” of catheter gradients by Doppler ultrasound in patients with aortic stenosis: a predictable manifestation of pressure recovery. J Am Coll Cardiol 1999;33:1655–61.

26. Garcia D, Dumesnil JG, Durand LG, Kadem L, Pibarot P. Discrepancies between catheter and Doppler estimates of valve effective orifice area can be predicted from the pressure recovery phenomenon: practical implications with regard to quantification of aortic stenosis severity. J Am Coll Cardiol 2003;41:435–42.

27. Bonow RO, Carabello BA, Kanu C et al. ACC/AHA 2006 guidelines for the management of patients with valvular heart disease: a report of the American College of Cardiology/American Heart Association Task Force on Practice Guidelines (writing committee to revise the 1998 Guidelines for the Management of Patients With Valvular Heart Disease): developed in collaboration with the Society of Cardiovascular Anesthesiologists: endorsed by the Society for Cardiovascular Angiography and Interventions and the Society of Thoracic Surgeons. Circulation 2006;114:e84–231.

28. Jamieson WRE, Cartier PC, Allard M et al. CCS Consensus Conference: Surgical Management of Valvular Heart Disease 2004.

29. Fernandes V, Olmos L, Nagueh SF, Quinones MA, Zoghbi WA. Peak early diastolic velocity rather than pressure half-time is the best index of mechanical prosthetic mitral valve function. Am J Cardiol 2002;89:704–10.

30. Zabalgoitia M. Echocardiographic recognition and quantitation of prosthetic valve dysfunction. In: CM Otto, (ed.) The Practice of Clinical Echocardiography. Philadelphia: Saunders, 2007:525–55.

31. O'Rourke DJ, Palac RT, Malenka DJ, Marrin CAS, Arbuckle BE, Plehn JF. Outcome of mild periprosthetic regurgitation detected by intraoperative transesophageal echocardiography. J Am Coll Cardiol 2001;38:163–6.

32. Rallidis LS, Moyssakis IE, Ikonomidis I, Nihoyannopoulos P. Natural history of early aortic paraprosthetic regurgitation: a five-year follow-up. Am Heart J 1999;138:351–7.

33. Davila-Roman VG, Waggoner AD, Kennard ED et al. Prevalence and severity of paravalvular regurgitation in the artificial valve endocarditis reduction trial (AVERT) echocardiography study. J Am Coll Cardiol 2004;44:1467–72.

34. Akins CW, Bitondo JM, Hilgenberg AD, Vlahakes GJ, Madsen JC, MacGillivray TE. Early and late results of the surgical correction of cardiac prosthetic paravalvular leaks. J Heart Valve Dis 2005;14:792–9.

35. Momplaisir T, Matthews RV. Paravalvular mitral regurgitation treated with an amplatzer septal occluder device: a case report and review of the literature. J Invasive Cardiol 2007;19:E46–50.

36. Vesey JM, Otto CM. Complications of prosthetic heart valves. Curr Cardiol Rep 2004;6:106–11.

37. Schoen FJ, Levy RJ. Calcification of tissue heart valve substitutes: progress toward understanding and prevention. Ann Thorac Surg 2005;79:1072–80.

38. Ruel M, Kulik A, Rubens FD et al. Late incidence and determinants of reoperation in patients with prosthetic heart valves. Eur J Cardiothorac Surg 2004;25:364–70.

39. Grunkemeier GL, Jamieson WRE, Miller DC, Starr A. Actuarial versus actual risk of porcine structural valve deterioration. J Thorac Cardiovasc Surg 1994;108:709–18.

40. Butany J, Leask R. The failure modes of biological prosthetic heart valves. J Long Term Eff Med Implants 2001;11:115–35.

41. Le Tourneau T, Vincentelli A, Fayad G et al. Ten-year echocardiographic and clinical follow-up of aortic Carpentier–Edwards pericardial and supraannular prosthesis: a case-match study. Ann Thorac Surg 2002;74:2010–5.

42. Puvimanasinghe JP, Takkenberg JJ, Edwards MB et al. Comparison of outcomes after aortic valve replacement with a mechanical valve or a bioprosthesis using microsimulation. Heart 2004;90:1172–8.

43. Vesely I. The evolution of bioprosthetic heart valve design and its impact on durability. Cardiovasc Pathol 2003;12:277–86.

44. Desai ND, Merin O, Cohen GN et al. Long-term results of aortic valve replacement with the St. Jude Toronto stentless porcine valve. Ann Thorac Surg 2004;78:2076–83.

45. Mohammadi S, Baillot R, Voisine P, Mathieu P, Dagenais F. Structural deterioration of the freestyle aortic valve: mode of presentation and mechanisms. J Thorac Cardiovasc Surg 2006;132:401–6.

46. Vesely I, Barber JE, Ratliff NB. Tissue damage and calcification may be independent mechanisms of bioprosthetic heart valve failure. J Heart Valve Dis 2001;10:471–7.

47. Sacks MS, Schoen FJ. Collagen fiber disruption occurs independent of calcification in clinically explanted bioprosthetic heart valves. J Biomed Mater Res 2002;62:359–71.

48. Manji RA, Zhu LF, Nijjar NK et al. Glutaraldehyde-fixed bioprosthetic heart valve conduits calcify and fail from xenograft rejection. Circulation 2006;114:318–27.

49. Farivar RS, Cohn LH. Hypercholesterolemia is a risk factor for bioprosthetic valve calcification and explantation. J Thorac Cardiovasc Surg 2003;126:969–75.

50. Nollert G, Miksch J, Kreuzer E, Reichart B. Risk factors for atherosclerosis and the degeneration of pericardial valves after aortic valve replacement. J Thorac Cardiovasc Surg 2003;126:965–8.

51. Briand M, Pibarot P, Despres JP et al. Metabolic syndrome is associated with faster degeneration of bioprosthetic valves. Circulation 2006;114:I512–7.

52. Bottio T, Thiene G, Pettenazzo E et al. Hancock II bioprosthesis: a glance at the microscope in mid-long-term explants. J Thorac Cardiovasc Surg 2003;126:99–105.

53. Antonini-Canterin F, Zuppiroli A, Popescu BA et al. Effect of statins on the progression of bioprosthetic aortic valve degeneration. Am J Cardiol 2003;92:1479–82.

54. Rahimtoola SH, Frye RL. Valvular heart disease. Circulation 2000;102:IV24–33.

55. Zegdi R, Khabbaz Z, Borenstein N, Fabiani JN. A repositionable valved stent for endovascular treatment of deteriorated bioprostheses. J Am Coll Cardiol 2006;48:1365–8.

56. Cianciulli TF, Lax JA, Cerruti FE et al. Complementary value of transthoracic echocardiography and cinefluoroscopic evaluation of mechanical heart prosthetic valves. Echocardiogr 2004;21:211.

57. Hendel PN. Bjork-Shiley strut fracture and disc escape: literature review and a method of disc retrieval. Ann Thorac Surg 1989;47:436–40.

58. Thorburn CW, Morgan JJ, Shanahan MX, Chang VP. Long-term results of tricuspid valve replacement and the problem of prosthetic valve thrombosis. Am J Cardiol 1983;51:1128–32.

59. Horstkotte D, Burckhardt D. Prosthetic valve thrombosis. J Heart Valve Dis 1995;4:141–53.

60. Roudaut R, Serri K, Lafitte S. Thrombosis of prosthetic heart valves: diagnosis and therapeutic considerations. Heart 2007;93:137–42.

61. Thomson LE, Chen X, Greaves SC. Entrapment of mitral chordal apparatus causing early postoperative dysfunction of a St. Jude mitral prosthesis. J Am Soc Echocardiogr 2002;15:843–4.

62. Shapira Y, Sagie A, Jortner R, Adler Y, Hirsch R. Thrombosis of bileaflet tricuspid valve prosthesis: clinical spectrum and the role of nonsurgical treatment. Am Heart J 1999;137:721–5.

63. Pibarot P, Dumesnil JG. Selection of the optimal prosthesis and long-term management. Circulation 2009;119:1034–48.

64. Botzenhardt F, Eichinger WB, Guenzinger R et al. Hemodynamic performance and incidence of patient-prosthesis mismatch of the complete supraannular perimount magna bioprosthesis in the aortic position. Thorac Cardiovasc Surg 2005;53:226–30.

65. Dalmau MJ, Gonzalez-Santos JM, Lopez-Rodriguez J, Bueno M, Arribas A, Nieto F. One year hemodynamic performance of the Perimount Magna pericardial xenograft and the Medtronic Mosaic bioprosthesis in the aortic position: a prospective randomized study. ICVTS 2007;6:345–9.

66. Dellgren G, Eriksson MJ, Brodin LA, Radegran K. Eleven years' experience with the Biocor stentless aortic bioprosthesis: clinical and hemodynamic follow-up with long-term relative survival rate. Eur J Cardiothorac Surg 2002;22: 912–21.

67. Garcia-Bengochea J, Sierra J, Gonzalez-Juanatey JR et al. Left ventricular mass regression after aortic valve replacement with the new Mitroflow 12A pericardial bioprosthesis. J Heart Valve Dis 2006;15:446–51.

68. Dossche K, Vanermen H, Daenen W, Pillai R, Konertz W. Hemodynamic performance of the PRIMA™ Edwards stentless aortic xenograft: early results of a multicenter clinical trial. Thorac Cardiovasc Surg 1996;44:11–4.

69. Jin XY, Dhital K, Bhattacharya K, Pieris R, Amarasena N, Pillai R. Fifth-year hemodynamic performance of the prima stentless aortic valve. Ann Thorac Surg 1998;66:805–9.

70. Chambers JB, Rimington HM, Rajani R, Hodson F, Shabbo F. A randomized comparison of the Cryolife O' Brien and Toronto stentless replacement aortic valves. J Thorac Cardiovasc Surg 2007;133:1045–50.

71. Koertke H, Seifert D, Drewek-Platena S, Koerfer R. Hemodynamic performance of the Medtronic ADVANTAGE prosthetic heart valve in the aortic position: echocardiographic evaluation at one year. J Heart Valve Dis 2003;12:348–53.
72. Bach DS, Sakwa MP, Goldbach M, Petracek MR, Emery RW, Mohr FW. Hemodynamics and early clinical performance of the St. Jude Medical Regent mechanical aortic valve. Ann Thorac Surg 2002;74:2003–9.
73. Chambers J, Ely JL. Early postoperative echocardiographic hemodynamic performance of the On-X prosthetic heart valve: a multicenter study. J Heart Valve Dis 1998;7:569–73.
74. Eichinger WB, Botzenhardt F, Gunzinger R et al. European experience with the Mosaic bioprosthesis. J Thorac Cardiovasc Surg 2002;124:333–9.

21 Infective Endocarditis

Andrew Wang and Christopher H. Cabell

CONTENTS

NATIVE VALVE ENDOCARDITIS

Epidemiology and Prevention

Infective endocarditis (IE) has been defined as an infection of the endocardium of the heart, usually with involvement of the valves. In addition to native valve infection, infection of prosthetic heart valves (termed prosthetic valve endocarditis, including mechanical, bioprosthetic, homograft valves) and implanted devices (termed cardiac device infection including pacemakers, implantable cardioverter defibrillators, and ventricular assist devices) may occur.

Several well-designed epidemiologic studies have estimated the incidence of IE at approximately 3–5 cases per 100,000 person-years *(1–3, 4)*. The incidence has not decreased over the past 30 years, yet the epidemiology has changed. Although previously recognized as a disease associated with poor dentition and rheumatic heart disease, many factors have altered the epidemiology of IE while maintaining its incidence: an aging population with degenerative valvular disease, injection drug use, increasing number of valve replacements, and medical interventions *(1, 2, 5, 6)*. Age is an important influence on the incidence of IE: for persons less than 50 years old, the median incidence is estimated at 3.6 per 100,000 persons per year, but increases to ≥ 15 cases per 100,000 persons per year for those older than 65 years *(4)*. Health-care-associated infection is another growing influence on the epidemiology of IE. The International Collaboration on Endocarditis – Prospective Cohort Study (ICE – PCS) found that *Staphylococcus aureus* was the most common pathogen throughout much of the world, with health-care-associated infection, with most acquisitions outside of the hospital setting, being the most common form of *S. aureus* IE *(5)*.

Recently, data have emerged related to predisposing cardiac conditions and the subsequent development of IE. Strom and colleagues utilized a population-based case–control study to quantify associations between certain predisposing risk factors and IE *(7)*. Strong associations were found in patients with previous valvular surgery, previous IE, rheumatic fever involving the heart, and mitral valve prolapse *(7)*, consistent with previous findings. Notably, there was no clear link between a previous dental procedure and subsequent development of IE *(7)*.

Despite recognition that certain cardiac diseases may increase the risk for developing IE, the utility of antibiotic prophylaxis given at the time of dental and other procedures remains controversial. Although bacteremia is recognized as the causative event for IE to develop, bacteremia may occur during many daily activities unrelated to dental or medical interventions, and prophylaxis for

From: *Contemporary Cardiology: Valvular Heart Disease*
Edited by: Andrew Wang, Thomas M. Bashore, DOI 10.1007/978-1-59745-411-7_21
© Humana Press, a part of Springer Science+Business Media, LLC 2009

all episodes of bacteremia is infeasible. After an extensive literature review and consensus process, the American Heart Association recently updated their endocarditis prophylaxis guidelines *(8, 9)*. This statement concluded that (1) only an extremely small number of cases of IE might be prevented by antibiotic prophylaxis for dental procedures even if such therapy was 100% effective; (2) endocarditis prophylaxis for dental procedures is recommended only for patients with underlying cardiac conditions associated with the highest risk of adverse outcome from IE; (3) for patients with these underlying cardiac conditions, prophylaxis is recommended for all dental procedures that involve manipulation of gingival tissue or the periapical region of teeth or perforation of the oral mucosa; (4) prophylaxis is not recommended based solely on an increased lifetime risk of acquisition of IE; and (5) administration of antibiotics solely to prevent endocarditis is not recommended for patients who undergo a genitourinary or gastrointestinal tract procedure *(9)* (*see* Chapter 16, Table 1).

Table 1
The Modified Duke Criteria and Case Definitions of Infective Endocarditis

Modified Duke criteria	Case definitions
Major criteria *Blood culture positive for IE* • Typical microbes consistent with IE from two separate blood cultures: viridans streptococci, *S. bovis*, HACEK group, *S. aureus*; community-acquired enterococci in absence of another focus • Microorganisms consistent with IE from persistently positive blood cultures defined as follows: at least two blood cultures drawn >12 h apart or all of three or majority of >4 separate blood cultures • Single positive blood culture for *Coxiella burnetti* or antiphase IgG antibody titer >1:800 *Evidence of endocardial involvement* Echo positive for IE defined as follows: • Oscillating intra-cardiac mass on valve or supporting structure • Abscess • New partial dehiscence of prosthetic valve • New valvular regurgitation **Minor criteria** • Predisposition; predisposing heart condition or injection drug use • Fever, temperature >38°C • Vascular phenomena, major arterial emboli, septic pulmonary infarcts, mycotic aneurysm, intracranial hemorrhage, conjunctival hemorrhage, and Janeway lesions • Immunologic phenomena; glomerulonephritis, Osler's nodes, Roth's spots, rheumatoid factor • Microbiological evidence: positive blood cultures but does not meet a major criterion as noted above, or serological evidence of active infection with organism consistent with causing IE	**Definite infective endocarditis** *Pathologic criteria* • Microorganisms demonstrated by culture or histologic examination of a vegetation, a vegetation that has embolized or an intracardiac abscess specimen • Pathologic lesions; vegetation or intra-cardiac abscess confirmed by histologic examination showing active endocarditis *Clinical criteria* • Two major criteria • One major and three minor criteria • Five minor criteria **Possible infective endocarditis** • One major criterion and one minor criterion • Three minor criteria **Rejected** • Firm alternate diagnosis explaining evidence of infective endocarditis • Resolution of infective endocarditis syndrome with antibiotic therapy for ≤4 days • No pathologic evidence of infective endocarditis at surgery or autopsy, with antibiotic therapy for <4 days • Does not meet criteria for possible infective endocarditis, as above

Adapted from Li JS et al. *(112)*.

Pathogenesis

The development of IE involves a complex interaction between the host and the invading microorganisms that includes the vascular endothelium, hemostatic mechanisms, cardiac anatomical and hemodynamic characteristics, the surface properties and the enzyme and toxin production by the microorganisms, and the host immune system *(4)*. The endothelial lining of the heart and valves is generally resistant to bacterial or fungal infection. A few highly virulent organisms, such as *S. aureus*, are capable of infecting apparently normal heart valves, but this is uncommon. The majority of patients who develop IE have pre-existing structural abnormalities of the cardiac valve *(10)*. Animal studies suggest that endothelial damage appears to be the initiating event. The role of endothelial damage as the inciting event is further supported by findings that the sites of vegetation formation are similar to those where blood flow injury is most likely to occur: on the ventricular side of semilunar valves and the atrial side of atrioventricular (i.e., mitral and tricuspid) valves *(11)*.

Once the inciting lesion on the endothelium has been formed, followed by platelet–fibrin deposition that provides a milieu for bacterial colonization, bacteremia must be present to colonize the vegetation, and organisms must adhere to the vegetation or the intact valve endothelium. Cell surface characteristics of the organism promote its adherence. These microbial proteins, collectively termed microbial surface components recognizing adhesive matrix molecules (MSCRAMMs), promote adhesion of the bacteria to areas of injured endothelium, where platelet and fibroblast activity may contribute to adhesion and development of a vegetation. Certain organisms appear to produce these adhesive surface molecules more commonly than others, promoting their infection of nascent nonbacterial vegetative lesion. For instance, streptococci that produce surface glucans and dextran appear to be more likely to cause endocarditis than those that do not *(12)*. Other proteins (e.g., fibronectin- and collagen-binding proteins) may also be involved depending on the organism. The cycle of adherence, organism growth, and platelet–fibrin deposition then repeats itself as the vegetation grows. Even after successful antimicrobial therapy, many sterile vegetations will persist indefinitely *(13)*.

Microbiology

A detailed description of the clinical microbiology is beyond the scope of this chapter. We will highlight the major microbiologic etiologic agents associated with native valve IE, focusing on aspects that may affect the management of a patient with IE.

GRAM-POSITIVE COCCI

Viridans Streptococci. Streptococcus viridans is the most common causative organism in community-acquired IE *(14)*. Although *S. viridans* IE is generally considered highly responsive to medical therapy, it has remained the leading causative organism in IE treated with surgery *(15)*.

Beta-Hemolytic Streptococci. Group D organisms include the enterococci and *Streptococcus bovis*. Enterococci are normal inhabitants of the gastrointestinal tract and occasionallythe anterior urethra. Enterococcal endocarditis, which typically affects older men with other comorbid medical conditions, is frequently associated with a genitourinary source of infection and may also be associated with recent health care contact *(16)*. Enterococcal IE is generally associated with complication of heart failure as opposed to embolic events.

Staphylococci. Staphylococci cause at least 30–40% of the cases of IE, and 80–90% of these are due to coagulase-positive *S. aureus*. This species is the causative agent in most cases of acute IE, but only a minority of patients (10–15%) with *S. aureus* bacteremia will have IE *(17)*. The organism may involve structurally normal heart valves in approximately one-third of IE cases. The course is often acute and fulminant when it involves the left-sided valves and may be complicated by metastatic infection. The increasing proportion of IE due to *S. aureus* has been associated with increasing health care contact. In a recent multinational cohort of 922 patients with definite IE *(5)*, *S. aureus* was the most common cause of IE, accounting for 36% of all cases, and among *S. aureus* cases, 46% were presumed to be health care associated *(5)*. Thus, health-care-associated *S. aureus* bacteremia should prompt an evaluation for possible underlying IE. Interestingly, nearly 40% of *S. aureus* cases in this cohort were community acquired in the absence of injection drug use *(5)*.

S. aureus IE is associated with higher rates of complications such as stroke, other systemic embolization, and persistent bacteremia, but with similar rates of intra-cardiac abscess and heart failure *(5)*. Despite the rate of complications, the rate of surgical intervention for *S. aureus* IE is lower than for other causes (38% vs. 52%), possibly related to patient characteristics such as injection drug use and other chronic diseases *(5)*.

Although coagulase-negative staphylococci, notably *Staphylococcus epidermidis*, are important agents in prosthetic valve endocarditis, it is increasingly recognized as a cause of native valve IE *(18)*. This organism has also been associated with recent health care contact, and despite similar rates of complications of IE as *S. aureus*, it has a much higher rate of surgical intervention *(18)*.

A number of reports of IE caused by a coagulase-negative staphylococcus called *Staphylococcus lugdunensis* have been published *(19)*. This organism tends to cause a substantially more virulent form of IE than that due to other coagulase-negative staphylococci, with high morbidity rates despite nearly uniform in vitro susceptibilities to most antibiotics, including penicillins and cephalosporins. These strains are frequently misidentified as *S. aureus*.

HACEK Gram-Negative Bacteria. The organisms within the HACEK group – *Haemophilus, Actinobacillus, Cardiobacterium, Eikenella, Kingella* – are slow growing in blood culture media and may require prolonged incubation. Only a small percentage of blood cultures will grow an organism in these cases of IE *(20)*. The clinical syndrome produced by these organisms is similar: large friable vegetations, frequent embolic events, and the development of CHF and often the eventual need for surgical intervention *(21)*.

Fungi. Most patients who have fungal endocarditis can be grouped into three categories: (1) narcotic addicts; (2) patients who have undergone reconstructive cardiovascular surgery; and (3) patients who are immunosuppressed, particularly after organ transplantation. *Candida albicans* is the most common fungal cause of IE. Recent evidence suggests an increase in health-care-associated cases of fungal IE. In a review of 152 cases between 1995 and 2000, IDU was an identified risk factor in only 4.1% of cases, while other predisposing factors such as cardiac abnormalities (47.3%), prosthetic valves (44.6%), and central venous catheters (30.4%) were more common *(22)*. In this case series, complicated IE, particularly embolic events and heart failure, were common in fungal IE, and surgical intervention was performed in two-thirds of cases *(22)*. The mortality rate was very high (56.6%) *(22)*. Other series have confirmed higher rates of complications, including myocardial abscess and persistent bacteremia *(23)*.

Other Microorganisms. IE due to *Coxiella burnetii* (the cause of Q fever) is generally chronic, with a history of an influenza-like illness occurring 6–12 months previously. There is a long delay from symptom onset to the diagnosis of IE, since this represents a form of "culture-negative" endocarditis. The aortic valve is involved in the majority of the cases. The diagnosis is best made serologically; a positive titer of antibody to the phase I antigen as measured by complement fixation or ELISA is indicative of chronic infection, whereas a fourfold rise in titer of antibody to the phase II antigen is associated with active current infection. A phase I antibody titer (generally IgG and/or IgA) greater than 1:200 is considered virtually diagnostic of Q fever endocarditis and may be useful to follow the response to therapy *(24)*.

"Culture-Negative" Endocarditis. Blood cultures are negative in only approximately 5–10% of patients with IE confirmed by strict diagnostic criteria *(25, 26)*. This may be due to several factors: (1) the prior administration of antibiotics; (2) cultures taken toward the end of a chronic course (longer than 3 months); (3) uremia supervening in a chronic course; (4) mural endocarditis as in ventricular septal defects, post-myocardial infarction thrombi, or infection related to pacemaker wires; (5) slow growth of fastidious organisms such as anaerobes; (6) subacute right-sided endocarditis; (7) fungal endocarditis; and (8) endocarditis caused by obligate intracellular parasites, such as rickettsiae, chlamydiae, *Tropheryma whippelii*, and perhaps viruses; or noninfective endocarditis or an incorrect diagnosis *(27)*.

Diagnosis

The diagnosis of IE is based upon clinical suspicion derived from signs and symptoms and, most importantly, the demonstration of associated bacteremia. In the late 1970s that Pelletier and Petersdorf developed a strict case definition based on a 30-year experience of caring for patients with IE in Seattle *(28)*. Although this case definition was highly specific for the diagnosis of IE, it lacked sufficient sensitivity for clinical use. A more refined diagnostic schema was developed in 1981, when von Reyn and colleagues published an analysis that provided four diagnostic categories in cases of suspected IE (rejected, possible, probable, and definite) *(29)*. These criteria, based upon broader clinical findings than the Pelletier and Petersdorf case definition, improved both the sensitivity and the specificity of the previous case definition, but did not incorporate imaging results from echocardiography.

In 1994, IE diagnostic criteria were refined further by Durack and colleagues from Duke University Medical Center. These criteria, which have come to be known as the Duke criteria, incorporated echocardiographic evidence of endocardial involvement *(30)*. These criteria had improved test performance characteristics when compared to previous criteria and have been validated subsequently by many other studies *(31–33)*. Recently, proposed modifications to enhance the sensitivity of these criteria have been published (Table 1) *(34)*.

Based upon the defined role of imaging in the diagnosis of IE, echocardiography is standard clinical practice in evaluating patients with suspected IE. Echocardiographic findings that provide specific evidence of IE include vegetations, evidence of periannular tissue destruction (abscess), aneurysm, fistula, leaflet perforation, and valvular dehiscence. Table 2 outlines specific definitions of these characteristic findings.

Table 2
Echocardiographic Findings in Infective Endocarditis

Echocardiographic finding	Description
Vegetation	– Irregularly shaped, discrete echogenic mass – Adherent to but distinct from endocardial surface or intra-cardiac device – Oscillation of mass (supportive, not mandatory)
Abscess	– Thickened area or mass within the myocardium or valve annulus – Evidence of flow into region (supportive, not mandatory)
Aneurysm	Echolucent space with thin surrounding tissue
Fistula	Blood flow between two distinct cardiac blood spaces or chambers through abnormal path/channel
Leaflet perforation	Defect in body of valve leaflet with flow through defect
Valve dehiscence	Prosthetic valve with abnormal rocking motion/excursion >15° in at least one direction

Adapted from Sachdev M et al. *(113)*.

Echocardiographic Findings in Endocarditis

With two-dimensional echocardiographic imaging in which the cardiac structures are viewed throughout the cardiac cycle, a vegetation is defined as an irregularly shaped, discrete echogenic mass. This mass must be adherent to, yet distinct from, the endothelial cardiac surface. Mass oscillation, high-frequency movement independent from that of intrinsic cardiac structures, is supportive but not mandatory for the echocardiographic diagnosis of a vegetation. Vegetations have the consistency of mid-myocardium (Fig. 1), but may also have areas of both echo-lucency and echo-density. Vegetations may also appear on nonvalvular intravascular structures, such as pacemaker leads.

Periannular extension of infection, or abscess formation, is one of the most serious complications of IE. On echocardiogram, a myocardial abscess can be defined as a thickened area or mass in the myocardium or annular region with an appearance that is generally non-homogeneous. If there is evidence of flow within the area then this is considered to be supportive of the diagnosis of abscess formation, but flow within the area is not mandatory for the diagnosis. With extension of infection into the myocardium, a fistula allowing abnormal flow between cardiac chambers may develop (Fig. 2).

There is little information available about valvular perforation formation, but it is generally accepted that this is either associated with a virulent microorganism, such as *S. aureus*, or occurs when the infection process continues for a substantial amount of time without detection. Once a perforation forms, a significant amount of valvular regurgitation may develop (Fig. 1). The endocarditis process can also involve the mechanical function of the valve to cause significant valvular regurgitation without perforation. This mechanical disruption can occur at the valve leaflets secondary to a physical impairment of proper leaflet coaptation or to the vegetative process. In addition, the mechanical disruption can involve the rupture of the chordae tendineae and possibly a flail leaflet.

Echocardiography in Patients with Suspected IE

Echocardiography is the imaging technology of choice for the diagnosis of IE and can detect cardiac involvement in a significant proportion of patients with clinically occult IE (35). Published diagnosis and treatment guidelines advocate the early use of echocardiography to establish the diagnosis of IE (36) but its optimal use is predicated on the appropriate pre-test probability of disease. Echocardiography may be overused in clinical scenarios with a low (<2–3%) pre-test probability of disease, where its diagnostic utility is minimal. The absence of five clinical criteria has been associated with zero probability of a transthoracic echocardiogram (TTE) showing evidence of IE (37): positive blood cultures; presence of central venous access; recent history of injection drug use; presence of prosthetic valve; and vasculitic/embolic phenomena.

Both transthoracic and transesophageal echocardiography (TEE) have an important role in the diagnosis and management of patients with suspected IE. In general, TTE is widely available and can provide rapid important diagnostic information, including the severity of valvular regurgitation in native valve IE. TEE imaging allows more proximal imaging of the heart and is typically performed using a higher ultrasonic frequency (6–7 MHz), providing greater spatial resolution of nearby structures including the cardiac valves. Under ideal conditions, TTE can reliably identify structures as small as 5 mm in diameter, while TEE can depict structures as small as 1 mm. It is generally accepted that the sensitivity and specificity are superior for TEE (93 and 96%, respectively) compared to TTE (46 and 95%, respectively) (27).

Recently, studies have shown that an initial strategy of TEE is more cost-effective than a staged procedure with TTE in the majority of clinical situations of suspected IE and is a optimal strategy over empiric antibiotic therapy alone (38). In this study, TEE imaging was optimal for patients who had a pre-test probability of IE endocarditis (4–60%) that is observed commonly in clinical practice and was associated with a lower cost per person compared with the use of transthoracic echocardiography. In

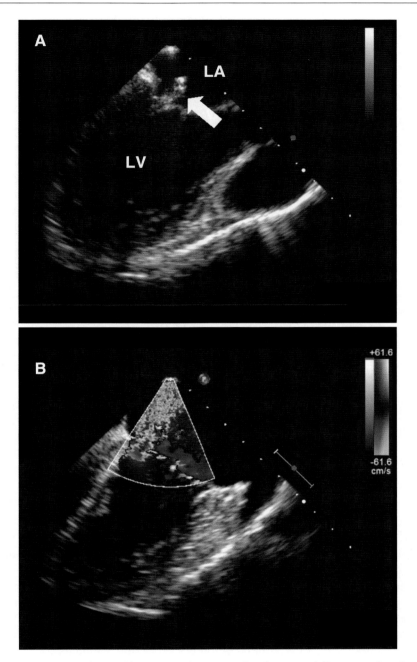

Fig. 1. Transesophageal echocardiographic images demonstrating large, mobile vegetation due to enterococcus on mitral valve leaflet (*Arrow*, **Panel A**) and leaflet perforation with severe mitral regurgitation (**Panel B**) (Courtesy of Cardiac Diagnostic Unit, Duke University Medical Center).

contrast, strategies that reserved the use of TEE for patients who had an inadequate transthoracic study provided similar quality-adjusted life years but had a modest increase in cost per patient *(38)*.

Similarly, the cost-effectiveness of TEE in establishing the duration of therapy for *S. aureus* bacteremia has been demonstrated *(39)*. Given the increasing frequency of *S. aureus* IE as a consequence of medical interventions, the differentiation between catheter-associated bacteremia and IE

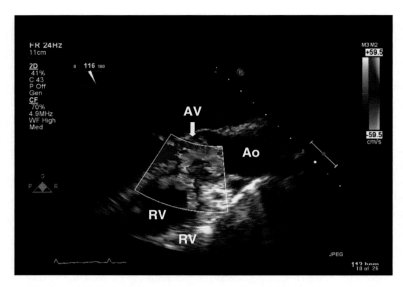

Fig. 2. Transesophageal echocardiogram of aorta to right ventricular fistula in aortic valve endocarditis (AV, aortic valve; Ao, aorta; RV, right ventricle). Courtesy of Cardiac Diagnostic Unit, Duke University Medical Center.

is important for treatment recommendations. In this study, three management strategies were compared: (1) empiric treatment with 4 weeks of antibiotics (long course); (2) empiric treatment with 2 weeks of antibiotic therapy (short course); and (3) TEE-guided therapy. In the case of the TEE strategy, a positive TEE dictated long-course therapy and a negative TEE dictated short-course therapy. The effectiveness of both an empiric long-course strategy and a TEE-guided strategy was superior to empiric short-course therapy. When costs were taken into account, the TEE-guided strategy was superior to the empiric long-course strategy *(39)*.

Clinical Management

GENERAL MANAGEMENT INCLUDING ANTIBIOTIC THERAPY

The management of IE has evolved over the last few decades with the improvements in diagnostic capabilities and therapy *(40, 30)*. Rapid diagnosis, early risk stratification, institution of appropriate bactericidal therapy, and prompt recognition and treatment of complications are key elements toward a good outcome. The appropriate management of these complex patients generally requires the involvement and close collaboration of multiple interdisciplinary teams including the general medicine team, infectious diseases specialists, cardiologists, and cardiothoracic surgeons.

Antibiotic therapy has improved survival in IE by 70–80% and has been shown to reduce the incidence of complications of IE. Detailed descriptions of antibiotic regimens for specific causative IE organisms are found in recent, comprehensive guidelines by the American Heart Association *(20)* and the European Society of Cardiology *(41)*. Although the choice of antimicrobial therapy is mainly guided by the infecting organism and its antibiotic susceptibilities, there are three basic tenets of antibiotic treatment for the eradication of native valve infection.

First, a prolonged course of antibiotic treatment (4–6 weeks) is necessary to eradicate infection because bacterial concentration within vegetations is as high as 10^9–10^{11} CFUs/g of tissue, and organisms deep within vegetations are inaccessible to phagocytic cells *(42, 43)*. Repeat sets of blood cultures after antibiotic initiation should be obtained every 24–48 h until the resolution of bacteremia is confirmed. If surgery for IE is performed, completion of the 4–6 week course of antibiotic therapy is generally favored to reduce the risk of recurrent IE.

Second, parenteral administration of antibiotic therapy is necessary to achieve adequate drug levels required to eradicate infection. Parenteral therapy is typically initiated in the hospital setting, and the patient may receive outpatient, parenteral treatment for the remaining duration after an initial period of observation to assess for clinical response to therapy (e.g., clearance of bacteremia and absence of complications).

Third, because of the need for prolonged therapy and rising antimicrobial resistance amongst organisms, combination therapy typically involving a beta-lactam and aminoglycoside antibiotic is recommended. Combination therapy has been shown to reduce the duration of bacteremia in *S. aureus* endocarditis *(44)*, although this more rapid resolution of bacteremia was not associated with an improved clinical response or outcome. Both antibiotics should be given temporally close together so that maximum synergistic killing effect is obtained *(20)*. In addition, careful monitoring of the dosage and renal function should be performed, as combination therapy has been associated with a higher rate of renal dysfunction *(44)*.

Antibiotic therapy should only be administered after obtaining at least three sets of blood cultures, since a high percentage of "culture-negative" endocarditis may be attributable to prior antibiotic therapy. In cases complicated by sepsis, valvular dysfunction, conduction disturbances, or embolic phenomena, empiric antimicrobial therapy, based on typical or suspected microorganisms for the clinical scenario, should be initiated after obtaining blood cultures *(41)*. After isolation of the specific causative microorganism from blood cultures, the antibiotic regimen should be adapted based on the minimal inhibitory concentration (MIC) required for bactericidal effect. Clinical efficacy studies support the use of antibiotic regimens described in the AHA and ESC recommendations and according to the type of valve infected, native vs. prosthetic valve involvement, the infecting organism, and its susceptibility to penicillin *(20, 41)*.

The issue of anti-coagulation in patients with IE is controversial. There is no demonstrable benefit of anti-coagulation in native valve IE. In patients with prosthetic valve endocarditis, continuation of oral anti-coagulation or switching to intravenous heparin has been advocated by some experts, while others have recommended discontinuation of all anti-coagulation in patients with *S. aureus* endocarditis and recent stroke until completion of 2 weeks of antibiotic therapy *(45)*, presumably to avoid hemorrhagic transformation *(46)*. Regarding anti-platelet therapy with aspirin, no beneficial effect on outcome has been found, and aspirin therapy has been associated with a higher risk of bleeding complication in IE *(47, 48)*.

Surgical Treatment: Indications and Outcome

Surgical intervention may be performed either in the acute/active phase of IE or after the eradication of infection. Surgery during the active phase is generally considered for (1) those patients in whom the likelihood of cure of infection with antibiotic therapy alone is low or (2) those in whom severe complications of IE have or will likely occur. Surgery after eradication of infection is predominantly performed for adverse hemodynamic effects of valvular regurgitation that result from valve damage (Table 3).

In native valve endocarditis, heart failure due to valvular regurgitation, which often develops and progresses rapidly due to ongoing valvular damage and the lack of ventricular adaptation in the acute setting, is a primary indication for urgent surgical intervention. In the absence of overt heart failure symptoms, hemodynamic evidence of severe regurgitation (such as premature closure of the mitral valve in severe aortic regurgitation or pulmonary hypertension in severe mitral regurgitation) should also prompt surgical intervention since valvular regurgitation, or rarely stenosis, is a mechanical or structural complication of IE that will not improve with antimicrobial therapy alone. For mitral valve regurgitation, surgical repair of the native valve without replacement of the valve with a prosthesis has been reported in a number of case series *(49, 50)*. However, the role of repair has not been evaluated

Table 3
Indications for Surgical Intervention in IE

Class I recommendation
- Heart failure
- Aortic regurgitation or mitral regurgitation with evidence of elevated left ventricular end-diastolic or left atrial pressure
- Fungal endocarditis
- Highly resistant organism (including persistently positive blood cultures despite ≥1 week of appropriate antibiotic therapy)
- Echocardiographic evidence of valve perforation, rupture, fistula, or large perivalvular abscess
- Prosthetic valve infection with evidence of heart failure, worsening valvular stenosis or regurgitation, valve dehiscence, or abscess formation

Class IIa recommendation
- Recurrent embolic events with persistent vegetations despite appropriate antibiotic treatment

Class IIb recommendation
- Mobile, large (>10 mm) vegetation with or without emboli

Adapted from Bonow RO et al. *(114)*.

in controlled studies and its feasibility will be limited by the extent of infection and valvular damage and the experience of the surgical team.

Intra-cardiac complications of IE such as abscess formation, valve perforation, or other evidence of tissue penetration (e.g., intra-cardiac fistula formation) necessitate surgical treatment as well. Persistent bacteremia despite appropriate therapy, fungal endocarditis, and infection with highly resistant organisms, as characteristics that suggest a lower likelihood of cure by antimicrobial therapy alone, are accepted indications for surgery. Finally, surgery may be considered for conditions with which additional complications may occur. Left-sided vegetations larger than 10 mm pose an increased risk of systemic embolization *(51, 52)*. This risk is particularly prominent with the involvement of the mitral valve and when staphylococcus is the infecting organism *(53)*. Thus large (>10 mm) mobile vegetations, particularly on the anterior mitral valve leaflet or persistent vegetation after systemic embolization, are potential indications for surgical intervention in active IE.

With valve conservation and improved surgical techniques, the surgical mortality rates have declined over time with recent reported rates in the range of 7–14% *(54, 55)*. Perioperative mortality is largely related to patient age, comorbidities, left ventricular dysfunction, presence of prosthetic valve, infecting organism especially *S. aureus*, and the extent of intra-cardiac and extra-cardiac complications *(50, 49, 56)*. The optimal timing of surgery in the setting of active endocarditis has not been well evaluated. In patients with serious, life-threatening complications, surgery should be performed emergently. A number of case series have shown that surgery in the active phase of IE can be performed with acceptable risk and without an obvious risk of prosthetic valve infection *(57)*. In patients with less urgent indications for surgery (e.g., recurrent emboli or large, mobile vegetation) in whom surgery is being considered for the prevention of complications, it is not known whether earlier surgery may reduce complications to a greater extent or perhaps improve the likelihood of valve repair rather than replacement.

A major controversy regarding cardiac surgery in IE is the potential risk of neurologic deterioration caused by cardiopulmonary bypass in patients who have experienced a cerebrovascular complication. In a retrospective, multicenter series from Japan, neurologic worsening occurred in 44% of patients having cardiac surgery within 7 days of cerebral infarction, but only in 2% if surgery occurred after 28 days *(58)*. A more recent, prospective study included 63/109 (58%) patients who underwent surgery for

IE after a cerebrovascular complication (transient ischemic attack or stroke). Only four (6%) patients (all having had symptomatic stroke rather than TIA or asymptomatic cerebral embolism) had post-operative neurologic worsening *(59)*.

An understanding of outcomes with surgical treatment of endocarditis is influenced by the inherent selection bias and the lack of randomized, controlled trials for this therapy. Our understanding of the role and impact of surgery for IE has been derived from studies involving various retrospective observational cohorts for patients with complicated IE. To adjust for differences in clinical characteristics between patients treated with surgery and those treated with medical therapy alone, propensity modeling has been used for those differences that may also impact treatment outcome. One recent, retrospective study of 513 cases of complicated, left-sided endocarditis found that valve surgery was independently associated with reduced 6-month mortality (HR, 0.40; 95% CI, 0.18–0.91; $P = 0.03$) in propensity-matched sub-groups. Patients with moderate to severe heart failure appeared to derive the greatest benefit from surgery, whereas surgical treatment had a neutral effect on mortality for patients without heart failure (Fig. 3) *(60)*. Other factors which have been related to a survival benefit from surgery include patients with aortic valve disease and prosthetic endocarditis *(61)*. Whereas surgical therapy has been found to improve the survival of patients with complicated IE (e.g., associated with heart failure), its role for the treatment of lower risk patients is unclear. For example, in-hospital survival for patients with a low propensity for surgery but who underwent surgical treatment suggested a higher mortality than medical therapy alone *(15)*.

This differential effect of surgery on outcome depending on the presence or absence of complications may simply reflect that surgery, as for many other interventions in medicine, confers the greatest clinical benefit or absolute risk reduction for patients at highest risk, but demonstrating a benefit for patients at lower risk or all patients with endocarditis is more challenging. Along these lines, when propensity score adjustment is used to assess the effect of surgery on outcome of IE as compared to medical therapy alone, studies have shown differing results, including survival benefit *(60)*, neutral

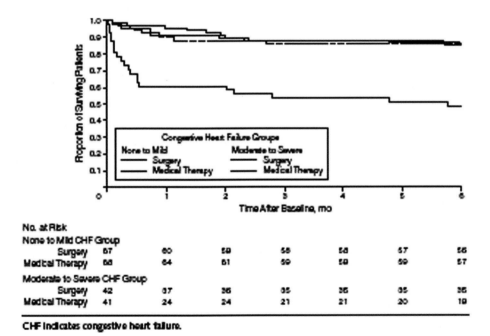

Fig. 3. Effect of surgery on 6-month survival in endocarditis complicated by heart failure (Reproduced with permission from Vikram et al. *(60)*.

effect *(15)*, and poorer survival *(62)* associated with surgery. These contrasting results likely reflect significant differences in the study cohorts, the clinical variables collected and included in the analyses, statistical methodologies, and the time points for the survival endpoint.

Complications and Outcome

In the absence of appropriate therapy, IE typically progresses to the development of various intra- and extra-cardiac complications. Cardiac complications are overwhelmingly common and affect up to 50% of patients *(63)*.

Heart failure or pulmonary edema is probably the most common complication, occurring in about one-third to one-half of patients with IE, as well as the deadliest complication and the most frequent indication for urgent surgery. Heart failure occurs as a result of valvular destruction and ensuing insufficiency, or in rare cases of large vegetations, as a result of valvular stenosis. Heart failure may result in the setting of moderate, rather than severe, regurgitation, particularly involving the aortic valve *(64)*, since the left ventricle is unable to compensate for the acute increase in preload and afterload in this condition. Heart failure is found to complicate aortic valve IE more frequently than mitral or tricuspid endocarditis.

The diagnosis of heart failure is subjective and most studies have not defined criteria for the presence or absence of heart failure, although validated criteria such as the Framingham criteria have been applied *(65)*. In addition to the clinical diagnosis of heart failure, echocardiography may be used to assess the severity of valvular regurgitation resulting from the infection as an early indicator of possible heart failure.

When heart failure occurs as a complication of IE, symptoms may be stabilized and improved acutely by supplemental oxygen, diuretic therapy, and the careful use of therapies for afterload reduction (thereby reducing the regurgitant volume). In the setting of severe mitral regurgitation, intra-aortic balloon pump may be employed for afterload reduction. Medical therapy alone is generally not sufficient for heart failure due to severe, acute aortic regurgitation, and intra-aortic balloon pump is contraindicated. Because acute aortic regurgitation is often progressive and poorly tolerated, delays in surgery to increase the duration of pre-operative antibiotic therapy may result in life-threatening pulmonary edema or cardiogenic shock and are generally discouraged *(41)*.

Spread of infection from valvular structures to the surrounding perivalvular tissue results in periannular complications that may place the patient at increased risk of adverse outcomes including heart failure and death. Intra-cardiac abscess complicates 30–40% cases of IE *(40)* and is a result of invasive infection that spreads generally along contiguous tissue planes, particularly with aortic valve infection. In the International Collaboration on Endocarditis (ICE) cohort, 22% cases of definite aortic valve IE were complicated by a periannular abscess *(66)*. These patients were more likely to have prosthetic valves and coagulase-negative staphylococcal infection. Abscess formation should be suspected in patients with persistent fever despite appropriate antibiotic therapy and those developing conduction abnormalities on the electrocardiogram. However, because the electrocardiogram is relatively insensitive for the diagnosis of an intra-cardiac abscess, transesophageal echocardiography is the diagnostic test-of-choice when an abscess is suspected clinically. An abscess is diagnosed by TEE as the visualization of a thickened area or mass with a heterogeneous echogenic or echolucent appearance *(40)*. Rarely, antibiotic therapy may be used to treat an intra-cardiac abscess, though this treatment is generally limited to patients who are poor surgical candidates. The vast majority of patients with an intra-cardiac abscess require cardiac surgery for debridement, as evidenced from a recent large study in which 86% of patients with periannular abscess underwent surgery *(66)*. In addition, surgery represents the gold standard for the diagnosis of abscess.

In rare cases, due to high systemic intravascular pressures and extension of intra-cardiac infection, these perivalvular cavities can form fistulous connections (aorto-atrial or aorto-ventricular), and even myocardial perforation. Fistula formation complicated endocarditis in 1.6% cases of native valve endocarditis and 3.5% cases of prosthetic valve endocarditis in a cohort of 4681 cases of IE. These occurred with similar frequency in the three sinuses of Valsalva and among all the cardiac chambers. Despite surgical intervention (87%), the mortality rate in this group of patients was 41% *(66)*. The development of cavitary fistulas thus heralds a poor outcome and must prompt surgical intervention.

Embolic phenomena frequently complicate the clinical course in endocarditis. Although clinical signs of embolization manifest in approximately one-third of patients with IE *(67)*, pathologic evidence of embolization has been found at much higher frequency in postmortem examinations. In the majority of cases, embolic events occur before the initiation of antibiotic therapy, whereas only 7% of events occur after treatment has begun *(52)*. In a subset of 66 patients with embolic complications among 178 patients with IE, the most frequent sites of embolic events were central nervous system (41%), lungs (18%), spleen (21%), peripheral artery (14%), and kidney (12%) *(68)*.

Factors including vegetation size, mobility, and location as well as the causative organism have been associated with the likelihood of embolic event. Vegetations larger than 10 mm in greatest diameter pose an increased risk of embolization *(51, 52)*. Causative organisms such as *S. aureus* and *S. bovis* confer an independent risk of embolization *(53)*. Similarly, there is a two to three times higher frequency of embolism in endocarditis caused by enterococci, Abiotrophia spp., fastidious gram-negative organisms (HACEK), and fungi as compared to streptococci *(69, 70)*. In addition to causing infarction of distal vascular beds, embolic events may result in metastatic sites of infection.

Cerebral embolization occurs in 10–35% and is at times complicated by meningitis, brain abscess, or intra-cerebral hemorrhage. In the ICE cohort, stroke complicated endocarditis in 15% of patients *(71)*. The risk of stroke dramatically decreases with initiation of antibiotic therapy, with a 65% reduction in stroke incidence by the second week of antimicrobial therapy *(71)*.

Given the low incidence of embolic event after initiation of antibiotic therapy, routine screening for emboli in patients with IE is not recommended. However, patients with persistent fever or bacteremia or localizing symptoms of possible infarction (e.g., focal neurologic deficit suggestive of cerebrovascular infarction, pleuritic chest pain suggestive of pulmonary infarction, left upper quadrant pain suggestive of splenic infarction) should undergo computed tomographic imaging with radiographic contrast for the diagnosis of embolic complications.

Embolic events have been found to be an independent predictor of in-hospital death in endocarditis *(65)*. In patients who experience recurrent embolic events, particularly if occurring after initiation of antibiotic therapy, surgical treatment is indicated. For the prevention of embolic events, surgery may be considered for patients with endocarditis who have large (greater than 10 mm), mobile vegetations, especially with involvement of left-sided heart valves. The greatest benefit of surgery to prevent additional emboli may be evident early in the treatment of endocarditis since the risk of embolization rapidly declines within 2 weeks of antibiotic therapy *(20)*.

Persistent bacteremia is a recognized complication which represents failure of antibiotic therapy. Importantly, patients with *S. aureus* may remain febrile for up to 2 weeks. All patients should have surveillance blood cultures obtained several days after initiation of antibiotic therapy to ensure that antimicrobial therapy is effective. Prolonged fever or recurrence of fever needs further evaluation as to whether the antibiotics are ineffective (persistent bacteremia), an abscess or metastatic site of infection has developed, or that a reaction to antibiotic therapy is the cause.

Mortality in Native Valve Endocarditis

Estimates of mortality rates for native valve endocarditis vary. Wallace et al. in their cohort of 208 patients noted an overall in-hospital mortality of 18% and a 6-month mortality of 27% *(72)*. Another recent study observed a similar 6-month mortality of 26% *(73)*. Such unacceptably high mortality rates despite therapeutic and diagnostic advances have prompted risk stratification of patients with IE

Among host factors, age, female sex, presence of diabetes mellitus, APACHE II score, elevated white blood cell count, serum creatinine level >2 mg/dL, and lower serum albumin have been associated with poor outcomes *(65, 72)*. Moderate to severe congestive heart failure, periannular abscess formation, vegetation length >10 mm, absence of surgical therapy, and infection with virulent organisms particularly *S. aureus* are disease factors related to embolic events and death *(72, 74, 75)*.

Recently, a prognostic classification system for mortality in left-sided IE consisting of five variables has been developed and validated. Abnormal mental status, Charlson comorbidity scale score ≥2, moderate–severe congestive heart failure, bacterial etiology other than *S. viridans* (particularly *S. aureus* and enterococcus), and medical therapy without valve surgery were associated with 6-month mortality in this retrospective cohort of 513 cases of IE. These five baseline predictive features were assigned point scores, and based on the scoring system, patients in the derivation cohort were classified into four groups with increasing risk for 6-month mortality: 5, 15, 31, and 59% ($P < 0.001$). In the validation cohort, a similar risk among the four groups was observed: 7, 19, 32, and 69% ($P < 0.001$) *(73)*.

PROSTHETIC VALVE ENDOCARDITIS

Epidemiology and Prevention

The first successful surgical replacements of cardiac valves in humans were performed in 1960 *(76–78)*. In 1963, Geraci et al. reported one of the first series of patients with infection of a valve prosthesis or prosthetic valve endocarditis (PVE) *(79)*. Since its early description, PVE, in addition to other potential complications such as prosthetic valve dysfunction, degeneration, and thromboembolism, has been recognized as an important clinical concern after valve replacement therapy. Despite major advances in the understanding of its pathogenesis, diagnosis, and treatment, this complication of valve surgery continues to have rates of morbidity and mortality in the contemporary era *(80)*.

PVE occurs at an overall rate of approximately 1% per year after prosthetic valve implantation *(81–83)*. PVE is classically differentiated as occurring "early" or "late" after valve implantation. This temporal classification is based on studies demonstrating marked differences in microbiologic causes of early and late PVEs *(84)*. Initial descriptions of early PVE utilized a definition of 60 days or less *(84)*. In these reports, early PVE accounted for approximately 30% of all PVE cases *(84)* and was predominantly caused by *S. aureus*, gram-negative bacilli, and coagulase-negative staphylococci.

In addition to infection of the prosthetic valve in the perioperative period as a cause of PVE, other risk factors for PVE have been described. Ivert et al. described 53 cases of PVE among 1465 consecutive patients undergoing prosthetic valve replacement in 1974–1979 and found that male gender, black race, antecedent native valve endocarditis, mechanical prosthesis (compared to biologic prosthesis in the initial 6 months after surgery), and prolonged cardiopulmonary bypass time were associated with PVE *(82)*. Active endocarditis at the time of valve replacement was similarly found to be associated with PVE in the Veterans Affairs Cooperative Study on Valvular Heart Disease (66 PVE cases in 1032 patients, 1977–1982), but type of valve prosthesis was not associated with PVE *(83)*. In another study of 116 cases of PVE among 2608 patients who underwent prosthetic valve replacement at a single center (1975–1982), mechanical prostheses had a higher rate of PVE development than biologic prostheses in the initial few months after implantation, but the rate of infection was not different at 5 years *(81)*. Multiple valve replacements were also associated with PVE, as was male gender among those patients undergoing aortic valve replacement *(81)*.

Recent studies have suggested a relationship between health care contact, bacteremia, and subsequent PVE *(80, 85)*. Intravascular catheters or devices and skin infections or wounds, were significant predisposing factors for PVE *(80, 85)*. Furthermore, these studies have suggested that PVE associated with health care contact was more likely to occur in the few months after valve implantation *(80, 85)*.

In 1963, Geraci et al. reported a 10% incidence of staphylococcal PVE in patients who had received no perioperative antibiotic therapy *(79)*. A subsequent cohort study from the same institution, including

4586 patients who received prophylactic antimicrobial therapy before and after valve replacement surgery, found that the incidence of PVE was 0.98% *(84)*. Short-term (2–3 days), perioperative, prophylaxis at the time of coronary artery bypass surgery with cephalosporin-based therapy has been shown to reduce the risk of wound infection but has an inconclusive effect on the rate of PVE *(86)*, likely related to the low incidence of PVE and underpowered studies.

Although prophylactic antibiotic therapy aimed primarily at reducing staphylococcal infection is now routinely used at the time of prosthetic valve implantation, few studies have evaluated prophylactic measures against the development of PVE. More broadly, only a few randomized, controlled trials have shown that systemic antibiotic prophylaxis significantly reduced the rate of infection of surgical implants *(87)*. For example, perioperative administration of anti-staphylococcal antibiotics has been found to reduce the rate of permanent pacemaker infection in a meta-analysis of seven small trials, although no single randomized study found evidence of benefit *(88)*. There are no prospective data comparing the efficacy of specific classes of antibiotic therapy, but the use of vancomycin for systemic prophylaxis is common given the increasing prevalence of methicillin-resistant staphylococcal species.

Antibiotic treatment of the prosthetic valve itself has been proposed to reduce the incidence of early PVE. Immersion of prosthetic valves into an antibiotic solution was found to reduce the incidence of early PVE in one non-randomized study *(89)*. Antimicrobial coating of the prosthetic valve with a silver alloy for the prevention of PVE was studied recently in a large, randomized trial *(90)*. However, after enrollment of 807 patients, or 18% of the estimated sample size, this trial was terminated due to a significantly higher rate of major paravalvular leakage *(91)*. Finally, given the association between intravascular catheters, bacteremia, and PVE, judicious use and care of these devices to prevent catheter-related infections are recommended in patients with prosthetic valves *(92)*.

Because the presence of a prosthetic heart valve is a predisposition to the development of endocarditis, antibiotic therapy, or prophylaxis, at the time of health-care-related procedures has been a mainstay of care of the patient with a prosthetic valve. However, prophylaxis is recommended only for patients with prosthetic heart valves prior to dental procedures, but not before gastrointestinal or genitourinary procedures *(9)*.

Pathogenesis and Microbiology

The pathogenesis of PVE is generally dependent on a series of events: bacterial adherence to the prosthetic valve, bacterial persistence and maturation of the vegetation, and tissue invasion *(4)*. Characteristics of the microorganisms, specifically the ability of organisms to adhere to the valve and resist host defenses, are important influences on the development of PVE. In addition, the ability of certain bacteria to form biofilm may contribute to poorer clearance of infection even with appropriate antibiotic therapy.

In addition, the pathogenesis of PVE may be dependent on the type of valve prosthesis. As discussed above, a number of studies have reported a higher incidence of PVE after mechanical valve replacement than biologic valve replacement in the initial few months after implantation. Although mechanical prostheses, made from materials such as pyrolytic carbon, do not allow adherence of microorganisms in the absence of thrombus, the sewing cuff or ring is a likely site of infection *(93)*, which may be more likely to occur before endothelialization after insertion. In support of this hypothesis, mechanical valves have been found to have a higher rate of PVE in the initial few months after insertion *(81, 82)* and commonly develop annular abscesses. Infection of bioprosthetic valves is often restricted to the cusps (Fig. 4), as in native valve IE, and, in comparison to mechanical prostheses, there is evidence of a delay in occurrence of PVE after implantation *(81, 82)*.

In contrast to previous studies which found coagulase-negative staphylococci to be the predominant cause of PVE *(81, 82, 94)*, a recent, large, contemporary study of PVE has found *S. aureus* to be the most frequent organism (23%), followed by coagulase-negative staphylococci (16%), enterococci

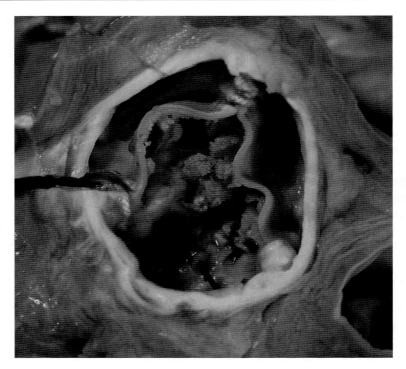

Fig. 4. Infection of a biologic prosthetic valve with multiple vegetations on valve leaflets and cusps (Courtesy of the Department of Pathology, Duke University Medical Center).

(13%), and viridans streptococci (12%) *(80)*. Although this change in pathogenesis may be influenced by referral bias to tertiary centers, the high prevalence of *S. aureus* PVE more likely represents the increase in health-care-associated infection as well as community-acquired *S. aureus* infections. In recent studies of IE, health-care-associated infection, including both nosocomial and non-nosocomial sources, was associated with *S. aureus* native *(5)* and prosthetic valve endocarditis *(80)*.

Health-care-associated infection in PVE has classically been described in the setting of PVE occurring soon after prosthetic valve implantation. In 1975, Wilson et al. described the Mayo Clinic experience with PVE from 1963 to 1974 in 45 patients. These investigators empirically differentiated between "early" (within 2 months post-operatively) and "late" onset infection (after 2 months). Using this classification, 36% of patients had early PVE, with the majority of early cases caused by *S. aureus* (44%) or gram-negative bacilli (37%). Among late PVE (64% of the cohort), streptococcal infection was the predominant cause (51%, including both viridans and group D streptococci), followed by gram-negative bacilli in 31%. In a later review *(94)* involving four separate studies of PVE (*n* = 184) *(94–97)*, the leading causes of PVE were coagulase-negative staphylococci (overall 24%, early 27%), gram-negative bacilli (overall 16%, early 19%), *S. aureus* (overall 15%, early 21%), and viridans streptococci (overall 18%, early 4%).

In 1985, Calderwood et al. reported on the incidence of PVE among 2608 patients who underwent valve replacement therapy and were followed for a mean duration of 40 months *(81)*. The results of this study showed that the rate of PVE development was greatest in the first year after prosthesis implantation *(81)*. In addition, the distribution of causative organisms was similar in patients with onset of infection within 2 months of surgery and between 2 and 12 months after surgery, and specifically coagulase-negative staphylococci caused 58% of PVE during the initial 2 months and 57% of PVE during the initial 12 months after surgery *(81)*. More recently, in a study of 172 patients with PVE, no differences in the microbiological profile of PVE occurring within 2 and 2–12 months were confirmed *(98)*. In comparison to the initial 12 months after implantation, PVE after 12 months was associated with a lower rate of staphylococcal infection (37 vs. 18%, respectively, $P = 0.005$) *(98)*. These microbiologic results, in conjunction with other results regarding health-care-associated PVE *(80)*, support conclusions that PVE within the initial 12 months after prosthetic valve implantation is more likely to be due to health care contact or exposure.

Diagnosis

The clinical presentation of PVE is similar to that of native valve endocarditis *(99)*, and fever and chills are the predominant symptoms in patients with PVE *(84, 94, 98, 100, 101)*. Given the high prevalence of *S. aureus* PVE, patients with PVE often have an acute presentation with fulminant symptoms, particularly in early PVE *(101)*. A new regurgitant murmur has been described in approximately 40–50% of patients with PVE *(84, 100)*. Heart failure symptoms occur in approximately one-third of PVE cases *(80)*, although the prevalence may be influenced by qualitative diagnostic findings and by the patients' underlying cardiac condition for which valve replacement was originally performed. Peripheral cutaneous manifestations of IE, including petechiae, Osler nodes, and Janeway lesions, are found in the minority of patients with PVE *(84, 100)*.

In the setting of a febrile illness in a patient with a prosthetic heart valve, blood cultures drawn from more than one peripheral venous site before the initiation of antibiotic therapy are the mainstay in the diagnosis of PVE. Bacteremia in IE is generally continuous, and the majority of patients with PVE have bacterial growth in multiple blood cultures. Culture-negative PVE may be more common soon after prosthetic valve implantation *(80)*, possibly related to routine perioperative antibiotic use.

Transesophageal echocardiography (TEE) is a necessary diagnostic tool in suspected PVE. The improved sensitivity of TEE compared to transthoracic echocardiography is marked in patients with prosthetic valves *(99, 102)* and apparent regardless of type or location of the prosthetic valve *(103)*. In addition to the presence of vegetations, which are found in 73% of PVE cases *(80)*, transesophageal, in comparison to transthoracic, echocardiography is more sensitive for the detection of prosthetic valve dysfunction *(104)* and for complications of PVE, particularly paravalvular regurgitation and intra-cardiac abscess *(40)*. These complications, which will also be discussed in the next section, are frequent sequelae of PVE that are prognostically significant and may influence therapeutic decision making in PVE *(80, 105)*. Because the anatomic findings of PVE may evolve or change during the index hospitalization, repeat TEE may be clinically useful in patients who initially do not meet criteria for definite PVE and in patients whom new complications of PVE are suspected, since these findings are likely to alter the treatment of the patient.

The Duke criteria *(30)* and the modified Duke criteria *(34)* for the diagnosis of IE have incorporated echocardiographic findings to enhance the sensitivity for identifying clinically definite cases of IE compared to other criteria (e.g., Beth Israel criteria). These criteria specify the visualization of an endocardial vegetation, periannular abscess, or new dehiscence of a prosthetic valve as major criteria for the diagnosis of IE. Furthermore, the modified Duke criteria, revised in 2000 to address limitations in the original criteria published in 1994, specifies transesophageal echocardiography as the diagnostic test-of-choice for suspected PVE *(34)*.

The sensitivity and specificity of these criteria have been evaluated in nearly 2000 patients with suspected IE in multiple cohorts and found to offer increased sensitivity compared to other, earlier diagnostic criteria *(20)*. However, few studies have evaluated the Duke criteria specifically in patients with suspected PVE. In 2000, the Duke and von Reyn *(29)* criteria were compared in a retrospective cohort of 76 surgically confirmed episodes of PVE *(100)*. In this study, the Duke criteria were found to be significantly more sensitive than the von Reyn criteria *(100)*. The Duke criteria classified 60/76

(79%) episodes as "definite" and 15 (20%) episodes as "possible" endocarditis compared to 36/76 (47%) episodes as "probable" and 24 (32%) as "possible" endocarditis *(100)*. Furthermore, application of the Duke criteria rejected only 1 episode of PVE, compared to 16 episodes by von Reyn criteria *(100)*.

In patients with a prosthetic heart valve and bacteremia, particularly staphylococcal bacteremia, a low threshold for performing TEE should therefore be maintained. Data from the Cleveland Clinic demonstrated that although the rate of bacteremia within 60 days of cardiac valve surgery was low (3%), 24% of these patients with early bacteremia, particularly in multiple blood cultures, were diagnosed with PVE *(106)*. Similarly, in another study of 51 patients with prosthetic heart valves and *S. aureus* bacteremia, PVE was diagnosed in 26 (51%) patients, with a similar percentage of PVE diagnosed before and after 12 months since valve implantation *(107)*.

Clinical Management of PVE and Its Potential Complications

Given the preponderance of staphylococcal and streptococcal infection in PVE, patients with suspected PVE should be treated with intravenous antibiotic therapy that is active against these species. In the setting of early or possible health-care-associated PVE, associated with a higher likelihood of penicillin-resistant staphylococcal infection, empiric treatment with vancomycin, rifampin, and gentamicin may be preferable until results of blood cultures and antibiotic susceptibility testing are available. When these microbiology results are determined, adjustment of the empiric antibiotic therapy may be required to maintain a bactericidal regimen for at least 6 weeks. High concentrations of antibiotic in the serum are required for diffusion into the vegetations, and long-term treatment is necessary to kill dormant bacteria *(4)*. Because the combination of antimicrobial agents is tailored to the culture and susceptibility results, specific recommendations for treatment will not be discussed but are available in a recent scientific statement from the American Heart Association *(20)*.

Close clinical assessments of the patient with PVE will typically guide additional diagnostic testing for complications of PVE, such as embolization, periannular extension of infection, sites of disseminated infection, and mycotic aneurysms. After the diagnosis of PVE, repeat TEE may be highly sensitive and useful to diagnose complications such as prosthetic valve dysfunction (regurgitation or stenosis), resultant changes in ventricular function or dilation, periannular extension of infection (intra-cardiac abscess or fistula formation), or involvement of other valves.

Because of difficulty in eradicating infection from prosthetic materials, all cases of prosthetic valve endocarditis should receive surgical consultation. Similar to the recommendations for native valve endocarditis, prosthetic valve endocarditis with evidence of heart failure, valve dehiscence, heart failure, increasing valve obstruction or regurgitation, or intra-cardiac complications are reasons to pursue surgical intervention. In addition, prosthetic valve endocarditis associated with persistent bacteremia, relapsing infection, or recurrent emboli despite appropriate antibiotic treatment may benefit from surgery.

Periannular infection is more common in PVE than native valve endocarditis, occurring in over 50% of patients *(108)*, because infection of a prosthetic valve generally involves the annulus or sewing cuff of the valve as opposed to the valve leaflets. Clinical signs, including persistent fever or bacteremia, heart failure, or new or changing regurgitant murmur, may suggest the presence of periannular extension. Electrocardiographic evidence of new atrioventricular block is an insensitive (45%) but specific marker of abscess formation *(109)*.

In addition to TEE, other imaging modalities may be utilized when clinical suspicion for remote complications of PVE is present. Complications such as emboli to the central nervous system, spleen, or kidneys or the development of intracranial mycotic aneurysms may be diagnosed by computed tomography or magnetic resonance imaging with contrast administration. Systemic embolization is a common complication in PVE, including stroke in 18% and other systemic embolization in 14% of cases *(80)*. The risk of embolization after initiation of antibiotic therapy declines, and the risk of new embolism after antibiotic therapy has not been found to be related to prosthetic valve type or location *(53)*. Although characteristics of the vegetation, namely length and mobility, have been associated with a higher risk of new embolic events, this association was not present for patients with PVE *(52)*.

In general, surgery for PVE is recommended for complications that are associated with higher mortality in PVE *(110)*:

- Heart failure
- Dehiscence of prosthetic valve
- Increasing valve dysfunction
- Periannular extension or abscess formation
- Persistent bacteremia or recurrent emboli despite appropriate antibiotic therapy

Outcome

In early series of PVE, the in-hospital mortality rates were approximately 50–60% *(84)*. In comparison, the contemporary in-hospital mortality rate was recently reported to be 23% in a large, multinational study *(80)*. Although this reduction in mortality represents a significant improvement in outcome, possibly related to earlier diagnosis and improvements in medical and surgical therapies, the mortality rate remains significant.

Because of the low incidence of PVE and limitations of previous studies to single center experiences, few studies have had adequate sample size to assess characteristics associated with higher mortality. In many early studies, PVE occurring within 60 days of valve implantation was significantly higher (>60%) than late PVE *(84, 96)*. However, more recent studies have found that long-term survival after the active phase of infection was similar for early and late PVEs (74 and 82% survival at 4 year follow-up) *(111)*.

In 1994, the Veterans Affairs Cooperative Study on Valvular Heart Disease reported that among 66 patients with PVE, baseline heart failure severity was the only predictor of death *(83)*. More recently, results of the International Collaboration on Endocarditis – Prospective Cohort Study (ICE – PCS) evaluated predictors of in-hospital mortality among 556 patients with definite PVE (Table 4) *(80)*. These results confirm that complications of heart failure, persistent bacteremia, abscess, and stroke are important, independent prognostic factors in PVE.

Table 4
Predictors of In-Hospital Mortality in PVE

Variable		Adjusted OR	95% CI
Age, years			
	<65	1 (Reference age group)	
	65–75	1.82	1.09–3.03
	>75	3.73	2.10–6.61
Health-care-associated infection		1.62	1.08–2.44
S. aureus		1.73	1.01–2.95
Persistent bacteremia		4.29	1.99–9.22
Congestive heart failure		2.33	1.62–3.34
Intra-cardiac abscess		1.86	1.10–3.15
Stroke		2.25	1.25–4.03

Adapted from Wang et al. *(80)*.

Recent guidelines support or recommend the use of surgery for PVE associated with these complications *(110)*. However, these recommendations have been based on observational studies of PVE, in which selection and treatment biases likely exist regarding the use of surgery. No randomized studies of surgery for IE have been performed, and many question whether such a trial would be ethical. In order to assess the effect of surgery on outcome of PVE, statistical adjustment for those clinical characteristics associated with surgical intervention can be performed using propensity analysis. In a large, retrospective, merged dataset of patients with PVE, surgery use was found to be associated with younger age, abscess, heart failure, and staphylococcal infection *(105)*. After propensity matching of 136/355 PVE patients (68 treated with antibiotic therapy alone and 68 treated with antibiotic therapy and surgery), only central nervous system emboli (OR, 11.1; 95% CI, 4.2–29.7) and *S. aureus* (OR, 3.7; 95% CI, 1.4–9.7), but not surgery (OR, 0.6; 95% CI, 0.2–1.4), were associated with in-hospital mortality *(105)*.

REFERENCES

1. Berlin JA, Abrutyn E, Strom BL, et al. Incidence of infective endocarditis in the Delaware Valley, 1988–1990. Am J Cardiol 1995;76(12):933–6.
2. Hoen B, Alla F, Selton-Suty C, et al. Changing profile of infective endocarditis: results of a 1-year survey in France. JAMA 2002;288(1):75–81.
3. Hogevik H, Olaison L, Andersson R, Lindberg J, Alestig K. Epidemiologic aspects of infective endocarditis in an urban population. A 5-year prospective study. Medicine (Baltimore) 1995;74(6):324–39.
4. Moreillon P, Que YA. Infective endocarditis. Lancet 2004;363(9403):139–49.
5. Fowler VG, Jr., Miro JM, Hoen B, et al. Staphylococcus aureus endocarditis: a consequence of medical progress. JAMA 2005;293(24):3012–21.
6. Friedman N, Kaye K, Stout J, et al. Health care-associated blood stream infections in adults: a reason to change the accepted definition of community-acquired infections. Ann Intern Med 2002;137:791–7.
7. Strom BL, Abrutyn E, Berlin JA, et al. Risk factors for infective endocarditis: oral hygiene and nondental exposures. Circulation 2000;102(23):2842–8.
8. Nishimura RA, Carabello BA, Faxon DP, et al. ACC/AHA 2008 guideline update on valvular heart disease: focused update on infective endocarditis: a report of the American College of Cardiology/American Heart Association Task Force on Practice Guidelines endorsed by the Society of Cardiovascular Anesthesiologists, Society for Cardiovascular Angiography and Interventions, and Society of Thoracic Surgeons. Catheter Cardiovasc Interv 2008;72(3): E1–12.
9. Wilson W, Taubert KA, Gewitz M, et al. Prevention of infective endocarditis. Guidelines from the American Heart Association. A Guideline From the American Heart Association Rheumatic Fever, Endocarditis, and Kawasaki Disease Committee, Council on Cardiovascular Disease in the Young, and the Council on Clinical Cardiology, Council on Cardiovascular Surgery and Anesthesia, and the Quality of Care and Outcomes Research Interdisciplinary Working Group. Circulation 2007:CIRCULATIONAHA.106.183095.
10. McKinsey DS, Ratts TE, Bisno AL. Underlying cardiac lesions in adults with infective endocarditis. The changing spectrum. Am J Med 1987;82(4):681–8.
11. Robard S. Blood velocity and endocarditis. Circulation 1963;22:18.
12. Moreillon P, Que YA, Bayer AS. Pathogenesis of streptococcal and staphylococcal endocarditis. Infect Dis Clin North Am 2002;16(2):297–318.
13. Vuille C, Nidorf M, Weyman AE, Picard MH. Natural history of vegetations during successful medical treatment of endocarditis. Am Heart J 1994;128(6 Pt 1):1200–9.
14. Tleyjeh IM, Steckelberg JM, Murad HS, et al. Temporal trends in infective endocarditis: a population-based study in Olmsted County, Minnesota. JAMA 2005;293(24):3022–8.
15. Cabell CH, Abrutyn E, Fowler VG, Jr., et al. Use of surgery in patients with native valve infective endocarditis: results from the International Collaboration on Endocarditis Merged Database. Am Heart J 2005;150(5):1092–8.
16. Fernandez-Hidalgo N, Almirante B, Tornos P, et al. Contemporary epidemiology and prognosis of health care-associated infective endocarditis. Clin Infect Dis 2008 Nov 15;47(10):1287–97.
17. Fowler VG, Jr., Olsen MK, Corey GR, et al. Clinical identifiers of complicated Staphylococcus aureus bacteremia. Arch Intern Med 2003;163(17):2066–72.
18. Chu VH, Woods CW, Miro JM, et al. Emergence of coagulase-negative staphylococci as a cause of native valve endocarditis. Clin Infect Dis 2008;46(2):232–42.

19. Anguera I, Del Rio A, Miro JM, et al. Staphylococcus lugdunensis infective endocarditis: description of 10 cases and analysis of native valve, prosthetic valve, and pacemaker lead endocarditis clinical profiles. Heart 2005; 91(2):e10.

20. Baddour LM, Wilson WR, Bayer AS, et al. Infective endocarditis: diagnosis, antimicrobial therapy, and management of complications: a statement for healthcare professionals from the Committee on Rheumatic Fever, Endocarditis, and Kawasaki Disease, Council on Cardiovascular Disease in the Young, and the Councils on Clinical Cardiology, Stroke, and Cardiovascular Surgery and Anesthesia, American Heart Association: endorsed by the Infectious Diseases Society of America. Circulation 2005;111(23):e394–434.

21. Ellner JJ, Rosenthal MS, Lerner PI, McHenry MC. Infective endocarditis caused by slow-growing, fastidious, Gram-negative bacteria. Medicine (Baltimore) 1979;58(2):145–58.

22. Pierrotti LC, Baddour LM. Fungal endocarditis, 1995–2000. Chest 2002;122(1):302–10.

23. Baddley JW, Benjamin DK, Jr., Patel M, et al. Candida infective endocarditis. Eur J Clin Microbiol Infect Dis 2008;27(7):519–29.

24. Marrie TJ, Raoult D. Update on Q fever, including Q fever endocarditis. Curr Clin Top Infect Dis 2002;22:97–124.

25. Hoen B, Selton-Suty C, Lacassin F, et al. Infective endocarditis in patients with negative blood cultures: analysis of 88 cases from a one-year nationwide survey in France. Clin Infect Dis 1995;20(3):501–6.

26. Tunkel AR, Kaye D. Endocarditis with negative blood cultures. N Engl J Med 1992;326(18):1215–7.

27. Bashore TM, Cabell C, Fowler V, Jr. Update on infective endocarditis. Curr Probl Cardiol 2006;31(4):274–352.

28. Pelletier LL, Jr., Petersdorf RG. Infective endocarditis: a review of 125 cases from the University of Washington Hospitals, 1963–72. Medicine (Baltimore) 1977;56(4):287–313.

29. Von Reyn CF, Levy BS, Arbeit RD, Friedland G, Crumpacker CS. Infective endocarditis: an analysis based on strict case definitions. Ann Intern Med 1981;94(4 pt 1):505–18.

30. Durack DT, Lukes AS, Bright DK. New criteria for diagnosis of infective endocarditis: utilization of specific echocardiographic findings. Duke Endocarditis Service. Am J Med 1994;96(3):200–9.

31. Cecchi E, Parrini I, Chinaglia A, et al. New diagnostic criteria for infective endocarditis. A study of sensitivity and specificity. Eur Heart J 1997;18(7):1149–56.

32. Hoen B, Beguinot I, Rabaud C, et al. The Duke criteria for diagnosing infective endocarditis are specific: analysis of 100 patients with acute fever or fever of unknown origin. Clin Infect Dis 1996;23(2):298–302.

33. Olaison L, Hogevik H. Comparison of the von Reyn and Duke criteria for the diagnosis of infective endocarditis: a critical analysis of 161 episodes. Scand J Infect Dis 1996;28(4):399–406.

34. Li JS, Sexton DJ, Mick N, et al. Proposed modifications to the Duke criteria for the diagnosis of infective endocarditis. Clin Infect Dis 2000;30(4):633–8.

35. Pedersen WR, Walker M, Olson JD, et al. Value of transesophageal echocardiography as an adjunct to transthoracic echocardiography in evaluation of native and prosthetic valve endocarditis. Chest 1991;100(2):351–6.

36. Bayer AS, Bolger AF, Taubert KA, et al. Diagnosis and management of infective endocarditis and its complications. Circulation 1998;98(25):2936–48.

37. Greaves K, Mou D, Patel A, Celermajer DS. Clinical criteria and the appropriate use of transthoracic echocardiography for the exclusion of infective endocarditis. Heart 2003;89(3):273–5.

38. Heidenreich PA, Masoudi FA, Maini B, et al. Echocardiography in patients with suspected endocarditis: a cost-effectiveness analysis. Am J Med 1999;107(3):198–208.

39. Rosen AB, Fowler VG, Jr., Corey GR, et al. Cost-effectiveness of transesophageal echocardiography to determine the duration of therapy for intravascular catheter-associated Staphylococcus aureus bacteremia. Ann Intern Med 1999;130(10):810–20.

40. Daniel WG, Mugge A, Martin RP, et al. Improvement in the diagnosis of abscesses associated with endocarditis by transesophageal echocardiography. N Engl J Med 1991;324(12):795–800.

41. Horstkotte D, Follath F, Gutschik E, et al. Guidelines on prevention, diagnosis and treatment of infective endocarditis executive summary; the task force on infective endocarditis of the European society of cardiology. Eur Heart J 2004;25(3):267–76.

42. Durack DT, Beeson PB. Experimental bacterial endocarditis. II. Survival of a bacteria in endocardial vegetations. Br J Exp Pathol 1972;53(1):50–3.

43. Hamburger M, Stein L. Streptococcus viridans subacute bacterial endocarditis; two week treatment schedule with penicillin. J Am Med Assoc 1952;149(6):542–5.

44. Korzeniowski O, Sande MA. Combination antimicrobial therapy for Staphylococcus aureus endocarditis in patients addicted to parenteral drugs and in nonaddicts: a prospective study. Ann Intern Med 1982;97(4):496–503.

45. Tornos P, Almirante B, Mirabet S, Permanyer G, Pahissa A, Soler-Soler J. Infective endocarditis due to Staphylococcus aureus: deleterious effect of anticoagulant therapy. Arch Intern Med 1999;159(5):473–5.

46. Salem DN, Daudelin HD, Levine HJ, Pauker SG, Eckman MH, Riff J. Antithrombotic therapy in valvular heart disease. Chest 2001;119(1 Suppl):207S–19S.

47. Anavekar NS, Tleyjeh IM, Anavekar NS, et al. Impact of prior antiplatelet therapy on risk of embolism in infective endocarditis. Clin Infect Dis 2007;44(9):1180–6.

48. Chan KL, Dumesnil JG, Cujec B, et al. A randomized trial of aspirin on the risk of embolic events in patients with infective endocarditis. J Am Coll Cardiol 2003;42(5):775–80.

49. Doukas G, Oc M, Alexiou C, Sosnowski AW, Samani NJ, Spyt TJ. Mitral valve repair for active culture positive infective endocarditis. Heart 2006;92(3):361–3.

50. Feringa HH, Shaw LJ, Poldermans D, et al. Mitral valve repair and replacement in endocarditis: a systematic review of literature. Ann Thorac Surg 2007;83(2):564–70.

51. Tischler MD, Vaitkus PT. The ability of vegetation size on echocardiography to predict clinical complications: a meta-analysis. J Am Soc Echocardiogr 1997;10(5):562–8.

52. Thuny F, Di Salvo G, Belliard O, et al. Risk of embolism and death in infective endocarditis: prognostic value of echocardiography: a prospective multicenter study. Circulation 2005;112(1):69–75.

53. Vilacosta I, Graupner C, San Roman JA, et al. Risk of embolization after institution of antibiotic therapy for infective endocarditis. J Am Coll Cardiol 2002;39(9):1489–95.

54. d'Udekem Y, David TE, Feindel CM, Armstrong S, Sun Z. Long-term results of surgery for active infective endocarditis. Eur J Cardiothorac Surg 1997;11(1):46–52.

55. Jassal DS, Hassan A, Buth KJ, Neilan TG, Koilpillai C, Hirsch GM. Surgical management of infective endocarditis. J Heart Valve Dis 2006;15(1):115–21.

56. Amrani M, Schoevaerdts JC, Rubay J, et al. Surgical treatment for acute native aortic valvular infective endocarditis: long-term follow-up. Cardiovasc Surg 1995;3(6):579–81.

57. Guerra JM, Tornos MP, Permanyer-Miralda G, Almirante B, Murtra M, Soler-Soler J. Long term results of mechanical prostheses for treatment of active infective endocarditis. Heart 2001;86(1):63–8.

58. Eishi K, Kawazoe K, Kuriyama Y, Kitoh Y, Kawashima Y, Omae T. Surgical management of infective endocarditis associated with cerebral complications. Multi-center retrospective study in Japan. J Thorac Cardiovasc Surg 1995;110(6):1745–55.

59. Thuny F, Avierinos JF, Tribouilloy C, et al. Impact of cerebrovascular complications on mortality and neurologic outcome during infective endocarditis: a prospective multicentre study. Eur Heart J 2007;28(9):1155–61.

60. Vikram HR, Buenconsejo J, Hasbun R, Quagliarello VJ. Impact of valve surgery on 6-month mortality in adults with complicated, left-sided native valve endocarditis: a propensity analysis. JAMA 2003;290(24):3207–14.

61. Vlessis AA, Hovaguimian H, Jaggers J, Ahmad A, Starr A. Infective endocarditis: ten-year review of medical and surgical therapy. Ann Thorac Surg 1996;61(4):1217–22.

62. Tleyjeh IM, Ghomrawi HM, Steckelberg JM, et al. The impact of valve surgery on 6-month mortality in left-sided infective endocarditis. Circulation 2007;115(13):1721–8.

63. Mansur AJ, Grinberg M, da Luz PL, Bellotti G. The complications of infective endocarditis. A reappraisal in the 1980s. Arch Intern Med 1992;152(12):2428–32.

64. Sexton DJ, Spelman D. Current best practices and guidelines. Assessment and management of complications in infective endocarditis. Cardiol Clin 2003;21(2):273–82, vii–viii.

65. Chu VH, Cabell CH, Benjamin DK, Jr., et al. Early predictors of in-hospital death in infective endocarditis. Circulation 2004;109(14):1745–9.

66. Anguera I, Miro JM, San Roman JA, et al. Periannular complications in infective endocarditis involving prosthetic aortic valves. Am J Cardiol 2006;98(9):1261–8.

67. De Castro S, Magni G, Beni S, et al. Role of transthoracic and transesophageal echocardiography in predicting embolic events in patients with active infective endocarditis involving native cardiac valves. Am J Cardiol 1997;80(8):1030–4.

68. Di Salvo G, Habib G, Pergola V, et al. Echocardiography predicts embolic events in infective endocarditis. J Am Coll Cardiol 2001;37(4):1069–76.

69. Salgado AV, Furlan AJ, Keys TF, Nichols TR, Beck GJ. Neurologic complications of endocarditis: a 12-year experience. Neurology 1989;39(2 Pt 1):173–8.

70. Steckelberg JM, Murphy JG, Ballard D, et al. Emboli in infective endocarditis: the prognostic value of echocardiography. Ann Intern Med 1991;114(8):635–40.

71. Dickerman SA, Abrutyn E, Barsic B, et al. The relationship between the initiation of antimicrobial therapy and the incidence of stroke in infective endocarditis: an analysis from the ICE Prospective Cohort Study (ICE-PCS). Am Heart J 2007;154(6):1086–94.

72. Wallace SM, Walton BI, Kharbanda RK, Hardy R, Wilson AP, Swanton RH. Mortality from infective endocarditis: clinical predictors of outcome. Heart 2002;88(1):53–60.

73. Hasbun R, Vikram HR, Barakat LA, Buenconsejo J, Quagliarello VJ. Complicated left-sided native valve endocarditis in adults: risk classification for mortality. JAMA 2003;289(15):1933–40.

74. Cabell CH, Pond KK, Peterson GE, et al. The risk of stroke and death in patients with aortic and mitral valve endocarditis. Am Heart J 2001;142(1):75–80.

75. Miro JM, Anguera I, Cabell CH, et al. Staphylococcus aureus native valve infective endocarditis: report of 566 episodes from the International Collaboration on Endocarditis Merged Database. Clin Infect Dis 2005;41(4):507–14.

76. Braunwald NS, Cooper T, Morrow AG. Complete replacement of the mitral valve. Successful clinical application of a flexible polyurethane prosthesis. J Thorac Cardiovasc Surg 1960;40:1–11.

77. Harken DE, Soroff HS, Taylor WJ, Lefemine AA, Gupta SK, Lunzer S. Partial and complete prostheses in aortic insufficiency. J Thorac Cardiovasc Surg 1960;40:744–62.

78. Starr A, Edwards ML. Mitral replacement: clinical experience with a ball-valve prosthesis. Ann Surg 1961;154:726–40.

79. Geraci JE, Dale AJ, Mc GD. Bacterial endocarditis and endarteritis following cardiac operations. Wis Med J 1963;62:302–15.

80. Wang A, Athan E, Pappas PA, et al. Contemporary clinical profile and outcome of prosthetic valve endocarditis. JAMA 2007;297(12):1354–61.

81. Calderwood SB, Swinski LA, Waternaux CM, Karchmer AW, Buckley MJ. Risk factors for the development of prosthetic valve endocarditis. Circulation 1985;72(1):31–7.

82. Ivert TS, Dismukes WE, Cobbs CG, Blackstone EH, Kirklin JW, Bergdahl LA. Prosthetic valve endocarditis. Circulation 1984;69(2):223–32.

83. Grover FL, Cohen DJ, Oprian C, Henderson WG, Sethi G, Hammermeister KE. Determinants of the occurrence of and survival from prosthetic valve endocarditis. Experience of the Veterans Affairs Cooperative Study on Valvular Heart Disease. J Thorac Cardiovasc Surg 1994;108(2):207–14.

84. Wilson WR, Jaumin PM, Danielson GK, Giuliani ER, Washington JA, II, Geraci JE. Prosthetic valve endocarditis. Ann Intern Med 1975;82(6):751–6.

85. Fang G, Keys TF, Gentry LO, et al. Prosthetic valve endocarditis resulting from nosocomial bacteremia. A prospective, multicenter study. Ann Intern Med 1993;119(7 Pt 1):560–7.

86. Bayer AS, Nelson RJ, Slama TG. Current concepts in prevention of prosthetic valve endocarditis. Chest 1990;97(5):1203–7.

87. Darouiche RO. Antimicrobial approaches for preventing infections associated with surgical implants. Clin Infect Dis 2003;36(10):1284–9.

88. Da Costa A, Kirkorian G, Cucherat M, et al. Antibiotic prophylaxis for permanent pacemaker implantation : a meta-analysis. Circulation 1998;97(18):1796–801.

89. Actis Dato A, Jr., Chiusolo C, Cicchitti GC, Actis Dato GM, Porro MC, Bello A. [Antibiotic pretreatment of heart valve prostheses]. Minerva Cardioangiol 1992;40(6):225–9.

90. Schaff H, Carrel T, Steckelberg JM, Grunkemeier GL, Holubkov R. Artificial valve endocarditis reduction trial (AVERT): protocol of a multicenter randomized trial. J Heart Valve Dis 1999;8(2):131–9.

91. Schaff HV, Carrel TP, Jamieson WR, et al. Paravalvular leak and other events in silzone-coated mechanical heart valves: a report from AVERT. Ann Thorac Surg 2002;73(3):785–92.

92. O'Grady NP, Alexander M, Dellinger EP, et al. Guidelines for the prevention of intravascular catheter-related infections. Infect Control Hosp Epidemiol 2002;23(12):759–69.

93. Piper C, Korfer R, Horstkotte D. Prosthetic valve endocarditis. Heart 2001;85(5):590–3.

94. Wilson WR, Danielson GK, Giuliani ER, Geraci JE. Prosthetic valve endocarditis. Mayo Clin Proc 1982;57(3): 155–61.

95. Block PC, DeSanctis RW, Weinberg AN, Austen WG. Prosthetic valve endocarditis. J Thorac Cardiovasc Surg 1970;60(4):540–8.

96. Dismukes WE, Karchmer AW, Buckley MJ, Austen WG, Swartz MN. Prosthetic valve endocarditis. Analysis of 38 cases. Circulation 1973;48(2):365–77.

97. Slaughter L, Morris JE, Starr A. Prosthetic valvular endocarditis. A 12-year review. Circulation 1973;47(6):1319–26.

98. Lopez J, Revilla A, Vilacosta I, et al. Definition, clinical profile, microbiological spectrum, and prognostic factors of early-onset prosthetic valve endocarditis. Eur Heart J 2007;28(6):760–5.

99. Schulz R, Werner GS, Fuchs JB, et al. Clinical outcome and echocardiographic findings of native and prosthetic valve endocarditis in the 1990s. Eur Heart J 1996;17(2):281–8.

100. Perez-Vazquez A, Farinas MC, Garcia-Palomo JD, Bernal JM, Revuelta JM, Gonzalez-Macias J. Evaluation of the Duke criteria in 93 episodes of prosthetic valve endocarditis: could sensitivity be improved? Arch Intern Med 2000;160(8):1185–91.

101. Chastre J, Trouillet JL. Early infective endocarditis on prosthetic valves. Eur Heart J 1995;16(Suppl B):32–8.

102. Lowry RW, Zoghbi WA, Baker WB, Wray RA, Quinones MA. Clinical impact of transesophageal echocardiography in the diagnosis and management of infective endocarditis. Am J Cardiol 1994;73(15):1089–91.

103. Daniel WG, Mugge A, Grote J, et al. Comparison of transthoracic and transesophageal echocardiography for detection of abnormalities of prosthetic and bioprosthetic valves in the mitral and aortic positions. Am J Cardiol 1993;71(2):210–5.

104. Daniel LB, Grigg LE, Weisel RD, Rakowski H. Comparison of transthoracic and transesophageal assessment of prosthetic valve dysfunction. Echocardiogr 1990;7(2):83–95.

105. Wang A, Pappas P, Anstrom KJ, et al. The use and effect of surgical therapy for prosthetic valve infective endocarditis: a propensity analysis of a multicenter, international cohort. Am Heart J 2005;150(5):1086–91.

106. Keys TF. Early-onset prosthetic valve endocarditis. Cleve Clin J Med 1993;60(6):455–9.

107. El-Ahdab F, Benjamin DK, Jr., Wang A, et al. Risk of endocarditis among patients with prosthetic valves and Staphylococcus aureus bacteremia. Am J Med 2005;118(3):225–9.

108. Fernicola DJ, Roberts WC. Frequency of ring abscess and cuspal infection in active infective endocarditis involving bioprosthetic valves. Am J Cardiol 1993;72(3):314–23.

109. Middlemost S, Wisenbaugh T, Meyerowitz C, et al. A case for early surgery in native left-sided endocarditis complicated by heart failure:results in 203 patients. J Am Coll Cardiol 1991;18(3):663–7.

110. Bonow RO, Carabello BA, Kanu C, et al. ACC/AHA 2006 guidelines for the management of patients with valvular heart disease: a report of the American College of Cardiology/American Heart Association Task Force on Practice Guidelines (writing committee to revise the 1998 Guidelines for the Management of Patients with Valvular Heart Disease): developed in collaboration with the Society of Cardiovascular Anesthesiologists: endorsed by the Society for Cardiovascular Angiography and Interventions and the Society of Thoracic Surgeons. Circulation 2006;114(5):e84–231.

111. Castillo JC, Anguita MP, Torres F, et al. Long-term prognosis of early and late prosthetic valve endocarditis. Am J Cardiol 2004;93(9):1185–7.

112. Li JS, Corey GR, Fowler VG. Infective Endocarditis. In: Topol EJ, Califf RM, ed. *Textbook of cardiovascular medicine*. Philadelphia: Lippincott Williams & Wilkins, 2007:xxix, 1628 p.

113. Sachdev M, Peterson GE, Jollis JG. Imaging techniques for diagnosis of infective endocarditis. Cardiol Clin. 2003;21:185–195.

114. Bonow RO, Carabello BA, Chatterjee K et al. ACC/AHA 2006 guidelines for the management of patients with valvular heart disease: a report of the American College of Cardiology/American Heart Association Task Force on Practice Guidelines (Writing Committee to Revise the 1998 guidelines for the management of patients with valvular heart disease) developed in collaboration with the Society of Cardiovascular Anesthesiologists endorsed by the Society for Cardiovascular Angiography and Interventions and the Society of Thoracic Surgeons. J Am Coll Cardiol 2006;48:e1–148.

22   Exercise and Noncardiac Surgery in Valvular Heart Disease

Stephen A. Hart and Richard A. Krasuski

CONTENTS

Exercise and noncardiac surgery are both significant stressors of the cardiovascular system, particularly within the unique hemodynamic milieu of valvular heart disease (VHD). Physical activity and noncardiac surgery are commonplace for patients with VHD, and overall risk can be significantly reduced with proper preparation and management. Regular physical exercise is an important component for health promotion, but patients with significant VHD typically have a decreased tolerance for exercise. In fact, exercise can cause significant hemodynamic perturbations that in extreme circumstances can result in syncope or pulmonary congestion. In a similar manner, the stress of noncardiac surgery can also impact the cardiovascular system. Anesthesia, fluid shifts, and positive pressure ventilation can all adversely affect the already comprised cardiovascular performance. This chapter discusses the changes in hemodynamics associated with exercise and noncardiac surgery for patients with valvular heart disease and, where appropriate, makes recommendations for optimal clinical care.

EXERCISE IN VALVULAR HEART DISEASE

The importance of regular physical activity is well established and increased exercise capacity routinely predicts improved clinical outcomes for patients with cardiovascular disease *(1)*. Exercise can result in systolic blood pressure reduction, weight loss, improved blood cholesterol levels, better glycemic control, and improved endothelial function. The American College of Sports Medicine/American Heart Association guidelines recommend all healthy adults aged 18–65 years to participate in moderate-intensity aerobic physical activity for 30 min/5 days each week or vigorous-intensity aerobic physical activity for 20 min/3 days each week *(1)*. Patients with VHD risk developing the consequences of a sedentary lifestyle, should they become overly cautious about their condition and avoid exercise. Similarly, patients with VHD who exert themselves past an acceptable limit may place themselves at risk for hypotension, syncope, and rhythm disturbances such as atrial fibrillation or ventricular tachycardia depending on their particular lesion. Recommending the appropriate exercise program to the VHD patient requires balancing these important risks and benefits.

The normal cardiovascular response to exercise involves an increase in blood flow to active muscles to meet increased metabolic demands. Increasing flow through stenotic valves generally results in increased flow resistance and transvalvular pressure gradients, while increased flow through regurgitant valves in most cases results in decreased regurgitant volume. The following is a review of the

From: *Contemporary Cardiology: Valvular Heart Disease*
Edited by: Andrew Wang, Thomas M. Bashore, DOI 10.1007/978-1-59745-411-7_22
© Humana Press, a part of Springer Science+Business Media, LLC 2009

normal cardiovascular response to exercise and detailed information regarding the physiologic effects of exercise on each unique valve lesion. Exercise hemodynamics in VHD have been well documented, but research investigating the long-term effects of exercise on the natural history of VHD is lacking.

General comments regarding the appropriate exercise program in VHD patients are contained within the American College of Cardiology/American Heart Association (ACC/AHA) 2006 Updated VHD Guidelines with the unique hemodynamics of each lesion in mind *(2)*. A detailed review of recommendations for competitive athletes with VHD may be found in the ACC/AHA 2005 Task Force 3 Report from the Bethesda Conference *(3)*.

Cardiovascular Response to Exercise

The physiologic response to exercise is mediated by the central nervous system and active skeletal muscle. The early response to exercise begins in the hypothalamus even before exercise begins. The hypothalamus directs the medulla to increase sympathetic output and decrease parasympathetic output. Globally, this increases cardiac output (CO) and produces vasoconstriction, transiently increasing the systemic vascular resistance (SVR). Locally, muscle metabolites eventually accumulate, leading to vasodilation in active muscle resulting in an overall decrease in SVR.

CO increases during exercise as a result of both increased heart rate (HR) and stroke volume (SV). Sympathetic β_1 adrenergic signaling has a positive chronotropic effect on the myocardium, which leads to increased contractility as intracellular concentration of Ca^{2+} builds. Increased contractility, along with a rise in preload, results in increased SV. To meet the demands placed on skeletal muscle during exercise, CO may increase up to four- or five-fold *(4)*. This is predominately mediated by rising HR, which increases nearly three-fold above resting levels, and to a lesser degree increased SV, which increases about 1.3-fold above resting levels (Fig. 1).

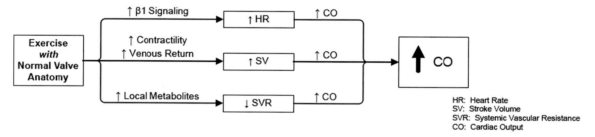

Fig. 1. Normal physiological response to exercise.

Selective vasoconstriction is mediated through sympathetic α_1 adrenergic signaling. Splanchnic, cutaneous, renal, and physically inactive muscle circulations are constricted, reducing fractional flow to these tissues. Despite this vasoconstriction, the absolute blood flow necessary to maintain normal physiological function is preserved by the general increase in CO *(4)*. Right ventricular preload is simultaneously augmented through alteration of venous return. This occurs by the contraction of skeletal muscles surrounding venous networks to propel blood toward the heart, and by the increase in sympathetic output, which induces venoconstriction and reduces unstressed circulatory volume.

After the early direction of the hypothalamus, exercise induces a delayed response consisting of vasodilation triggered by muscle metabolites, which eventually dominates over sympathetically mediated vasoconstriction. Lactate, potassium, and adenosine concentrations increase in the interstitial space surrounding active muscles *(4)*. These locally released metabolites increase blood flow to active muscles by dilating and recruiting capillary beds. Decreased resistance with the simultaneous increase in CO can increase resting capillary flow up to 20-fold *(4)*. As stroke volume increases during exercise, flow rates through the mitral and aortic valves increase. Interestingly, increased blood flow across the aortic valve is mainly mediated through increased velocity, while increased blood flow across the mitral valve is primarily augmented through increased diastolic mitral valve orifice size *(5, 6)*.

When exercise ends, a rapid reversal of the sympathetic/parasympathetic balance takes place. The parasympathetic system again becomes dominant as resting tone is restored. HR and CO return to basal levels within minutes. Despite this, SVR remains depressed for a prolonged period after exercise ends *(7)*. Blood pressure (BP) is directly related to both CO and SVR. Since CO returns to normal resting values while SVR remains depressed, BP will be reduced below pre-exercise levels *(8)*.

The hemodynamic adaptation to exercise above is characteristic of isotonic, or "dynamic", exercise such as running or cycling. Isotonic exercise occurs when muscle contraction involves a movement and the force generated within the muscle remains constant throughout muscle shortening. Isometric, or "static", exercise occurs when muscle contraction results in no movement *(4)*. Weight lifting is often used to describe isometric exercise; however, the actions of lifting weights are a combination of isotonic and isometric exercises. The distinction between isotonic and isometric exercises is important in VHD because isotonic exercise results in increased CO and decreased BP while isometric exercise results in only a slightly increased CO and increased BP *(7)*. The implications of the differing hemodynamic effects will be discussed below when appropriate.

Aortic Stenosis

During the isovolumic contraction phase of systole, pressure builds in the left ventricle (LV). Once the pressure exceeds aortic pressure, the valve opens to permit blood flow into the aorta. A stenotic valve produces an increased resistance to opening, and a pressure gradient is generated as the ventricle attempts to maintain adequate CO across the narrowed valve. The hemodynamics produced by aortic stenosis (AS) cause energy dissipation across the stenotic valve and result in a tendency toward higher LV pressures and lower arterial pressures, with this difference becoming particularly exaggerated during exercise (Fig. 2).

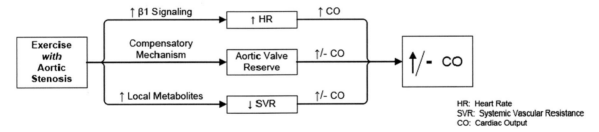

Fig. 2. Response to exercise with aortic stenosis.

In one study challenging asymptomatic AS patients with maximal treadmill exercise, Doppler measurements demonstrated that cardiac output increased from 6.5 ± 1.7 to 10.2 ± 4.4 L/min *(9)*. As expected, the transvalvular pressure gradient and aortic jet velocity increased to generate the necessary increase in CO. Interestingly, the increase in CO appeared to be mediated solely by HR. Stroke volume actually decreased slightly, concurrent with the shortened systolic ejection period. In another study challenging asymptomatic AS patients with exercise, Burwash and colleagues also demonstrated that SV had little effect on maintaining CO *(10)*.

Typically, asymptomatic AS patients retain normal CO at rest and with exercise. With severe AS, however, the ability to augment CO during exercise diminishes, and eventually becomes nearly fixed. Coronary blood flow may also become inadequate as the increased LV end systolic pressures generated by the stenotic valve results in decreased coronary perfusion pressure *(11)*. The compensatory response of LV hypertrophy maintains cardiac function at the cost of inadequately perfused coronary arteries.

The additional muscle mass must be perfused and the hypertrophied tissue also abnormally compresses the coronary arteries in the subendocardium *(12)*. Patients may present with angina pectoris, which is often compounded by concurrent coronary artery disease *(13)*.

By comparing the increase in mean systolic pressure gradient with the increase in aortic flow, Bache and colleagues demonstrated that exercise in asymptomatic AS patients results in an apparent increase in aortic valve area. They found that the increase in the transvalvular gradient was less than that predicted by the increase in aortic flow and concluded that the valve area had increased with exercise *(14)*. More recent studies have also demonstrated an increase in valve area with physiologic or pharmacologic exercise *(14–19)*. Otto has also demonstrated that those patients with less severe disease have greater increases in valve area with exercise. One possible mechanism for this relationship is that the valve leaflets are more compliant early in the disease and become stiffer as AS progresses *(20)*.

According to the ACC/AHA 2005 Task Force 3 Report, exercise testing should not be performed in patients believed to be symptomatic from their aortic stenosis, but testing in asymptomatic patients appears relatively safe and may yield additional information to the clinical evaluation *(3, 21)*. In particular, supervised exercise testing may help guide physicians to recommend the most appropriate level of normal exercise *(22)*. Prior to initiating any exercise regimen or undergoing an exercise test, the degree of stenosis should be accurately assessed. Exercise testing should be stopped for any fall in blood pressure, excessive ST-segment depression, significant arrhythmias or the development of AS-related symptoms such as dyspnea, angina, or syncope *(23)*. With close supervision, asymptomatic patients with mild AS tolerate exercise without complications and may even be able to participate in competitive sports *(3, 24)*. Patients with moderate to severe AS, however, have a lower threshold of tolerated exercise due to decreased coronary blood flow, and should not be allowed to participate in sports that involve high dynamic or static muscular demands. These patients should be evaluated in a controlled setting to determine the appropriate exercise program.

Patients with low flow/low gradient AS typically have advanced disease and physical activity is generally symptom limited. These patients should undergo a pharmacological provocation such as a dobutamine infusion to determine the true severity of the stenosis prior to considering a surgical intervention or participating in a strenuous physical activity *(17)*.

Aortic Insufficiency

An insufficient aortic valve results in diastolic LV volume overload and increased stroke volume. LV dilatation ensues to compensate for the increased wall stress. Acute aortic insufficiency (AI), however, results in decreased stroke volume as the LV muscle does not have sufficient time to compensate. In this situation tachycardia becomes the prominent compensatory mechanism. Exercise usually induces CO and HR to increase and SVR to decrease. This leads to a drop in regurgitant volume for at least two reasons: as HR increases, LV filling time decreases reducing regurgitation time, additionally the drop in systemic vascular resistance causes a decrease in afterload *(25–27)*. Reduced regurgitant volume also leads to increased coronary perfusion and increased peripheral filling, both of which are beneficial to the patient with AI (Fig. 3).

In a study performed by Thompson et al., patients with AI were subjected to exercise in order to measure LV volume and net SV *(26)*. While all patients with AI exhibited elevated LV volume, only those patients with severe AI (ejection fraction of 0.44 ± 0.09 at rest) demonstrated increased LV size as exercise progressed. Patients with less severe AI, similar to controls, demonstrated decreased LV size as exercise progressed. Patients with preserved myocardial function exhibited identical net SV to controls and significantly higher net SV than those with the most severe AI. Furthermore, net SV for patients with good myocardial performance increased as exercise progressed in a normal manner. A similar study later confirmed these findings and demonstrated reduction in regurgitant fraction leading to increased net SV *(27)*.

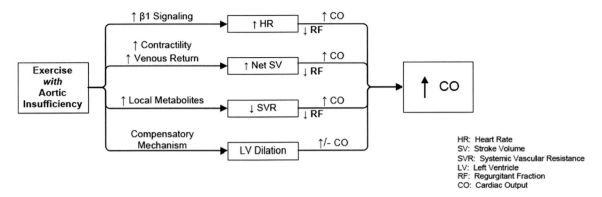

Fig. 3. Response to exercise with aortic insufficiency.

At this time there is no evidence to suggest that asymptomatic patients with AI who regularly exercise experience progression in LV dysfunction. Therefore, asymptomatic patients may participate in normal physical activities including isotonic exercise. More than mild isometric exercises, however, should be avoided by patients with significant AI to avoid increasing afterload. Supervised exercise testing to at least the level of physical activity anticipated in an exercise program should be conducted to ensure patient safety *(2)*. Eliciting symptoms with exercise testing may help quantify the functional capacity of the patient with AI *(28)*. Despite the seemingly beneficial physiologic effects of exercise on AI, there is insufficient data to formulate recommendations regarding long term or more strenuous exercise *(3)*.

Mitral Stenosis

Mitral stenosis (MS) causes increased resistance to LV filling during diastole, necessitating increased left atrial (LA) pressures to overcome the obstruction. Elevated LA pressures can lead to pulmonary hypertension and dyspnea, particularly during exercise *(29)*. Elevated HR during exercise decreases diastolic filling time and further limits flow across the stenotic valve.

Although LA pressure normally increases with exercise, pulmonary artery pressure appears to increase excessively and inappropriately in patients with MS *(30)*. Some of this may be related to vasoconstriction resulting from alveolar hypoxia during exercise, and it has been postulated to serve a protective role in preventing pulmonary congestion *(31)*. Elevated pulmonary vascular resistance results in excessive afterload on the right ventricle and can lead to strain and dilatation. This can exacerbate tricuspid regurgitation and further impair exercise intolerance *(32)* (Fig. 4).

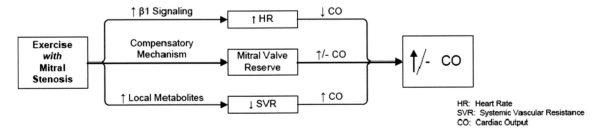

Fig. 4. Response to exercise with mitral stenosis.

Atrial fibrillation (AF) occurs in up to 40% of MS patients. While the etiology of AF in MS is debatable *(33)*, exercise capacity clearly becomes depressed when AF develops *(34)*. Both the hemodynamic influences of MS and inflammatory process of rheumatic valvular disease may lead to LA enlargement which appears to be a major factor in the etiology of AF *(35)*. Aside from the increased tendency toward thromboembolism, AF places a larger burden on the right heart to fill the LV. Although exercise capacity in MS patients with AF is primarily dictated by hemodynamics, AF significantly compounds exercise intolerance *(36)*. MS patients at most risk for atrial fibrillation are typically older and have more advanced disease *(37)*. Hemodynamic perturbations associated with MS, such as transvalvular pressure gradient and pulmonary artery pressure, do not necessarily correlate with AF suggesting an alternate etiology *(34)*. Furthermore, recent studies suggest that valvuloplasty, which leads to a significant reduction in hemodynamic burden, may not prevent the development of AF *(38)*, implying a nonhemodynamic component in the etiology of AF in patients with MS.

Exercise induced increases in CO for normal patients are primarily mediated by increasing mitral valve area, also referred to as "mitral valve reserve." The same principle holds true for patients with mitral stenosis. The paradoxical situation of an enlarging stenotic valve may be explained by the morphology of the valve lesion *(39)*. Stenoses that are purely fibrous may be more pliable than calcified valve leaflets and allow normal physiological enlargement. One study of MS patients demonstrated that more pliable leaflets resulted in greater valve area with exercise *(40)*. Interestingly, mitral valve reserve cannot be accurately predicted at rest from other hemodynamic indicators such as transmitral pressure gradient or CO *(39, 41)*. Exercise induced mitral valve reserve can only be measured with physiologic or pharmacologic stress testing.

Asymptomatic patients at rest with mild to moderate MS are able to exercise to symptom limitation and some patients may remain asymptomatic with strenuous activity *(2)*. Patients with severe MS will generally be symptom limited but do risk developing pulmonary edema from acute increases in LA and pulmonary vasculature pressures during exercise *(42)*. Patients are also at risk for developing AF, which further compromises exercise capacity. Similar to other valve lesions, supervised stress testing should be conducted in patients with mild to moderate MS to determine exercise capacity prior to beginning an exercise program or participating in competitive athletics. The severity of stenosis may only be accurately assessed with stress testing, since mitral valve reserve is only induced on exertion.

Mitral Regurgitation

Mitral regurgitation (MR) is defined by the abnormal ejection of blood from the LV to the LA during systole which increases the volume load on the LV *(43)*. Chronic volume overload leads to compensatory dilatation. LV dilatation maintains adequate CO for mild to moderate regurgitation but eventually becomes inadequate as the disease progresses or during exercise. Regurgitation may also lead to elevated LA pressure and pulmonary hypertension, which further limits the normal rise in CO with exercise.

The body responds to exercise by decreasing SVR in order to increase peripheral tissue perfusion. As SVR drops, the afterload on the LV also drops reducing the regurgitant fraction (RF), regurgitant volume, and effective regurgitant orifice (ERO) for patients with MR and normal ventricular function. Despite the drop in RF, the total regurgitant flow which is the product of HR and RF always increases because of elevated HR *(44)*. Exercise-induced increases in HR and BP may even result in substantial increases in regurgitation leading to pulmonary vascular pressure elevation and congestion *(3)*.

Progression of MR typically leads to dilatation and hypertrophy of the left ventricle, ultimately resulting in ventricular systolic dysfunction. MR with systolic ventricular dysfunction is also common in the context of ischemic heart disease *(45)*. Once ventricular dysfunction develops with MR, adaptation to exercise becomes further impaired. ERO in the presence of ventricular dysfunction increases instead of the usual decrease. The beneficial drop in RF and regurgitant volume that occur with exercise in the MR patient with intact ventricular function is eliminated *(44)*. In this situation, SV remains static during exercise inhibiting normal CO and exercise capacity *(46)* (Fig. 5).

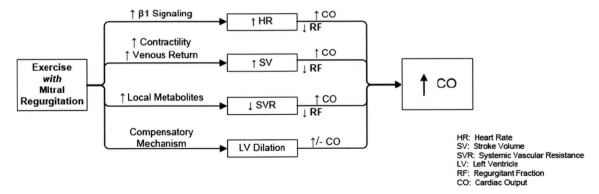

Fig. 5. Response to exercise with mitral regurgitation.

Madaric and colleagues showed that exercise capacity and cardiopulmonary function significantly improved in patients with severe MR who underwent successful minimally invasive mitral valve repair *(47)*. Although all patients in the study had evidence of severe MR and exercise limitation on testing, only 20% reported having any prior symptoms or limitations. This study suggests that patients who claim to be asymptomatic may have such gradual onset of limitations that their symptoms are not self-detectable or that patients may limit their activity and thereby mask their symptoms. Since the genesis of ventricular dysfunction begins well before symptoms manifest, stress testing is important to detect which patients may require intervention before overt symptoms develop. The importance of exercise testing prior to beginning an exercise program is highlighted by the demonstration that the ERO at rest cannot predict changes in ERO with exercise *(45)*. The true severity of the lesion with exercise therefore might be underestimated with ERO measurement at rest.

Isometric exercises such as weight lifting which increase SVR should generally be avoided by patients with significant MR. Patients with mild to moderate MR and normal LV size, rhythm, and pulmonary artery pressure may undertake dynamic exercise and competitive sports. As signs of disease progression increase, such as LV enlargement or pulmonary hypertension, the intensity of exercise should be reduced. Patients experiencing atrial fibrillation or having a history of atrial fibrillation should not participate in any contact sports *(3)*. Exercise does not produce significant hemodynamic changes in patients with mild to moderate MR; however, exercise testing is particularly useful in identifying patients with latent ventricular dysfunction and diminished contractile reserve *(48)*.

Pulmonic Stenosis

Pulmonic stenosis (PS) results in elevated RV pressure which increases further during exercise. RV hypertrophy results from long-standing pressure overload and eventually leads to diastolic dysfunction and exercise intolerance. Ikkos reported on 46 patients with PS and stratified them according to valve area. Patients with the most severe lesions demonstrated the lowest exercise tolerance *(49)*. However, in the Second Natural History of Congenital Heart Defects Study, there was no association between the degree of stenosis and exercise tolerance. The main reason for this, however, was that some patients had undergone prior valvotomy and all patients had transvalvular gradients <20 mmHg, far below where symptoms would be expected to occur *(50)*.

A study comparing the hemodynamic effects of exercise between children and adults with PS showed that while children with mild to moderate PS demonstrate an appropriate hemodynamic response to exercise, adults with similar valve obstructions do not. When the stenosis became severe, both children and adults exhibited abnormal responses to exercise including abnormally elevated RV end diastolic pressure *(51)*.

For most patients with significant PS, exercise will generally be symptom limited, and regular activity poses minimal additional risk. Exercise testing is important in this population to identify reduced cardiac performance which may only be detected during exertion as well as to determine the continued efficacy of prior valvuloplasty *(52)*.

Pulmonic Insufficiency

Chronic, significant pulmonary insufficiency (PI) is unusual and generally limited to patients with prior tetralogy of Fallot repair or valvotomy for pulmonic stenosis. It is a slowly progressing disease and exertional symptoms may be the first indication of any problem in these patients. PI generates elevated RV volumes leading to RV diastolic and eventually systolic dysfunction over the course of many years. The resulting ventricular dilatation can result in tricuspid regurgitation, which further compounds the RV dysfunction. Ventricular wall stretch and dilatation decreases conduction velocity and increases the likelihood of ventricular tachycardia and sudden cardiac death *(53)*, both of which may present serious risks to exercise.

Roest observed a decrease in regurgitant fraction on exercise with repaired tetralogy of Fallot patients with PI *(54)*. This could be caused by at least three mechanisms *(54)*. RV pressure normally drops with exercise, but patients with long-standing PI sustain increased RV pressure with exercise. Since regurgitation depends on relatively low RV pressure, patients with PI exhibit a decreased RF *(54, 55)*. Elevated pulmonary artery pressure could also contribute to an unfavorable gradient, but this has generally not been found *(56)*. Finally, exercise results in tachycardia which decreases diastolic filling time and the available regurgitation time.

Exercise testing should be used to establish a safe threshold of exertion for patients with significant PI. Exercise testing may also be an important technique to identify patients with early indications of RV dysfunction, which if left uncorrected could eventually become irreversible *(53)*.

Tricuspid Stenosis

Patients with primary tricuspid stenosis (TS) should undergo supervised exercise testing to determine exercise capacity. Asymptomatic patients are generally allowed to participate in exercise training programs. In most cases, TS is seen in the context of rheumatic heart disease together with mitral valve involvement. These patients should adhere to the exercise recommendations presented for MS *(3)*.

Tricuspid Regurgitation

Exercise may lead to RV overload and diastolic dysfunction in patients with primary tricuspid regurgitation (TR). Asymptomatic patients with primary TR may participate in exercise programs so long as there is absence of RA pressure greater than 20 mmHg or significant elevation of the RV systolic pressure *(3)*.

Special Conditions

Patients with a bicuspid aortic valve often have concomitant connective tissue disorders that result in a dilated aortic root or ascending aorta *(57)*. These patients appear to be at risk for aortic dissection with aortic roots even smaller than 50 mm^2 *(58)*. According the recommendations of the Bethesda Conference, patients with aortic roots <40 mm and no significant AS or AI may participate in athletic competition. Patients with aortic root dilation between 40 and 45 mm may participate in competitive athletics not involving the potential for collision or trauma. Patients with aortic root dilation >45 mm should only participate in low-intensity athletics *(3)*. Patients with BAV are likely to develop AS, AI, or both *(57)*. Exercise recommendations for these patients should merge the recommendations for isolated bicuspid aortic valve and the recommendations for the additional lesion(s) *(3)*.

Aortic root diameter and function generally limit the degree of physical activity for Marfan syndrome patients. Patients with aortic root diameters <40 mm with less than mild to moderate aortic regurgitation and no family history of dissection may participate in athletic competition. When aortic root diameter increases beyond 40 mm and significant AI develops, patients will need to limit their participation to low-intensity, noncontact athletics, and nonisometric exercises *(59)*.

NONCARDIAC SURGERY IN VALVULAR HEART DISEASE

Cardiovascular complications comprise 25–50% of all complications following noncardiac surgery. In 1977, Goldman published the first study describing the process of risk assessment in patients undergoing noncardiac surgery *(60)*. The study followed 1001 patients who underwent noncardiac surgery and the investigators compiled nine variables that conferred increased risk for postoperative cardiac complications. The original nine variables were revised in 1986 by Detsky, improving the prediction of postoperative complications by combining the complication rate of a given surgical procedure with the individual risk factors of the patient *(61)*. In addition, the cardiovascular effects of the anesthetic agent must also be taken into account when determining surgical risk *(62)*.

Cardiovascular Response to Anesthesia

General anesthetics typically result in decreased myocardial contractility and vasodilation. Vasodilation causes SVR to decrease, thereby reducing blood pressure and afterload on the heart. In addition, baroreceptor control and sympathetic tone are reduced. Since cardiac output is a function of HR, preload, afterload, and contractility, the hemodynamic effect is complex. The depression in myocardial performance is dependent on the particular anesthetic used; however, all anesthetics have known cardiovascular effects which should be carefully evaluated. Regional anesthetics also present unique risks. Peripheral nerve blocks have the advantage of having limited hemodynamic effects, while spinal anesthesia causes similar sympathetic blockade as general anesthetics. This method may cause depressed BP and HR which could provoke ischemia *(63)*.

Unfortunately there is no "best" anesthetic technique or agent that carries the lowest cardiovascular complication rate. The condition of the patient and the surgical procedure, regardless of anesthetic used, appear to be the major determinants for complications *(62)*. The choice of anesthetic agent should be considered in concert with the unique hemodynamic milieu of VHD patients. The primary focus of preoperative evaluation should be to establish the severity of the valve lesion and underlying myocardial dysfunction – two important determinants of cardiac output under stress.

Aortic Stenosis

Studies by Goldman and subsequent investigation by Detsky have established AS as a significant, independent risk factor for noncardiac surgery *(64)*. AS confers perioperative risks that depend on the complexity and timing of the procedure, concomitant heart disease, and the severity of stenosis *(65)*. The use of anesthesia causes systemic vasodilation and can result in hypotension. Acute hypotension may compromise flow across an already highly resistant valve and can result in hemodynamic collapse.

Kertai et al. showed that patients with moderate to severe AS have a five-fold increased risk of perioperative mortality and nonfatal myocardial infarction *(66)*. Rohde et al. also showed an increase (seven-fold) in risk of cardiovascular events for patients with aortic stenosis undergoing noncardiac surgery *(67)*. Kertai and colleagues further stratified patients and found that those patients with a revised cardiac risk index of 0 (1 point assigned for each of the following – high-risk surgery, ischemic heart disease, history of heart failure, history of cerebrovascular disease, insulin therapy for diabetes, and preoperative serum creatinine level >2.0 mg/dL) had no additional incidence of perioperative events but, as the revised risk ratio increased, the incidence of perioperative events increased exponentially. As a conclusion to their study, they suggest that symptomatic patients with AS be considered for valve replacement with or without revascularization (for concomitant CAD) prior to noncardiac surgery *(66)*.

In contrast, a number of more recent studies have shown that even with severe AS, noncardiac surgery may be conducted under close perioperative supervision with adverse event risks of 0–7% *(68–70)*. One study also showed that patients with unrecognized AS had much higher rates of complications than those who had undergone a preoperative echocardiogram *(68)*. Improvements in AS assessment through the years, particularly the widespread availability of echocardiography, have led to a more accurate evaluation of surgical risk for patients with AS.

All patients with suspected AS should undergo echocardiography to determine the severity of the stenosis prior to noncardiac surgery. Symptomatic AS patients should be considered for valve replacement prior to noncardiac surgery. Palliative valvuloplasty should be considered when patients are not candidates for valve replacement *(71)*. This reduces symptoms prior to undergoing noncardiac surgery or serves as a bridge to eventual valve replacement when other, more pressing medical issues have been addressed. Percutaneous techniques to implant prosthetic valves are increasing in popularity and may eventually provide an additional therapeutic option in such patients. Symptomatic patients with AS and concomitant CAD should be carefully evaluated for revascularization and valve replacement prior to noncardiac surgery *(65)*. Patients without signs or history of CAD may undergo noncardiac surgery with acceptable risk, provided that the operative team is aware of the stenosis and maintains careful hemodynamic control. Awareness of the stenosis is particularly important during emergent procedures where surgical risks increase (Fig. 6).

Aortic Insufficiency

Patients with AI are susceptible to volume overload. Perioperative attention should be focused on maintaining appropriate volume and avoiding bradycardia. The regurgitant fraction may increase as diastolic filling time increases. Patients with severe AI may benefit from afterload reduction therapy such as ACE-inhibitors or calcium channel blockers, though this remains controversial *(7, 72)*. Patients with AI who have not developed underlying ventricular dysfunction may safely undergo noncardiac surgery *(65)*. If ventricular dysfunction is mild to moderate, surgery should be delayed 4–6 weeks to allow for treatment optimization *(73)*. Large fluid shifts should be closely monitored, and efforts should be made to reduce afterload throughout the procedure. Valve replacement or surgical alternatives should be considered for patients with severe ventricular dysfunction *(73)* (Fig. 8).

Mitral Stenosis

Patients with MS are particularly vulnerable to tachycardia. Avoiding tachycardia prevents elevated LA pressure and pulmonary hypertension. Pulmonary vasoconstriction also presents a challenge in MS patients and should be avoided if possible. Hypoxia, hypercarbia, and acidosis all increase pulmonary vascular resistance and further compound pulmonary hypertension *(74)*.

Noncardiac surgery may be performed in patients with mild to moderate MS without significant additional risk. Again, to maintain adequate CO it is necessary for strict HR control, as tachycardia

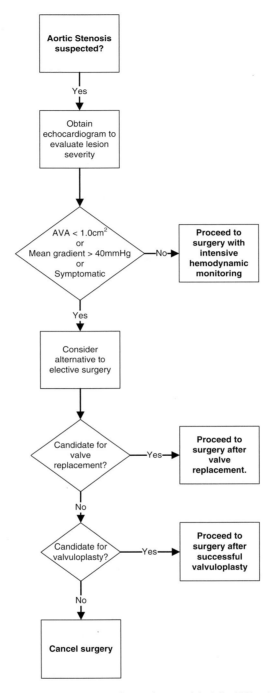

Fig. 6. Noncardiac surgical assessment for patients with AS. AVA: Aortic Valve Area.

may lead to pulmonary congestion and cardiogenic shock *(65,73)*. Severely stenotic lesions require balloon valvuloplasty or surgical replacement if balloon intervention is not feasible prior to noncardiac surgery *(75)*. Valvuloplasty, surgical commissurotomy, or valve replacement should be considered for any symptomatic patient with a valve area <1.5 cm² prior to noncardiac surgery *(2)* (Fig. 7).

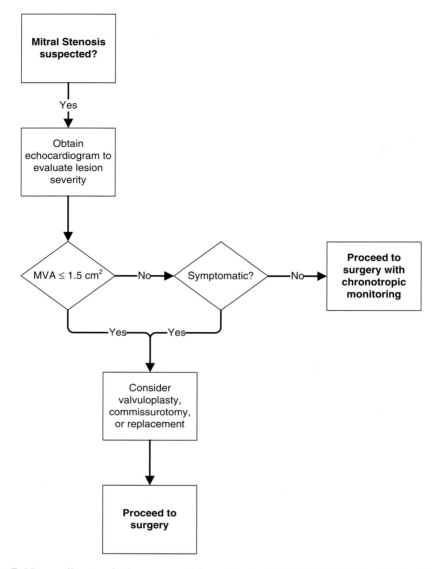

Fig. 7. Noncardiac surgical assessment for patients with MS. MVA: Mitral Valve Area.

Mitral Regurgitation

Similar to patients with AI, the hemodynamics of patients with severe MR are believed to be best stabilized when afterload is reduced and volume status is optimized *(65)*. Identification of the cause of MR is important to unmask concurrent disease such as coronary artery disease which may confound the preoperative evaluation *(7)* (Fig. 8).

Right Heart Valve Lesions

There is a lack of data concerning patients with primary lesions of the pulmonic and tricuspid valves and noncardiac surgery. The hemodynamics of these cases should be evaluated on a case-by-case basis,

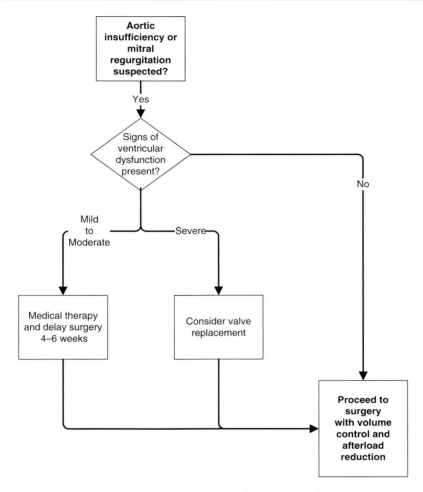

Fig. 8. Noncardiac surgical assessment for patients with AI or MR.

but no data currently suggests any problems regarding noncardiac surgery unless there is underlying pulmonary hypertension.

REFERENCES

1. Haskell WL, Lee IM, Pate RR, et al. Physical activity and public health. Updated recommendation for adults from the American College of Sports Medicine and the American Heart Association. Circulation 2007;116(9):1081–93.
2. Bonow RO, Carabello BA, Chatterjee K, et al. ACC/AHA 2006 Guidelines for the Management of Patients with Valvular Heart Disease: A Report of the American College of Cardiology/American Heart Association Task Force on Practice Guidelines (Writing Committee to Revise the 1998 Guidelines for the Management of Patients with Valvular Heart Disease): Developed in Collaboration with the Society of Cardiovascular Anesthesiologists: Endorsed by the Society for Cardiovascular Angiography and Interventions and the Society of Thoracic Surgeons. Circulation 2006;114: e84–231.
3. Bonow RO, Cheitlin MD, Crawford MH, Douglas PS. Task Force 3: valvular heart disease. J Am Coll Cardiol 2005;45:1334–40.
4. Boulpaep EL. Integrated control of the cardiovascular system. In: Boron WF, Boulpaep EL, (ed.) Medical physiology: a cellular and molecular approach. Philadelphia, PA: W.B. Saunders, 2003, 2005:582–585.
5. Rassi A Jr, Crawford MH, Richards KL, Miller JF. Differing mechanisms of exercise flow augmentation at the mitral and aortic valves. Circulation 1988;77:543–51.

6. Stewart WJ, Jiang L, Mich R, Pandian N, Guerrero JL, Weyman AE. Variable effects of changes in flow rate through the aortic, pulmonary and mitral valves on valve area and flow velocity: impact on quantitative Doppler flow calculations. J Am Coll Cardiol 1985;6:653–62.

7. Fuster V, O'Rourke RA, Walsh RA, Poole-Wilson P. Hurst's The Heart. New York: McGraw-Hill Book Company, 2008.

8. Pescatello LS, Fargo AE, Leach CN, Scherzer HH. Short-term effect of dynamic exercise on arterial blood pressure. Circulation 1991;85:1557.

9. Otto CM, Pearlman AS, Kraft CD, Miyake-Hull CY, Burwash IG, Gardner CJ. Physiologic changes with maximal exercise in asymptomatic valvular aortic stenosis assessed by Doppler echocardiography. J Am Coll Cardiol 1992;20:1160–7.

10. Burwash IG, Pearlman AS, Kraft CD, Miyake-Hull C, Healy NL, Otto CM. Flow dependence of measures of aortic stenosis severity during exercise. J Am Coll Cardiol 1994;24:1342–50.

11. Johnson LL, Sciacca RR, Ellis K, Weiss MB, Cannon PJ. Reduced left ventricular myocardial blood flow per unit mass in aortic stenosis. Circulation 1978;57:582–90.

12. Vinten-Johansen J, Weiss HR. Oxygen consumption in subepicardial and subendocardial regions of the canine left ventricle. The effect of experimental acute valvular aortic stenosis. Circ Res 1980;46:139–45.

13. Marcus ML, Doty DB, Hiratzka LF, Wright CB, Eastham CL. Decreased coronary reserve: a mechanism for angina pectoris in patients with aortic stenosis and normal coronary arteries. N Engl J Med 1982;307:1362–6.

14. Bache RJ, Wang Y, Jorgensen CR. Hemodynamic effects of exercise in isolated valvular aortic stenosis. Circulation 1971;44:1003–13.

15. Burwash IG, Thomas DD, Sadahiro M, et al. Dependence of Gorlin formula and continuity equation valve areas on transvalvular volume flow rate in valvular aortic stenosis. Circulation 1994;89:827–35.

16. Ettinger PO, Frank MJ, Levinson GE. Hemodynamics at rest and during exercise in combined aortic stenosis and insufficiency. Circulation 1972;45:267–76.

17. deFilippi CR, Willett DL, Brickner ME, et al. Usefulness of dobutamine echocardiography in distinguishing severe from nonsevere valvular aortic stenosis in patients with depressed left ventricular function and low transvalvular gradients. Am J Cardiol 1995;75:191–4.

18. Martin TW, Moody JM Jr, Bird JJ, Slife D, Murgo JP. Effect of exercise on indices of valvular aortic stenosis. Cathet Cardiovasc Diagn 1992;25:265–71.

19. Lin SS, Roger VL, Pascoe R, Seward JB, Pellikka PA. Dobutamine stress Doppler hemodynamics in patients with aortic stenosis: feasibility, safety, and surgical correlations. Am Heart J 1998;136:1010–6.

20. Otto CM, Burwash IG, Legget ME, et al. Prospective study of asymptomatic valvular aortic stenosis. Clinical, echocardiographic, and exercise predictors of outcome. Circulation 1997;95:2262–70.

21. Peidro R, Brion G, Angelino A. Exercise testing in asymptomatic aortic stenosis. Cardiology 2006;108:258–64.

22. Alborino D, Hoffmann JL, Fournet PC, Bloch A. Value of exercise testing to evaluate the indication for surgery in asymptomatic patients with valvular aortic stenosis. J Heart Valve Dis 2002;11:204–9.

23. Pierard LA, Lancellotti P. Stress testing in valve disease. Heart 2007;93:766–72.

24. Carabello BA. Aortic stenosis. N Engl J Med 2002;346:677–82.

25. Dehmer GJ, Firth BG, Hillis LD, et al. Alterations in left ventricular volumes and ejection fraction at rest and during exercise in patients with aortic regulation. Am J Cardiol 1981;48:17–27.

26. Thompson R, Ross I, Leslie P, Easthope R. Haemodynamic adaptation to exercise in asymptomatic patients with severe aortic regurgitation. Cardiovasc Res 1985;19:212–8.

27. Kawanishi D, McKay C, Chandraratna P, et al. Cardiovascular response to dynamic exercise in patients with chronic symptomatic mild-to-moderate and severe aortic regurgitation. Circulation 1986;73:62–72.

28. Bekeredjian R, Grayburn PA. Valvular heart disease: aortic regurgitation. Circulation 2005;112:125–34.

29. Rosendorff C. Essential Cardiology: Principles and Practice. Totowa, NJ: Humana Press, 2005, p. 865.

30. Song JK, Kang DH, Lee CW, et al. Factors determining the exercise capacity in mitral stenosis. Am J Cardiol 1996;78:1060–2.

31. Wood P. Pulmonary hypertension with special reference to the vasoconstrictive factor. Br Heart J 1958;20:557–70.

32. Johnston DL, Kostuk WJ. Left and right ventricular function during symptom-limited exercise in patients with isolated mitral stenosis. Chest 1986;89:186–91.

33. Carabello BA. Modern management of mitral stenosis. Circulation 2005;112:432–7.

34. Kabukcu M, Arslantas E, Ates I, Demircioglu F, Ersel F. Clinical, echocardiographic, and hemodynamic characteristics of rheumatic mitral valve stenosis and atrial fibrillation. Angiology 2005;56:159–63.

35. Krasuski RA, Bush A, Kay JE, et al. C-reactive protein elevation independently influences the procedural success of percutaneous balloon mitral valve commissurotomy. Am Heart J 2003;146:1099–104.

36. Ueshima K, Myers J, Ribisl PM, et al. Hemodynamic determinants of exercise capacity in chronic atrial fibrillation. Am Heart J 1993;125:1301–5.

37. Alpert JS, Dalen JE, Rahimtoola SH. Valvular Heart Disease. Philadelphia: PA, Lippincott Williams & Wilkins, 2000; p. 478.

38. Krasuski RA, Assar MD, Wang A, et al. Usefulness of percutaneous balloon mitral commissurotomy in preventing the development of atrial fibrillation in patients with mitral stenosis. Am J Cardiol 2004;93:936–9.

39. Voelker W, Berner A, Regele B, et al. Effect of exercise on valvular resistance in patients with mitral stenosis. J Am Coll Cardiol 1993;22:777–82.

40. Dahan M, Paillole C, Martin D, Gourgon R. Determinants of stroke volume response to exercise in patients with mitral stenosis: a Doppler echocardiographic study. J Am Coll Cardiol 1993;21:384–9.

41. Voelker W, Karsch KR. Exercise Doppler echocardiography in conjunction with right heart catheterization for the assessment of mitral stenosis. Int J Sports Med 1996;17 (Suppl 3):S191–5.

42. Rahimtoola SH, Durairaj A, Mehra A, Nuno I. Current evaluation and management of patients with mitral stenosis. Circulation 2002;106:1183–8.

43. Otto CM. Clinical practice. Evaluation and management of chronic mitral regurgitation. N Engl J Med 2001;345:740–6.

44. Armstrong GP, Griffin BP. Exercise echocardiographic assessment in severe mitral regurgitation. Coron Artery Dis 2000;11:23–30.

45. Lancellotti P, Lebrun F, Pierard LA. Determinants of exercise-induced changes in mitral regurgitation in patients with coronary artery disease and left ventricular dysfunction. J Am Coll Cardiol 2003;42:1921–8.

46. Takano H, Adachi H, Ohshima S, Taniguchi K, Kurabayashi M. Functional mitral regurgitation during exercise in patients with heart failure. Circ J 2006;70:1563–7.

47. Madaric J, Watripont P, Bartunek J, et al. Effect of mitral valve repair on exercise tolerance in asymptomatic patients with organic mitral regurgitation. Am Heart J 2007;154:180–5.

48. Leung DY, Armstrong G, Griffin BP, Thomas JD, Marwick TH. Latent left ventricular dysfunction in patients with mitral regurgitation: feasibility of measuring diminished contractile reserve from a simplified model of noninvasively derived left ventricular pressure-volume loops. Am Heart J 1999;137:427–34.

49. Ikkos D, Jonsson B, Linderholm H. Effect of exercise in pulmonary stenosis with intact ventricular septum. Br Heart J 1966;28:316–30.

50. Driscoll DJ, Wolfe RR, Gersony WM, et al. Cardiorespiratory responses to exercise of patients with aortic stenosis, pulmonary stenosis, and ventricular septal defect. Circulation 1993;87:I102–13.

51. Krabill KA, Wang Y, Einzig S, Moller JH. Rest and exercise hemodynamics in pulmonary stenosis: comparison of children and adults. Am J Cardiol 1985;56:360–5.

52. Steinberger J, Moller JH. Exercise testing in children with pulmonary valvar stenosis. Pediatr Cardiol 1999;20:27,31; discussion 32.

53. Bouzas B, Kilner PJ, Gatzoulis MA. Pulmonary regurgitation: not a benign lesion. Eur Heart J 2005;26:433–9.

54. Roest AA, Helbing WA, Kunz P, et al. Exercise MR imaging in the assessment of pulmonary regurgitation and biventricular function in patients after tetralogy of Fallot repair. Radiology 2002;223:204–11.

55. Cumming GR. Maximal supine exercise haemodynamics after open heart surgery for Fallot's tetralogy. Br Heart J 1979;41:683–91.

56. Jonsson H, Ivert T, Jonasson R, Holmgren A, Bjork VO. Work capacity and central hemodynamics thirteen to twenty-six years after repair of tetralogy of Fallot. J Thorac Cardiovasc Surg 1995;110:416–26.

57. Braverman AC, Guven H, Beardslee MA, Makan M, Kates AM, Moon MR. The bicuspid aortic valve. Curr Probl Cardiol 2005;30:470–522.

58. Svensson LG, Kim KH, Lytle BW, Cosgrove DM. Relationship of aortic cross-sectional area to height ratio and the risk of aortic dissection in patients with bicuspid aortic valves. J Thorac Cardiovasc Surg 2003;126:892–3.

59. Maron BJ, Ackerman MJ, Nishimura RA, Pyeritz RE, Towbin JA, Udelson JE. Task Force 4: HCM and other cardiomyopathies, mitral valve prolapse, myocarditis, and Marfan syndrome. J Am Coll Cardiol 2005;45:1340–5.

60. Goldman L, Caldera DL, Nussbaum SR, et al. Multifactorial index of cardiac risk in noncardiac surgical procedures. N Engl J Med 1977;297:845–50.

61. Detsky AS, Abrams HB, Forbath N, Scott JG, Hilliard JR. Cardiac assessment for patients undergoing noncardiac surgery. A multifactorial clinical risk index. Arch Intern Med 1986;146:2131–4.

62. Eagle KA, Brundage BH, Chaitman BR, et al. Guidelines for perioperative cardiovascular evaluation for noncardiac surgery. Report of the American College of Cardiology/American Heart Association Task Force on Practice Guidelines. Committee on Perioperative Cardiovascular Evaluation for Noncardiac Surgery. Circulation 1996;93:1278–317.

63. Libby P, Bonow RO, Mann DL, Zipes DP. Braunwald's Heart Disease: A Textbook of Cardiovascular Medicine. Philadelphia, PA: W.B. Saunders, 2007.

64. Christ M, Sharkova Y, Geldner G, Maisch B. Preoperative and perioperative care for patients with suspected or established aortic stenosis facing noncardiac surgery. Chest 2005;128:2944–53.

65. Fleisher LA, Beckman JA, Brown KA, et al. ACC/AHA 2007 Guidelines on Perioperative Cardiovascular Evaluation and Care for Noncardiac Surgery: Executive Summary: A Report of the American College of Cardiology/American

Heart Association Task Force on Practice Guidelines (Writing Committee to Revise the 2002 Guidelines on Perioperative Cardiovascular Evaluation for Noncardiac Surgery): Developed in Collaboration With the American Society of Echocardiography, American Society of Nuclear Cardiology, Heart Rhythm Society, Society of Cardiovascular Anesthesiologists, Society for Cardiovascular Angiography and Interventions, Society for Vascular Medicine and Biology, and Society for Vascular Surgery. Circulation 2007;116:1971.

66. Kertai MD, Bountioukos M, Boersma E, et al. Aortic stenosis: an underestimated risk factor for perioperative complications in patients undergoing noncardiac surgery. Am J Med 2004;116:8–13.

67. Rohde LE, Polanczyk CA, Goldman L, Cook EF, Lee RT, Lee TH. Usefulness of transthoracic echocardiography as a tool for risk stratification of patients undergoing major noncardiac surgery. Am J Cardiolz 2001;87:505–9.

68. Torsher LC, Shub C, Rettke SR, Brown DL. Risk of patients with severe aortic stenosis undergoing noncardiac surgery. Am J Cardiol 1998;81:448–52.

69. O'Keefe JH Jr, Shub C, Rettke SR. Risk of noncardiac surgical procedures in patients with aortic stenosis. Mayo Clin Proc 1989;64:400–5.

70. Raymer K, Yang H. Patients with aortic stenosis: cardiac complications in non-cardiac surgery. Can J Anaesth 1998;45:855–9.

71. Wang A, Harrison JK, Bashore TM. Balloon aortic valvuloplasty. Prog Cardiovasc Dis 1997;40:27–36.

72. Evangelista A, Tornos P, Sambola A, Permanyer-Miralda G, Soler-Soler J. Long-term vasodilator therapy in patients with severe aortic regurgitation. N Engl J Med 2005;353:1342–9.

73. Potyk D, Raudaskoski P. Preoperative cardiac evaluation for elective noncardiac surgery. Arch Fam Med 1998;7:164–73.

74. Barash PG, Cullen BF, Stoelting RK. Clinical Anesthesia 5th Edition. Philadelphia, PA: Lippincott Williams & Wilkins, 2006;1:1595.

75. Reyes VP, Raju BS, Wynne J, et al. Percutaneous balloon valvuloplasty compared with open surgical commissurotomy for mitral stenosis. N Engl J Med 1994;331:961–7.

23 Valvular Heart Disease and Pregnancy

Cary Ward and Andra H. James

CONTENTS

INTRODUCTION

During the course of a normal pregnancy, the cardiovascular system of the mother is required to adapt to significant alterations in hemodynamics, including an almost 50% increase in cardiac output. This change in cardiac output is mediated by an increase in heart rate, a change in blood volume, and a significant increase in vasodilatation. While these changes are well tolerated in normal young women, mothers with pre-existing valvular disease may not have the cardiovascular reserve required to adapt to the rapid changes in their hemodynamic profile, leading to congestive heart failure for the mother or decreased perfusion of the fetus. Recent work by Hameed et al. reviewed both the maternal and fetal outcomes of 66 women with valvular heart disease when compared to 66 matched controls from 1979 to 1998. Although the incidence of maternal mortality was rare (occurring in one patient with severe congenital heart disease), the incidence of congestive heart failure (38%) and hospitalization (15%) was significantly higher in mothers with valvular heart disease *(1)*. The incidence of fetal complications was also increased with a 23% increase in preterm delivery and a 21% increase in intrauterine growth delay *(1)*. Nevertheless, with careful monitoring and prenatal care many mothers with valvular heart disease can have successful and healthy pregnancies. This chapter will review the important aspects of caring for these patients, both before and after pregnancy, and the medicines and procedures that are available to help both mother and baby.

PHYSIOLOGIC CHANGES ASSOCIATED WITH PREGNANCY

The initial hemodynamic change associated with pregnancy is a decrease in systemic vascular resistance *(2)*. This decrease in vascular tone is sensed by the kidney and induces compensatory mechanisms to increase plasma volume and cardiac output. The decreased systemic vascular resistance is mediated by vasoactive prostaglandins and enhanced nitric oxide (NO) production. NO is an important vasodilator produced by the endothelium, and recent work notes an increase in NO production in pregnant mammals. This increase in NO metabolites has also been confirmed in humans, and the

From: *Contemporary Cardiology: Valvular Heart Disease*
Edited by: Andrew Wang, Thomas M. Bashore, DOI 10.1007/978-1-59745-411-7_23
© Humana Press, a part of Springer Science+Business Media, LLC 2009

Table 1
Commonly Used Cardiovascular Drugs in Pregnancy

Drug	Possible adverse effect to fetus	FDA Risk category	Breast feeding
Amiodarone	IUGR, prematurity, thyroid disease, bradycardia, prolonged QT in newborn	C	Not recommended
ACE inhibitors	IUGR, prematurity, oligohydramnios, neonatal hypotension, renal failure, anemia, death, patent ductus arteriosus, limb and skull deformities	C	Not recommended
Beta-blockers	Bradycardia, low placental weight, IUGR, hypoglycemia	B, C, D	Compatible
Calcium channel antagonists (diltiazem, verapamil)	Limited data	C	Compatible
Digoxin		C	Compatible
Diuretics	Hypovolemia resulting in decreased uteroplacental perfusion, hypoglycemia; thiazides can inhibit labor and suppress lactation	C	Compatible
Heparin		C	Compatible
Hydralazine		C	Compatible
Sotalol	Limited data	B	Compatible
Warfarin	Fetal hemorrhage in utero, embryopathy, central nervous system abnormalities	X	Compatible

FDA pregnancy risk category: C = studies in animals have revealed adverse effects on fetus, or studies not available; X = studies in animals or humans have demonstrated fetal abnormalities. IUGR = intrauterine growth retardation.
Adapted from *(23)*.

syncytiotrophoblast is known to be an important site of NO synthesis. Placental production of NO maintains vasodilatation of the uterine vessels and ensures a high-flow/low-pressure fetoplacental and uteroplacental system *(2)*. In addition to the reduced afterload created by the low-pressure uterine circulation, there is also a reduced response to vasoconstrictors such as norepinephrine and angiotensin II during pregnancy *(3)*. The mechanism by which this reduced responsiveness occurs is not well understood but does not appear to be mediated by estrogen or progesterone *(4)*. This overall vasodilatory effect leads to a decrease in mean arterial blood pressure and activates the renin–angiotensin system and production of vasopressin to increase plasma volume.

When measuring plasma volume by Evans blue dye dilution, Bernstein et al. found that plasma volume had increased by 14% at 12 weeks of gestation *(5)*. The increase in plasma volume continues until the 34th week of gestation. The expansion of blood volume is accompanied by a 7–8 L increase in total body fluid volume distributed between the fetus, amniotic fluid, and the intracellular and extracellular space *(2)*. This increase in plasma volume is one factor responsible for the increase in cardiac output that occurs with normal pregnancy (Fig. 1). A recent study which used echocardiography to assess changes in the hemodynamics of 35 healthy pregnant women found a 46% increase in cardiac output at 37 weeks gestation when compared to postpartum values, with a mean cardiac output of 6.94 L/min at term. Although the mean cardiac output continued to increase throughout pregnancy until term, statistically significant changes occurred in the mid-second trimester and late second trimester. The increase in cardiac output was mediated by both an increase in heart rate (15%) and an increase in stroke volume (24%) *(6)*. A similar study from Hennesey et al. calculated the cardiac output of 26

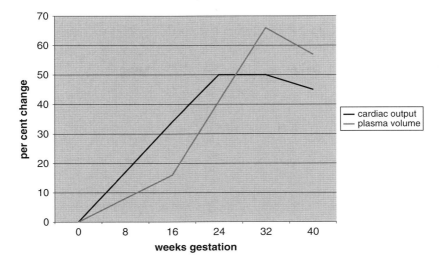

Fig. 1. Physiologic changes in pregnancy plotted as percent change from baseline.

pregnant patients by echocardiographic measurements. In this study the cardiac output peaked at 32 weeks gestation at 49% above control values but then began to decrease until term *(7)*. For young women with pre-existing valvular disease, adjustments to these dramatic hemodynamic changes may not be easily made, resulting in volume overload, pulmonary edema, and shortness of breath. Therefore, pregnant women must be carefully monitored by both cardiologists and obstetricians as these changes occur.

EVALUATION

The initial cardiac evaluation will ideally take place prior to conception and should include a detailed history, assessment of the patient's exercise capacity, and review of the medical regimen to avoid teratogenic medications whenever possible. It is important to record a detailed physical exam as the increased cardiac output and high-flow state of pregnancy result in many physical findings that are also found in cardiac failure such as distended neck veins, presence of an S3, and peripheral edema. In addition, an echocardiogram must be obtained to assess severity of the valvular disease. In patients with valvular disease and advanced heart failure symptoms (NYHA class III or IV) prior to conception, pregnancy poses a high risk to both the mother and the fetus. Therefore, pregnancy should not be recommended in such patients until the underlying valve disease has been treated and symptoms have improved. In patients with borderline valvular lesions or those with a questionable functional capacity, an exercise test may be useful *(8)*. Once these baseline data are obtained, the patient can proceed with pregnancy or have the procedures necessary to make pregnancy safe for mother and baby. The patient can then be followed intermittently by her cardiologist unless symptoms or signs of congestive heart failure are present. However, the patient must be closely evaluated toward the end of the second trimester when plasma volume and cardiac output are peaking *(7, 8)* and again at the time of delivery.

STENOTIC LESIONS

Mitral Stenosis

Stenotic lesions are the least well tolerated during pregnancy since a major increase in cardiac output is required in the face of a fixed obstruction. Unfortunately, rheumatic mitral stenosis (MS) is the valvular disease most commonly encountered in young women of childbearing age. Therefore, mitral stenosis represents the most common clinically significant valvular abnormality in pregnant women. Women who have unlimited exercise tolerance prior to pregnancy may present with dyspnea, pulmonary edema, or atrial fibrillation as cardiac output and left atrial pressure rise. The increase in heart rate that occurs with pregnancy reduces the diastolic filling period and the time that the left atrium has to empty, leading to further increases in left atrial pressure *(9)*. Obviously, these symptoms are more likely to occur during late second trimester, as volume status and cardiac output reach their peak levels.

Silversides et al. followed 74 women with varying degrees of mitral stenosis between 1986 and 2000. At baseline, 11% of the women studied had a mitral valve area of less than 1.0 cm^2 corresponding to severe mitral stenosis, and 14% had pulmonary hypertension with an estimated right ventricular systolic pressure of greater than 50 mmHg. Eleven percent of the women were symptomatic before pregnancy. Although there were no maternal deaths, the rate of complication was significant with 35% of women having a cardiac event (defined as pulmonary edema or arrhythmia) *(10)*. The complication rate was highest in the group with severe mitral stenosis, as almost 70% of these women had a cardiac event *(10)*. The overall rate of fetal/neonatal complication was 30%, driven by the incidence of premature birth. Other complications that occurred included respiratory distress in the neonate, small for gestational age babies, and fetal death *(10)*. Interestingly, no statistically significant difference in either the maternal or the fetal complication rate was found between patients who were symptomatic prior to pregnancy versus those who were asymptomatic. The only independent predictors of cardiac morbidity identified were moderate or severe MS as determined at baseline echocardiogram and a history of cardiac events prior to pregnancy.

In a similar study, Barbosa et al. examined the records of 41 pregnant patients with mitral stenosis from 1991 to 1999. The population in this study was slightly more symptomatic with 35.9% described as functional class II (only 11% in Silversides study) and 5% described as functional class III. The event rate was higher for women who were symptomatic prior to pregnancy, since the majority of women in the "uneventful" group began pregnancy as a functional class I (83%), while the majority of women in the "eventful" group were functional class II (57%) *(11)*. Nearly 50% of women in this study progressed to functional class III/IV. This decrease in functional class led to a significant number of interventions, with 35.5% requiring a balloon mitral valvotomy and 7% requiring surgery *(11)*. There was one maternal death. As in the Silversides study, the rate of complication was higher in women with smaller mitral valve areas *(11)*. Together, these studies indicate that women with mitral stenosis face a cardiac event rate of at least 30% and that this event rate is higher in women with smaller valve areas and women with symptoms prior to pregnancy. Fortunately, the complications that occur are most commonly pulmonary edema and atrial arrhythmias. Maternal death is rare. Therefore, in patients with mitral stenosis who present with symptoms or severe MS by valve area, we recommend treatment prior to pregnancy. In patients who are asymptomatic but have significant MS by echocardiographic measurement, an objective assessment of their exercise tolerance may be useful prior to clearing them for pregnancy.

Pulmonary hypertension is a common complication of mitral stenosis and has special significance in pregnancy since it can place women at much higher risk of complications. The pulmonary hypertension associated with MS is secondary to both the elevated wedge and the pulmonary vasoreactivity, and this vasoreactivity may worsen as pregnancy progresses. In a Japanese study of 1033 women with mitral stenosis and pregnancy, all women with an estimated right ventricular systolic pressure over 50 mmHg deteriorated clinically *(12, 13)*. In addition, the severity of pulmonary hypertension prior to pregnancy correlated with the risk of developing congestive heart failure during pregnancy *(14)*. Therefore, women with known pulmonary hypertension in the setting of mitral stenosis are at even greater risk of maternal complications during pregnancy and must be counseled appropriately to avoid pregnancy until they have had definitive therapy for their valve disease.

For women who are already pregnant and are found to have significant MS, optimal medical therapy is required for the purpose of reducing left atrial pressure. Diuretics can be used to treat volume overload, but they must be used cautiously since the increase in volume as a physiologic mechanism to maintain uteroplacental perfusion and hypovolemia must be avoided. Left atrial pressure can also be reduced by a decrease in the heart rate which allows more time for the left atrium to empty. Al-Kasab et al. used beta-blockers to treat symptomatic pregnant women with a mean valve area of 1.1 cm^2 (Table 1). Symptomatic improvement was obtained in 92% of patients, and fetal heart rate remained within the normal range (15). Beta-blockers are relatively safe during pregnancy although beta-1 selective agents are preferred since they have less effect on uterine relaxation. In addition, atenolol has been associated with lower birth weights and higher incidence of preterm delivery, especially in women taking the medication early in pregnancy and for long durations (16). Therefore, metoprolol may be the beta-blocker of choice for pregnant women. An alternative method of reducing heart rate is to restrict physical activity.

Atrial fibrillation commonly occurs in these patients secondary to elevated left atrial pressure and left atrial enlargement. In a patient who relies on diastolic filling time, the tachycardia that ensues may quickly worsen pulmonary edema and decrease cardiac output to the fetus. Therefore, rapid therapy may be required. Rate control can be achieved using a beta-blocker, digoxin, or a non-dihydropyridine calcium channel blocker (17). If chemical cardioversion is necessary, quinidine has a good safety profile in pregnancy, although other agents including sotalol and amiodarone have been used previously (17, 18). Electrical cardioversion may be safely used if hemodynamic instability is present. Anticoagulation must be considered in patients with sustained atrial fibrillation.

For women who remain very symptomatic despite maximal medical therapy or have signs of clinical heart failure, balloon mitral valvuloplasty (BMV) may be required. Although the procedure carries the risk of radiation exposure to the fetus, these risks can be reduced by waiting until after the 14th week of gestation when organogenesis is complete, by using minimal fluoroscopy time, and by abdominal shielding of the mother. Multiple studies have demonstrated that the technique is safe and effective for pregnant women and is certainly an improvement over cardiopulmonary bypass which carries a 15–30% risk of fetal mortality (19–22). Current ACC/AHA guidelines recommend BMV as the treatment of choice for patients who have persistent heart failure despite maximal medical therapy (23).

Recent investigation into the long-term outcome of BMV in pregnancy by Esteves et al. included 71 women who were NYHA functional class III or IV despite maximal medical therapy. All patients were ≥ 28 weeks gestation and had favorable valve morphology for BMV (52% with Wilkins echocardiographic valve score ≤ 8 (24)). Women were excluded if they had more than moderate MR. A successful outcome was defined as a post-valvuloplasty valve area of ≥ 1.5 cm^2 or an increase in valve area of >25%, and BMV was successful in all patients at the 48 hour time point. Only one maternal death occurred secondary to conditions unrelated to the procedure. At a mean follow-up of 44 months, the combined event rate of death, mitral valve replacement or repair, and repeat BMV occurred in only 14% of women (21). The mean gestational age at delivery was 38 weeks, with preterm delivery in 13% of patients. At long-term follow-up, all children showed normal growth and development (21). In a similar study, Mangione et al. followed 30 pregnant patients who underwent BMV at an earlier gestational age (mean of 25 weeks). All patients were functional class III or IV prior to the procedure, and 91% remained functional class I or II at follow-up of 5 years. Although there were two fetal deaths, these were not directly related to the procedure, and the other 21 children showed normal growth and development at 5 years (22). In summary, BMV represents a safe and effective technique for pregnant women with severe MS according to multiple different series. Although elective BMV is safely performed after the first trimester, it can be performed sooner in cases of severe maternal distress.

Aortic Stenosis

In young women of childbearing age, the most common etiology of aortic stenosis (AS) is a congenital bicuspid aortic valve. Other causes of congenital AS include subaortic membrane and subvalvular obstruction *(25)*. Aortic stenosis may also be seen in women with rheumatic heart disease. Early studies demonstrated a high rate of cardiac complications associated with pregnancy in women with AS secondary to the elevated LVEDP that occurs as the cardiac output increases. Current guidelines recommend that women with moderate to severe AS consider therapy for the obstructed valve prior to conception *(23)*. In one recent study, 22% of women with congenital AS had been counseled against pregnancy secondary to increased risk of cardiac complications *(26)*.

However, two more recent studies demonstrate improved outcomes for pregnant women with AS. Silversides reviewed 39 women with 49 pregnancies in the setting of congenital aortic stenosis. Ninety percent of the women had bicuspid aortic valves and 59% were classified as severe AS with peak gradients as high as 67 mmHg. In the group with severe AS there were only three events (defined as pulmonary edema, arrhythmia, or maternal death): two women with pulmonary edema and one with atrial arrhythmias. There were no maternal deaths *(27)*. In the women with mild to moderate AS there were no cardiac events during the antepartum and peripartum period, but four women in this group did experience a significant deterioration in their functional class *(27)*. There was a not-unexpected rate of obstetric and fetal complications in this study as six pregnancies (12%) resulted in premature birth, one a small for gestational age baby, or respiratory distress syndrome and no fetal deaths *(27)*.

Yap et al. reviewed 53 pregnancies in women with congenital aortic stenosis and a mean aortic jet velocity of 3.3 m/s (range 1.7–5.3 m/s). Left ventricular function was normal in all women. Cardiac events including heart failure, arrhythmia, and stroke occurred in five women (9.4% of pregnancies). Two women in the severe AS group had an episode of congestive heart failure requiring medical therapy *(26)*. Again, there was the usual incidence of obstetric complications with 7.5% of pregnancies resulting in premature labor and 13.2% of babies born prematurely, but 11.5% of pregnancies were complicated by hypertensive disorders of pregnancy and there was a 4% incidence of placental abruption. In summary, these data indicate that in the majority of women with aortic stenosis, pregnancy is well tolerated, although the risk of obstetric and perinatal complications may be increased *(26)*. Improvements in both cardiac and obstetric care may account for the difference between these results and earlier studies which demonstrated a high rate of both maternal and fetal mortality *(28)*. Obviously, it is critical that pregnant women with significant AS be closely followed by both cardiologists and obstetricians, and they should deliver at a medical center with the capability of delivering aggressive cardiac and perinatal care.

For women with aortic stenosis who develop signs and symptoms of congestive heart failure, the options for therapy are limited. Medical therapy includes judicious use of diuretics and bed rest. There are multiple reports of aortic valve replacement in pregnant women, but the rate of fetal mortality in these reports is high at 39% *(29)*. As in the case of mitral stenosis, pregnant women can undergo aortic valvuloplasty, and there are case reports indicating that this technique is effective *(30)*. However, there are no large series of patients reported in the literature to confirm the safety of this technique in pregnant women.

Pulmonic Stenosis

Pulmonic stenosis (PS) in young women can be an isolated congenital abnormality or found as part of a spectrum of anomalies such as tetralogy of Fallot *(8)*. As with other obstructive lesions, PS is a potential problem in pregnancy since it limits the output of the right heart. Therefore, women with known pulmonic stenosis, symptoms and a gradient from right ventricle (RV) to pulmonary artery

(PA) over 30 mmHg, or asymptomatic women with a gradient from RV to PA over 40 mmHg should undergo percutaneous balloon valvuloplasty prior to conception (23). Although there is little in the literature regarding this situation, women who conceive in the setting of known pulmonic stenosis are thought to tolerate pregnancy quite well (23). In 2004, Hameed et al. reported on 17 patients with PS and compared them to controls matched in age, ethnicity, and year of delivery (31). Only one patient had deterioration in her functional class (NYHA class I to NYHA class II). There was no statistically significant difference in obstetric or fetal complications when the patients were compared to the control group. In addition, there was no difference in outcome between the groups with severe PS and those with milder PS (31). In the rare patient who has symptoms that are refractory to medical therapy, percutaneous valvuloplasty is possible (23).

REGURGITANT LESIONS

Mitral Regurgitation

In general, the regurgitant lesions are much better tolerated than those that involve stenosis since the reduction in afterload that occurs during pregnancy works to improve forward cardiac output. Mitral regurgitation, usually the result of a prolapsing valve or rheumatic disease, is rarely a problem in pregnant women with a normal ventricle and requires little therapy (8). Lesniak et al. evaluated 44 women with varying grades of MR; 24 of the women were functional class I at the beginning of pregnancy and 20 were functional class II. Only seven women had adverse cardiac events later in pregnancy, including three women with congestive heart failure and four with supraventricular tachycardia. All were treated medically (32). There was a small incidence of fetal complications including one baby born prematurely and three babies with intrauterine growth retardation. Thus, the incidence of maternal or fetal complications is low when compared to mitral or aortic stenosis. If left ventricular dysfunction is also present, there may be more risk of pulmonary congestion and a decrease in functional capacity. Medical therapy includes gentle diuresis to avoid pulmonary edema. The use of angiotensin-converting enzyme (ACE) inhibitors is contraindicated during pregnancy since they are known to be teratogenic, but if systemic hypertension is present, hydralazine and nitrates may be used for afterload reduction (8, 23). Careful monitoring of patients is required in the first 24–48 hours after delivery, since the sudden increase in vascular resistance and the abrupt changes in volume status may result in volume overload requiring aggressive diuresis (33).

Aortic Regurgitation

Similar to MR, aortic insufficiency (AI) in the setting of a normal ventricle is also fairly well tolerated during pregnancy secondary to the decrease in vascular resistance and the increase in heart rate. The most common etiologies in this age group include congenital abnormalities of the aortic valve, rheumatic disease, infective endocarditis, and diseases of the aortic root (34). The presence of a dilated aortic root in a young woman bears special notice, since it could be the result of previously unrecognized Marfan syndrome. Pregnant patients with Marfan syndrome are at especially high risk of spontaneous aortic dissection secondary to the considerable activation of the collagenolytic system that occurs in preparation for delivery. Although women with Marfan syndrome and aortic roots over 40 mm are at a greater risk of dissection (35), current guidelines recommend that any woman with Marfan syndrome be advised of the risks associated with pregnancy, since the risk of catastrophic aortic dissection is present even in the setting of a normal-sized aortic root (23). Some experts argue that women with a dilated aortic root secondary to congenital heart disease are similarly at risk (36).

For women with AI not associated with a dilated root, symptoms generally occur only in the setting of depressed ventricular function. Lesniak followed women with aortic regurgitation and found that

19/22 tolerated pregnancy without difficulty. Three women described a decrease in their functional class and received diuretic therapy during the third trimester, but all three women had a dilated left ventricle and depressed left ventricular ejection fraction *(32)*. Medical treatment for these patients included diuretics and afterload reduction using nitrates and hydralazine *(8)*. As in the case of MR, close monitoring after delivery is required, since the abrupt changes in hemodynamics may result in acute pulmonary edema.

Pulmonary Regurgitation

As in the case of pulmonic stenosis, significant pulmonary regurgitation in young women is most often the result of congenital abnormalities and is seen commonly after complete repair of tetralogy of Fallot *(37)*. Usually performed in infancy, the technique involves enlargement of the right ventricular outflow tract through the use of a transannular patch leaving the patient with an incompetent pulmonary valve. In 10–15% of patients, this pulmonary insufficiency (PI) leads to progressive right ventricular dilatation and dysfunction and may require pulmonary valve replacement later in life *(37)*. Multiple studies have reviewed the outcome of pregnancy in patients with repaired tetralogy and show favorable results, although they included small numbers of patients, not all of whom had pulmonary valve dysfunction *(38, 39)*. Singh et al. evaluated 44 pregnancies in 24 women with repaired tetralogy and found no maternal or perinatal complications, although one infant was found to have pulmonary atresia. More recently Meijer et al. evaluated 50 pregnancies in women with a history of repaired tetralogy of Fallot *(37)*. Severe PI was present in 14 of the 50 pregnancies (28%), and 2 of the 5 women who experienced a cardiac event during pregnancy were from the group with severe PI. Both these patients developed right-sided heart failure and supraventricular tachycardia late in pregnancy and were treated medically *(37)*. There were no maternal deaths. In addition, in a recent review of pregnancy outcomes in congenital heart disease, Khairy et al. found that the presence of severe PI was an independent predictor of primary cardiac events during pregnancy with an odds ratio of 4.6 *(40)*. Again, the most common cardiac event in this study was heart failure which responded to medical therapy without need for further intervention *(40)*. There were no maternal deaths. Therefore, in summary, the data suggest that although women with severe pulmonary regurgitation are at risk for right-sided heart failure and arrhythmia, they respond well to medical therapy, with no other adverse outcomes.

PROSTHETIC HEART VALVES

For women who have already undergone valve replacement and are contemplating pregnancy, there are multiple issues. In women with bioprosthetic valves, there is a considerable debate as to whether pregnancy causes structural valve deterioration and may accelerate the need for a second operation. In women with a mechanical prosthesis, anticoagulation during pregnancy is a challenge and the risk of thromboembolism not insignificant *(41)*. Although the majority of these women have normal valvular function and normal hemodynamics, they face as many challenges with pregnancy as their counterparts who have ongoing valve disease and require a high level of care from cardiologists as well as obstetricians who are familiar with the issues at hand.

Structural Valve Deterioration and Bioprostheses

Bioprosthetic valves are often used in women of childbearing age, since they avoid the need for anticoagulation and the risk of thromboembolism during pregnancy. However, early studies suggested that the rate of structural valve deterioration was significantly accelerated by pregnancy. From 1975 to 1987 Badduke et al. compared the outcomes of 17 women with bioprosthetic valves who became pregnant versus 60 women who did not. Structural valve deterioration (SVD) occurred in 47.1% of the pregnant group but in only 14.3% of the nonpregnant group (a statistically significant difference). The freedom from structural valve deterioration at 10 years was 23.3% ± 14% for the pregnant group and 74.2% ± 8.5% for the nonpregnant group *(42)*. Although these results were concerning, later studies have failed to show similar outcomes. Jamieson et al. evaluated 255 women who received bioprostheses from 1972 to 1992, 52 of whom had 94 pregnancies. Although there was a trend toward a higher incidence of SVD in the pregnant group (50.9%) versus the nonpregnant group (40.6%), the difference was not statistically significant *(43)*. There was also a higher rate of reoperation in the women who had pregnancies, but again this was not a statistically significant difference *(43)*. The authors concluded that pregnancy did not adversely affect valve survival in women with bioprosthetic valves. In a similar but broader study, North et al. evaluated the long-term survival and complication rates in young women with all types of cardiac valve replacements (bioprosthetic, mechanical, and homografts) *(44)*. Their results demonstrated that valve survival was highest in women with mechanical valves. However, the group with bioprosthetic valves had a higher 10-year survival rate of 84% versus 70% in the group with mechanical prostheses. Interestingly, the group who had undergone valve replacement with a homograft had the highest 10-year survival rate at 96% *(44)*. When they compared the outcomes of women with valve replacements who had pregnancies to those who had not, there was no evidence that pregnancy accelerated valve loss with any type of graft *(44)*. Thus, bioprosthetic valve grafts, both xenografts and homografts, are acceptable for use in young women and provide them with the opportunity for a healthy and successful pregnancy.

Mechanical Valves and Anticoagulation

In the study by North et al., the rate of valve loss either secondary to valve replacement or valve-related death was lowest in women with mechanical prostheses at only 29%. However, they also had the lowest 10-year survival rate at only 70% *(44)*. The durability of mechanical valves is well documented, but the reason for decreased survival in this group is less clear. Women with mechanical valve prostheses had a higher rate of thromboembolic complications, with nearly 50% of women suffering a thromboembolic event within 5 years. There was also a higher rate of hemorrhagic complication in women with mechanical valves *(44)*. The high incidence of these complications becomes critically important when evaluating a pregnant patient with a mechanical valve, since appropriate anticoagulation is even more of a challenge in this group.

During pregnancy, anticoagulation with coumadin is limited by its teratogenic effects. Warfarin embryopathy is characterized by nasal hypoplasia and stippled epiphyses and is thought to occur in up to 30% of infants exposed during the first trimester *(45, 46)*. Treatment with warfarin later in pregnancy is associated with central nervous system abnormalities and the risk of fetal hemorrhage *(45, 46)*. Although these complications occur at low rates, many physicians avoid treatment with warfarin in pregnancy altogether. Heparins, both unfractionated and of low molecular weight, do not cross the placenta and are therefore the best option for anticoagulation with respect to fetal safety. However, the dosing of both medicines is difficult during pregnancy and the risk of valve thrombosis with unfractionated heparin is approximately 30% with a 40–50% mortality rate when it occurs *(45, 47, 48)*. Although there was initial concern over the safety of low-molecular-weight heparin (LMWH), a recent review of the literature examined 76 cases of women with mechanical heart valves in which LMWH was used for anticoagulation *(45)*. In this series, there were 17 thrombotic events (22%), indicating a rate of thrombosis similar to that established in women with mechanical valves on unfractionated heparin *(45)*. This data led to the FDA lifting the "black box warning" against the use of LMWH in prosthetic valves. Since low-molecular-weight heparins achieve a more consistent level of anticoagulation than unfractionated heparin, they can be dosed using a weight-based formula and may require less frequent blood work to ensure adequate dosing. Because of the challenges surrounding adequate anticoagulation and the risks to mother and baby that result, many women with mechanical heart valves are advised not to pursue pregnancy. If they do become pregnant, most centers recommend the use of unfractionated or low-molecular-weight heparin until the 12th week of gestation when organogenesis is complete. They are then switched to warfarin therapy until late in the third trimester at which point they are changed back to heparin in preparation for delivery. Women who elect to avoid warfarin for the duration of pregnancy are maintained on subcutaneous heparin or LMWH with supplemental low-dose aspirin and frequent monitoring to ensure adequate anticoagulation *(23, 45)*.

PERIPARTUM CARE

Labor and delivery is a time for vigilance in pregnant women with valvular heart disease since it is a time of increases in hemodynamic stress and significant shifts in volume status. Labor may be difficult since pain induces tachycardia and uterine contractions increase venous return and therefore pulmonary congestion. Women with valvular heart disease should be given adequate pain control to avoid tachycardia, and medicines such as beta-blockers can be used to reduce the adrenergic stimulation *(1, 10)*. In most cases, a vaginal delivery is best since cesarean section is associated with increased blood loss and greater fluid shifts. However, mothers with heart disease may not tolerate the work of pushing in the second stage. A prolonged second stage can be avoided by the use of a low forceps or vacuum delivery. Cesarean section is reserved for obstetric indications *(8, 33)*. In the immediate postpartum period, women are at risk for volume overload as afterload increases and the blood volume from the placenta returns to the maternal circulation. Therefore, hemodynamic monitoring in an ICU setting is necessary in the 12–24 hours following delivery *(8)*. Finally, although the AHA/ACC practice guidelines have not included antibiotic prophylaxis for women undergoing uncomplicated vaginal deliveries, recent evidence indicates that there is a significant risk of bacteremia *(49)*. Thus, most centers routinely use antibiotic prophylaxis during delivery in women with valvular heart disease *(8, 33)*.

REFERENCES

1. Hameed A, Karaalp IS, Tummala PP, et al. The effect of valvular heart disease on maternal and fetal outcome of pregnancy. Journal of the American College of Cardiology 2001;37(3):893–9.
2. Carbillon L, Uzan M, Uzan S. Pregnancy, vascular tone, and maternal hemodynamics: a crucial adaptation. Obstetrical & Gynecological Survey 2000;55(9):574–81.
3. Chesley LC. Hypertension in pregnancy: definitions, familial factor, and remote prognosis. Kidney International 1980;18(2):234–40.
4. Novak J, Reckelhoff J, Bumgarner L, Cockrell K, Kassab S, Granger JP. Reduced sensitivity of the renal circulation to angiotensin II in pregnant rats. Hypertension 1997;30(3 Pt 2):580–4.
5. Bernstein IM, Ziegler W, Badger GJ. Plasma volume expansion in early pregnancy. Obstetrics and Gynecology 2001;97(5 Pt 1):669–72.
6. Desai DK, Moodley J, Naidoo DP. Echocardiographic assessment of cardiovascular hemodynamics in normal pregnancy. Obstetrics and Gynecology 2004;104(1):20–9.
7. Hennessy TG, MacDonald D, Hennessy MS, et al. Serial changes in cardiac output during normal pregnancy: a Doppler ultrasound study. European Journal of Obstetrics, Gynecology, and Reproductive Biology 1996;70(2):117–22.
8. Elkayam U, Bitar F. Valvular heart disease and pregnancy part I: native valves. Journal of the American College of Cardiology 2005;46(2):223–30.
9. Reimold SC, Rutherford JD. Clinical practice. Valvular heart disease in pregnancy. The New England Journal of Medicine 2003;349(1):52–9.
10. Silversides CK, Colman JM, Sermer M, Siu SC. Cardiac risk in pregnant women with rheumatic mitral stenosis. The American Journal of Cardiology 2003;91(11):1382–5.
11. Barbosa PJ, Lopes AA, Feitosa GS, et al. Prognostic factors of rheumatic mitral stenosis during pregnancy and puerperium. Arquivos Brasileiros de Cardiologia 2000;75(3):215–24.

12. Sugishita Y, Ito I, Kubo T. Pregnancy in cardiac patients: possible influence of volume overload by pregnancy on pulmonary circulation. Japanese Circulation Journal 1986;50(4):376–83.
13. Weiss BM, Hess OM. Pulmonary vascular disease and pregnancy: current controversies, management strategies, and perspectives. European Heart Journal 2000;21(2):104–15.
14. Weiss BM. Managing severe mitral valve stenosis in pregnant patients – percutaneous balloon valvuloplasty, not surgery, is the treatment of choice. Journal of Cardiothoracic and Vascular Anesthesia 2005;19(2):277–8.
15. Al Kasab SM, Sabag T, Al Zaibag M, et al. Beta-adrenergic receptor blockade in the management of pregnant women with mitral stenosis. American Journal of Obstetrics and Gynecology 1990;163(1 Pt 1):37–40.
16. Lydakis C, Lip GY, Beevers M, Beevers DG. Atenolol and fetal growth in pregnancies complicated by hypertension. American Journal of Hypertension 1999;12(6):541–7.
17. Walsh CA, Manias T, Patient C. Atrial fibrillation in pregnancy. European Journal of Obstetrics, Gynecology, and Reproductive Biology 2007;138:119–120.
18. Fuster V, Ryden LE, Cannom DS, et al. ACC/AHA/ESC 2006 Guidelines for the Management of Patients with Atrial Fibrillation: a report of the American College of Cardiology/American Heart Association Task Force on Practice Guidelines and the European Society of Cardiology Committee for Practice Guidelines (Writing Committee to Revise the 2001 Guidelines for the Management of Patients with Atrial Fibrillation): developed in collaboration with the European Heart Rhythm Association and the Heart Rhythm Society. Circulation 2006;114(7):e257–354.
19. Sivadasanpillai H, Srinivasan A, Sivasubramoniam S, et al. Long-term outcome of patients undergoing balloon mitral valvotomy in pregnancy. The American Journal of Cardiology 2005;95(12):1504–6.
20. Nercolini DC, da Rocha Loures Bueno R, Eduardo Guerios E, et al. Percutaneous mitral balloon valvuloplasty in pregnant women with mitral stenosis. Catheterization and Cardiovascular Interventions 2002;57(3):318–22.
21. Esteves CA, Munoz JS, Braga S, et al. Immediate and long-term follow-up of percutaneous balloon mitral valvuloplasty in pregnant patients with rheumatic mitral stenosis. The American Journal of Cardiology 2006;98(6):812–6.
22. Mangione JA, Lourenco RM, dos Santos ES, et al. Long-term follow-up of pregnant women after percutaneous mitral valvuloplasty. Catheterization and Cardiovascular Interventions 2000;50(4):413–7.
23. Bonow RO, Carabello BA, Kanu C, et al. ACC/AHA 2006 guidelines for the management of patients with valvular heart disease: a report of the American College of Cardiology/American Heart Association Task Force on Practice Guidelines (writing committee to revise the 1998 Guidelines for the Management of Patients with Valvular Heart Disease): developed in collaboration with the Society of Cardiovascular Anesthesiologists: Endorsed by the Society for Cardiovascular Angiography and Interventions and the Society of Thoracic Surgeons. Circulation 2006;114(5): e84–231.
24. Wilkins GT, Weyman AE, Abascal VM, Block PC, Palacios IF. Percutaneous balloon dilatation of the mitral valve: an analysis of echocardiographic variables related to outcome and the mechanism of dilatation. British Heart Journal 1988;60(4):299–308.
25. Yap SC, Takkenberg JJ, Witsenburg M, Meijboom FJ, Roos-Hesselink JW. Aortic stenosis at young adult age. Expert Review of Cardiovascular Therapy 2005;3(6):1087–98.
26. Yap SC, Drenthen W, Pieper PG, et al. Risk of complications during pregnancy in women with congenital aortic stenosis. International Journal of Cardiology 2007;126:250–246.
27. Silversides CK, Colman JM, Sermer M, Farine D, Siu SC. Early and intermediate-term outcomes of pregnancy with congenital aortic stenosis. The American Journal of Cardiology 2003;91(11):1386–9.
28. Arias F, Pineda J. Aortic stenosis and pregnancy. The Journal of Reproductive Medicine 1978;20(4):229–32.
29. Parry AJ, Westaby S. Cardiopulmonary bypass during pregnancy. The Annals of Thoracic Surgery 1996;61(6):1865–9.
30. Myerson SG, Mitchell AR, Ormerod OJ, Banning AP. What is the role of balloon dilatation for severe aortic stenosis during pregnancy? The Journal of Heart Valve Disease 2005;14(2):147–50.
31. Hameed A. Effect of severity of pulmonic stenosis on pregnancy outcome: a case control study. American Journal of Obstetrics and Gynecology 2004;191:93.
32. Lesniak-Sobelga A, Tracz W, KostKiewicz M, Podolec P, Pasowicz M. Clinical and echocardiographic assessment of pregnant women with valvular heart diseases – maternal and fetal outcome. International Journal of Cardiology 2004;94(1):15–23.
33. Stout KK, Otto CM. Pregnancy in women with valvular heart disease. Heart 2006;93:552–558.
34. Roberts WC, Ko JM, Moore TR, Jones WH, 3rd. Causes of pure aortic regurgitation in patients having isolated aortic valve replacement at a single US tertiary hospital (1993 to 2005). Circulation 2006;114(5):422–9.
35. Rahman J, Rahman FZ, Rahman W, al-Suleiman SA, Rahman MS. Obstetric and gynecologic complications in women with Marfan syndrome. The Journal of Reproductive Medicine 2003;48(9):723–8.
36. Immer FF, Bansi AG, Immer-Bansi AS, et al. Aortic dissection in pregnancy: analysis of risk factors and outcome. The Annals of Thoracic Surgery 2003;76(1):309–14.
37. Meijer JM, Pieper PG, Drenthen W, et al. Pregnancy, fertility, and recurrence risk in corrected tetralogy of Fallot. Heart 2005;91(6):801–5.

38. Singh H, Bolton PJ, Oakley CM. Pregnancy after surgical correction of tetralogy of Fallot. British Medical Journal (Clinical Research ed) 1982;285(6336):168–70.
39. Lewis BS, Rogers NM, Gotsman MS. Successful pregnancy after repair of Fallot's tetralogy. South African Medical Journal = Suid-Afrikaanse tydskrif vir geneeskunde 1972;46(27):934–6.
40. Khairy P, Ouyang DW, Fernandes SM, Lee-Parritz A, Economy KE, Landzberg MJ. Pregnancy outcomes in women with congenital heart disease. Circulation 2006;113(4):517–24.
41. Elkayam U, Bitar F. Valvular heart disease and pregnancy: Part II: prosthetic valves. Journal of the American College of Cardiology 2005;46(3):403–10.
42. Badduke BR, Jamieson WR, Miyagishima RT, et al. Pregnancy and childbearing in a population with biologic valvular prostheses. The Journal of Thoracic and Cardiovascular Surgery 1991;102(2):179–86.
43. Jamieson WR, Miller DC, Akins CW, et al. Pregnancy and bioprostheses: influence on structural valve deterioration. The Annals of Thoracic Surgery 1995;60(Suppl 2):S282–6; discussion S7.
44. North RA, Sadler L, Stewart AW, McCowan LM, Kerr AR, White HD. Long-term survival and valve-related complications in young women with cardiac valve replacements. Circulation 1999;99(20):2669–76.
45. James AH, Brancazio LR, Gehrig TR, Wang A, Ortel TL. Low-molecular-weight heparin for thromboprophylaxis in pregnant women with mechanical heart valves. Journal of Maternal-Fetal and Neonatal Medicine 2006;19(9):543–9.
46. Bates SM. Treatment and prophylaxis of venous thromboembolism during pregnancy. Thrombosis Research 2002;108(2–3):97–106.
47. Sadler L, McCowan L, White H, Stewart A, Bracken M, North R. Pregnancy outcomes and cardiac complications in women with mechanical, bioprosthetic and homograft valves. BJOG 2000;107(2):245–53.
48. Chan WS, Anand S, Ginsberg JS. Anticoagulation of pregnant women with mechanical heart valves: a systematic review of the literature. Archives of Internal Medicine 2000;160(2):191–6.
49. Furman B, Shoham-Vardi I, Bashiri A, Erez O, Mazor M. Clinical significance and outcome of preterm prelabor rupture of membranes: population-based study. European Journal of Obstetrics, Gynecology, and Reproductive Biology 2000;92(2):209–16.

Subject Index

From: *Contemporary Cardiology: Valvular Heart Disease*
Edited by: Andrew Wang, Thomas M. Bashore, DOI 10.1007/978-1-59745-411-7,
© Humana Press, a part of Springer Science+Business Media, LLC 2009